Essentials in
Gynecology
for Undergraduate Medical Students

Essentials in
Gynecology
for Undergraduate Medical Students

Snehamay Chaudhuri
MBBS, MD, DNB

Associate Professor
Department of Obstetrics and Gynecology
NRS Medical College
Kolkata, India

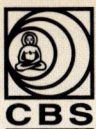

CBS

CBS Publishers & Distributors Pvt Ltd

New Delhi • Bengaluru • Chennai • Kochi • Kolkata • Mumbai
Bhopal • Bhubaneswar • Hyderabad • Jharkhand • Nagpur
• Patna • Pune • Uttarakhand • Dhaka (Bangladesh)

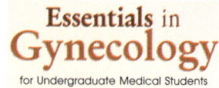

ISBN: 978-81-239-2601-8

Copyright © Author and Publisher

First Edition: 2015
Reprint: 2019

Published by Satish Kumar Jain and Produced by Varun Jain for
CBS Publishers & Distributors Pvt Ltd
4819/XI Prahlad Street, 24 Ansari Road, Daryaganj, New Delhi 110 002, India.
Ph: 23289259, 23266861, 23266867   Fax: 011-23243014   Website: www.cbspd.com
e-mail: delhi@cbspd.com; cbspubs@airtelmail.in.
Corporate Office: 204 FIE, Industrial Area, Patparganj, Delhi 110 092, India
Ph: 4934 4934   Fax: 4934 4935   e-mail: publishing@cbspd.com; publicity@cbspd.com

Branches

• **Bengaluru:** Seema House 2975, 17th Cross, K.R. Road, Banasankari 2nd Stage, Bengaluru 560 070, Karnataka
  Ph: +91-80-26771678/79   Fax: +91-80-26771680   e-mail: bangalore@cbspd.com
• **Chennai:** 7, Subbaraya Street, Shenoy Nagar, Chennai 600 030, Tamil Nadu
  Ph: +91-44-26260666, 26208620   Fax: +91-44-42032115   e-mail: chennai@cbspd.com
• **Kochi:** 42/1325, 1326, Power House Road, Opp KSEB Power House, Ernakulam 682 018, Kochi, Kerala
  Ph: +91-484-4059061-65   Fax: +91-484-4059065   e-mail: kochi@cbspd.com
• **Kolkata:** No. 6/B, Ground Floor, Rameswar Shaw Road, Kolkata-700014 (West Bengal), India
  Ph: +91-33-2289-1126, 2289-1127, 2289-1128   e-mail: kolkata@cbspd.com
• **Mumbai:** 83-C, Dr E Moses Road, Worli, Mumbai-400018, Maharashtra
  Ph: +91-22-24902340/41   Fax: +91-22-24902342   e-mail: mumbai@cbspd.com

Representatives

• **Bhopal**	0-8319310552	• **Bhubaneswar**	0-9911037372	• **Hyderabad**	0-9885175004
• **Jharkhand**	0-9811541605	• **Nagpur**	0-9421945513	• **Patna**	0-9334159340
• **Pune**	0-9623451994	• **Uttarakhand**	0-9716462459		
• **Dhaka (Bangladesh)**	01912-003485				

Printed at Magic International Pvt. Ltd., Greater Noida, UP, India

to

---

my parents, teachers and my family

Foreword

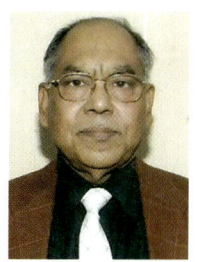

This book has evolved out of historical necessities. I have witnessed the gradual transformation in medical education for the last 50 years, first as a student, then as a practitioner, and lastly as a teacher. We inherited an archaic and fossilized curriculum of unnecessary details which taxed the young minds and hindered their natural growth. As students we were attracted by huge tomes of elaborate treatise written by British and American authors. Only later we realized their negative impact on our overall understanding of the subject.

The system was faulty but not disastrous because in the early post-World War era in Great Britain (where our aspiring specialists mainly went for higher studies) the state of the society and medical education were not much different from our own.

Gradually the Western society rebuilt itself and its education system changed to stay relevant. Unfortunately due to apathy and inertia we lagged behind. This I realized during my stint in subdivisional and district hospitals.

Fortunately from early eighties of the last century, a wave of fresh thinking in medical education resulted in extensive restructuring of its course and curriculum. And then we found that the Western textbooks were no longer relevant as an instrument of learning. A spate of homegrown textbooks arrived.

This treatise by my beloved student Prof Snehamay Chaudhuri is latest in this line of very useful textbooks. It is meant not only for undergraduate students but also useful for postgraduate students and busy practitioners. As the title suggests, it concentrates on 'essentials' and is put in an extremely readable and easy to remember format. It deliberately leaves out certain topics which are not strictly necessary for undergraduates.

In this age of 'explosion' of information via internet, the role of this type of concise, no-nonsense textbooks cannot be overemphasized. I was an expectant onlooker during the preparation of the manuscript. I know how hard the author worked to make this book worthy.

I wish the author all the best and his textbook a grand success. I urge every student and practitioner to go through it. It will be value both for their time and money.

Prof Partha Kumar Bhattacharyya

Ex-Head, Department of Obstetrics and Gynaecology
Eden Hospital, Medical College
Kolkata
West Bengal

Preface

Scientific knowledge is ever expanding but the student's time to assimilate this knowledge is limited. Challenged with a vast syllabus of MBBS curriculum, a student often finds it difficult what really he/she needs to learn. Moreover, the current standard textbooks do not orient the student for both theoretical and practical aspects of examination in Indian universities. Keeping these problems in mind, I decided to go with an original idea to write a textbook that will not only provide core knowledge of gynecology but also help the student to solve practical problems of gynecology as well as prepare them for theory and practical examination from one book at a time.

Essentials in Gynecology has been written by keeping all these aspects in mind which make it suitable for undergraduate students. The text is described in 37 chapters and covers the gynecological aspects of women from conception to old age. The book has been written in simple and easy to understand language. Each chapter is presented in a highly accessible style with many headings, subheadings, illustrations, tables, flowcharts and photographs which make it easy to read, understand and reproduce.

A note to the students

This textbook is unique due to following reasons:

1. To answer the question 'what a student really needs to know?' clear **learning objectives** are established in each chapter. The aim is to define breadth and depth of knowledge a student needs at undergraduate level.

2. Each new chapter begins with a typical example of **clinical presentation** that a student is likely to encounter as a health care professional. A question is added with the clinical presentation to make the student curious about the topic.

3. Each chapter covers the core knowledge a student needs to have. The text includes the latest and most **uptodate information**. Considering context of a developing country, the recommendations of Government of India, World Health Organization (WHO), FIGO are adopted more than that of European or American Scientific Societies. The volume of every chapter is weighed against the need of the student and the element of personal bias is kept aside to the maximum.

4. In each topic, clinically important information is highlighted as **fact sheet** to make the reading interesting and **clinical pearls** are added so that students remember the important clinical information during their practice in professional life.

5. At the end of each chapter, technical words that might be difficult to understand for undergraduate students are explained as **keywords.**

6. An extensive number of **questions** is provided as **exercises** at the end of each chapter to test the understanding of important concepts. The questions that are likely to be asked in theory paper are provided as long questions, short notes, fill in the blanks, justify/criticize. Questions for oral tables are also provided at the end of exercise as questions from instruments, X-rays, specimens, contraceptives. As a part of self-directed learning, each chapter closes with a set of questions from the clinical presentation which is provided at

the beginning of the chapter. These are the typical questions which are commonly asked in long and short cases during practical examination. Thus the objective to help the student to prepare for both theory and practical examination at a time is fulfilled.

7. For further reading and references, a bibliography is incorporated in each chapter.
8. Postgraduate students (MD/MS/DNB/DGO courses) will also find this textbook helpful as the postgraduate training is always deficient without a solid knowledge of basic facts. They will also be benefited in the preparation of their theory and practical examination.

Snehamay Chaudhuri
snehamay_chaudhuri_dr@yahoo.com

Acknowledgements

First and foremost, I would like to thank my teacher Prof Partha Kumar Bhattacharyya, FRCOG from whom I have learnt gynecology and who has been my source of inspiration, motivation and encouragement in writing this book.

I also take this opportunity to remember my teachers Prof Manab Kumar Sanyal, Prof Mumtaz Sanghamita and Prof Hiranmay Das without whose blessings I would not have become a gynecologist. I also remember my seniors Prof Joydeb Mukherjee, Prof Tapan Kumar Lahiri, Prof Sudip Saha, Prof Pranati Sinha, Prof Rekha Datta, Prof Sudhir Adhikary, Prof Sibani Sengupta, Prof Rupkamal Das, (Late) Prof Balaram Samanta, Dr Goutam Chaterjee, Dr Ujjal Mandal and Dr SS Panja from whom I have learnt obstetrics and gynecology in my younger days.

I express my sincere gratitude and thanks to Prof Manju Banerjee, Principal; Prof SA Amam, Medical Superintendent cum Vice Principal and Prof Nabendu Bhattacharyya, Head, Department of Obstetrics and Gynecology, NRS Medical College, for allowing me in using clinical material utilised in this book.

I am indebted to Prof Debasis Banerjee, ex-Head, Department of Obstetrics and Gynecology, NRS Medical College; Prof Srikanta Purakayastha, ex-Principal, NRS Medical College and Prof Hiralal Konar for their constant support and encouragement in my professional life.

I express my sincere thanks to Prof Sankar Nath Mitra, Prof Malay Mundle, Prof Pranab Kumar Biswas, Prof Pradip Kumar Banerjee, Prof Chandana Das, Prof Sarmila Kundu, Prof Joydeb Roy Chowdhury, Dr Anjan Dasgupta, Dr Debasis Chaterjee, Dr Apurba Mondal, Dr Samares Malo, Dr Sarmistha Ganguly, Dr Sanjeeb Mondal for their participation in many of my research projects and became constant source of inspiration in my professional life.

I must mention the names of Dr Abantika Konar, Dr Ansuman Sarkar, Dr Sumita Bhuiya, Dr Sumit Poddar, Dr Sibram Chaterjee, Prof Sritanu Bhattcharya, Prof Tapan Kumar Maity, Prof Swapan Jana, Dr Abhimanyu Gayen, Dr Priyadarshi Mondal, Dr Popli Bhattacharyya, Dr Reena Dey, Dr Arnab Koley, Dr Sumita Mukherjee, Dr Sanjay Show and Mr Mani Mohan Ghosh for inspiring me in writing this book.

Two of my postgraduate students, Dr Sumana Nath and Dr Soham Chowdhury, have captured all the photographs used in this book and no word of appreciation is enough for them.

I keep my head down in front of Eden Hospital, Medical College, Kolkata, where I have learnt gynecology, and Department of Obstetrics and Gynecology, NRS Medical College, where I have practised gynecology. I express my gratitude to all the patients who have allowed me to learn gynecology.

I would like to thank my wife Rupa for standing beside me throughout my career and writing this book. I also thank my wonderful son Srinjay for understanding my long nights at the computer. I remain indebted to my uncle Dr Asok Kumar Chowdhury for his support and encouragement. My family, including my in-laws, have always supported me throughout my career and authoring this book and I really appreciate it.

Last, but not the least, I express my sincere thanks to CBS Publishers & Distributors, New Delhi, for their sincere efforts in publishing this book within a very short time.

Snehamay Chaudhuri

Contents

- Approach to a patient with postmenopausal bleeding par vagina   313
- Differential diagnosis   313
- Investigations   314
- Treatment   315

33. Contraception   318
- Introduction   318
- Counselling   318
- Contraceptive methods   319
- Contraceptive effectiveness   320
- Behavioural methods   320
- Barrier methods   321
- Hormonal contraception   323
- Combined oral contraceptive   323
- Contraceptive patch   328
- Contraceptive vaginal ring   328
- Combined injectable contraceptive   328
- Progestogen-only contraception   329
- Progestogen-only pill (POP)   329
- Progestogen injections   330
- Implant   331
- Intrauterine devices   331
- Female sterilization   337
- Male sterilization   340
- Emergency contraception (postcoital contraception)   342

34. Common Minor Gynecological Operations   347
- Dilatation and curettage   347
- Hysterosalpingography   351
- Cervical biopsy   353

35. Major Operations in Gynecology   357
- Consent for surgery   357
- Hysterectomy   358
- Steps of abdominal hysterectomy   359
- Steps of vaginal hysterectomy   360
  - Postoperative management of hysterectomy patient   361
- Complications of hysterectomy   361
- Myomectomy   362
- Laparoscopy   363
- Hysteroscopy   367

36. Medical Termination of Pregnancy (MTP)   370
- Introduction   370
- Medical Termination of Pregnancy Act   370
- Methods of MTP   372
  - Methods of MTP first trimester   372
    - Medical abortion   372
    - Surgical termination of pregnancy   374
  - Methods of MTP in second trimester   376
    - Medical methods   376
    - Surgical methods   378
    - Complications of MTP   378

37. Instruments, Specimens and X-rays   382
- Instruments   382
- Specimens   389
- X-ray plates   393

Index   395

Applied Anatomy of the Female Genital Organs

The urethral opening, the vaginal opening and the anus are all close together in the vulva. What do you think is the clinical importance of this close relationship for the woman?

In this chapter we will learn:
- Name of different organs of female genital tract
- Description of each genital organ in terms of appearance, blood supply, lymphatic drainage and functions
- To draw and label external genitalia of a female
- To draw a sagittal section diagram of uterus, cervix and vagina to show their relationship to the bladder, urethra and rectum
- Description of major supports of uterus

The female genital organs can be subdivided into the external and internal genitalia.

External genitalia: All the structures which are visible externally, surrounding the urethral and vaginal openings, make the **external female genitalia.** These structures are collectively named the **vulva.** The boundaries of vulva include the mons pubis anteriorly, the rectum posteriorly, and the genitocrural folds (thigh folds) laterally. The vulva consists of the following organs: mons pubis, labia minora and majora, hymen, clitoris, vestibule, urethra, Skene glands, greater vestibular (Bartholin) glands, and vestibular bulbs.

Internal genitalia: Internal genital organs are:
1. Vagina
2. Uterus
3. Fallopian tubes
4. Ovaries

Structures closely related to genital structures are:
1. Urethra and urinary bladder
2. Ureter
3. Pelvic colon
4. Rectum and anus.

External Female Genitalia

Vulva: The vulva is the external female genitalia (Fig. 1.1) and is composed of:
- *Mons pubis:* The **mons pubis** is a thick, hair-covered, fatty and semi-rounded area overlying the *symphysis pubis*. The function of the fatty tissue in the mons pubis is to protect the woman's pubic area from bruising during the sex act.

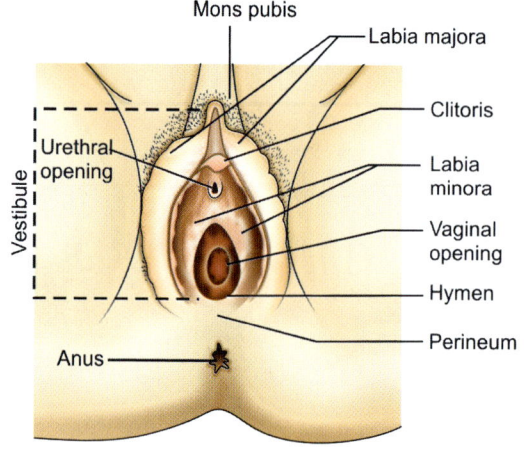

Fig. 1.1: The external female genitalia (or vulva)

- *Labia majora:* The **labia majora** are two elongated, hair-covered, fatty skin folds that enclose and protect the other organs of the external female genitalia. They contain apocrine, sebaceous and sweat gland. They are analogous to the male scrotum.

- The **labia minora** are two thick skin folds that contain no fat or hair. They protect the opening of the vagina and the urethra. The labia minora normally have an elastic nature, which enables them to distend and contract during sexual activity, and labour and delivery. The labia minora enclose the clitoris anteriorly. They also enclose the vagina and fused posteriorly forming the fourchette. The labia minora are homologous to the male penile urethra.

Fact sheet: In African countries, the labia minora and the clitoris (described below) may be removed by female genital mutilation, one of the harmful traditional practices.

- *Vestibule:* The **vestibule** is the area between the labia minora, and consists of the clitoris, urethral opening and the vaginal opening.

- The **clitoris** is a short (2 cm) erectile organ at the top of the vestibule, which has a very rich nerve supply and blood vessels. The clitoris is made up of 2 crura, which attach to the periosteum of the ischiopubic rami. Its function is sexual excitation and it is very sensitive to touch. Its anatomical position is similar to the position of the male penis.

- The **urethral opening** is the opening of the urethra, which is a small tubular structure that drains urine from the bladder. A female urethra ranges in length from 3.5 to 5.0 cm (average 4 cm).

- The **vaginal opening** is the entrance to the vagina. Hymen is a thin and incomplete membrane covering the vaginal orifice in a virgin. The hymen has one or more openings. The hymenal openings can be annular, crescent, septate or cribriform. The hymenal opening allows menstrual blood to escape during menstruation. The hymen is torn during intercourse and/or child birth. The tags of torn hymen are known as 'curunculae myrtiformes'. A woman with intact hymen is said to be virgin.

- *Bartholin's gland and Skene's gland:* Bartholin's glands are responsible for secreting lubrication to the vagina, with openings just outside the hymen, bilaterally, at the posterior aspect of the vagina. Each gland is small, similar in shape to a kidney bean. The Bartholin's duct is homologous to male Cowper's duct. The Skene's glands also secrete lubrication at the opening of the urethra.

- *Vestibular bulbs:* The vestibular bulbs are 2 masses of erectile tissue that lie deep to the bulbocavernosus muscles bilaterally.

- *Perineum:* The skin-covered muscular area between the vaginal opening and the anus is called the **perineum**. It has strong muscles and its own nerve supply, and it helps to support the contents of the pelvic cavity.

Vulval blood supply: The vulva is highly vascularised and it gets its blood supply from:
1. Vaginal artery which is a branch of internal iliac artery.

2. Superficial pudendal artery which is a branch of the femoral artery.

Vulval lymphatic drainage: The main drainage site of the vulva is the superficial inguinal lymph nodes. The lymphatic drainage extends to the deep inguinal lymph nodes, then to external iliac lymph nodes and the common iliac lymph nodes. There is a contralateral lymphatic drainage of the labia.

Internal Female Genitalia

Vagina: The vagina is the tube like passage connecting the vulva and the uterus. The vagina is lined with rugae which allow it to expand during sexual intercourse and childbirth. The structure of the vagina is a network of connective, membranous, and erectile tissues. The vagina is always moist, the fluid being derived from cervical secretions and Bartholin's glands. This fluid has an acidic reaction (pH 3.5–4.5) making it capable of resisting infection (*see* physiological vaginal discharge—Chapter 14). The vagina is divided into four areas in relation to the cervix. The four vaginal areas are called fornices.

1. Anterior fornix is shallowest of the fornices and the length of anterior vaginal wall measures around 7.5–9 cm in an adult female.
2. Posterior fornix is the deepest of all fornices and the length of posterior vaginal wall measures around 9–11 cm in adult female.
3. Two lateral fornices

The **relationship** of the vagina with surrounding structures is as shown in Fig. 1.3:
1. Anteriorly there is the urethra and urinary bladder.
2. Posteriorly there is perineal body, rectum and peritoneum of the Pouch of Douglas.
3. Laterally there are sphincter vaginae (pubococcygeal muscles act as a sphincter for the vagina), Levator ani muscles, Bartholin's glands. The lateral fornix of the vagina is related to the ureter and uterine artery.
4. Superiorly is the cervix.

The vagina has three **functions:**
1. It is a receptacle for the penis, where sperm are deposited during sexual intercourse.
2. It is the outlet for the menstrual flow every month in the non-pregnant woman.
3. It is the passage way down which the baby passes at birth.

Vaginal blood supply: The vagina gets its blood supply from the vaginal artery, branches of the pudendal artery and twigs from middle and inferior rectal artery.

Vaginal lymphatic drainage: The lower one-third of vagina has the same lymphatic drainage as the vulva while upper two-thirds have the same lymphatic drainage as that of cervix.

Nerve supply of vagina: The nerve supply to the vagina is primarily from the autonomic nervous system. Sensory fibers to the lower vagina arise from the pudendal nerve, and pain fibers are from sacral nerve roots.

THE UTERUS

The uterus is the thick walled, hollow pear-shaped female reproductive organ that lies within the pelvis between the bladder and the rectum. In an adult female it is 9 cm long, 3 cm thick and 6 cm broad at its widest part. The average weight of a nonpregnant, nulliparous uterus is approximately 40–50 g. A multiparous uterus may weigh slightly more than this, with an upper limit of approximately 110 g. A menopausal uterus is small and atrophied and typically weighs much less.

The uterus can be divided into 3 parts:
- *Body:* The major portion, which is the upper two-thirds of the uterus (corpus uteri). Body extends from the fundus to a constriction known as the isthmus which corresponds with internal os of cervical canal.
- *Fundus:* The domed area at the top of the uterus, above the insertion of the two

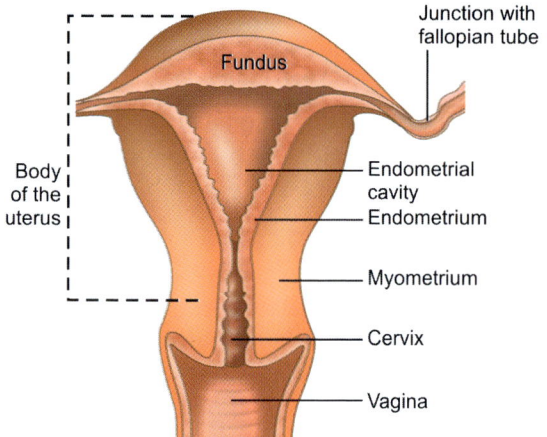

Fig. 1.2: Structure of the empty uterus, showing the main regions

fallopian tubes. Fundus is the part of the body.

- *Cervix:* Cervix lies below the isthmus. The cervix may be subdivided in two parts:
  1. A supravaginal portion superior to the limits of the vagina and
  2. A vaginal portion, which projects into the cavity of the vagina. The region between the body and cervix is referred to as the isthmus, a short area of constriction. During pregnancy, it is known as the "lower uterine segment." The cavity of the isthmus is called the "internal os."

The wall of the uterus has three layers of tissue, two of which are shown in Fig. 1.2:

1. The **perimetrium:** The outermost thin membrane layer covering the uterus.
2. The **myometrium:** The thick, muscular, middle layer in Fig. 1.2.
3. The **endometrium:** The thin, innermost layer of the uterus, which thickens during the menstrual cycle. This is the tissue that builds up each month in a woman of reproductive age, under the influence of the female reproductive hormones. There are two layers—a superficial functional layer which is shed monthly and a basal layer which is not shed and from which new functional layer is regenerated.

The cavity of the uterus is flattened and triangular and is around 6–7 cm in length. The uterine tubes enter the uterine cavity bilaterally in the superolateral portion of the cavity.

The body of the uterus is usually angled forward in relation to the cervix (anteflexion), while the uterus and cervix as a whole lean forward from the upper vagina (anteversion). The normal anatomical position of uterus is anteflexion and anteversion. In about 15% women the uterus is retroverted and in most instances retroversion is an asymptomatic variant of normality.

The peritoneum is reflected from the front of uterus over the superior surface of bladder and forms the uterovesical pouch. The posterior surface of the uterus is completely covered by peritoneum, which passes down over the posterior fornix of the vagina into the pouch of Douglas. Anteriorly peritoneum is reflected off the uterus at a much higher level onto the superior surface of bladder.

The relationship of the uterus to its surrounding organs (Fig. 1.3) is as follows:

- Anteriorly there is the uterovesical peritoneum and urinary bladder.
- Posteriorly there is pouch of Douglas and coils of intestine .
- Laterally is the parametrium. Uterine artery crosses over the ureter (water under the bridge) 2 cm lateral to the cervix.

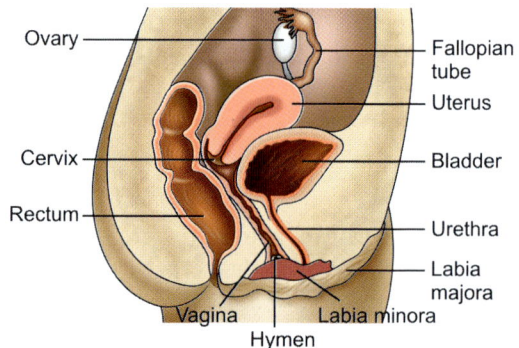

Fig. 1.3: The uterus and vagina and their relationship with adjacent organs

- Superiorly there are coils of intestine and omentum.
- Inferiorly is the vagina.

Blood supply of the uterus: The uterus gets its main blood supply from the uterine artery which is branch of anterior division of internal iliac artery. The ovarian artery which is a branch of the abdominal aorta also nourishes the uterus. The arteries anastomose along the fallopian tube.

Lymphatic Drainage

From the fundus and upper part of the body
1. Most of the lymphatic vessels drain into pre-aortic and lateral aortic lymph nodes following the ovarian blood vessels.
2. A few lymphatic vessels from lateral angles drain into superficial inguinal lymph nodes passing along the round ligamants of uterus.

Uterine supports: Uterine supports which prevent the uterus from prolapsing, are seen in pairs:
- The cardinal ligaments, also known as trans-verse cervical ligaments or Mackenrodt's ligaments. These are strongest of all uterine supports. The cardinal ligaments are essentially dense condensations of connective tissue around the venous and nerve plexuses which extends from the pelvic side walls toward the genital tract. Medially they are firmly fused with the fascia surrounding the cervix and upper part of the vagina. They pass upwards and backwards towards the root of the internal iliac vessel. These condensation of fibrous and elastic tissue, together with plain muscle fibers, are sometimes referred as parametrium. They support the upper vagina and cervix, helping to maintain, helping to maintain anteflexion. Inferiorly they are continuous with the fascia on the upper surface of the levator ani muscle.
- *Uterosacral ligaments:* The uterosacral ligaments pass upwards and backwards from the posterior aspect of the cervix toward the lateral part of the second piece of the sacrum. In their lower part they contain plain muscle along with fibrous tissue and autonomic nerve fibres. In their upper part they dwindle to shallow peritoneal folds. The ligaments divide the pouch of Douglas from the para rectal fossa from each side.
- Pubocervical ligaments are the weakest. These are a pair of thin fibrous bands which extend from the cervix to the pubic bones along the inferolateral surfaces of the bladder. The ligaments pull the cervix forward countering the pull of uterosacral ligament backwards.

Apart from the above mentioned ligaments there are other ligaments, the round ligaments (Prevent the uterus from axial rotation and maintain its anteflexion state) and the broad ligaments through which blood vessels nourishing the uterus and fallopian tubes pass. The levator ani muscles which act as pelvic floor support and prevent the uterus from prolapsing (for more details *see* Chapter 27).

Clinical pearl: The vagina and cervix can be inspected through a speculum in the vagina. Digital examination per vagina may be combined with palpation through the anterior abdominal wall by the other hand (bimanual examination).

The Cervix

The cervix connects the uterus and vagina, and projects into the upper vagina. The 'gutter' surrounding the projection comprises the **vaginal fornices—lateral, anterior and posterior.** The cervix is 2.5 cm long. Vaginal part is 1.25 cm and supravaginal part is 1.25 cm. The endocervical canal is fusiform in shape between the external and internal os. After child birth external os looses its circular shape and resembles a transverse slit. **The epithelial lining of the canal is a columner mucous membrane** with an anterior and posterior longitudinal ridge, from which shallow palmate fold extends, hence the name arbor vitae.

There are numerous glands secreting mucus which becomes more abundant and less viscous at the time of ovulation in mid cycle. **The vaginal surface of the cervix is covered with stratified squamous epithelium.** The squamo columner junction commonly does not correspond to the anatomical os. This 'tidal zone' within which epithelial junction migrates at different stages of life, is termed the **transformation zone** (for more details see Chapter 22). The shifting of the squamo columner junction is influenced by the estrogenic stimulation. In the newborn female and in pregnancy this outgrowth is vey common, forming a bright pink rosette around the external os. This appearance has been misnamed as **erosion** but the epithelium covering, though delicate, is intact. In cases , where the cervix has under gone deep bilateral laceration during childbirth, the resulting anterior and posterior lips tend to evert, exposing the glandular epithelium of the canal widely. This appearance is termed **ectropion**.

Lymphatic Drainage of Cervix

On each side the lymphatic drain in three directions:

a. Laterally some vessels pass through parametric tissue and drain into external iliac and obturator lymph nodes. A few lymphatic vessels are intercepted by para cervical lymph nodes which are situated at the crossing of the ureter and uterine artery.

b. Posterolaterally, the lymphatics pass along the lateral pelvic wall and drain into internal iliac nodes.

c. Posteriorly some of the lymphatics pass along the uterosacral ligaments and drain into sacral lymph nodes.

Clinical Aspects

- The endometrium and uterine cavity can be examined by hysteroscopy. The tubal ostia can be seen. Because the anterior and posterior wall are normally in contact, the cavity must be inflated with gas or fluid to obtain an adequate view of surfaces.

- It is specially important to distinguish retroversion from anteversion before introducing a sound or similar instrument into the uterine cavity to avoid perforation of uterine wall.

- Because the uterus lies behind the bladder, and between the lower parts of ureters, particular care must be taken not to damage these structures during hysterectomy.

- The transformation zone is typically the area where precancerous change occurs. This can be detected by microscopic assessment of cervical cytological smear.

- If the duct of a cervical gland is occluded, gland distends with mucous to form a retention cyst (Nabothian follicle).

Fallopian Tubes

There are two fallopian tubes each of which measures about 10 cm long. Each fallopian tube is divided in four major parts:

- *Interstitial* portion is the part of fallopian tube (1.25 cm) which is within uterine muscle. The interstitial portion opens into the uterine cavity. It is the narrowest part of the fallopian tube.

- *The isthmus* extending out of the cornu for about 2.5–3 cm is also narrow.

- *Ampulla:* It is thin walled, dilated and tortuous, and measures about 5 cm.

- *Infundibulum:* It is trumpet like and about 1.25 cm long. The bottom of the infundibulum presents pelvic ostium, the circumference of which is provided with the fimbriae.

Blood supply: The fallopian tube has a dual blood supply, the medial half from the tubal branch of uterine artery and lateral half from the tubal branch of ovarian artery.

Clinical Aspects

- The fallopian tube is derived from the cranial end of the müllerian duct and its lumen is therefore continuous with the uterine cavity and the cervical canal. Sperms can thus easily travel upwards through the cervix and uterus into the tubal lumen to fertilize the ovum.
- At the time of ovulation the fimbriae grasp the ovary in the area where the stigma (or point of follicular rupture) is forming. Usually, therefore, the ovum is discharged into the infundibulum and carried by tubal peristalsis into the ampulla of tube, which is where fertilization occurs.
- Sterilization is effected by occluding both tubes preferably in narrow isthmic portion using clips, sutures, diathermy, or rings.
- Patency of the tubes can be tested by injecting a watery dye (methylene blue) through the cervix and observing spill from abdominal ostia by laparoscopy.
- The contours of the tubal lumen and uterine cavity may also be demonstrated with radio opaque fluid during a hysterosalpingogram.
- When the outer portion of the tube distends with pus (pyosalpinx) or serous fluid (hydrosalpinx), these tubo-ovarian masses are felt in the posterolateral quadrant of pelvis.

The Ovary

The ovaries form the gonads of the female. Each ovary is ovoid structure measuring about 3.5 cm × 2 cm × 1.5 cm. They are a dull white and are attached to the superior aspect of the broad ligament by a short peritoneum fold called meso-ovarium. Follicle or corpus leuteal cysts may be seen on surface of the ovary.

Its lateral border is free but anteriorly is attached to the broad ligament at the hilum through which ovarian vessels and nerves enter or leave the organ. Medially the ovarian ligament connects it to the uterine cornu and laterally ovarian fimbriae of the tube.

Blood supply: The blood supply of ovary is through the ovarian artery, a branch of abdominal aorta and uterine artery and numerous anastomosis. The venous drainage is through the pampiniform plexus to the ovarian veins. The right ovarian vein drains into the inferior vena cava and left ovarian vein drains into the left renal vein.

Lymphatic drainage: Primarily through the aortic nodes. Rarele they may drain through iliac lymph nodes.

Clinical Aspects

- The tubes and ovaries often collectively called uterine adnexa and are so intimately related that when the tube is inflamed the ovary is also affected resulting in salpigo-oophoritis.
- The ovary is most common site of endometriosis and rarely become seat of extra-uterine gestation.
- Besides providing ova, it is an important endocrine gland producing estrogen, progesterone and androgens.
- Its histology and histogenesis is of interest in understanding of complex varities of ovarian neoplasms.

EXERCISES

1. Answer the following questions

- Name the structures forming external genitalia of female.
- What is the boundary of vulva?
- What is the composition of labia majora?
- What is the composition of labia minora?
- What is the composition of clitoris?
- What are Bartholin's glands?
- What is the lymphatic drainage of vulva?
- What are the organs of female internal genitalia?
- What is the relationship of uterus with other pelvic organs?
- What are the parts of uterus?
- What is the uterine cervix?

- What is the uterine corpus?
- What are the ligaments of uterus and cervix?
- What are the uterosacral ligaments?
- What are the cardinal ligaments?
- What is the blood supply of uterus?
- What is the blood supply of ovary?
- What is the lymphatic drainage of ovaries?

2. Write short notes on

- Supports of uterus
- Transformation zone

3. Explain or justify the following statements

- Determination of anatomical position of uterus is important at the time of intrauterine instrumentation.
- Knowledge of anatomical relation of uterus with adjacent structures is important for not to damage these structures during hysterectomy.

4. Fill in the blanks with appropriate word/s

- Length of female urethra is _____ cm.
- Bartholin's duct opens at _____ .
- The pH of the vagina is _____ .

- The length of the uterine cavity is _____ cm
- Uterine artery crosses the uterus _____ cm lateral to the isthmus.
- Uterine artery is a branch of _____ artery.
- Length of fallopian tube is _____ cm.
- Left renal vein drains into _____ .
- Ovarian artery is a branch of _____ .

Bibliography

1. Clinical Gynecology. K Bhaskar Rao, NN Roy Chowdhury. Orient Longman Limited, 4th edition 1999.
2. Clinical Obstetrics and Gynecology 2nd edition. B Magowan, P Owen, J Drife. Saunders Elsevier 2009.
3. Essentials of Obstetrics and Gynecology for Clinical Officers. Mbilu J NK.
4. Graziottin A, Giraldi A. Anatomy and physiology of Women's Sexual Function in: Porst H. Buvat J. (eds), ISSM (International Society of Sexual Medicine) Standard Committee Book, Standard practice in Sexual Medicine, Blackwell, Oxford, UK, 2006, p. 289–304.
5. Van Anh T. Ginger and Claire C. Yang. Functional Anatomy of the Female Sex Organs. P. Mulhall et al. (eds.), Cancer and Sexual Health, Current Clinical Urology, DOI 10.1007/978-1-60761-916-1_2, © Springer Science+Business Media, LLC 2011.

Development of Female Genital Organs and Its Congenital Anomalies

A 25-year-old married woman has presented in outpatient department with history of three consecutive spontaneous abortions each at 5 months of gestation. During her investigations for mid trimester pregnancy losses, hysterosalpingogram revealed a bicornuate uterus with bilateral tubal spillage of dye (see Fig. 2.4). How she should be treated?

In this chapter we will learn:
- Development of gonad and sexual differentiation
- Development of uterus, cervix, fallopian tubes and vagina
- Development of external genitalia
- Congenital abnormalities, clinical presentation and management

Introduction

The development of the normal female genital tract is a complex process. The undifferentiated gonad differentiates to the ovary. The mesonephros, wolffian and müllerian ducts differentiate in a coordinated manner to form the uterus, vagina and lower urinary tract. Abnormalities in differentiation can result in congenital anomalies of female reproductive tracts, renal tract and lower intestines. A knowledge of normal embryology is essential for an understanding of congenital anomalies as they are encountered in clinical practice .

Development of the Gonads

1. *Indifferent gonadal phase:* In the fifth week of intrauterine life gonadal development starts. The mesothelium medial to the mesonephros of the developing kidneys thickens and forms the paired gonadal (urogenital) ridges (Fig. 2.1a). Transient epithelial finger-like structures, referred to as the primary sex cords, form and extend into the supporting mesenchyme. The gonadal ridges remain similar in both male and female fetuses until the seventh week.

2. *Gonadal sex differentiation:* Under the influence of two X-chromosomes the cortex of the indifferent gonad is developed in the female embryo than the male. The cortex gives rise to the secondary sex cords (cortical cords) which extend from the surface epithelium to the mesenchyme (Fig. 2.1c). The secondary sex cords sustain and regulate ovarian cortical follicular development. The undifferentiated gonads persist until around the tenth week, at which time the ovaries first become identifiable. A male fetus will develop in the presence of a

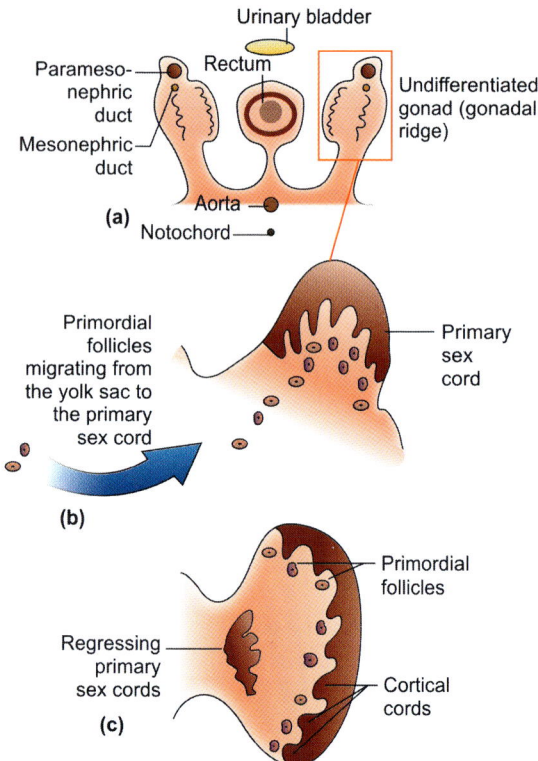

Fig. 2.1: Development of the ovaries from the undifferentiated (indifferent) gonads: **(a)** The indifferent gonads appear as primitive longitudinal streaks in the intermediate mesoderm adjacent to the mesonephros. **(b)** Magnified view of the undifferentiated gonad during 5–6 fetal weeks. The primordial follicles develop in the yolk sac and migrate to the gonadal ridge and are sustained by the primary sex cords. **(c)** The primary cords are transitory and regress by 8 weeks. The cortical (secondary cords) maintain ovarian follicular development. The ovaries are identifiable by 10 weeks

Y-chromosome which encodes the SRY protein. The SRY protein enables testicular differentiation and the production of androgens including testosterone. The medulla of the indifferent gonad in males differentiates into the testis, the cortex involutes giving rise to vestigial remnants. In addition to the SRY protein and androgens a third factor is required for male development, anti-müllerian hormone (AMH). AMH prevents female genital ductal differentiation. An immature female will develop in the absence of these three factors.

3. *Development of ovaries (gonadal differentiation):* The primordial germ cells migrate from the yolk sac to the genital ridge via the dorsal mesentery and undergo successive mitotic divisions. The primordial germ cells divide repeatedly and produce a population of primary oocytes surrounded by follicle cells—the primordial follicles. By 5–6 months gestation the ovaries contain 6–7 million primordial follicles. The fate of an oocyte is determined once meiosis begins and no further mitotic division is possible thereafter. The vast majority of oocytes eventually degenerate over time; the remaining oogonia enter a dormant state referred to as meiotic arrest (first phase of meiosis). First meiosis will not complete until the onset of ovulation. Ovulatory follicles complete meiotic differentiation. At birth, between 2 and 4 million follicles remain. Around 400,000 follicles are present at menarche (Baker, 1963) and less than 500 will proceed to ovulation.

4. *Pelvic descent of the ovaries:* The ovaries in part undergo descent from the posterior abdominal wall into the pelvis due to the marked growth of the upper abdomen relative to the pelvis. By the third month the maturing ovaries descend into the pelvis guided by the gubernaculum into the ovarian fossae. The gubernaculum is a peritoneal fold which attaches the caudal aspect of the ovary to the uterus, eventually forming the utero-ovarian and round ligaments.

Fact sheet: 'Gonad' is the general name for the organ which produces or will produce, gametes, and can be applied to both sexes.

Developments of Fallopian Tubes, Uterus, Cervix and Vagina

In females the paramesonephric (müllerian) ducts arise from the mesoderm lateral to the mesonephric ducts in the seventh week of intrauterine life. The paramesonephric ducts are the precursors of the uterus, fallopian tubes, cervix and upper vagina.

The paramesonephric ducts grow caudally, coursing lateral to the urogenital ridges. The paramesonephric ducts fuse together (müllerian organogenesis) and represents the initial stage in the development of the upper two-thirds of the vagina, the cervix, uterus and both fallopian tubes (Fig. 2.2). The cranial end of the fused ducts forms the future uterus. The ducts contain mesoderm that will form the uterine endometrium and myometrium. The unfused cranial ends of the paramesonephric ducts assume a funnel shaped configuration and remain open to the future peritoneal cavity as the fimbrial portions of the fallopian tubes. The caudal end of the fused ducts will form the upper two-thirds of the vagina.

Clinical pearl: Since the paramesonephric ducts (Müllerian) develops alongside the renal system, when one system is abnormally formed, an abnormality in other is frequently present. For example, the kidney should also be evaluated, since renal anomalies (i.e., agenesis or ectopia) frequently accompany müllerian duct anomalies because of the close embryogenic relationship. Conversely, despite the functional connection between ovaries and fallopian tubes, an absence of one does not indicate probable absence of other.

Development of Lower Genital Tract

The primary urogenital sinus develops into the definitive urogenital sinus (UGS). The UGS

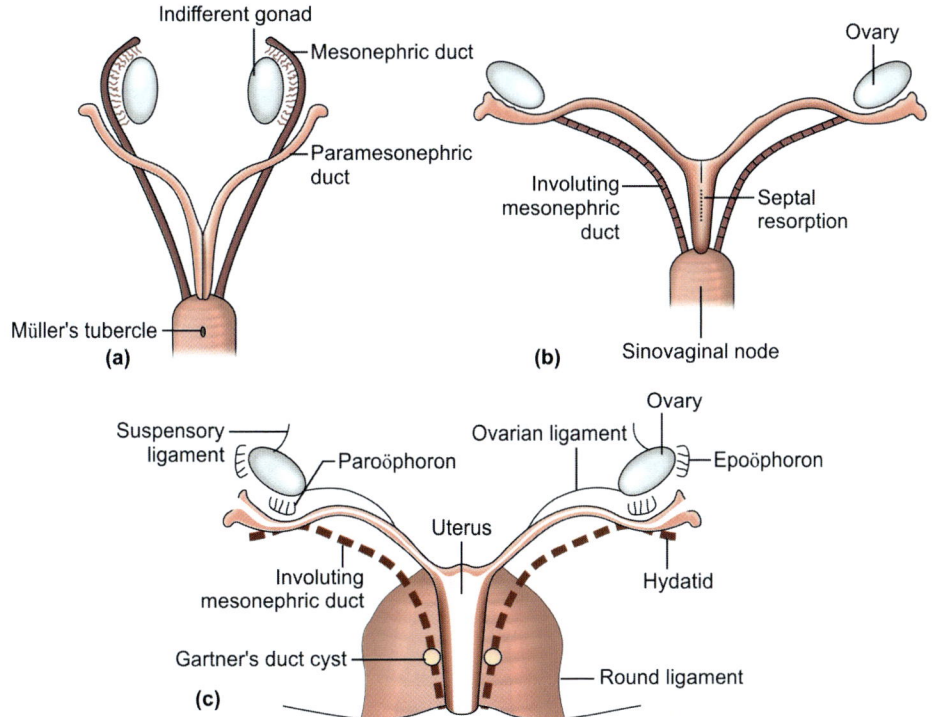

Fig. 2.2: Differentiation of the paramesonephric (müllerian) ducts: **(a)** Indifferent phase with both mesonephric and paramesonephric ducts present. Female internal genital development proceeds in the absence of the male SRY protein. **(b)** At 7 weeks the paramesonephric ducts differentiate whilst the mesonephric ducts involute. The medial portions of the paramesonephric ducts fuse to form the uterus and upper vagina (lateral fusion 9–11 weeks), the lateral portions give rise to fallopian tubes. Müllerian organogenesis is complete by 5 months with uterine septal resorption. **(c)** The female internal genitalia at 5 months. Occasionally remnants of the mesonephric duct may persist

Table 2.1: Vestigial remnants and postnatal derivatives of the genitourinary tract

Embryonic structure	Female	Male counterpart
Gonad	Ovary	Testis
Paramesonephric duct	Hydatid of morgagni, fallopian tubes, uterus, cervix, upper vagina	Appendix of testis
Urogenital sinus	Urethra, urethral, paraurethral and greater vestibular glands, urinary bladder, lower vagina, hymen	Urethra, prostate utricle, prostate and bulbourethral gland
Genital tubercle	Clitoris	Penis
Urogenital folds	Labia minora	Ventral aspect of penis
Labioscrotal swelling	Labia majora	Scrotum
Mesonephric tubule	Epöphoron, paröphoron	Ductuli efferentes

consists of a caudal phallic portion and a pelvic portion. The urethral groove and phallic (distal) portion of the UGS enlarge to form the vaginal introitus (vestibule). This is closed off externally by the urogenital membrane which perforates in the seventh week. The narrow pelvic (proximal) segment of the definitive urogenital sinus contributes to the short distal female urethra and lower third of the vagina.

Development of External Genitalia

The external genitalia develop from the same primordia in both sexes. In girls the unfused parts of the labioscrotal (genital) folds give rise to the labia majora. The folds fuse anteriorly to form the mons pubis and anterior labial commissure, and posteriorly the posterior labial commissure. The urethral folds fuse posteriorly to form the frenulum of the labia minora. The unfused urethral (urogenital) folds give rise to the labia minora. The unfused genital swellings enable the urogenital sinus to open into the anterior (urethral) part of the vagina and the vaginal vestibule. The genital tubercle becomes the clitoris and is recognizable.

Congenital Abnormalities

Vulva

- Rarely there may be congenital enlargement of labia minora

- If the female fetus is exposed to androgens in intrauterine life, there may be labial fusion with clitoral hypertrophy.

Treatment: Girls with clitoral hypertrophy and labial fusion should be treated with cliteroplasty and separation of labia.

Uterus, Cervix, Vagina and Fallopian Tubes

i. Uterine anomaly

Müllerian duct anomalies are classified according to the system established by the American Fertility Society (*see* Table 2.2 and Fig. 2.3)

Class I: Hypoplasia or agenesis. Failure of normal development of the müllerian ducts causes uterine agenesis or hypoplasia. In uterine agenesis uterus is felt as a small nodule or ridge at the vault of vagina. There is absence of endometrium and the girl suffers from primary amenorrhea. In hypoplasia of uterus the uterus is small in size or may be infantile where the cervix is long in relation to the body of uterus. The women may present with amenorrhea or hypomenorrhea and/or dyspareunia.

Class II: Unicornuate. Agenesis of a unilateral müllerian duct causes a single, so-called banana-shaped uterus with a single fallopian tube. Some patients have a rudimentary horn on the contralateral side. When the rudimentary horn is noncommunicating, endometrial

Table 2.2: AFS classification of patients based on the anatomy of the female genital system, especially uterine anomaly

Classification	Anomaly
Class I Hypoplasia and agenesis	(a) Vaginal, (b) cervical, (c) fundal, (d) tubal
Class II Unicornuate	(a) Communicating, (b) noncommunicating, (c) no cavity, (d) no horn
Class III Didelphys	Didelphys
Class IV Bicornuate	(a) Partial, (b) complete
Class V Septate	(a) Partial, (b) complete
Class VI Arcuate	Arcuate
Class VII DES drug-related	DES related

AFS: American Fertility Society
DES: Diethylstilbestrol
Source: Classification of female genital anomalies. Fertil Steril 2010.

tissue expelled retrogradely through the fallopian tube during menstruation results in an increased frequency of endometriosis. This makes surgical resection of the horn necessary. Spontaneous abortion and premature labor may occur in pregnancies with a unicornuate uterus, and the poorest fetal survival among all uterine anomalies has been reported.

Class III: Didelphus. Complete failure of fusion of the two müllerian ducts results in two complete uteri, each with its own cervix and vagina. Among all uterine anomalies, uterus didelphys is associated with the highest possibility of successful pregnancy, except for arcuate uterus.

Class IV: Bicornuate. Partial fusion of two Müllerian ducts results in a bicornuate uterus with one cervix. The external uterine contour is concave or heart shaped, and the uterine horns are widely divergent.

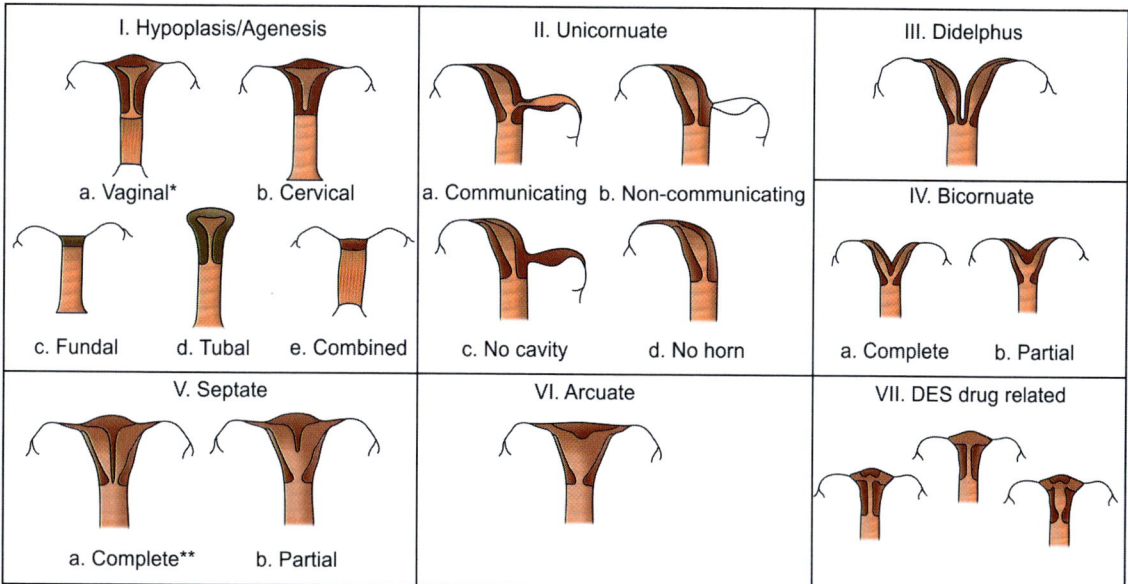

Fig. 2.3: American Fertility Society classification of müllerian duct anomalies. DES: diethylstilbestrol, * uterus may be normal or take a variety of abnormal forms, ** may have two distinct cervices.

Class V: Septate. Septate uterus results from failure of resorption of a septum after complete fusion of the müllerian ducts. The septum may be a combination of both fibrous tissue and muscle. The external uterine contour is normally convex, flat, or minimally indented by less than 1 cm, in contrast to that of a bicornuate uterus. Most patients evaluated for repeated abortions and found to have a uterine anomaly will have a septate uterus Metroplasty is a surgical procedure used for treatment of this anomaly and may enhance fetal survival.

Class VI: Arcuate. Arcuate uterus should be considered a normal variant, with a small indentation of the fundal endometrial canal and a normal external contour. There is no presence of septum inside the uterine cavity. It has no effect on fertility.

Class VII: Diethylstilbestrol related. Diethylstilbestrol is a synthetic estrogen that was used to prevent miscarriage in the 1940s to 1970s. Exposure of the female fetus to diethylstilbestrol results in uterine anomalies including T-shaped uterus, irregular constrictions, and hypoplasia. Diethylstilbestrol-related anomalies are associated with an increased rate of spontaneous abortions, preterm deliveries, and ectopic pregnancies.

Clinical Features

The girl with rudimentary, infantile or absence of uterus presents with primary amenorrhea. In hypoplastic uterus women may have amenorrhoea, scanty menstruation and may have infertility. In all other abnormalities of uterus, the women will have normal menstruation. Rarely there may be menorrghagia in uterine anomaly (bicornuate uterus) because of increased surface area of endometrium. In most women pregnancy may occur in either horn. There is increased chance of abortion (may be recurrent), preterm delivery, malpresentation. Occasionally rudimentary horn may obstruct labour.

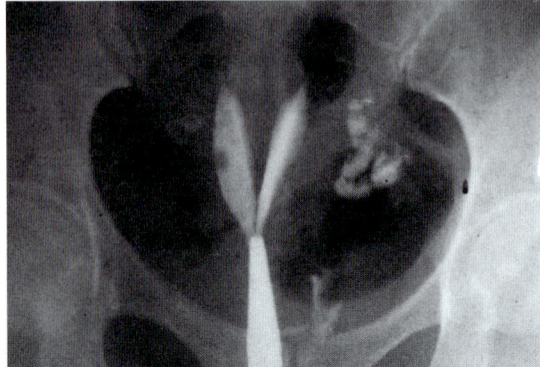

Fig. 2.4: HSG shows bicornuate uterus with patent fallopian tubes

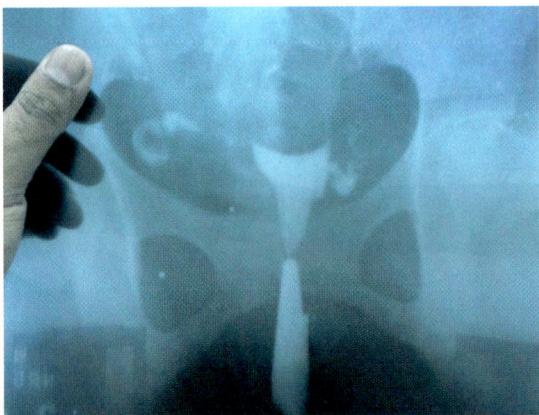

Fig. 2.5: HSG shows arcuate uterus with patent fallopian tubes

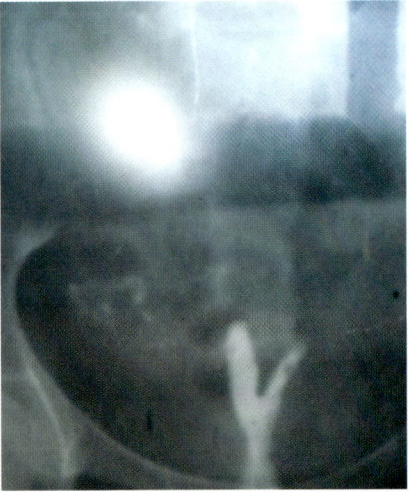

Fig. 2.6: HSG shows septate uterus with patent fallopian tubes

Pregnancy may occur in the rudimentary horn. The pregnancy may be continued till 16 weeks because of thick muscular wall, however, eventually ruptures resulting in acute abdomen.

Diagnosis

The diagnosis of congenital malformation is suspected on history (recurrent abortion, preterm birth), pelvic examination, during exploration of uterus (e.g. manual removal of placenta), or during caesarean section. Hysterosalpingogram will be able to demonstrate any abnormality of the uterus. Occasionally, bicornuate uterus and septate uterus are difficult to differentiate on hysteron salpingography alone. Laparoscopy combined with hysteroscopy will help to reach correct diagnosis. Ultrasonography may also help in diagnosis. MRI will give a clear picture of all uterine anomaly, however, it is costly.

Treatment

Hypoplastic uterus estrogen therapy has been tried but it is not of much help.

Rudimentary uterine horn: Excision is done if ectopic pregnancy occurs in ruduimentary horn or if rudimentary horn is responsible of obstructed labor.

Bicornuate uterus: Unification of the bicornuate uterus and removal of the septum is indicated in presence of recurrent abortion and preterm labor. Bicornuate uteus is repaired by the Strassman's operation.

Septate uterus: Uterine septum is removed by a hysteroscope, if available. This is a much simpler procedure than the open surgery. In open surgery, the uterine wall is incised to open the cavity and septum is excised and then stitching makes it a high risk for future vaginal delivery.

Complete müllerian agenesis or MRKH syndrome is discussed in detail in Chapter 10 of primary amenorrhoea.

ii. Vagina

Vaginal atresia, imperforate hymen, or complete septum may lead to cryptomenorrhea and the conditions are discussed in Chapter 10 of Primary amenorrhea.

iii. Fallopian tubes

Fallopian tubes may be absent in one or both sides if the uterus is absent or other anomaly is present. The tube may be too long or too short or may have congenital diverticulae . Occasionally, ostia are duplicated or an accessory tube may be present. These may have a little clinical significance except it may result in an ectopic pregnancy.

Parovarian/fimbrial cysts may arise as developmental remnants (wolffian duct, epoöphoron or paroöphoron). These are usually symptom less and have no clinical significance. Sometimes parovarian cysts may attain a large size and may be misdiagnosed as ovarian cysts. Excision of cyst is advised in these cases.

Ovaries

Disorders of sex development (DSD)

It is surprisingly difficult to define 'femaleness' or 'maleness'. Neither law nor medicine seems to have a well-established definition. However, it seems that at least 4 criteria must be taken into account:

1. *Genetic sex*
   - Female—46XX
   - Male—46XY
2. *Gonadal sex*
   - A normal female has 2 intra-abdominal ovaries
   - A normal male has 2 extra-abdominal testes
3. *Phenotypic sex:* The form of the external and internal genitalia and general body form. *Female:* The female has relatively wide hips compared with shoulder span; a vulval cleft with urethral and vaginal openings, labia majora and minora, and a small imperforate clitoris; at puberty the breasts develop, the

pubic hair has a horizontal upper margin, the forehead hairline is straight and facial hair inconspicuous; subcutaneous fat is deposited generously over hips and thighs

Male: The male has relatively narrow hips compared with shoulder span, and a penis conveying the urethra to its tip. At puberty, males develop conspicuous facial hair, pubic hair which extends to the umbilicus and a greater amount of body hair compared with the female. Later in life, the forehead hairline recedes and baldness may appear.

4. *Psychological sex*

A psychological libido usually directed towards members of the other sex.

Thus, for a person to be a 'normal' woman or a 'normal' man, each of the four criteria listed above should correspond to one sex only. If one or more does not match, the condition is known as disorder of sex development or 'intersex'.

The disorders in sex development in relation to abnormality in ovary may result from (a) chromosomal abnormality and (b) gonadal abnormality.

a. Chromosomal Abnormality

The sex chromosomes act primarily on the gonads. The Y chromosome is dominant and testis-producing, but if it is accompanied by more than one chromosome, development of a normal testis is prevented. Disorders of the sex chromosomes generally arise during the meiotic divisions of gametogenesis, but errors of mitosis may occur during embryonic development to give mosaicism, i.e.: an embryo with two or more cell populations, each with a different chromosomal complement. In addition to anomalies in the number of whole chromosomes, it is possible to have localised anomalies of a single sex chromosome sufficient to disrupt normal development. On the other hand, the presence of seemingly normal sex chromosomes does not guarantee development of a normal gonad; true

hermaphrodites with both testicular and ovarian tissues have been found to have apparent normal chromosomal constitutions.

1. *Turner's syndrome (45 XO):* The condition is described in detail in Chapter 10.
2. *Triple X female (47 XXX):* Sometimes called 'super female', however the condition may be associated with amenorrhea, under-developed breasts, infantile external genitalia, and learning difficulties.

b. Gonadal Abnormality

True hermaphroditism

1. Ovarian and testicular tissues are present in the same person. The possibilities are:
   - Testes and ovary
   - Testes and ovotestes
   - Ovo testes and ovo testes

   The external genitalia may be male-like or female-like or ambiguous. There are no exclusive characteristic features to distinguish true hermaphrodites. The majority are reared as boys, but most develop breasts at puberty. The karyotype is usually 46 XX, but XX/XY mosaics occur. The only treatment is hormone therapy and plastic surgery to enhance any phenotypic tendency.

2. *Gonadal dysgenesis:* In gonadal (ovarian) dysgenesis with normal XX karyotype, patients present with a female phenotype but fail to proceed to puberty and do not develop female secondary characteristics. They have elevated gonadotrophins and streak gonads. The streak gonads are similar to those found in patients with Turner's syndrome; however, patients with gonadal dysgenesis do not have short stature or other stigmata associated with Turner's syndrome.

Keywords

SRY protein: SRY (Sex-determining region Y) is a sex-determining gene on the Y chromosome. SRY protein initiates male sex determination.

Mullerian duct: Müllerian ducts (or paramesonephric ducts) are paired ducts that pass along the sides of the urogenital ridge and terminate at the mullerian eminence in the primitive urogenital sinus. In the female, they will develop to form the fallopian tubes, uterus, cervix, and the upper two-thirds of the vagina.

DSD (disorder of sex development): Intersex is a group of conditions where there is a discrepancy between the external genitals and the internal genitals (the testes and ovaries).

The older term for this condition, hermaphroditism, came from joining the names of a Greek god and goddess, Hermes and Aphrodite. Hermes was a god of male sexuality (among other things) and Aphrodite a goddess of female sexuality, love, and beauty.

Although the older terms are still used, they have been replaced by most experts (and patients and families) because they are misleading, confusing, and insensitive. Increasingly this group of conditions is being called disorders of sex development (DSD).

EXERCISES

Answer the following questions

1. Describe the development of ovaries and sex differentiation.
2. Describe the development of uterus, fallopian tubes.
3. Name the different types of uterine anomaly.
4. What are the clinical significances of different müllerian anomaly?

Write short notes on

1. Bicornuate uterus
2. Development of vagina

Explain or justify/criticize the following statements

1. Müllerian duct anomaly may be associated with urinary tract abnormality.
2. Gonadal differentiation to ovary is under genetic control.

Fill in the blanks with appropriate word/s

1. Ovary is developed from _____ .
2. The caudal end of the fused müllerian ducts form _____ .

3. Lower third of vagina is developed from _____ .
4. Genital tubercle forms the _____ .
5. Strassman's operation is done for repair of _____ .

Questions for practical (Read the case summary at the begining of chapter before answering following questions)

1. Describe the HSG plate.
2. How do you differentiate bicornuate and septate uterus?
3. Apart from abortion what other pregnancy complication she might develop?
4. Name some uterine anomaly other than bicornuate uterus that can lead to abortion?
5. Apart from HSG what other investigations you consider for this patient?
6. How she should be treated?

Bibliography

1. Clinical Gynecology Kruger Botha.
2. Eleni K, Papathanasiou A, Skordis N. Sex determination and disorders of sex development according to the revised nomenclature and classification in 46,XX individuals HORMONES 2010, 9(3):218–231.
3. Healy A. Embryology of the female reproductive tract G. Mann et al (eds). Imaging of Gyneco-logical Disorders in Infants and Children, Medical Radiology Diagnostic Imaging, DOI: 10.1007/174_2010_128, Springer-Verlag Berlin Heidelberg 2012.
4. Hegazy AM. Lectures on human embryology genital ducts.
5. Marino AT. Development of the urogenital system Langman's Medical Embryology chp. 15; pp 272–311.
6. Muckle CW, Feinberg EC Developmental abnormalities of the female reproductive organs GLOWM.
7. Neas FJ. Reproductive system development, Ch 27. The reproductive system, Embryology atlas.
8. Postgraduate gynecology Prassanakumari.
9. Textbook of Gynecology, Bhargava.
10. Textbook of Gynecology, Rao.

Gynecological Examination

Introduction

Taking history is the first step of physician patient relationship. History taking forms the basis for subsequent gynecological examination, investigations and treatment. Gynecological examination is indicated for both screening of diseases and diagnosis of ailments. A complete gynecological examination screens for infections as well as cervical, breast, uterine, and ovarian cancer. Symptoms commonly evaluated with gynecological history taking and examinations include vaginal discharge, alteration of menstrual pattern, dyspareunia, pain and lump in lower abdomen, breast lump or pain.

GYNECOLOGICAL HISTORY TAKING

The complete gynecological history taking may include deeply personal issues and may provoke emotional responses of woman. It is important to obtain history in a relaxed and personal setting (Table 3.1). Ideally gynecological history should be obtained without observer and when the patient is still dressed. In order to increase a patient's level of comfort

Table 3.1: Elements of gynecological history

- Identification
- Chief complaint
- History of present illness
- Menstrual history
- Obstetric history
- Past medical history
- Past surgical history
- Family history
- Social history
- Personal history
- Sexual history

during the history taking, questions should be asked in an open-ended and nonjudgmental way. Assumptions should not be made about aspects of the patient's background such as sexual orientation. Aspect of comprehensive history include:

Identification

Date of admission:
Date of examination:
Name:
Age:

Religion:
Address:
Marital status:
Parity:
Social status:

Chief Complaints

The patients main complains with duration are recorded in chronological sequence.

History of Present Illness

The patient is asked to describe any symptoms in her own words. Additional information about the nature of the problem can then be obtained by asking specific questions. It is helpful to know:

1. The circumstances at the time the problem began, including activities that the patient was engaged in, medical problems that she was experiencing at the time, and any medications that she was taking around that time.
2. The time course of the problem. Was this a transient problem, or has this been chronic, recurrent, or persistent? Are the symptoms temporally related to the menstrual cycle?
3. Is this a new problem, or has the patient experienced similar symptoms in the past? If the problem involves disruption of an otherwise normal function (such as amenorrhea), did the patient have normal function at some point in the past?
4. Characteristics of the problem, and associated symptoms. In the case of pain, this would include questions about the location, severity, nature (e.g., sharp, dull, cramp-like), exacerbating factors, relieving factors, and whether the pain radiates to another location. With respect to bleeding, this would include the frequency, amount, and duration of flow, and whether the patient is experiencing fatigue or light headedness. For complaint of vaginal discharge this should include color, odor, amount, presence of blood, relation to the period and associated itching and irritation.

5. To what extent is the problem interfering with the patient's usual activities?
6. Has the patient undergone any previous evaluation or treatment for the problem? If so, it is helpful to obtain the patient's permission to request these medical records.
7. Why did the patient seek evaluation of the problem at this point? Have the symptoms changed or increased in severity?

Menstrual History

1. *Age at menarche*—age of onset of first menstruation. Average age of menarche is 12–13 years.
2. *Last menstrual period* (LMP)—by convention, the first day of the last menstrual period is recorded.
3. *Cycle length*—the cycle length is the interval from the first day of one menstrual period to the first day of the next menstrual period. The median cycle length is 28 days with a normal range of 21–35 days.
4. Regularity of cycle
5. *Duration of flow*—menses commonly last for 3–5 days, with a range of 2–7 days.
6. Amount of flow—scanty/average/excessive
7. *Moliminal symptoms?* Many women experience predictable physical and emotional symptoms during the late luteal (premenstrual) phase of ovulatory menstrual cycles. Symptoms typically begin a few days before menses and resolve with the onset of bleeding. Commonly reported symptoms include breast tenderness, abdominal distension, weight gain, food cravings or increased appetite, irritability, and lability of mood.
8. Associated pain (dysmenorrhea, mittelschmerz)
9. Intermenstrual bleeding or discharge per vagina

If the patient is postmenopausal
- Age of onset of menopause
- Menopausal symptoms if any
- Previous menstrual pattern

No	Year and date	Pregnancy events	Labor events	Mode of delivery	Puerperium	Baby-living or not, duration of breast feeding/ immunization status

Table 3.2: Components of obstetric history

Obstetric History

The obstetric history includes both live births as well as spontaneous and elective abortions. The details are to be enquired as given in Table 3.2.

Past Medical History

The patient should be asked to list any major medical illnesses that she has had, or has currently, and any hospitalizations.

Past Surgical History

The patient should be asked to list all gynecologic and non-gynecologic surgical procedures that she has undergone, the dates of these procedures, and any complications that she experienced.

Family History

Illnesses experienced by family members should be listed, including cancer, diabetes mellitus, tuberculosis, cardiovascular diseases, hyperlipidemia, osteoporosis, and other hereditary disorders. It is helpful to know which family members are affected, and the age at which each diagnosis was made.

Social History

Pertinent aspects of a patient's social history include family income, marital status, level of education, and occupation.

Sexual History

The sexual history includes an assessment of the type of sexual activity that the patient is having and whether the patient has any questions or concerns about this. It is appropriate to ask whether the patient has any concerns about libido, and if she is having intercourse, whether she experiences dyspareunia. Sexual history has special importance in women with infertility, reproductive tract infections (RTI).

Personal History

Personal history should include patients desire for fertility, present and past use of contraceptives, intake of any medication or allergy, addiction, bowel habit, sleep and appetite.

Clinical pearl: Take a detailed history. Do not leave a stone unturned.

General and Systemic Examination

General examination: Build-Obese/thin/ average

Nutrition—well nourished/malnourished

Height:

Weight:

Pallor:

Pulse rate:

Blood pressure:

Respiratory rate:

Oedema:

Temperature:

Jaundice:

Cyanosis:

Neck veins:

Neck glands:

Systemic examination:

Cardiac examination: Heart should be examined thoroughly for apex beat, heart sounds, murmurs and click.

Pulmonary examination: Lung fields should be examined systematically for breath sounds, wheezes, ronchi and crepitations.

The Gynecological Examination

General considerations

- The gynecological examinations include examination of breasts, abdomen and pelvic examinations.
- Women are often apprehensive of pelvic examination. It is often helpful to describe the process in detail including seeing of speculum. The patient's verbal consent must be obtained prior examination.
- A female attendant should be present. Apart from providing medicolegal protection she may help in positioning of the woman.
- Patient should be asked to empty her bladder prior examination. This will help to palpate the pelvic organs easily without possible discomfort during examination.
- Patient should be properly positioned with adequate exposure under good light sourcing. However, patient's privacy should be maintained by covering the other areas apart from examination area with a sheet or Gown.
- Patient is examined standing on right side.
- Equipment required for the examination such as gloves, speculum of proper size and water soluble lubricants should be available prior hand.

Clinical pearl: *Voiding before pelvic examination helps to decrease possible discomfort and make the pelvic organ more easily palpable.*

Performance of the Gynecological Examination

Examination of breast: Breasts are inspected for asymmetry in shape, nipple inversion, bulging, and dimpling. Although size difference is common, each breast should have a regular contour. The breast is palpated with the patient seated and again with the patient supine, the ipsilateral arm above the head, and a pillow under the ipsilateral shoulder. An underlying cancer is sometimes detected by having the patient press both hands against the hips or the palms together in front of the forehead (Fig. 3.1). In these positions, the pectoral muscles are contracted, and a subtle dimpling of the skin may appear if a growing tumor has entrapped a Cooper's ligament. The nipples are squeezed to check for discharge.

The breast should be palpated with the palmar surfaces of the 2nd, 3rd, and 4th fingers, moving systematically in a small circular pattern from the nipple to the periphery. The axillary and supraclavicular lymph nodes are most easily examined with the patient seated or standing. Supporting the patient's arm during the axillary examination allows the arm to be fully relaxed so that nodes deep within the axilla can be palpated (Fig. 3.1e).

Abdominal Examination

Abdominal examination comprises inspection, palpation, percussion and if appropriate, auscultation.

Inspection

Prerequisites:

a. Bladder should be emptied (Only exception is history suggestive of stress incontinence).

b. The patient should lie flat on her back with legs extended.

c. The whole abdomen from nipple above to the saphenous openings below should be completely exposed.

d. Examination should be carried out in good light preferably in day light. Inspection to be done first from the side then tangentially and finally from either ends of bed.

e. The physician usually stands on right side.

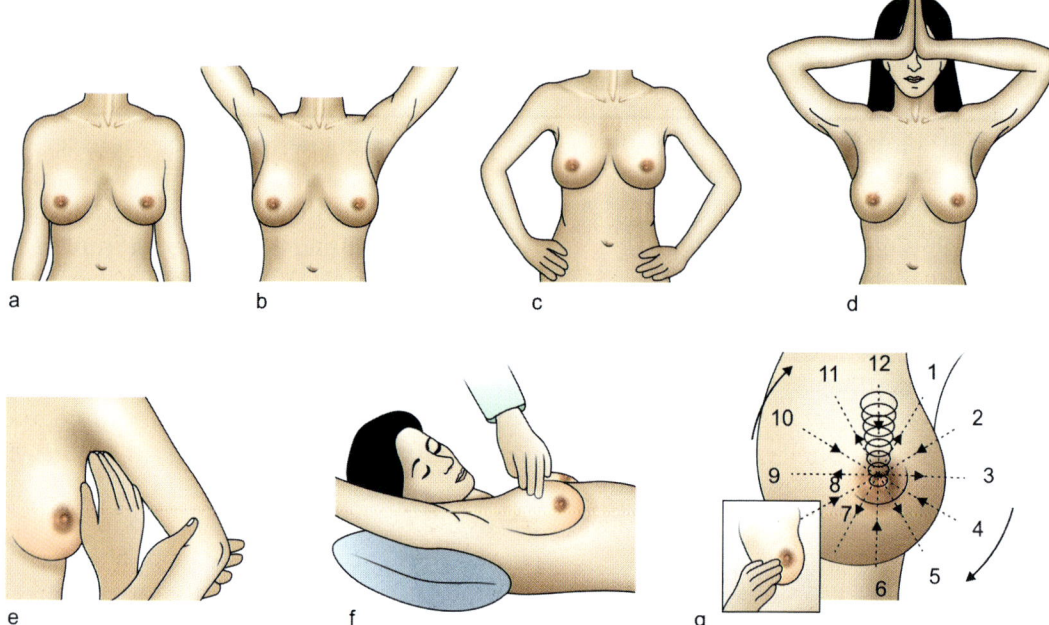

Fig. 3.1: Positions include patient seated or standing **(a)** with arms at sides; **(b)** with arms raised over the head, elevating the pectoral fascia and breasts; **(c)** with hands pressed firmly against hips; or **(d)** with palms pressed together in front of the forehead, contracting the pectoral muscles. **(e)** Palpation of axilla; arm supported as shown, relaxing the pectoral muscles. **(f)** Patient supine with pillow under the shoulder and with the arm raised above the head on the side being examined. **(g)** Palpation of breast in circular pattern from the nipple outward. (*Courtesy:* The Merck Manual - Breast disorder and breast examination)

Skin and subcutaneous tissue: Look carefully for any visible swelling—if any swelling is present note whether the skin is shining, tense, red or pigmented. Are there any scar marks? Specifically examine umbilicus for any laparoscopy scar or just above the symphysis for Pfannenstiel scar. Whether it is linear scar (healing by first intention) or broad and irregular scar (indicating wound infection). Are there any engorged veins? Are there any linea nigra or stria gravidarum?

Position of swelling: Position of the swelling is to be described in relation to nine anatomical region of the abdomen.

Umbilicus: The umbilicus is displaced upwards by swelling arising from the pelvis or downwards by ascites. Any swelling on one side of abdomen will push the umbilicus to opposite side. The umbilicus may be everted (ascites, pregnancy)

Contour of the abdomen: Normal abdomen is neither retracted nor distended. Symmetrical distention may be due to fat, fluid flatus, fetus faeces (Fig. 3.2). Distention due to obesity to be differentiated from other intra-abdominal causes. In obesity umbilicus is deeply inverted but in other conditions umbilicus shows varying degree of eversion.

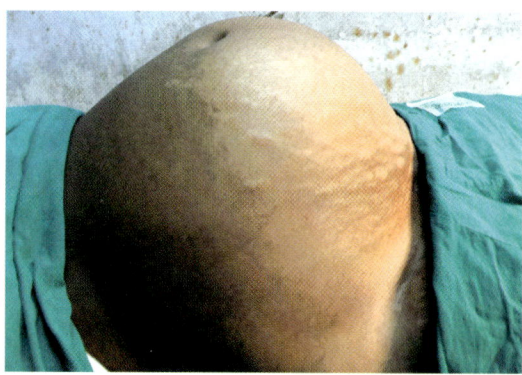

Fig. 3.2: Symmetrical distention of the abdomen

Movements

a. *Respiratory:* Localized limitation of respiratory movement is indicative of subjacent inflammation.

b. *Peristaltic:* Peristalsis will be visible in intestinal obstruction.

c. *Pulsatile:* Pulsatile swelling in abdomen means a tumour in front of abdominal aorta or aortic aneurysm.

The patient should be asked to raise her head and cough, any hernia or divarication of the rectus abdominis muscle will be evident.

Palpation

During palpation patient's confidence must be gained. Under no circumstances she should be hurt. Otherwise, abdominal muscle will go into spasm and important findings will be missed.

1. The patient should lie flat on her back comfortably with a pillow under her head. She is asked to flex the hips and knees to relax the abdominal muscles.

2. Routine palpation of the abdomen should be carried out with flat of the hand using mainly flexor surfaces of fingers. The fingers must not be held vertical and poke the abdominal wall.

3. If the patient is having abdominal pain she should be asked to point to the site. This area should not be examined until the end of palpation. For example, if the pain is in rignt eliac fossae, commence palpating the left hypochondrium and after palpating each quadrant in turn reach the affected area last.

4. The patient is asked to breath quietly and deeply with her mouth open.

5. In winter the hands of clinician must be kept warm same as patient's skin by rubbing one hand against the other.

6. While palpating different regions of abdomen keep an eye on patient's face to know her reaction. She may wince at palpation of a region where she did not complain pain and this may be valuable to reach to diagnosis.

7. Palpation should include examination of masses, liver, spleen, gall bladder, kidneys, caecum and colon.

8. The patient should also be examined for inguinal lymph nodes.

9. When the hand is over particular area mind should visualize particular structure deep to it.

Palpation—the abdomen is palpated by superficial and deep palpation.

Temperature: This examination should be done first in palpation, as manipulation of swelling during subsequent examination may increase the temperature without definite reason. Temperature of the swelling is best felt by the back of the fingers. Local temperature is raised due to infection or excessive vascularity of swelling.

Tenderness: To elicit tenderness one should be very gentle and to keep an eye on patient's facial expression while palpating the lump to note whether it is giving rise to pain or not.

Site of swelling: To be noted in relation to the different abdominal quadrants.

Size: The vertical and horizontal dimensions of swelling are expressed in centimeters.

Shape: Shape may be circular, pyriform or oval or globular, etc.

Surface: This may be smooth or irregular.

Consistency: The swelling may be soft, cystic, firm or hard. Same consistency may be present throughout the swelling or variable consistency at different parts of swelling. Ovarian tumor may be cystic, tense cystic or firm (solid). Fibroids are firm, may be cystic in cystic degeneration. In case of cystic swelling test for fluid thrill should be performed.

Margin: Whether lower border of lump can be reached or not should be elicited. In general lower border can not be reached if lump is of pelvic origin, but in ovarian tumor with a long pedicle one can go below the lower margin.

Movements

a. Is the swelling movable in all directions? Uterine lump is mobile from side to side but mobility is restricted from above downwards. Ovarian lump is also freely mobile side to side but restricted from above down unless the pedicle is long. Mobility may be restricted if the lump is very large or adhesions are present surrounding the lump. A mesenteric cyst moves freely at right angle to attachment of mesentery but not so along the line (the line of attachment of mesentery is 1 inch left to midline and one inch below transpyloric plane and extending downwards and to right for about six inches).

b. Is the swelling ballotable? A renal swelling is ballotable. One hand is placed behind the loin and the other hand in front of the abdomen and the swelling is moved anteroposterior between the two hands.

c. Does the swelling move with respiration or not? Swelling associated with liver, gall bladder, spleen and stomach moves with respiration. This is up and down movement and can be tested by asking the patient to take deep breath and placing the hands over swelling.

Parietal or intra-abdominal: This can be tested by making the abdominal muscles taut by asking the patient:

1. To raise the shoulders from bed with the arms folded over the chest—rising test.
2. To raise both the extended legs from the bed—leg lifting test.

If the swelling disappears or becomes smaller when the abdominal muscles are made taut, the swelling is intra-abdominal (hand will be placed over the swelling to note this change). If the swelling is parietal, the swelling will be more prominent and freely mobile when the abdominal muscle is made taut. If the swelling is parietal but fixed to abdominal muscle the swelling will not be moveable when the muscles are made taut, e.g. desmoid tumor (recurrent fibroid of Paget) and hematoma of rectus muscle.

Is the swelling pulsatile or not? A swelling in front of abdominal aorta is pulsatile and an aneurism of abdominal aorta is also pulsatile, to differentiate between "transmitted" and "expansile" pulsatiom one may put two index fingers of each hand over the swelling. When the two index fingers are not only raised but separated the pulsation will be: "expansile" one. When the two fingers are only raised but not separated the pulsation is "transmitted".

A swelling at any of the hernia sites should be tested for expansible impulse on coughing and reducibility. These tests are positive in hernia.

Lastly palpate the liver, spleen, kidney, gallbladder, caecum and colon to ascertain relationship of the tumor with these organs.

Percussion

1. Presence of free fluid in the peritoneal cavity can be demonstrated by shifting dullness. Percussion should be started from the center of the abdomen and is carried down to one flank (Fig. 3.3). At the

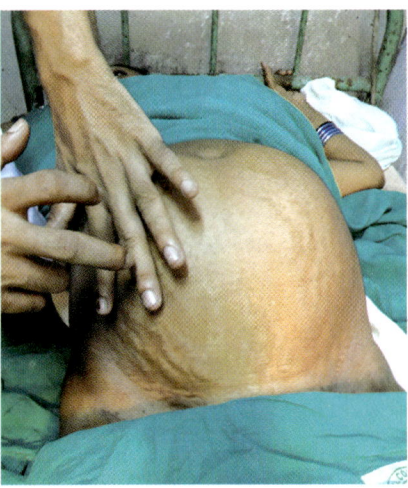

Fig. 3.3: Percussion of the abdomen

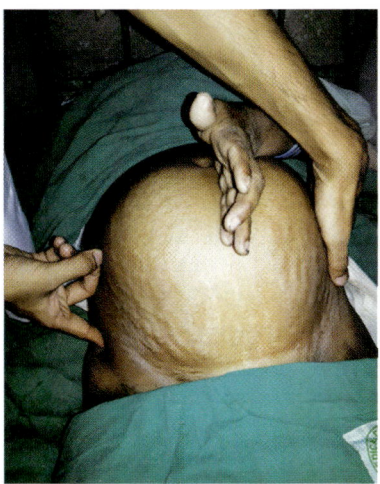

Fig. 3.4: Demonstration of fluid thrill

point where dullness starts the finger is kept in its position and the patient is asked to turn to opposite side. That particular area is again percussed after waiting for a few minutes to allow the fluid to gravitate down. If the area now become resonant, indicate presence of free fluid in abdomen.

A swelling arising from a solid organ is dull in percussion if the swelling is quiet superficial. If the coils of intestine overlie the swelling the percussion note will be resonant even if the swelling is solid one. Differentiation of ovarian cyst and the ascites can be made by percussion. In ascites there is resonance anteriorly and dullness in the flanks whereas in an ovarian cyst there is dullness anteriorly and resonance in flanks. Further, shifting dullness can be elicited in ascites but not in ovarian cyst.

2. *Fluid thrill:* Ask the patint to position her hand in midline of abdomen and flik the abdomen to test for transmitted thrill. In presence of ascites a fluid thrill can be demonstrated but in presence of ovarian cyst fluid thrill is absent (Fig. 3.4).

Pelvic Examination

The pelvic examination has three components: External examination, speculum examination and the bimanual examination.

Prerequisites

1. The patients verbal consent should be obtained. In case of minor, the consent and presence of a parent or guardian is necessary.
2. A female attendant should be present.
3. Bladder should be emptied.
4. The patient's privacy should be maintained.
4. Examination should be made in adequate light.
5. For general pelvic examination the patient should be placed in dorsal position with buttock at the edge of table and with knees flexed. The gynecologist should stand on right side.
6. Occasionally she may be examined in lithotomy position appropriately draped. The gynecologist can thereby complete the pelvic examination as well as can collect material for cytological examination or other examination.

a. Inspection of External Genitalia

Inspection should be started with vulva to note whether it is healthy, ulcerated, or leucoplakic, to determine the size of clitoris, and to look for perineal tears or relaxation. Discharge of any kind from urethral meatus, vaginal or hymenal orifice or Bartholins duct should be noted. The patient is asked to cough or strain to note any cystocele or prolapsed uterus. If hymen is intact or the patient is virgins, further vaginal examination does not proceed. If necessary, rectal examination or examination under anesthesia is carried out. If the woman is having symptom of stress urinary incontinence, she should be examined in full bladder and asked to cough to see any urine leakage through urethra.

b. Speculum Examination

This is carried out to visualize the cervix and vagina to note whether they are healthy or diseased. This is also necessary to collect smears for cytology and for cervical biopsy. In many clinics speculum examination is done

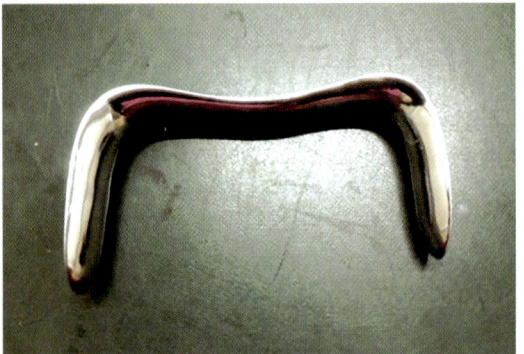

Fig. 3.5: Sims double bladed posterior vaginal speculum

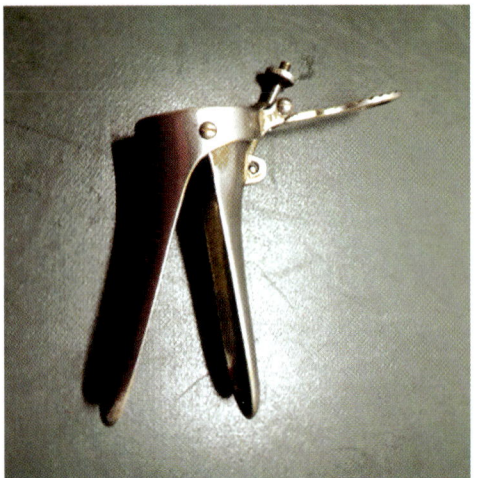

Fig. 3.6: Cusco's bivalve self retaining adjustable vaginal speculum

routinely before bimanual examination but in some clinics speculum examination is done in selected cases. When the complaint is white discharge or blood stained discharge per vagina or post menopausal bleeding, a speculum examination should be performed before bimanual examination. Initially if smears are to be obtained from cervix or posterior fornix for cytology or other study, vaginal discharge has to be obtained by speculum examination before bimanual examination.

There are several types of specula such as Sims', Cusco's, Ferguson's and Graves. In India Sims' and Cusco's speculum are most popular (Figs 3.5 and 3.6).

Insertion of Cusco's speculum: The speculum examination includes entry, positioning, opening, use and removal.

The speculum is moistened with warm water before insertion. The labia is gently separated with gloved left hand to expose the introitus. Then, the speculum is inserted with the blades closed nearly in the vertical plane (at about 1 and 7 o'clock) and thereby avoiding pressure over sensitive urethra. The speculum is fully inserted toward the cervix, then rotated by almost 90° so that the handle is down, and gently opened; it is pulled back as needed to visualize the cervix.

The vagina and cervix are inspected for lesions. The size, shape, color of the cervix and any adherent secretions should be carefully assessed. The nulliparous os is small and round. Following vaginal delivery, the cervical os normally increases in size and becomes transverse slit like and irregular in contour. The ectocervix is typically covered by squamous epithelium, whereas the endocervix is lined with columnar epithelium. The junction between the pale pink of the squamous epithelium and the red color of the columnar epithelium is most commonly located just inside the cervical os. In some young women the columnar epithelium may extend from the cervical canal well onto the ectocervix (an "ectropion" or "cervical ectopy") and appear as a red and beefy area. Nabothian cysts are a common, normal finding in reproductive age women. The cysts often appear in clusters over the surface of the cervix with only a section of the cyst visible above the cervical surface (Fig. 3.7). Cervical or endometrial polyps can protrude from the cervix, and sometimes are a cause of bleeding or discharge. The cervix should be examined for gross abnormalities of the epithelium, such as ulcers, leukoplakia, or cancerous growth. A minimal amount of mucoid discharge within the cervical os may be normal; a significant volume of purulent discharge from the os can signify cervical infection or upper

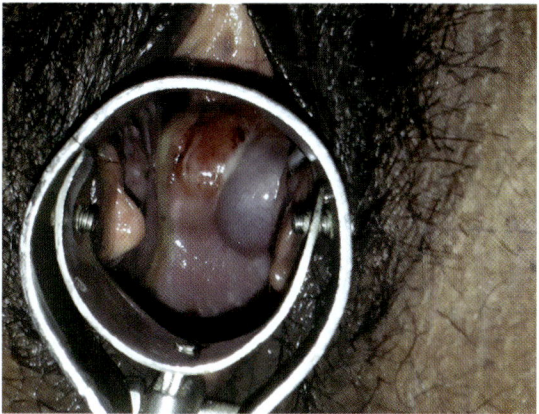

Fig. 3.7: Cusco's speculum is used to visualize Nabothian cyst (1 o'clock position)

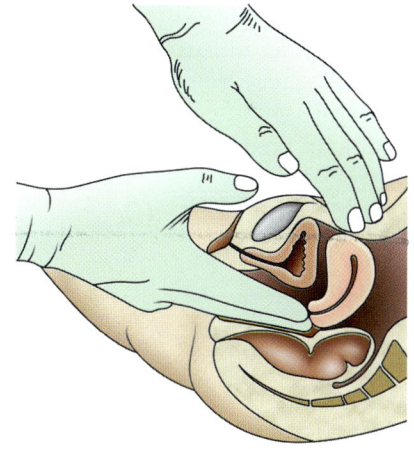

Fig. 3.8: Bimanual examination

reproductive tract infection (pelvic inflammatory disease).

The vagina is also inspected for the presence or absence of rugae to assess the level of estrogen present. The examiner assesses any vaginal discharge that is present for normalcy in appearance, color, consistency, and odor. Physiologic vaginal discharge is scant in amount, flocculent, and white. The pH of the normal vagina is less than 4.5.

Before the metal speculum is removed, the screw should be loosened so the speculum blades can partially close. The speculum should gradually partially close upon withdrawal. The examiner should take care to keep a finger between the two metal blades to prevent complete apposition, which could pinch the patient's mucosa.

Sims' Speculum Examination

Sims speculum allows inspection of the cervix and vaginal walls for pelvic organ prolapse and vesicovaginal fistula. It is best used in Sims' position. In Sims' position, position of the woman should be in left lateral position with chest prone to bed and legs partly curled up. The patient is asked to lift upper thigh using her hand (exaggerated left lateral position). Insert speculum into vagina from behind, with one end pressing on the posterior wall so can assess anterior wall of vagina.

Repeat with one end pressing on anterior wall so can assess posterior wall of vagina. Ask patient to cough. Alternately, the instrument can be introduced in lithotomy position in a similar way that of Cusco's speculum.

c. Bimanual Examination

The bimanual examination provides information about the uterus and adnexa (ovaries and fallopian tubes). During this portion of examination urinary bladder should be kept empty. The labia are separated and gloved, lubricated index and middle fingers of the dominant hand are inserted into the vagina to just below the cervix. The other hand is placed just above the pubic symphysis (Fig. 3.8) and gently presses down to determine the size, position, and consistency of the uterus. Tenderness with lateral movement of the cervix (cervical motion tenderness) is assessed along with its consistency, size and contour. The adnexa are palpated. Any masses that are appreciated are assessed for size, location, mobility, tenderness, and contour. The posterior cul-de-sac and uterosacral ligaments are checked for nodularity and masses.

Normally, the uterus is about 6 cm by 4 cm and anteverted but it may be retroverted to various degrees. The uterus may also be bent at an angle anteriorly (anteflexion) or posteriorly (retroflexion). The uterus is movable and smooth; irregularity suggests uterine leiomyomas. Normally, the ovaries are about 2 cm by 3 cm in young women and are not palpable in postmenopausal women.

Fact sheet: A parous woman may have a larger uterus than a nulliparous woman because uterine size increases with each pregnancy and does not fully return to its prepregnant state.

d. Rectal and Rectovaginal Examination

Some believe that a rectal examination is an important element of every gynecologic examination. Others feel that it is only necessary in the age group for whom colon cancer screening is recommended for routine preventative health care (beginning at age 50). A reasonable middle-ground approach involves including a rectovaginal examination when the bimanual examination alone has been insufficient to fully assess the pelvic anatomy, when one suspects endometriosis or a pelvic mass, or if there are symptoms attributable to the rectal area.

In rectal examination, the examiner palpates the rectovaginal septum by inserting the index finger in the rectum. A slow, single-digit insertion, allowing the rectal sphincter to relax, decreases the discomfort of the rectal examination. Rectal sphincter tone should be noted and any mucosal lesion should be recorded. Rectal examination is important for evaluating the parametrium in women with cervical cancer. Rectal examination may be essential in differentiating between a rectocele and an enterocele.

In rectovaginal examination the examiner inserts an index finger into the vagina, and utilizing lubricant, inserts the middle finger into the rectum. The examiner palpates the rectovaginal septum and again places the opposite hand on the patient's lower abdomen to palpate the previously assessed structures. The uterosacral ligaments may be palpated more easily with the rectovaginal examination than the bimanual examination. The rectum is assessed for masses.

Clinical pearl: The vaginal examination assesses the anterior pelvis, whereas the rectal/recovaginal examination is directed at the posterior pelvis.

Keyword

Sims' speculum: *Sims' speculum is named after James Marion Sims of USA. Sims; surgical discoveries include the Sims speculum and the sims position, and the use of silver sutures to prevent internal infections (Sims triad). These innovations eventually enabled him to repair a vesicovaginal fistula.*

EXERCISES

1. Answer the following questions

- What are the elements of gynecological history taking?
- What do you mean by menarche and LMP?
- Name the different components of menstrual history.
- Name the different elements of general examination.
- Name the prerequisites to be fulfilled prior gynecological examination.
- Why voiding prior gynecological examination is necessary?
- How breasts are examined?
- What are the prerequisites of abdominal examination?
- Name the points you note at the time of inspection of abdomen?
- What are the components of superficial palpation?
- Which points you record at the time of palpation of a pelvic lump?
- How do you know the lump is abdominal or parietal by clinical examination?
- Describe the methods of percussion?
- What are the components of pelvic examination?
- How do you carry out speculum examination?
- Name some common types of speculum that are used in clinical practice?

- How do you perform a bimanual examination?
- How do you perform rectovaginal examination?

2. Write short notes on

- Leg lifting test
- Shifting dullness
- Fluid thrill

3. Explain or justify the following statement

- Cervical pathologies are readily detected during speculum examination

4. Fill in the blanks with appropriate word/s

- The gynecological examinations include examination of _____ , _____ and _____ .
- Clinically _____ can differentiate between ascites and ovarian cyst.
- _____ and _____ speculum are commonly used in India.

5. Questions for practical. Look at Figure 3.6 before answering the following questions

- Identify the instrument.
- Why you use this instrument?
- How do you use it?

- Name the lesions that can be diagnosed with use of this instrument?
- How do you sterilize it?

Look at Figure 3.5 before answering the following questions

- Identify the instrument?
- Who invented this instrument?
- How do you use this instrument and when?
- What is Sims triad?

Bibliography

1. Ashhouse S. History taking in obstetrics and gynecology.
2. Barad HD General Gynecologic Evaluation The Merck Manual.
3. Bowdler, N, Elson, M, Glob. libr. women's med., (ISSN: 1756-2228) 2008; DOI 10.3843/GLOWM. 10003.
4. Case files obstetrics and gynecology.
5. Charney P. The gynecologic examination Practical Gynecology.
6. Clinical gynecology. Bhaskar Rao.
7. Clinical obstetrics and gynecology a problem based approach.
8. Gambone J C. Clinical approach to the patient.
9. Obstetrics and Gynecology. Charles RB Beckmann.
10. Womens Gynocologic health Kerry Durnell.

Puberty and Its Abnormalities

A young girl of 15 years of age has presented with Tanner stage 3 development of breast and pubic hair and absence of menstruation. Is it normal?

In this chapter we will learn:
- **Definition of puberty and adolescence**
- **Physical changes in puberty**
- **Hormonal changes in puberty**
- **Abnormalities in pubertal development**

Definition

From a biological perspective, puberty is the stage of physical maturation in which an individual becomes physiologically capable of sexual reproduction. During this period sex steroid production will ensure the appearance and maintenance of sexual characteristics and the capacity for reproduction. So in strict sense puberty refers to physical changes of sexual maturation rather than psychosocial aspect of development. However, adolescence is the period of physical, psychological and social transition between childhood and adulthood. Thus it is the period of life between beginning of puberty and adulthood (roughly from 11 to 19 year of age). So adolescence largely overlaps the period of puberty, but its boundaries are less precisely defined and it refers as much to the psychosocial and cultural characteristics of development during the teen years as to the physical changes of puberty.

Fact sheet: The average age at which the onset of puberty occurs has dropped significantly since 1840. Researchers refer to this drop as the 'secular trend'. In every decade from 1840 to 1950 there was a drop of four months in the average age of menarche among Western European females. Scientists believe the phenomenon could be linked to obesity or exposure to chemicals in the food chain, and is putting girls at greater long-term risk of breast cancer.

PHYSICAL CHANGES IN PUBERTY

Puberty proceeds through five stages from childhood to full maturity (P1 to P5) as described by Marshall and Tanner. It takes place in an orderly predictable sequence that includes growth acceleration, breast development, pubic and axillary hair development (maximum growth rate), menarche and ovulation. The initial event is accelerated growth, however this may be subtle and breast budding is easier to detect as the first event. The end results of pubertal maturation are:

1. Secondary sexual development
2. The attainment of immediate capacity of reproduction
3. Attainment of adult stature.

Female Secondary Sex Characteristics

Secondary sexual development in girls involves the enlargement of the ovaries, uterus, vagina, labia, and breasts and growth of pubic and axillary hair. Puberty usually begin with breast development (8–9 yrs) as first sign. This follows a prepubertal slowing of growth kinetics. Between 11 and 14.5 years of age, the typical adolescent growth spurt takes place, and acne is frequent. Breasts usually do not grow much after 16 years. It is not uncommon of one breast to begin to grow before the other. The breasts may develop unevenly; one breast may be bigger than the other and this is normal (Fig. 4.1). If breast development has not started by 14 years of age, is abnormal and needs investigation.

Development of body hair varies greatly and depends largely on heredity. Pubic hair is usually noticeable with start of puberty (within 6 months). Axillary hair begins to grow a year or two later (12–13 yrs) With progressive increase in breast size, sexual hair, and genital development the vaginal mucosa becomes more humid, darker pink color. Whitish secretions appear as normal effect of estrogen The uterus increases in size up to stage P4 when the first menstruation occurs, and the maximal growth rate is reached.

Most girls reach menarche around 12.5 to 13 years of age; however, its occurrence may be as early as 10 or as late as 16 years of age in otherwise-normal girls.

First ovulatory cycles usually occur at a median age of 9 to 10 months after menarche. However, the time sequence in the appearance of sex characteristics may vary. Puberty is completed usually within 3 to 4 years of its onset, and the final height resulting from

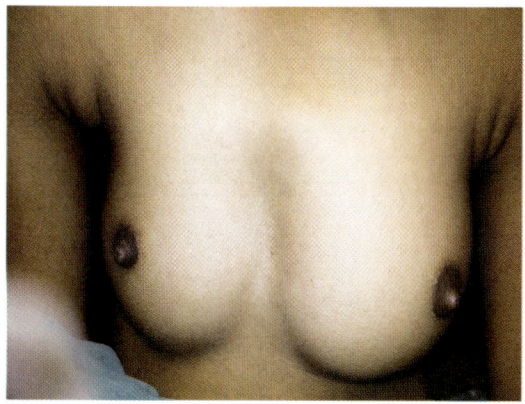

Fig. 4.1: Uneven development of breast

complete fusion of the epiphyses occurs within approximately 2 years after menarche.

Definitions of Puberty Terminology

Characteristic physical changes occur during puberty. These include:

1. *Adrenarche:* Activation of the adrenal cortex with increased production of adrenal androgens which lead to development of axillary and pubic hair.
2. *Puberche:* The appearance of pubic hair
3. *Thelerche:* The appearance of breast tissue
4. *Menarche:* The first menstrual bleeding

Tanner Stages

Puberty follows a fairly consistent sequence in girls. A series of predictable physical changes was noted and studied by several groups. In 1970, Dr WA Marshall and Dr JM Tanner published a landmark paper standardizing this sequence, and the series of changes have subsequently been known as the Tanner stages. Tanner stages have been developed as a way to classify the time, course, and progress of changes that occur during puberty. Girls who do not show any physical changes of puberty are at Tanner stage I. Adults who have completed puberty are at Tanner stage V. Tanner staging is done to assess both breast and pubic hair changes. The sequential stages of sexual maturity are listed below (Fig. 4.2).

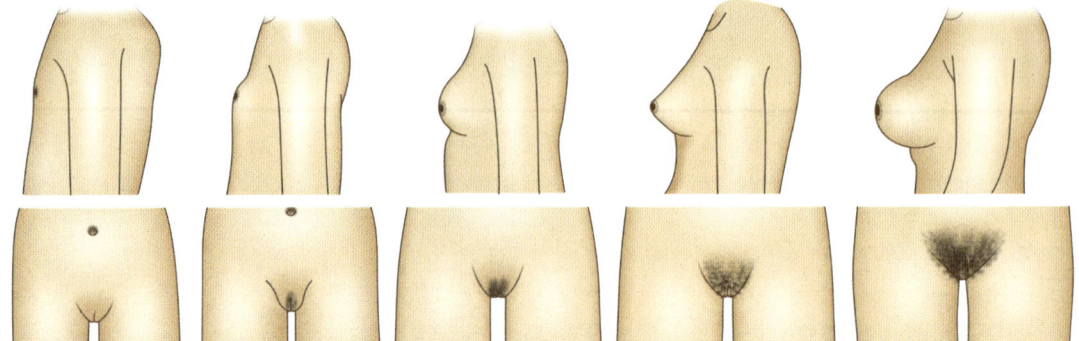

Fig. 4.2: Tanner stages (I—V) of breast (above) and pubic hair (below) development

Tanner I: Preadolescent breast, absent pubic hair.

Tanner II: Devolopment of breast bud as a small mound with onset of areolar enlarge-ment. Sparse longitudinal labial pubic hair in midline of mons pubis.

Tanner III: Increase in breast tissue volume and areolar enlargement and so as to resemble a small adult breast. Coarser and curlier pubic hair spreads sparsely over the symphysis pubis.

Tanner IV: Adult breast shape and elevation of the nipple and areola to produce a secondary projection. Thickening and broader distribution of pubic hair like adult but does not cover entire triangle. Upper lateral corners of the triangle still require to be filled in. No spread to medial surface of thighs.

Tanner V: Mature adult breast shape and rounded contour. Adult pubic hair character and distribution with typical triangular distribution.

HORMONAL CHANGES OF PUBERTY

Gonadotrophin-releasing Hormone

The physical changes that are described above, occur as a result of hormonal changes. The primary triggering mechanism that initiates the activation of the hypothalamic-pituitary-ovarian axis at puberty is still hypothetical. One of the important neuro-endocrine mechanisms that control the onset of puberty is probably an increase in the frequency of GnRH pulse stimulation of the pituitary. Whatever the mechanism, the process is not abrupt but develops over several years, as evidenced by slowly rising plasma concentrations of the gonadotropins and estrogens.

Gonadotropins

The release of FSH and LH tends to occur at night in early puberty, and as menarche approaches, the level of release becomes equal day and night. As puberty progresses, the frequency and amplitude of LH secretory peaks increase. Circulating FSH levels increase progressively from 10 to 11 years of age (stage P2), approximately 1 year prior to those of LH. Thereafter, gonadotropins continue to increase throughout puberty, but important fluctuations are observed in relation to the menstrual cycle (Fig. 4.3).

Prolactin

Serum prolactin concentrations increase modestly during puberty. The physiological role of prolactin in the course of puberty, if any, is unknown.

Adrenal Steroids

Two adrenal hormones, dehydroepiandro-sterone (DHEA) and dehydroepiandrosterone sulfate (DHEAS) increase as early as 6 to 7 years of age. Androstenedione starts increasing within 1–2 years after that.

The adrenal androgens are responsible for the appearance of axillary hair and, in part, for the appearance of pubic hair in the adolescent; however they do not appear to play a decisive role in determining the initiation of puberty.

Ovarian Development

The rising levels of plasma gonadotropins stimulate the ovary to produce increasing amounts of estradiol. Estradiol is responsible for the development of secondary sexual characteristics, that is, growth and development of the breasts and reproductive organs, fat redistribution (hips, breasts), and bone maturation.

The prepubertal uterus is tear-drop shaped, with production of estrogen the uterine body increases in length and thickness proportionately more than the cervix and it becomes pear shaped.

During puberty, plasma estradiol levels fluctuate widely, probably reflecting successive waves of follicular development that fail to reach the ovulatory stage. The uterine endometrium is affected by these changes and undergoes cycles of proliferation and regression, until a point is reached when substantial growth occurs so that withdrawal

of estrogen results in the first menstruation (menarche). Plasma progesterone remains at low levels even if secondary sexual characteristics have appeared. A rise in progesterone after menarche is, in general, indicative that ovulation has occured. The first ovulation does not take place until 6–9 months after menarche because the positive feedback mechanism of estrogen is not developed.

Role of GH, IGF-I, and Insulin in Puberty

There is accumulating evidence that growth hormone (GH) plays a role in pubertal development.

Growth hormone-releasing factor (GRF) levels and GH secretion increase considerably during puberty, mainly at night. The amplitude of GH peaks increases early in puberty. IGF-I is an important modulator of growth during childhood and adolescence. Adrenal androgens seem to have no physiological role in normal growth. The characteristic pubertal growth spurt results mainly from the synergetic effect of gonadal sex steroids, growth hormone, and IGF-I production, with all showing a significant increase at the time of pubertal growth acceleration.

Insulin is also important for normal growth. Plasma insulin levels increase throughout childhood, but the rise is particularly pronounced during puberty with a strong positive correlation with IGF-I.

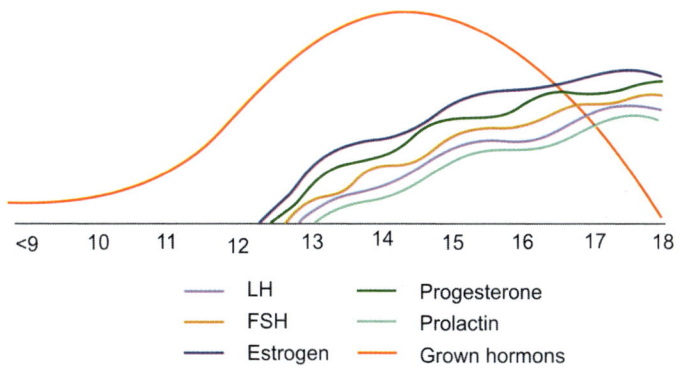

Fig. 4.3: Hormonal changes in puberty

ABNORMAL PUBERTAL DEVELOPMENT

Abnormal pubertal development includes precocious puberty, primary amenorrhea, delayed sexual maturation and incomplete sexual maturation (*see* Chapter 10 for primary amenorrhea, delayed sexual maturation and incomplete sexual maturation). Puberty is considered precocious if pubertal changes are noted prior to 8 years of age and is considered delayed when such changes do not occur prior to 14 years of age. If breast development, pubic and/or axillary hair, and menses occur earlier than normal variations from the mean, the terms premature thelarche, pubarche and/ or adrenarche, and menarche are used.

Precocious puberty: Precocious puberty means onset of menarche or appearance of any secondary sexual character before age of 8 years. Precocious puberty is caused by either GnRH dependent or GnRH independent sex hormone production.

Types

a. *True (central or cerebral) precocious puberty:* It is due to increased production of pituitary ganodotrophins.

b. *False or pseudoprecocious puberty:* It is due to production of sex hormones (estrogen or androgens) which is not due to increased pituitary gonadotrophins (as in estrogen or androgen producing ovarian tumours). Thus it is of peripheral origin. False precocious puberty again may be of two types, isosexual or heterosexual, depending upon type of sex hormone production. A girl who feminizes early is defined as having isosexual precocious puberty. A girl who virilize early is defined as having heterosexual precocious puberty or female pseudo-hermaproditism.

c. *Incomplete precocious puberty:* In this condition only one pubertal change such as breast development occur before age of 8 years and other pubertal changes occur at normal age. Incomplete form of

precocious puberty include premature thelarche (unilateral or bilateral), premature pubarche and premature adrenarche with development of pubic and axillary hair.

Etiology

1. *Constitutional or idiopathic (90%):* For unknown reasons hypothalamus stimulates pituitary gland to secrete gonadotrophins.

2. Organic lesions of brain such as meningitis, encephalitis, brain abscess, brain tumour such as glioma, craniopharyngioma, and hamartomas.

3. McCune-Albright syndrome, see below.

4. *Adrenal causes:* Congenital adrenal hyperplasia, adrenal adenoma, adrenal carcinoma, Cushing syndrome lead to precocious puberty in male direction, i.e. heterosexual precocious puberty. Estrogen secreting adrenal tumour is very rare.

5. *Ovarian causes:*
   i. Estrogen producing tumors such as granulosa cell tumor or theca cell tumor.
   ii. Androgen producing tumor such as androbastoma.
   iii. Choriocarcinoma, because it secretes HCG which might stimulate ovaries to secrete estrogen.
   iv. Dysgerminoma if it secretes HCG

6. *Juvenile hypothyroidism:* Lack of thyroxin results in increased TSH secretion and the pituitrary gonadotrophin secretion may also be increased.

7. *Drugs:*
   a. Iatrogenic-may follow oral or local application of estrogen preparation.
   b. A long course of estrogen cream for treatment of vulvovaginitis of children may lead to breast development or vaginal bleeding.

8. *Silver syndrome:* Short stature, retarded bone age and increased gonadotrophin level.

Diagnosis

History:

i. It excludes iatrogenic source of estrogen and androgen

ii. It differentiates between isosexual and heterosexual precocious puberty.

Physical Examination

i. It diagnoses McCune-Albright syndrome

ii. Neurologic and ophthalmic examination excludes organic lesions of brain.

Investigations

Investigations are carried out depending upon the history and clinical findings. These include:

i. X-ray examination of non dominant hand and wrist to determine bone age. Estrogen stimulates growth of bone but early fusion of epiphysis. So the child is taller than her peer in childhood but she is short in adult life. However, hypothyroidism retards bone age and only condition of precocious puberty in which bone age is retarded.

ii. Hormone assay includes FSH, LH, TSH, prolactin, estradiol, testosterone, 17-hydroxy progesterone estimation and in selected cases human chorionic gonadotrophin estimation to diagnose choriocarcinoma.

iii. Ultrasonography to diagnose ovarian and adrenal tumour.

iv. CT/MRI to diagnose organic lesion in brain or adrenal. Idiopathic precocious puberty is diagnosed after excluding all other causes.

Treatment

Objectives of treatment are:

i. Arrest maturation until normal pubertal age.

ii. Attenuate and diminish established precocious characteristics.

iii. Maximize adult height.

iv. Avoid abuse, reduce emotional and social problems.

Specific Treatment

i. *Treatment of the cause:* Thyroxin for the hypothyroidism and removal of ovarian or adrenal tumour.

ii. In incomplete form of precocious puberty no treatment is required as estrogen production is not increased.

iii. Idiopathic type is treated with explanation and reassurance and by giving one of the following drugs which inhibits secretion of gonadotrophins.

a. Gonadotrophn releasing hormone analogues which are given daily nasal spray or intramuscular or subcutaneous injections every 4 weeks.

b. Medroxy progesterone tablets or Injections

c. Danazole capsule

d. Cyproterone acetate tablets.

McCune-Albright Syndrome

The disease is characterized by a triad of

i. Precocious puberty

ii. Cystic changes in bone and

iii. Cafe au lait patches of skin (Fig. 4.4). The cause of precocious puberty is autonomous production of estrogen from ovary, FSH, LH levels are low. The treatment is with Testolactone oral tablets which inhibit production of ovarian hormones.

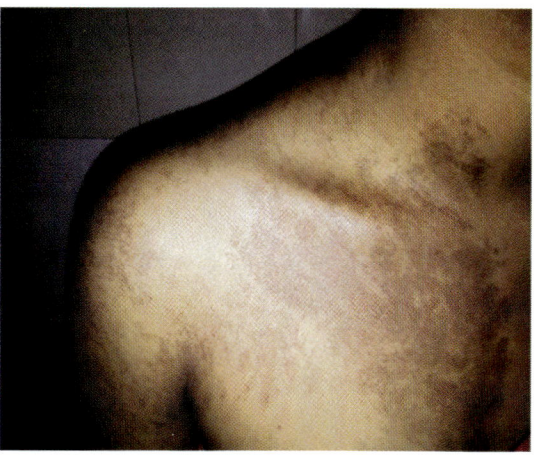

Fig. 4.4: Cafe au lait patches

EXERCISES

1. Answer the following questions

- Differentiate puberty and adolescence.
- What type of physical changes occur in puberty?
- What is meant by following terms? Thalarche, pubarche menarche.
- What is typical sequence of events in puberty in girls?
- When does puberty starts and what is its average time duration?
- What are Tanners stages? Describe Tanner stages for breast and pubic hair development.
- What happens to external genitalia in puberty?
- What happens to uterus during puberty?
- Describe the pattern of growth occurs in puberty.

2. Fill in the blanks

- Puberty usually begins with _____ development.
- Most girls reach menarche at _____ age.
- Tanner staging is done to assess _____ and changes.
- Adrenal androgens are responsible for development of _____ and _____.
- Pubertal changes are precocious if are noted prior _____ years of age.

3. Write shot notes on

- Hormonal changes in puberty
- Precocious puberty

4. Explain or justify the statement

- Adolescence largely overlaps puberty.
- Puberty follows a consistent pattern of physical changes.

5. Questions for practical

- What do you mean by adrenerche, thelarche, pubarche?
- What are the sequences of growth changes during puberty?
- How do you assess breast and sexual hair changes in adolescent girls?
- When puberty is called precocious and when it is delayed?
- What are the causes of precocious puberty?
- How do you treat precocious puberty?

Bibliography

1. Fauda A, Puberty available at www. obgyn.net /educational tutorials/article/12124 accessed on 16/12/2011.
2. Reindollar RH, Davis A J Abnormalities of female pubertal development available at www. endoteext.org /female accessed on 25/6/2011.
3. Sanfilippo J, Jammison M Physiology of puberty Glob. libr. women's med., (ISSN: 1756-2228) 2008; DOI 10.3843/GLOWM.10286

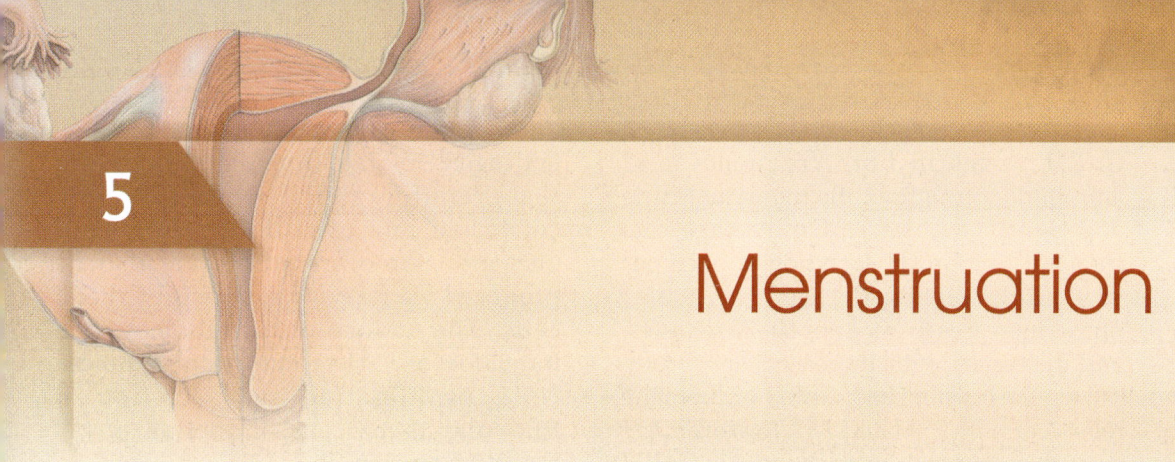

5

Menstruation

A woman is having menstrual cycle length of 33 days with duration of menstruation 2 days. Is it normal?

In this chapter we will learn:
- Definition of menstruation
- Hormones that regulate menstrual cycle
- Hypothalamopituitary ovarian axis
- Hormone changes in menstrual cycle
- Ovarian cycle—Follicular phase, ovulation, leuteal phase
- Uterine cycle—Proliferative phase, secretory phase, menstrual phase
- Clinical aspects and management of menstruation

Definition

Menstruatuion (Greek word, men-month) is defined as visible manifestation of cyclic uterine bleeding due to shedding of the endometrium as a result of hormonal changes operated through hypothalamopituitary ovarian axis.

Fact sheet

Overt menstruation (menstrual bleeding from uterus comes out through vagina) found primarily in humans and close evolutionary relatives such as chimpanzees. The females of other placental mammal species have estrous cycles, in which the endometrium is re absorbed by the animal (covert menstruation) at the end of its reproductive cycle.

HORMONES OF MENSTRUAL CYCLE

There are five main hormones that are involved in the regulation of menstrual cycle

1. Gonadotropin releasing hormone (GnRH)
2. Follicle stimulating hormone (FSH)
3. Luteinizing hormone (LH)
4. Estrogen
5. Progesterone.

GnRH is secreted by the hypothalamus, the gonadotropins FSH and LH are secreted by the anterior pituitary gland, and estrogen and progestin are secreted from the ovary.

GnRH stimulates the release of LH and FSH from the anterior pituitary, which in turn stimulate release of estrogen and progestin at the level of the ovary.

a. *Gonadotropin releasing hormone (GnRH)* is a decapeptide, secreted from the hypothalamus in a pulsatile manner throughout the menstrual cycle. To maintain the menstrual cycle normal, GnRH must be released in pulses. The pulsatile release of

GnRH varies in both frequency and amplitude throughout the menstrual cycle and tightly regulated. On average, the frequency of GnRH secretion is once per 90 minutes during the early follicular phase, increases to once per 60–70 minutes, and decreases with increased amplitude during the luteal phase. GnRH induces the release of both FSH and LH; however, LH is much more sensitive to changes in GnRH levels.

b. *Follicle stimulating hormone (FSH)* is secreted by the anterior pituitary gland and is essential for follicular growth until the antrum develops. FSH secretion is highest and most critical during the first week of the follicular stage of the menstrual cycle. FSH stimulates granulosa cells in newly recruited follicles and produce increasing quantities of estrogen and inhibin blood serum levels of two hormones rise progressively and produces a negative feedback effect on pituitary FSH secretion and serum FSH levels progressively declines. FSH further induces the expression of LH receptors on granulosa cells.

c. *Luteinizing hormone (LH)* is secreted by the anterior pituitary gland and is required for both growth of preovulatory follicles and luteinization and ovulation of the dominant follicle. During the follicular phase of the menstrual cycle, LH stimulates (proliferation and differentiation) theca cells for androgen synthesis and androgen is then transported to the granulosa cells for conversion into estrogens. The preovulatory LH surge drives the oocyte into the first meiotic division and initiates luteinization of thecal and granulosa cells. The resulting corpus luteum produces high levels of progesterone and some estrogen.

d. *Estrogen:* Estradiol is the most potent and abundant estrogen produced from ovary. Other types are estrone and estriol. Estradiol is primarily derived from androgens produced by theca cells. The androgens migrate from the theca cells to the granulosa cells, where they are converted into estradiol by aromatase enzyme. Some estradiol can also be produced via de novo synthesis by thecal cells. The actions of estradiol include induction of FSH receptors on granulosa cells, proliferation and secretion of follicular theca cells, induction of LH receptors on granulosa cells, and proliferation of endometrial stromal and epithelial cells. At low circulating levels (at early follicular phase), estrogens exert negative feedback on LH and FSH secretion; however, at very high levels (prior ovulation) estrogens exert positive feedback on LH and FSH secretion. In the uterine endometrial cycle, estrogen induces proliferation of the endometrial glands, increases motility of fallopian tubes and have other effects on breast, behavior.

e. *Progesterone progestin* is secreted at the level of the ovary, primarily by corpus luteum. Progestin levels increase just prior to ovulation and peak five to seven days postovulation. The first step in progestin synthesis requires P450 enzyme and the two circulating forms of progestin are progesterone and 17-hydroxyprogesterone. Progestins stimulate the release of proteolytic enzymes from thecal cells that ultimately prepare for ovulation. Progestins further induce migration of blood vessels into the follicle wall and stimulate prostaglandin secretion in follicular tissues. During the luteal phase, progestins induce swelling and increased secretion of the endometrium.

According to the two-cell-two-gonadotrophin theory, the ovary has two cellular compartments that are driven independently by LH and FSH to produce ovarian steroids. LH stimulates the theca cell segment of the follicle and induces production of androgens from cholesterol, while FSH is responsible for promoting conversion of androgen precursors to estrogens in the granulosa cell compartment.

HYPOTHALAMOPITUITARY OVARIAN AXIS

In the presence of a GnRH pulse, the pituitary and ovarian hormones exert mutual control over the circulating levels of one another. The complex interactions between pituitary and ovarian hormones involve forward control, positive feedback and negative feedback mechanisms, and serve to sustain a self-perpetuating monthly endocrine cycle (Fig. 5.1).

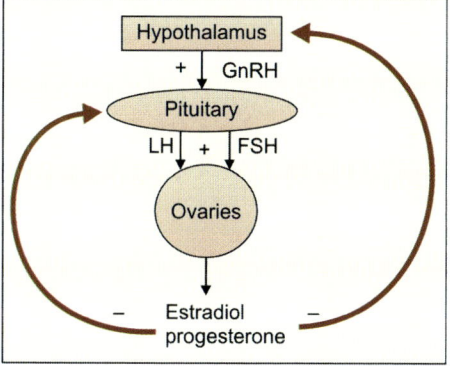

Fig. 5.1: Hypothalamopituitary ovarian axis

HORMONAL CHANGES IN MENSTRUAL CYCLE

The interplay between pituitary and ovarian hormones gives rise to a stereotyped pattern of hormone levels during the menstrual cycle. Figure 5.2 shows relative hormone levels in an average 28-day cycle. The sequence of events in the menstrual cycle is determined by the relative hormone levels at each stage.

For better understanding, menstrual cycle can be classified in different ways.

1. On the basis of changes that occur in the ovaries (ovarian cycle)
   a. Follicular pahase
   b. Ovulatory phase
   c. Luteal phase
2. On the basis of changes that take place in the linings of the uterus (uterine cycle/ endometrial cycle)
   a. Proliferative phase
   b. Secretory phase
   c. Menstrual phase
1a. *The follicular phase* of the menstrual cycle starts from the first day of

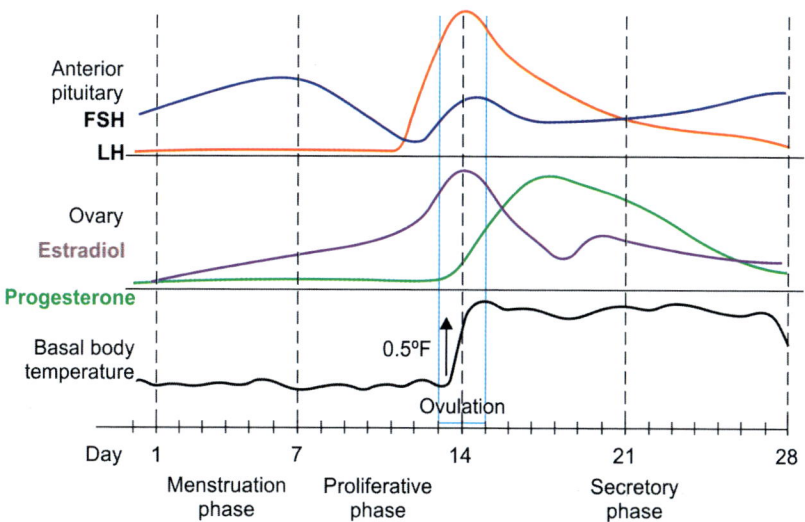

Fig. 5.2: Hprmonal changes and change in body temperature during menstrual cycle

menstruation until ovulation. The primary goal during the follicular phase is to develop a follicle which will undergo ovulation. The early events of the follicular phase are initiated by a rise in FSH levels at the first day of the cycle. The rise in FSH levels can be attributed to a decrease in progesterone and estrogen levels at the end of the previous cycle. FSH stimulates the development of 15–20 follicles each month and stimulates follicular secretion of estradiol by inducing the aromatase enzyme receptor on granulosa cells. As estradiol levels increase under the influence of FSH, estradiol inhibits the secretion of FSH and FSH levels decrease.

Under normal circumstances, one follicle evolves into the dominant follicle, destined for ovulation, while the remaining follicles undergo atresia. The fully mature graffian follicle just prior to ovulation measures about 20 mm. It is currently not known how the dominant follicle is selected; yet it has been observed that the dominant follicle always expresses an abundance of FSH receptors. The dominant follicle, with its high concentration of FSH receptors, continues to acquire more FSH even as FSH levels decrease. The dominant follicle can continue to synthesize estradiol, which is essential for its complete maturation. The remaining, poorly FSH receptor-endowed follicles can not produce the requisite amount of estradiol. These follicles cease to develop and ultimately undergo atresia. The dominant follicle matures and secretes increasing amounts of estrogen. Estrogen levels peak towards the end of the follicular phase of the menstrual cycle. At this critical moment (serum estradiol level 200 pg/ml persisting approximately 50 hrs), estrogen exerts positive feedback on LH, generating a dramatic preovulatory LH surge.

Estrogen can only exert positive feedback on LH at this precise stage in the menstrual cycle; if estrogen is artificially provided earlier in the cycle, ovulation will not be induced.

b. *Ovulation:* The LH surge is the key event for ovulation. Under the influence of LH, the primary oocyte enters the final stage of the first meiotic division and divides into a secondary oocyte and the first polar body. The LH surge induces release of proteolytic enzymes, which degrade the cells at the surface of the follicle, and stimulates angiogenesis in the follicular wall and prostaglandin secretion. These effects of LH cause the follicle to swell and rupture. At ovulation, the oocyte and corona radiata are expelled into the peritoneal cavity. The oocyte adheres to the ovary and muscular contractions of the fallopian tube bring the oocyte into contact with the tubal epithelium to initiate migration through the oviduct. Ovulation occurs approximately 10–16 hours of LH peak and 32–36 hours after the onset of LH surge.

c. The *luteal phase* is defined by the luteinization of the components of the follicle which were not ovulated and is initiated by the LH surge. The granulosa cells, theca cells, and some surrounding connective tissue are all converted into the corpus luteum, which eventually undergoes atresia. The major effects of the LH surge are the conversion of granulosa cells from predominantly androgen-converting cells to predominantly progesterone-synthesizing cells. This results in increased progesterone secretion with some estrogen secretion. Progesterone secretion by the corpus luteum peaks between five and seven days postovulation and can be used as presumptive sign that ovulation has occurred. High progesterone levels exert negative feedback on GnRH and subsequently GnRH pulse frequency decreases. As GnRH pulse frequency decreases, FSH and LH secretion also decreases. Lacking stimulation by FSH and LH, after 14 days corpus luteum undergoes atresia and begins evolving into the corpus albicans. With the decline of both estrogen and progesterone levels, an important negative feedback control on FSH is removed and FSH levels rise once again to initiate the next menstrual cycle.

Clinical indicators of ovulation

i. Secretory pattern in endometrium seen on biopsy.
ii. Rise in basal body temperature (BBT). BBT is the temperature taken on awakening and before activity. Persistent elevation of 0.5°–1.0° F reflects ovulation

d. *Follicular development*: During embryogenesis, primordial germ cells develop from mesoderm in the allantois, migrate to the ovary, and then proliferate and differentiate into primordial follicles. Primordial follicles are arrested in growth until menarche, and some remain so until menopause. At the beginning of each menstrual cycle, between 15 and 20 primordial follicles develop into primary follicles. Under the influence of gonadotropins and ovarian hormones, primary follicles grow; ultimately, however, only one primary follicle develops into a graafian follicle and the remaining follicles undergo atresia. The graafian follicle is ovulated, expelling the oocyte and corona radiate into the peritoneum while the zona granulosa cells remain in the ovary. The zona granulosa and surrounding theca cells develop into the corpus luteum, which in turn becomes atretic after 14 days. After several months, the corpus luteum has fully devolved into the corpus albicans (Fig. 5.3).

2. *Uterine or endometrial cycle:* Cyclical changes in the endometrium prepare for implantation in the event of fertilization and necessitate menstruation in the absence of fertilization. The endometrium is divided into two portions which are stratum functionalis and stratum basalis. The functionalis undergoes changes throughout the menstrual cycle and is shed during menstruation while the basalis remains constant during the menstrual cycle and regenerates the functionalis each month.

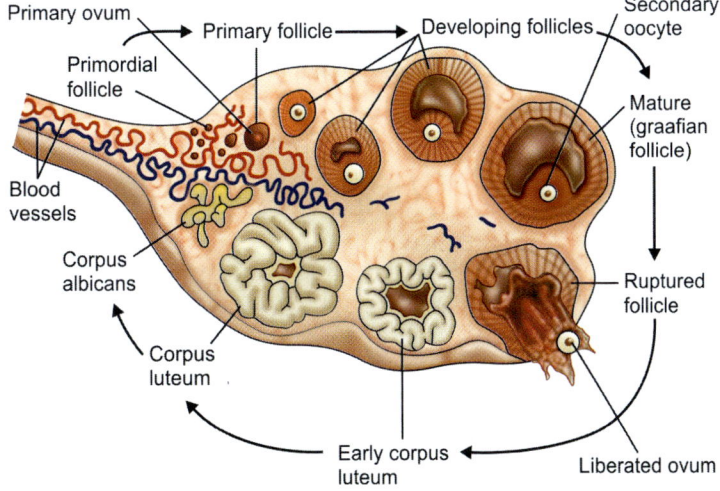

Fig. 5.3: Ovarian cycle

a. *Proliferative phase:* The proliferative phase, spans from the end of the menstruation until ovulation. Increasing levels of estrogen induce proliferation of the functionalis from stem cells of the basalis, proliferation of endometrial glands, and proliferation of stromal connective tissue. Endometrial glands are elongated with narrow lumens and their epithelial cells contain some glycogen. Glycogen, however, is not secreted during the follicular phase. Spiral arteries elongate and span the length of the endometrium (Fig. 5.4).

b. *Secretory phase:* The luteal, or secretory phase, begins at ovulation and lasts until the menstrual phase of the next cycle. At the beginning of the secretory phase, progesterone induces the endometrial glands to secrete glycogen, mucus, and other substances. These glands become tortuous and have large lumens due to increased secretory activity. The spiral arteries extend into the superficial layer of the endometrium (Fig. 5.4). In the absence of fertilization by day 23 of the menstrual cycle, the corpus luteum begins to degenerate and consequently ovarian hormone levels decrease. As estrogen and progesterone levels decrease, the endometrium undergoes involution. Days 25–26 of the menstrual cycle, endothelin and thromboxin begin to mediate vasoconstriction of the spiral arteries. The resulting ischemia may cause some early menstrual cramps. By day 28 of the menstrual cycle, intense vasoconstriction and subsequent

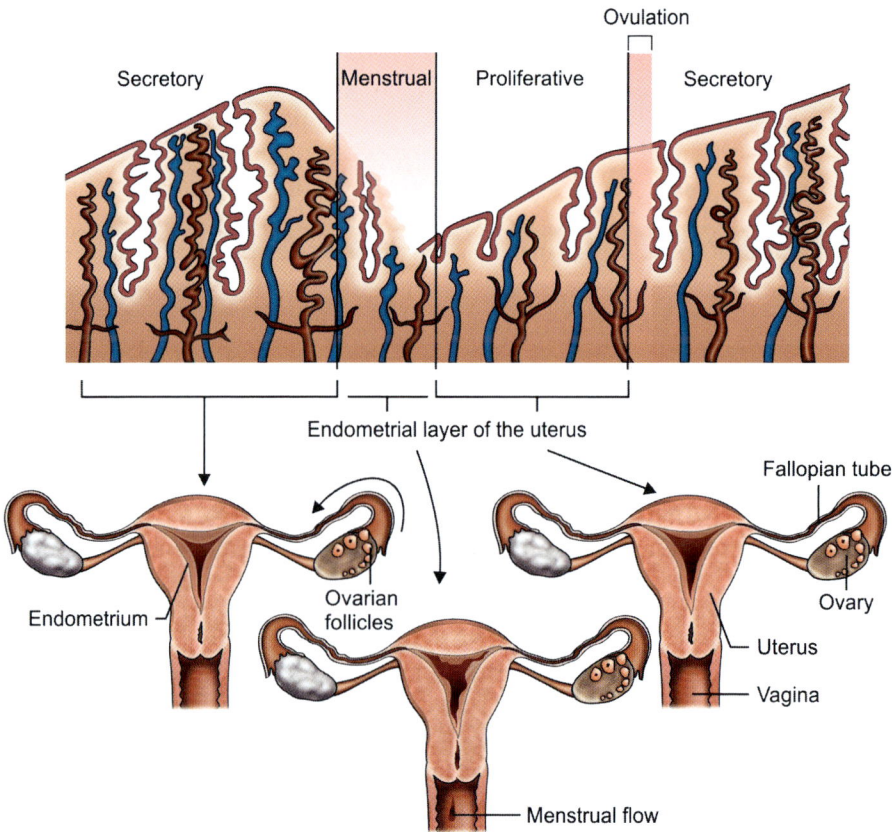

Fig. 5.4: Uterine or endometrial cycle

ischemia cause mass apoptosis of the functionalis.

c. *Menstrual phase:* The menstrual phase begins as the spiral arteries rupture secondary to ischemia, releasing blood into the uterus, and the apoptosed endometrium is sloughed off and usually lasts four days. During this period, the functionalis is completely shed. Arterial and venous blood, remnants of endometrial stroma and glands, leukocytes, and red blood cells are all present in the menstrual flow.

SUMMARY OF MENSTRUAL CYCLE REGULATION (Fig. 5.5)

1. GnRH is secreted from the hypothalamus in pulsatile fashion and reaches to anterior pituitary through portal circulation.

2. Ovarian follicular development moves from a period of gonadotrophin independent to a phase of FSH dependence.

3. As the corpus luteum of previous cycle degenerates, luteal production of progesterone and inhibin decreases, allowing FSH level to rise.

4. In response to FSH stimulus, follicles grow and differenciate and secrete increasing amount of estrogen.

5. Estrogen stimulates growth and differentiation of functional layer of the endometrium, which prepares for implantation.

6. Two cell two gonadotrophion theory dictates that with LH stimulation of the ovarian theca cells will produce

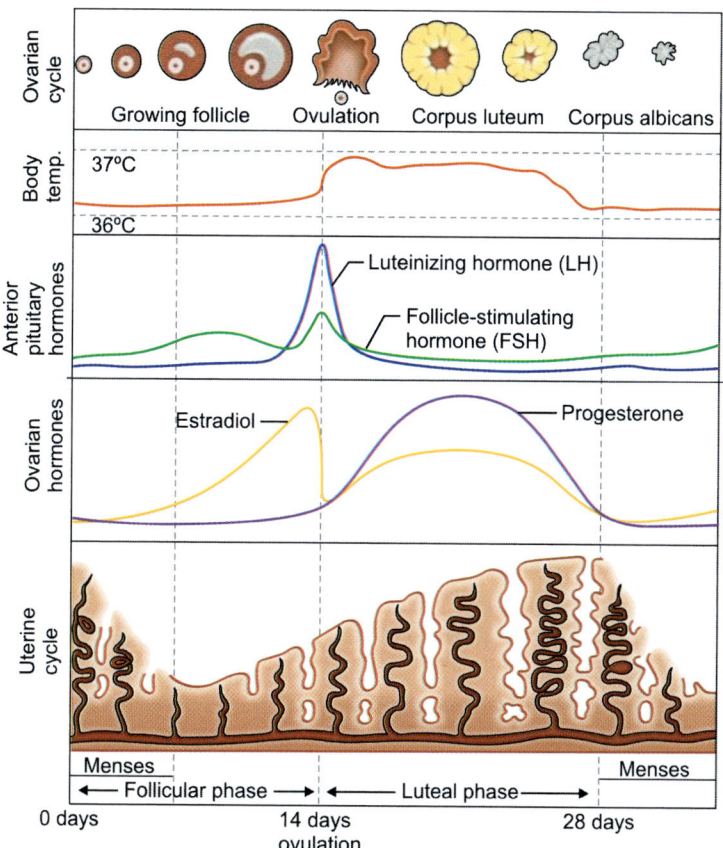

Fig. 5.5: Menstrual cycle regulation

androgens that are converted by the granulosa cells into estrogen under the stimulus of FSH.

7. Rising estrogen level negatively feedback on the pituitary gland and the hypo-thalamus and decrease the secretion of FSH.

8. The one follicle destined to ovulate each cycle is called the dominant follicle. It has relatively more FSH receptors and produce a large concentration of estrogens than the follicles that will undego atresia. It is able to continue to grow despite falling FSH levels.

9. Sustained high estrogen level will cause a surge in pituitary LH secretion that triggers ovulation, progesterone produc-tion and the shift to the secretory or luteal phase.

10. Luteal function is dependent on the presence of LH. Without continued LH secretion, the corpus luteum will regress after 14 days.

11. If pregnancy occurs, trophoblast secretes hCG, which mimic the action of LH by sustaining the corpus luteum. The corpus luteum continue to secrete progesterone and the supports the secretory endo-metrium, allowing the pregnancy to continue to develop.

Normal Limits of Menstruation

- The first menstruation (menarche) occurs between 10 and 16 years with a mean of 13 years.
- Once menstruation starts, it continues cyclically at intervals of 21–35 days with a mean of 28 days.
- Normal menstrual cycle is considered to be between 21 and 35 days long with any irregularity being less than 7 days.
- Duration of menstrual flow is normal between 2 and 7 days.
- Only 15% of women have a 28 day cycle.
- Length of the menstrual cycle is determined by the follicular phase.
- Luteal phase is fairly fixed at 14 days.

- Normal menstrual loss is around 35 ml (20–60 ml).
- Above 80 ml is considered excessive.

CLINICAL ASPECTS AND MANAGEMENT OF MENSTRUATION

Clinical Features

Menstruation is physiological function of body. Most women will have menstrual bleeding for 3–5 days with no discomfort. However around one-fourth women get menstrual discomforts, known as menstrual molimina. These discomforts do not interfere with usual day's activity and require no treatment. Only 5–10 percent develops during some part in their about 30 years menstrual life, painful mens interfering day's activities (dysmenorrhoea). The menstrual molimina are as follows:

Symptoms

1. Feeling of heaviness and discomfort in the pelvis, lower abdomen and in the back.
2. Feeling of pricking and fullness in the breasts.
3. Frequency of urination and constipation.
4. Feeling of lassitude, irritability, and headache. Above symptoms vary in severity from individual to individual. Rarely, bleeding from nose may occur as vicarious menstruation.

Signs

1. Sudden drop in temperature of about 1° but with individual variations.
2. Pulse rate and blood pressure tend to drop.
3. Gain in weight occurs during premenstrual fortnight up to about 1 kg due to retention of water and salt; it occurs in about half of women. There is loss of weight with the onset of flow.
4. Menstrual loss (mens). The vaginal men-strual bleeding mainly arterial, partly venous is a dark reddish liquid (not clotted) blood with shed endometrial tissue bits.

The discharge has disagreeable smell due to the secretion of vulvar sebaceous glands and decomposition of blood elements. Menstrual blood is deficient in prothrombin, and fibrinogen but rich in calcium. Microscopically, it contains red cells, large number of leucocytes, vaginal epithelium, cervical mucus, fragments of endometrium with macrophages, histiocytes, mast cells and bacteria, menstrual discharge also contains cholesterol, oestrogen, lipids and prostaglandins. Menstrual blood from the endometrium clots in the uterine cavity by its thromboplastic property. The clots are dissolved by the fibrinolysins released from the endometrium. Fibrin degradation products therefore circulate in increased amount during menstruation. In general menstrual blood does not clot. Clots are passed when menstrual bleeding becomes excessive.

Interval and Duration

The menstrual cycle lasts on an average 28 days. A deviation of 2 to 3 days can be frequently encountered. The extremes of 21 and 35 days interval may also be found. In any woman's menstrual life, the interval can vary. The usual duration is 3 to 5 days with essentially normal extremes of 2 and 7 days.

Blood Loss

The average total blood loss during menstruation has been estimated as 35 ml (range 5–60 ml); average loss of iron was found as 12 mg. A rough clinical estimate is that normally not more than three fresh pads are necessary in the 24 hours, two during the day and one at night, thus requiring total 12–15 pads during a mens. This loss widely varies and becomes greater in women living in warm climate than those living in cold climate.

Clinical pearl: A menstrual history that includes normal cycle length with regularity and associated with menstrual molimina virtually guarantees ovulatory physiology.

Management

Proper education on menstruation is important. Women should be educated that menstruation is not the drainage of noxious blood from the body but a normal manifestation of womanhood. During menses, she should carry on her usual activities including daily bathing, playing games. Personal hygiene is maintained by changing regularly sanitary pads. Intravaginal tampons can be used by the married provided she does not forget to leave it behind. Healthy couple can have sexual intercourse during menses.

Postponement or Advancement of Menstruation

This becomes at times necessary for important social reason like marriage. This is not to be advocated on flimsy ground. The hormone therapy employed is the following:
1. Progesterone—Norethisterone one tab thrice daily starting from 20th day of menstrual cycle till beyond the date of postponement.
2. Oestrogen progestogen contraceptive pills, two a day is started from the 20th day. Menstrual flow is expected 2 to 3 days after the treatment is suspended. Menstruation can be prematurely brought by starting hormone therapy from 5th day of mens for 14 days, The therapy is (a) oestrogen ethinyl oestradiol 0.05 mg tds or (b) oestrogen progestogen oral pill once daily. Anovular menstrual flow is likely to begin within 2–3 days of the cessation of therapy.

Keywords

Menstruation: Visible manifestation of cyclic uterine bleeding due to shedding of the endometrium.

Progestin: A natural or synthetic progestational substance that mimics some or all of the actions of progesterone.

Cytochrome P450 enzymes are present in most tissues of the body, and play important roles in hormone synthesis and breakdown (including estrogen and testosterone synthesis and metabolism), cholesterol synthesis, and vitamin metabolism.

HPO axis = As Hypotahalamus, Pituitary and ovary behave in cooperation, physiologists and endocrinologist find it convenient to call them as a single system, HPO axis.

Follicular phase from the first day of menstruation until ovulation.

Ovulation: Expulsion of the oocyte and corona radiata into the peritoneal cavity.

Luteal phase: Begins with formation of corpus leuteum and ends with onset of mentruation

Proliferative phase: Starts from the end of the menstruation until ovulation.

Secretory phase begins at ovulation and ends at onset of menstrual phase of the next cycle.

Menstrual phase: The phase of the menstrual cycle during which the lining of the uterus is shed (the first day of menstrual flow is considered day 1 of the menstrual cycle).

Molimina: Menstrual molimina is appearance of menstrual symptoms (both physical and psychological) that does not interfere with normal daily routines. The onset of menstrual molimina indicates the occurrence of ovulation.

EXERCISES

1. Answer the following questions:

a. Define menstruation.
b. Name the hormones regulating menstrual cycle.
c. What is ovulation? Describe the mechanism of ovulation.
d. Compare the roles of estrogen and progesterone in menstrual cycle.
e. What is the functional significance of the rise of FSH at the end of luteal phase?
f. LH surge is the key event during the ovulatory cycle. What is the mechanism that brings it out?
g. Mention the histological changes in proliferative and secretory phase of endometrium.
h. Describe the limits of normal menstruation.
i. What causes variability of menstrual cycle?
j. Describe the hormonal regulation involved in menstrual cycle.

k. What is happening in ovary?
l. What is the function of Corpus leuteum?

2. Fill in the blanks

a. GnRH is released in _____ fashion.
b. Inhibin inhibits production of ____ hormone.
c. Three main estrogens are estradiol and estriol _____ .
d. Proliferative phase is under the influence of _____ hormone.
e. Secretory phase is due to effect of _____.
f. Corpus luteum secretes large quantities of _____ and _____.

3. Write short notes on

a. Two cell two gonadotrophin theory
b. Menstrual molimina

4. Explain or justify

a. Menstrual blood does not clot.
b. Endometrial changes are related with hormonal changes of menstruation cycle.
c. Postponement of menstruation is possible with medications.

5. Questions for practical

a. What is menarche?
b. What is the normal cycle length of menstruation?
c. What is the normal duration of menstruation?
d. What is the amount of blood loss in normal menstruation?
e. From menstrual history how will you assume that the woman is ovulatory?

Bibliography

1. Ferin, M, Glob. libr. women's med.,(ISSN: 1756–2228) 2008; DOI 10.3843/GLOWM.10283.
2. The menstruation anatomy and physiology Prosono 2008 available at www jimbaun.com accessed on 25/7/2011.
3. The normal menstrual cycle and control of ovulation Sabir NK.2005 availble at www endotext.com accessed on 25/5/2011.

6

Disorders of Menstruation—Abnormal Uterine Bleeding

A 37-year-old, P 2+0 woman has presented with a history of persistent vaginal bleeding for last 2 weeks. Over the last year her periods have been longer and irregular. She is sexually active and had tubectomy following her last child birth 5 years ago. Her general examination is un remarkable except mild pallor. Bimanual examination reveals an enlarged uterus equivalent to 8 weeks pregnant uterus and mild uterine bleeding. How should her case be managed?

In this chapter we will learn:
- Types of menstrual disorders
- Definition of abnormal uterine bleeding (AUB)
- Causes of abnormal uterine bleeding
- Types of abnormal uterine bleeding
- Clinical presentation and Investigations in cases of AUB
- Treatment of abnormal uterine bleeding

Introduction

If we consider the complexities and varieties that control menstrual cycle, it is not surprising that abnormal uterine bleeding would occur even in absence of obvious disease. Menstruation has three clinical characteristics: the menstrual interval or cycle length, the duration of flow and the amount of flow. The mean cycle length is 28 days, although a menstrual interval of 21–35 days can be considered normal. A menstrual interval shorter than 21 days is defined as polymenorrhoea. A menstrual interval longer than 35 days is defined as oligomenorrhoea. A duration of menstrual flow of 2–7 days is considered normal. A duration of flow less than 2 days is defined hypomenorrhoea and duration more than 7 days is menorrhagia. Average amount of blood loss is 20–60 ml. However blood loss upto 79 ml is considered normal and a blood loss of more than 80 ml is called menorrhagia.

Apart from these abnormalities some women may develop excessive pain during menstruation (dysmenorrhea) or cyclical physical and mental disturbances related with menstruation (PMS) Thus menstrual abnormalities may be of following types.

TYPES OF MENSTRUAL DISORDERS

- Abnormal uterine bleeding (AUB)
- Dysmenorrhea

Fact sheet: The primitive woman had fewer menstrual periods because of the fact that women were more often pregnant or lactating. Today, women experience approximately 400 menstrual cycles. It has been postulated that an increase in the number of menstrual cycles has contributed to an increased magnitude of menstrual disorders.

- Premenstrual syndrome (PMS)
- Premenstrual dysphonic disorder (PMDD)

Abnormal Uterine Bleeding

Definition: Abnormal uterine bleeding (AUB) means abnormality in menstrual period frequency, duration or amount of blood flows as well as bleeding between cycles. Thus abnormal uterine bleeding may be defined as any deviation in normal frequency, duration or amount of menstruation in women of reproductive age. Terms used to describe patterns of abnormal uterine bleeding are shown in Table 6.1. Dysfunctional uterine bleeding (DUB), defined as abnormal uterine bleeding not caused by pelvic pathology, medications, systemic disease or pregnancy, is the most common cause of abnormal uterine bleeding but remains a diagnosis of exclusion (*see* Chapter 7).

Causes: Abnormal uterine bleeding that occurs from adolescence through perimenopause can be broadly divided in three categories: anovulatory, ovulatory and anatomic. Anovulatory bleeding is characterized by irregular or infrequent periods, with flow ranging from light to excessively heavy. Terms commonly associated with anovulatory menstruation include amenorrhea (absence of menstruation for more than three cycles or six months), oligomenorrhea, metrorrhagia and dysfunctional uterine bleeding. Anovulatory bleeding occurs more frequently in extreme of reproductive age and in obese women.

In contrast to anovulatory patterns, ovulatory abnormal uterine bleeding occurs at regular intervals (every 21–35 days) and with excessive volume (> 80 ml) or duration of more than seven days (menorrhagia). Excessive menstrual bleeding is identified by need to change sanitary pads every one to two hours, passage of clots greater than one inch (2.54 cm) and/or heavy periods as reported by the patient. It is commonly associated with low Hb and ferritin level. Table 6.2 summarizes characteristics of anovulatory and ovulatory abnormal uterine bleeding.

Uterine leiomyoma, endometrial and fibroid polyps, adenomyosis are common antomic causes of abnormal uterine bleeding. These women might present with abnormal bleeding, pain anemia and occasionally infertility. Some medications can also cause abnormal uterine bleeding (*see* Table 6.2).

FIGO Classification: Causes of Abnormal Uterine Bleeding

The International Federation of Gynecology and Obstetrics (FIGO) has approved a new classification system (PALM-COEIN; pronounced "pahm-koin") for causes of abnormal uterine bleeding (AUB) in non-

Table 6.1: Terminology used to describe abnormal uterine bleeding

Term	Definition
Menorrhagia	Prolonged or excessive menstrual bleeding at regular intervals
Metrorrhagia	Irregular, frequent uterine bleeding of varying amounts but not excessive
Menometrorrhagia	Prolonged or excessive menstrual bleeding at irregular intervals
Polymenorrhea	Regular menstrual bleeding at intervals of less than 21 days
Oligomenorrhea	Menstrual bleeding at intervals greater than every 35 days
Amenorrhea	No uterine bleeding for at least 6 months
Intermenstrual	Uterine bleeding between regular cycles

Table 6. 2: Characteristics of abnormal uterine bleeding

Causes	Characteristics
Anovulatory	Unpredictable cycle length; irregular often infrequent periods
	Unpredictable bleeding pattern, flow ranges from absent or minimal or excessive
	Frequent spotting
	Infrequent heavy bleeding
	Monophasic temperature curve
	Progesterone deficient/estrogen dominant state
	Increased risk to endometrial hyperplasia or carcinoma
Ovulatory	Regular cycle length with excessive bleeding or duration greater than seven days
	Presence of premenstrual symptoms
	Dysmenorrhea
	Breast tenderness
	Change in cervical mucous
	Mittelschmertz
	Biphasic temperature curve
Anatomic	Caused by uterine leiomyoma, polyp, adenomyosis, endometrial
	Hyperplasia, carcinoma
	Often heavy bleeding, pain
	Uterus might be enlarged
Medications	Anticoagulants, hormone therapy, tamoxifen, corticosteroids, phenothiazines, acetylsalicylic acid, contraceptives, antidepressants

pregnant women of reproductive age (Fig. 6.1). Of the 9 categories in the new FIGO classification system (PALM-COEIN), the first 4 are defined as visually objective structural criteria

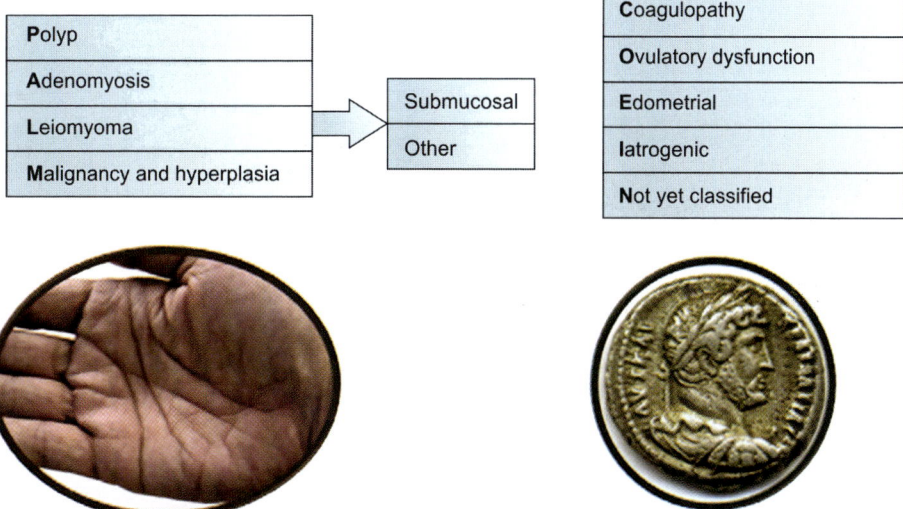

Fig. 6.1: FIGO classification of causes of AUB (*Adapted from* FIGO Classification system (PALM- COIEN) for causes of abnormal uterine bleeding in non-gravid women of reproductive age by Munro M, Critchley H, Border M, Fraser I Int J Gynecology Obstetrics 113:2011;3–13)

(PALM: polyp, adenomyosis, leiomyoma, and malignancy and hyperplasia). The second 4 are unrelated to structural abnormalities (COEI: coagulopathy, ovulatory dysfunction, endometrial, and iatrogenic), and the final category is for entities that are not yet classified (N). FIGO classification suggests the term dysfunctional uterine bleeding should be replaced by coagulopathy, endometrial dysfunction, and ovulatory disorders. FIGO classification also suggests the descriptive terms "heavy menstrual bleeding" and "intermenstrual bleeding" should replace the terms "menorrhagia" and "metrorrhagia". However, in this chapter we continue to use previous terminologies (FIGO recommended terminologies are mentioned within parenthesis—*see* below) because of their wide spread use among gynecologists and gynecologic literature till now.

Polyp (AUB-P): Endocervical and endo-metrial polyps are epithelial proliferations comprise a variable vascular, glandular and fibromuscular and connective tissue component and often contribute to genesis of AUB. Polyps in the endometrium are diagnosed by clinical examination, ultrasound or hysteroscopy.

Adenomyosis (AUB-A): Adenomyosis is another common condition associated with abnormal uterine bleeding (*see* Chapter 18) Adenomyosis can be most accurately diagnosed on the basis of tissue analysis of a hysterectomy specimen, but in everyday clinical practice, ultrasound is commonly used to establish the diagnosis.

Leiomyomas (AUB-L): It can be solitary or multiple, can be located close to the cavity (submucosal), in the myometrium (intra-mural), close to the outer surface (subserosal), or independent of the uterus (parasitic). On the basis of these characteristics, further subcategories have been created as submucosal and others. Because it is generally considered that submucous lesions are most likely to contribute to the genesis of AUB.

Malignancy (AUB-M): It includes hyperplasia and endometrial cancer. The diagnosis requires the histologic analysis of a biopsy sample.

Coagulopathy (AUB-C): It is a cause of AUB in adolescent age group. Most abnormalities are the result of von Willebrand disease and idiopathic thrombocytopenia.

Ovulatory (AUB-O) dysfunction: In which cycle length and volume of flow are unpredictable.

Endometrial (AUB-E): When AUB occurs in the context of predictable and cyclic menstrual bleeding, typical of ovulatory cycles, and particularly when no other definable causes are identified, the mechanism is probably a primary disorder of the endometrium.

Iatrogenic (AUB-I) causes: There are commonly the result of exogenous hormone administration or anticoagulant therapy.

Nonclassified (AUB-N) causes such as arteriovenous malformations and myometrial hypertrophy.

Some specific types of abnormal uterine bleeding are discussed below.

MENORRHAGIA (HEAVY MENSTRUAL BLEEDING)

Menorrhagia is defined as menstruation at regular cycle intervals but with excessive flow or duration or both. Clinically, menorrhagia is said to be present when total blood loss exceeding 80 mL per cycle or menses lasting longer than 7 days. In clinical practice, however, measurement of menstrual blood loss is not possible. Thus, the diagnosis is usually based upon the patient's history. As such menorrhagia is not a disorder by itself but is a symptom of some underlying pathology.

Causes

Numerous underlying pathology has been attributed to the excessive flow and duration of menstruation. The causes can be categorized as pelvic, systemic and other causes.

Pelvic Causes

1. Uterine leiomyoma
2. Adenomyosis
3. Endometrial polyp, hyperplasia and cancer
4. Early tubercular endometritis
5. Endometriosis
6. Pelvic inflammatory disease
7. Tubo-ovarian mass
8. IUCD in utero
9. Arteriovenous malformation of uterus
10. Granulosa cell tumour of ovary
11. PCOS

Systemic Causes

1. Liver dysfunction (coagulopathy)
2. Renal disease
3. Hypothyroidism
4. Hyperthyroidism
5. Bleeding disorders such as von Willebrand disease, ITP, leukemia, aplastic anemia.

Other Causes

1. Dysfunctional uterine bleeding
2. Iatrogenic causes such as use of chemotherapy agents, anticoagulants.

Diagnosis

During the evaluation of menorrhagia, history and examination findings often helps to find out the cause of menorrhagia.

History—Age

1. Young patients, from menarche to the late-teen years, most commonly have anovula-tory bleeding due to the immaturity of their hypothalamic-pituitary axis.
2. Women aged 30–50 years may have systemic or structural abnormalities. Leiomyomas or polyps are frequent anatomical findings. Systemic causes can be anything from thyroid dysfunction to renal failure.

Parity

Adenomyosis may be associated with multi parity.

History of Present Illness

1. Fatigue, dyspnea on exertion may suggest pallor.
2. Cold intolerance, weight gain, hair and skin changes may suggest hypothyroidism.
3. Easy bruissing, gum bleeding, epistaxis may suggest coagulation disorder. If menstrual bleeding is excessive since menarche consideration of a bleeding disorder is heightened.

Menstrual History

Quantity is a very subjective issue when considering menstrual bleeding. Amount of blood loss can be assessed from the rate of change of sanitary pads during full flow, total number of pads used, size and number of clots greater than 1 inch passed during menstruation and sign, symptoms of anemia.

Menstrual irregularity and absent signs of ovulation may indicate anovulatory bleeding.

Medication History

Possible iatrogenic causes include IUCD use, Anticoagulants, hormone therapy, tamoxifen use.

Clinical pearl: Bleeding at a rate of soaking a pad in an hour for at least 2 consecutive hours implies PROFUSE bleeding. Orthostatic hypotension implies hemodynamic instability. Urgent evaluation is imperative!!

General Examination

- *Pallor:* Varying degree of pallor may be present depending upon severity and duration of menorrhagia.
- Obesity, hair loss, brittle nail, nonpitting edema may suggest hypothyroidism.
- Enlarged thyroid gland may be associated with hypothyroidism.
- Obesity, hirsutism, acnthosis nigricans, acne may raise the suspicion of PCOS.
- Jaundice, hepatomegaly, ecchymoses, and other stigmata of liver disease may indicate hepatic dysfunction and coagulopathy.

Gynecological Examination

Abdominal examination may reveal a lump arising from uterus or adnexae.

Speculum examination may reveal structural cervical or endometrial lesion such as polyp, cervical carcinoma.

Bimanual examination may reveal genital tract pathology such as uterine leiomyoma, or adnexal masses .

Uterine size, shape, and contour: An enlarged irregularly shaped uterus suggests uterine leiomyoma. Uniformly enlarged uterus may be due to adenomyosis, or leiomyoma.

Cervical motion tenderness: This is a common symptom of pelvic inflammatory disease (PID) that usually is caused by gonorrhea or Chlamydia.

Adnexal tenderness or masses: An enlarged, tender mass felt through fornices may be due to chocolate cyst of ovary or Tubo-ovarian mass following PID. Hormone producing ovarian tumor may present with menorrhagia.

Differential Diagnosis

Differential diagnosis of menorrhagia will include the conditions which are associated with abnormal vaginal bleeding such as pregnancy complication (such as abortions, ectopic pregnancy, molar pregnancy), cevical lesions such as cervical cancer, cervical polyp.

Investigations

Choice of investigations for a patient with menorrhagia depends upon the provisional diagnosis and deferential diagnosis for the cause of menorrhagia. A full blood count (FBC) is helpful for evaluating the extent of anemia. Hormonal and other laboratory testing is necessary when signs and symptoms suggest hormonal imbalance or coagulation disorders. Imaging studies are employed based on suspicion of structural or mass lesions. Endometrial assessment with hysteroscopy and/or biopsy are typically the final diagnostic step, when imaging and laboratory studies have not revealed specific pathology.

Following investigations are usually considered:

- *Full blood count:* A complete hemogram is useful to evaluate for the presence of anemia. Use the platelet count in conjunction with a peripheral smear if a coagulation defect is suspected.
- *TSH* is indicated when weight gain, cold intolerance, and other factors raise suspicion for hypothyroidism. It is reasonable to consider this test in women of childbearing age, even without the classic symptoms.
- *Coagulation study:* PT/aPTT may indicate coagulopathy, but is rarely sufficient to rule-in most bleeding disorders. Study of coagulation factors are used to rule out von Willebrand disease; and factors II, V, VII, or IX deficiency. These tests should be ordered sparingly because they are expensive tests for rare disorders (usually in the adolescent age group).
- A *urine pregnancy test* is the first test performed in sexually active women of child-bearing age to exclude pregnancy related vaginal bleeding.
- *Liver function tests:* Liver function tests (LFTs) are considered when liver disease is suspected, such as in persons with alcoholism or hepatitis.

- *Hormone assays:* LH, FSH, and androgen levels help to diagnose patients with suspected PCOS.

Imaging—Ultrasonography

Pelvic ultrasound is the best noninvasive imaging study to assess uterine shape, size, and contour; endometrial thickness; and adnexal areas. Ultrasonography is helpful in excluding underlying structural lesion s such as uterine leiomyoma or polyp.

Sonohysterography (saline-infusion sonography)

Fluid infused into the endometrial cavity enhances intrauterine evaluation. One advantage is the ability to differentiate polyps from submucous leiomyomas (i.e. fibroids).

Endometrial Biopsy

This procedure is used in women who are at risk for endometrial carcinoma, polyps, or hyperplasia. The histologic type of endometrium (proliferative or secretory) may help in confirming the diagnosis of anovulatory or ovulatory dysfunctional uterine bleeding (DUB), respectively. This may be of value in determining the most appropriate type of treatment.

Hysteroscopy

Hysteroscopy is indicated when endometrial cavity pathology is suspected (e.g., endometrial polyp, submucous leiomyomas, or endometrial cancer). With pathologic examination, it is the most sensitive and specific diagnostic test for diagnosing uterine cavity disorders. A biopsy sample should be taken, regardless of the endometrial appearance.

Clinical pearl: History should focus on the type of abnormal bleeding: ovulatory, anovulatory, or anatomic. The rest of the investigation should be guided by this classification and can include ultrasound (transvaginal) scans and endometrial biopsy.

Treatment

Principle of Treatment

The goals of treatment of menorrhagia are:

1. To control acute bleeding
2. To maintain an adequate hemoglobin level
3. To prevent future abnormal bleeding and to minimize the risk of endometrial carcinoma.

In choosing an appropriate treatment of menorrhagia the following points are taken into consideration

1. The cause of the bleeding
2. Age of the patient
3. Patients desire regarding future fertility
4. Patients desire regarding future menstruation.

In general, if there is no evidence of neoplasia, nonsurgical treatment should be the first step in management. The options available are both nonhormonal and hormonal, and the choice of drug should take into account the amount of bleeding, any associated pain, existing conditions, and potential side effects of treatment. If medical therapy is ineffective or inappropriate, treatment options progresses to less invasive (e.g. endometrial ablation) to more invasive surgical treatment (e.g. hysterectomy).

General Measures

Many women with menorrhagia are anemic due to blood loss. General treatment involves:

1. Rest during bleeding phase
2. A nutritious diet
3. Correction of anemia with oral iron and vitamin therapy. In some cases blood transfusion may be needed to correct severe anemia.

Medical Treatment

Treatment of severe or acute menorrhagia (Hb < 10 gm%): Management of these patients will include stoppage of acute bleeding, correction of shock, if any, and correction of anemia. In

Table 6.3: Treatment options for acute menorrhagia without bleeding disorder

First line
- Antifibrinolytic agents: Tranexamic acid 1.3 gm orally or 10 mg/kg IV 8 hrly for 5 days
- Hormonal agents (IV conjugated estrogen 25 mg 4–6 hr/COC one tablet PO 6 hrly/norethindrone acetate 5–10 mg PO 4 hrly/medroxyprogesterone 10 mg PO 4 hrly)
- Balloon tamponade

Second line treatment (depending on desire of fertility)
- Dilatation and curettage (D&C)
- Endometrial ablation (if no desire of fertility)
- Uterine artery embolization
- Recombinant factor VIII
- Hysterectomy

Maintenance therapy (once stabilized)
Hormonal agents—combined oral contraceptives, progestin only contraceptive including LNG IUS
IV—intravenous
PO—per oral
COC—combined oral contraceptive

Adapted from James AH, et al. Evaluation and management of acute menorrhagia in women with and without bleeding disorders: consensus from an international expert panel European Journal of Obstetrics and Gynecology and Reproductive biology 2011.

severe acute bleeding (signs and symptoms such as fainting or change in blood pressure or pulse; hematocrit < 30%), hospitalization, stabilization with intravenous fluid, blood transfusion, if necessary, is indicated. Algorithm for the management of acute menorrhagia have been developed from an International expert panel (Table 6.3). A range of first line treatment options was devised. The options for first line therapy include hormonal, surgical and hemostatic treatment. Whether they should be used alone or in combination is dependent on clinical judgment and social and cultural aspects.

Treatment of menorrhagia (chronic): Medical therapy for menorrhagia should be tailored to the individual (Table 6.4).

Nonsteroidal Anti-inflammatory Drugs

Nonsteroidal anti-inflammatory drugs (NSAIDs) are the first-line medical therapy in ovulatory menorrhagia.Studies show an average reduction of 20–46% in menstrual blood flow. NSAIDs reduce prostaglandin levels by inhibiting cyclooxygenase and increasing the ratio of prostacyclin to thromboxane. NSAIDs are ingested for only 5 days of the entire cycle, limiting their most common adverse effect of stomach upset.

Oral Contraceptive Pills

Oral contraceptive pills (OCPs) are a popular first-line therapy for women who desire contraception. Menstrual blood loss is reduced as effectively as NSAIDs secondary to endometrial atrophy. OCPs suppress pituitary gonadotropin release, preventing ovulation. Common adverse effects include breast tenderness, breakthrough bleeding, nausea, and, possibly, related weight gain in some individuals.

Progestin Therapy

Progestin is the most frequently prescribed medicine for menorrhagia. Therapy with progestin results in a significant reduction in menstrual blood flow when used alone. Progestin works as an antiestrogen by minimizing the effects of estrogen on target

Table 6.4: Recommended dose of medical therapy

Medical therapy	Dosage
Tranexamic acid	1 gm every 6 hrs for the first four days
NSAIDs D1–D5 or until cessation of menses	Mefenamic acid 500 mg TDS
Oral contraceptive pills (COC)	COC containing 30 microgram ethinyl estradiol
Progesterone day 5–25	Norethisterone 15 mg daily or medroxyprogesterone 30 mg daily
Danazol	100–200 mg daily for 3 months

cells, thereby maintaining the endometrium in a state of down-regulation. Common adverse effects include weight gain, headaches, edema, and depression.

Levonorgestrel Intrauterine System

Reduces menstrual blood loss by as much as 97%. Comparable to transcervical resection of the endometrium for reduction of menstrual bleeding. Adverse effects of LNG-IUS (Mirena) include uterine bleeding or spotting, headache, ovarian cysts, vaginitis, and breast tenderness.

Gonadotropin-releasing Hormone Agonists

These agents are used on a short-term basis due to high costs and severe adverse effects. GnRH agonists are effective in reducing menstrual blood flow. They inhibit pituitary release of FSH and LH, resulting in hypo-gonadism. A prolonged hypoestrogenic state leads to bone demineralization and reduction of high-density lipoprotein (HDL) cholesterol.

Danazol

Danazol competes with androgen and progesterone at the receptor level, causing amenorrhea in 4–6 weeks. Androgenic effects cause acne, decreasing breast size, and, rarely, hoarse voice.

Tranexamic Acid

Tranexamic acid inhibits the activation of plasminogen to plasmin and thereby prevents fibrinolysis and the breakdown of clots during heavy bleeding. Common adverse effects include menstrual discomfort, headache, and back pain.

Surgical Treatment

Surgical management has been the standard of treatment in menorrhagia due to organic causes (e.g. fibroids) or when medical therapy fails to alleviate symptoms. Surgical treatment ranges from a simple D&C to a full hysterectomy.

i. Dilatation and Curettage

A D&C should be used for diagnostic purposes, however it can be used for treatment because it provides only short-term relief, typically 1–2 months. It is contraindicated in patients with known or suspected pelvic infection. Risks include uterine perforation, infection, and Asherman syndrome.

ii. Endometrial Ablation Techniques

Endometrial ablation is an outpatient procedure that removes or destroys the endometrial layers. The opposing walls of the myometrium collapse onto each other, and the damaged tissue contracts and develops into a scar. Endometrial ablation is used to treat menorrhagia in women who failed standard therapy. It is considered a less invasive alternative to hysterectomy; however, as with hysterectomy, the procedure is not recommended for women who wish to preserve their fertility. Endometrial ablation techniques are generally classified into hysteroscopic/resectoscopic techniques (e.g., Nd: YAG laser and electrosurgical rollerball) and non-hysteroscopic techniques (e.g., cryosurgical and radiofrequency [RF] ablation).

> **Clinical pearl:** The endometrium can be destroyed by several different techniques but reoperation rate at five years may be up to 40 percent with roller ball ablation. This should be reserved for the woman who has finished her childbearing and is aware of the risk of recurrent bleeding. (IA)

iii. Surgical Techniques

Myomectomy: Myomectomy is useful in women with leiomyoma (fibroid uterus) who wish to retain their uterus and/or fertility. Since myomectomy can be associated with large blood loss, this procedure is often reserved for cases of a single or few myomas. Risks include large blood loss or recurrence.

Hysterectomy: Hysterectomy provides definitive cure for menorrhagia. However, this procedure results in greater morbidity than ablative procedures. The mortality rate ranges from 0.1–1.1 cases per 1000 procedures. The morbidity rate is usually 40%. Risks include those usually associated with major surgery.

METRORRHAGIA
(INTERMENSTRUAL BLEEDING)

Definition: Metrorrhagia is irregular acyclic bleeding from the uterus. (However, any irregular bleeding from any part of uterus is included in metrorrhagia.)

Causes: Uterine polyp (fibroid polyp or endometrial polyp), submucous leiomyoma, dysfunctional uterine bleeding, IUCD in uterus, ovular bleeding, endometrial carcinoma, mucous polyp of cervix, cervical carcinoma, cervical tuberculosis, cervical endometriosis, break through bleeding during oral contraceptive pill use, decubitous ulcer in prolapsed uterus.

Investigations: Investigations depend upon provisional and differential diagnosis. In younger women pelvic ultrasonography is often helpful. In elderly women, Pap test, hysteroscopy, dilatation and curettage, saline infusion sonography often helpful to diagnose the cause.

Management: Treatment of all except bleeding at the time of ovulation is necessary. It is described in respective chapter.

OLIGOMENORRHEA
(INFREQUENT MENSTRUAL BLEEDING)

Definition: Menstrual bleeding occurring more than 35 days apart and remains constant at that frequency. Even though the menses are irregular, it may not affect fertility of the women in most cases.

Causes: During adolescence and pre menopause due to anovulatory cycles. Polycystic ovarian syndrome, tubercular endometritis, hyperprolactinemia, hyper- and hypothyroidism, ovarian and adrenal tumors.

Treatment: Oligomenorrhea in absence of underlying pathology does not require any treatment. However, if menstrual periods are erratic and infrequent, it should be evaluated and treated as in secondary amenorrhea. In case of underlying pathologies, they should be treated appropriately.

POLYMENORRHEA

Definition: Menstrual bleeding occurs frequently at cycle length less than 21 days. Polymenorrhea when associated with menorr-hagia is known as polymenorrhagia.

Causes: It is common at extremes of age groups. Common causes are anovulatory cycle, pelvic infection, stressful situation.

Treatment: Treatment with oral contraceptive pill facilitates the return of to normal menstrual cycle in absence of any underlying pathology. Presence of pelvic pathology requires specific treatment.

HYPOMENORRHEA

Definition: Hypomenorrhea is defined as diminution of flow and shortening of duration of menstruation to less than 2 days. It is not considered to be pathological if menstrual cycle remains regular.

Causes: Hypo plastic uterus, oral contraceptive use, genital tuberculosis, premenopausal period, thyroid dysfunction.

Treatment: No treatment is required in absence of pelvic pathology. In presence of any abnormality detected, cause to be treated.

Keywords

Resectoscopic endometrial ablation techniques

a. *Transcervical resection of the endometrium:* This procedure requires the use of a resectoscope (i.e., hysteroscope with a heated wire loop), and it requires time and skill. The primary risk is uterine perforation.

b. *Roller-ball endometrial ablation:* In roller-ball endometrial ablation a heated roller ball is used to destroy the endometrium. It has the same requirements, risks, and outcome success as TCRE.

c. *Endometrial laser ablation:* Endometrial laser ablation requires Nd:YAG equipment and optical fiber delivery system. The laser is inserted into the uterus through the hysteroscope while transmitting energy through the distending media to warm and eventually coagulate the endometrial tissue.

Nonresectoscopic endometrial ablation techniques

a. *Thermal balloon therapy:* A balloon catheter filled with isotonic sodium chloride solution is inserted into the endometrial cavity, inflated, and heated to 87°C for 8 minutes. Uterine balloon therapy cannot be used in irregular uterine cavities because the balloon will not conform to the cavity. Studies report a 90% satisfaction rate and a 25% amenorrhea rate. Long-term studies are ongoing.

b. *Heated free fluid:* HydroThermAblator® (HTA) is an office procedure in which normal saline is infused into the uterus via the hysteroscope. The solution is heated to 194°F (90°C) for 10 minutes under direct visualization. This procedure requires only local anesthesia. HTA may be used in patients with irregularly shaped endometrial cavities and/or fibroids. Vaginal and skin burns are the most reported complications.

c. *Cryoablation:* Cryoablation is the use of liquid nitrogen to freeze the endometrium. The procedure is performed in approximately 10 minutes under ultrasonographic guidance. Patients usually experience 1 week of watery vaginal discharge postprocedure. Risks include perforation and suboptimal ablation of the entire uterine cavity.

d. *Microwave endometrial ablation alternative:* Microwave endometrial ablation (MEA) uses high-frequency microwave energy to cause rapid but shallow heating of the endometrium. Microwaves are selected so that they do not destroy beyond 6 mm in depth. MEA requires 3 minutes of time and only local anesthetic. It is proving to be as effective as TCRE.

e. *Radiofrequency electricity:* NovaSure system is a detailed microprocessor-based unit with a bipolar gold mesh electrode array. It contains a system for determining uterine integrity based upon the injection of CO_2. The device is placed transcervically, the array is opened and electrical energy is applied for 80–90 seconds, desiccating the endometrium.

EXERCISES

Answer the following questions

1. Name the different types of menstrual disorders.
2. What is considered excessive blood loss during menstruation?
3. What is abnormal uterine bleeding?
4. Differentiate anovulatory and ovulatory abnormal uterine bleeding.
5. Describe the patterns of abnormal uterine bleeding—oligomenorrhea, polymenorrhea, menorrhagia, metrorrhagia, menometrorrhagia, hypomenorrhea.
6. Enumerate the causes of abnormal uterine bleeding.
7. What are the causes of menorrhagia?
8. How do you investigate and treat a case of menorrhagia?
9. How do you treat acute severe menorrhagia?

Write short notes on

1. Medical treatment of menorrhagia.
2. PALM-COIEN classification of causes of AUB

Explain or justify the following statements

1. Details of menstrual history is essential for diagnosis of menorrhagia.
2. Several terminologies are used to describe abnormal uterine bleeding.

Fill in the blanks with appropriate word/s

1. Most common cause of abnormal uterine bleeding is _____ .
2. Two common causes of abnormal uterine bleeding in adolescent girls are _____ and _____ .
3. Two menstrual cycle length disorders are _____ and _____ .

Questions for practical (read the case summary at the beginning of the topic before answering the questions)

1. Which type of AUB this woman is suffering from?
2. How age is related with AUB?
3. What are the probable causes of bleeding in this patient?
4. Name the investigations that can be considered for her and why?
5. How she should be treated?

Bibliography

1. Albers JR, et al. Abnormal uterine bleeding Am Fam Physician 2004;69:1915-26; 1931–2.
2. Ely WJ, et al. Abnormal uterine bleeding- a management algorithm JABFM November-December 2006 Vol. 19 No. 6.
3. Frase IS, Chritchley HOD, Malcom GM. Abnormal uterine bleeding: getting our terminology straight. Current Opinion in Obstetrics and Gynecology 2007, 19:591–595.
4. James AH, et al. Evaluation and manage-ment of acute menorrhagia in women with and without underlying bleeding disorders: consensus from an international expert panel. Eur J Obstet Gynecol 2011, doi:10.1016/j.ejogrb.2011.04.025.
5. Management of acute abnormal uterine bleeding in nonprgnanat reproductive age women. Committee opinion no 557 Committee on gynecologic practice ACOG April 2013.
6. Managemet of menorrhagia Clinical Practice Guideline, Ministry of Malaysia 2004.
7. Mattison KA. Nonsurgical Management of Heavy Menstrual Bleeding. A Systematic Review Obstet Gynecol 2013;121:632–43.
8. Munro MG, et al. FIGO classification system (PALM-COEIN) for causes of abnormal uterine bleeding in nongravid women of reproductive age. International Journal of Gynecology and Obstetrics 113; 2011: 3–13.
9. Oriel K. Abnormal uterine bleeding Am Fam Physician. 1999 Oct 1;60(5):1371–1380.
10. Sokkary, et al. Management of heavy menstrual bleeding in adolescents. Curr Opin Obstet Gynecol 2012, 24:275–280.
11. Sweet MG, et al. Evaluation and Management of Abnormal Uterine Bleeding in Premeno-pausal Women Am Fam Physician. 2012; 85(1):35–43.
12. Telner D, et al. Approach to diagnosis and management of abnormal uterine bleeding Canadian Family Physician Vol 53; 58–64: 2007.

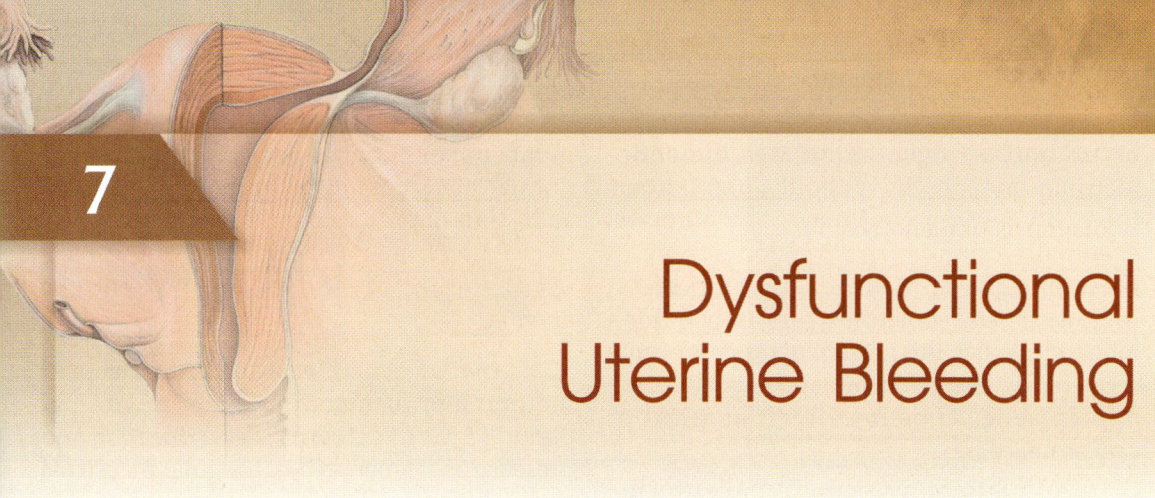

7

Dysfunctional Uterine Bleeding

A 16-year-old girl presents to the emergency room with history of excessive menstrual bleeding that started yesterday and has been increasing since early morning. She had her first period (Menarche) at 13 years of age and since then her periods have been irregular and unpredictable. She looks pale, however, her vital signs are stable. Examination reveals significant uterine bleeding that soaks one pad every 2 hours. She is admitted to the hospital. How her bleeding should be controlled?

In this chapter we will learn:
- What is dysfunctional uterine bleeding
- What are its causes
- Clinical presentation of patients with dysfunctional uterine bleeding
- Investigations and treatment of DUB

Definition

Dysfunctional uterine bleeding (DUB) is defined as abnormal uterine bleeding in the absence of organic disease. This means that even after thorough clinical examination and other investigations (e.g. ultrasonography), the cause of uterine bleeding cannot be attributed *the usual* causes of uterine bleeding (structural gynecologic abnormalities, cancer, inflammation, systemic disorders, complications of pregnancy, use of oral contraceptives or certain drugs). Thus DUB is diagnosis made by exclusion of other causes of uterine bleeding. Dysfunctional uterine bleeding (DUB), the most common cause of abnormal uterine bleeding, occurs most often in women > 45 (> 50% of cases) and in adolescents (20% of cases).

Classification

DUB may be classified into anovulatory DUB and ovulatory DUB. However, some experts restrict the term to anovulatory DUB.

AUB and DUB

AUB is often due to anatomical lesion of uterus and exogenous hormones. However, DUB results from endogenous hormonal etiology. The pathophysiology underlying DUB depends upon ovulatory status. Thus all DUBs are a variety of AUB but all AUB are not DUB.

Pathophysiology

During an anovulatory cycle, the corpus luteum does not form. Thus, the normal cyclical secretion of progesterone does not occur, and estrogen stimulates the endometrium unopposed. Without progesterone, the endometrium continues to proliferate, eventually outgrowing its blood supply; it then sloughs and bleeds incompletely, irregularly, and sometimes profusely or for a long time. When this abnormal process occurs repeatedly, the endometrium can become hyperplastic, sometimes with atypical or cancerous cells.

In ovulatory dysfunctional uterine bleeding, bleeding occurs cyclically, and menorrhagia is thought to originate from defects in the control mechanisms of menstruation. It is thought that, in women with ovulatory dysfunctional uterine bleeding, there is an increased rate of blood loss resulting from vasodilatation of the vessels supplying the endometrium due to decreased vascular tone, and prostaglandins have been strongly implicated. Therefore, these women lose blood at rates about 3 times faster than women with normal menses.

Clinical pearl: Random breakdown of the endometrial lining (DUB) does NOT occur when the endometrium has been adequately primed with estrogen and stabilized with progesterone.

Diagnosis

An accurate history and detailed physical examination are enough to achieve a provisional diagnosis of DUB in more than two-thirds of the cases. Most likely the patient will present with chief complaint of AUB. Most organic causes of AUB can be ruled out with history and physical examination.

History

Complaint: Patients often present with complaints of amenorrhea, menorrhagia, metrorrhagia, or meno metrorrhagia. The amount and frequency of bleeding and the duration of symptoms, as well as the relationship to the menstrual cycle, should be established. Ask patients to compare the number of pads or tampons used per day in a normal menstrual cycle to the number used at the time of presentation. Assess the severity of bleeding from passage of clots, no. of pads used, soiling of clothes and presence of anemia.

Menstrual history: Menstrual history should include age of menarche, last menstrual period (LMP), regularity, flow, duration and presence of dysmenorrhea. Irregular menstrual cycle, absence of premenstrual molimina (e.g. breast fullness and tenderness, weight gain, and mild mood swings), are clues for anovulation and anovulatory DUB.

Obstetric history: Previous abortion or recent termination of pregnancy.

Medical history: Bleeding disorders and other associated complaints are important to exclude, particularly in young post-puberty patients. Endocrine disorders such as thyroid problems may be a cause of irregular menses.

Menopausal symptoms: These are important clues in women late in their reproductive life. DUB in these patients may be related to menopause.

Sexual activity: The possibility of pregnancy should be considered in all patients and excluded.

Physical Examination

Signs of anaemia: Acute bleeding may present with unstable vital signs, and chronic bleeding may be associated with non-specific manifestations of chronic iron deficiency anaemia, such as dyspnoea, pallor on examination.

Abdominal and pelvic examination: In presence of DUB, abdominal and pelvic examination will reveal no abnormality and will exclude anatomical causes of abnormal uterine bleeding.

Diagnosis: DUB is a diagnosis of exclusion; other conditions that can cause similar bleeding must be excluded. Pregnancy should be excluded in sexually active women. Coagulation disorders should be considered, particularly in adolescents who have anemia or require hospitalization for bleeding. Regular cycles with prolonged or excessive bleeding (possible ovulatory DUB) suggest structural abnormalities.

Investigations

Several tests are typically done but more important tests that are done initially are:

- *Complete blood count (CBC):* CBC is routinely done to exclude anemia.
- *Urine pregnancy test:* When evaluating a woman of reproductive age with vaginal bleeding, pregnancy must always be ruled out by urine human chorionic gonadotropin.
- *Ultrasonography:* Ultrasound is the initial imaging test which will determine uterine wall and uterine cavity disorders such as endometrial polyps and leiomyomas. An endometrial thickness > 15 mm warrants further evaluation with endometrial biopsy and hysteroscopy.
- *TSH, prolactin and progesterone level:* In patients with suspected endocrine disorders, thyroid function tests and prolactin levels are usually measured because thyroid disorders and hyperprolactinemia are common causes of abnormal bleeding. To determine whether bleeding is anovulatory or ovulatory, some clinicians measure serum progesterone levels during the luteal phase. A level of ≥ 3 ng/mL (≥ 9.75 nmol/L) suggests that ovulation has occurred.
- *Coagulation profile:* Coagulation studies and platelet function tests should be considered in adolescent girls when presenting with menorrhagia.

Other tests are done depending on results of the history and physical examination and initial investigation findings. Subsequent tests may include the following:

- *Dilatation and curettage:* Endometrial biopsy is done to exclude more serious underlying pathology such as endometrial hyperplasia and endometrial cancer. The histological type of endometrium (proliferative or secretory) may help in confirming the diagnosis of anovulatory or ovulatory DUB, respectively.
- *Hysteroscopy* is recommended when endometrial cavity pathology is suspected, such as endometrial polyp, submucous leiomyomas, or endometrial cancer.
- *Hysterosalpingography (HSG) and saline infusion sonography (SIS)* of the uterus further evaluates the presence of endometrial or uterine pathology. Distending the uterine cavity with infusion of saline under ultrasound imaging is helpful in detecting endometrial cavity irregularity caused by uterine polyps and uterine leiomyomas that bulge into the uterine cavity. Presence of active bleeding contraindicates HSG and saline infusion sonography.
- *Testosterone and dehydroepiandrosterone sulfate (DHEAS)* levels are measured if polycystic ovary syndrome is suspected.
- *Follicle-stimulating hormone (FSH) and estradiol levels* are measured if ovarian failure is a possibility.

If all clinically indicated tests are normal, the diagnosis is DUB.

Treatment

The aim of treatment in DUB is to restore normal menstrual bleeding pattern and to treat associated complications, most commonly anemia.

a. *General consideration:* Before any treatment other pathology must be excluded. Exclusion of pregnancy or underlying pelvic or systemic diseases is the most important initial step. Where there is systemic disease, treat accordingly or refer to the appropriate specialist. Iron therapy, usually oral, is prescribed if iron deficiency anemia is diagnosed.

b. *Medical treatment*

- *Emergency treatment of excessive uterine bleeding:* DUB sometimes presents in the form of excessive uterine bleeding that requires immediate hospital admission and emergency treatment as described previously in treatment of menorrhagia (Chapter 6— Table 6.4).

- *Anovulatory or ovulatory DUB*

  i. *Progestogens:* Progestogens are the first-line treatment for DUB, particularly when associated with anovulation. Progestogens are used cyclically but can be used continuously. In anovulatory DUB they are prescribed in leuteal phase from day 15 to day 25. In ovulatory DUB progestogen is prescribed from day 5 to day 25. However, progestogen may be delivered through progesterone-containing IUDs and contraceptive implants.

  ii. *Antifibrinolytic agents:* Tranexamic acids is an antifibrinolytic agent that reduces endometrial fibrinolytic enzymes that are increased in DUB. Menstrual blood loss is reduced by 40–60%. Tranexamic acid is prescribed only on the heavy days of menstrual flow usually on the first five days. The dose prescribed is 1 gm 3–4 times per day. Side effects are infrequent and include nausea and leg cramps. Tranexamic acid is appropriate first line treatment for ovulatory DUB.

  iii. *Combined oral contraceptive pill:* Combined oestrogen and progestogen is a second-line therapy that can be used when a progestogen alone is not associated with an adequate response. It has the added advantage of reducing dysmenorrhoea and providing contraception. It can be used in all patients except in those with contraindications for oestrogen, such as history of thromboembolic disorders or conditions predisposing for thrombo-embolism (e.g., smoking, particularly in women > 35 years). Both monophasic and triphasic combined contracptive pill are used in restoring menstrual bleeding (withdrawal bleeding) in most cases of DUB whether anovulatory or ovulatory.

Table 7.1: Treatment regimen for chronic anovulatory DUB

Drug	Dose	Purpose	Side effects
Oral medroxyprogesterone	5–10 mg/day 10 days/month	Cycle regulation Prevention of endometrial hyperplasia	Mood changes, irritability, depression, weight gain, oedema, bloating, nausea, breast tenderness
Oral norethidrone acetate	5–10 mg 10 days/month		Norethidrone, norethidrone acetate, norgestrel lower HDL cholesterol level and exhibit androgenic effects
Oral micronized progesterone	200–300 mg /day 10–12 days /m		
IM medroxy progesterone	150 mg every 3 month	Contraception	
Levonorgestrel intrauterine device		Contraception	
Combined oral contraceptive	1 oral tablet per day for 21 days	Contraception, cycle regulation, prevention of endometrial hyperplasia	Bloating, nausea, weight gain, acne, oedema, breasts changes, cholelithiasis
Clomiphene	50 mg/day for 5 days	Induction of ovulation	Ovarian hyperstimulation, multiple pregnancy

Table 7.2: Treatment regimen for ovulatory DUB

Drug	Dose	Purpose	Side effects
NSAIDs mefenamic acid Ibuprofen Naproxen	500–1500 mg/day in divided doses 600–1200 mg/day in divided doses 270 mg 7 hrly after a loading dose of 550 mg	Reduction in amount/duration in menstrual flow, pain relief	GI irritation Contraindicated in peptic ulcer disease and renal failure
Antifibrinolytics– Epsilon amino caproic acid Tranexamic acid	18 g/day × 3 days then 12 g, 9 g, 6 g, 3 g on successive days 1 g 4 times daily for days 1–4 of cycle	Reduction in amount/ duration of menstrual flow	Nausea, dizziness, diarrhea, headache, abdominal pain, allergic reactions Contraindicated in renal failure and pregnancy
Progestin or LNG IUS IM Medroxy progesterone Combined oral contraceptive	See Table 7.1 See Table 7.1	Reduction in menstrual flow Reduction in amount/duration of flow, contraception	See Table 7.1 See Table 7.1

Sometimes higher doses are needed initially, for example, 2 or 3 pills every day during the first few days until bleeding stops.

iv. *NSAIDs:* Because prostaglandins are believed to play a significant role in mediating the pathophysiology of uterine bleeding, anti-prostaglandins, such as non-steroidal anti-inflammatory drugs (NSAIDs), have been suggested as possible useful treatment, particularly when the use of oestrogens and progestogens are contraindicated. They are usually helpful for DUB presenting as mild uterine bleeding, and may be particularly useful for ovulatory DUB. They are contraindicated in peptic ulcer disease and bronchial asthma.

v. *Other therapies:* Danazol has been found to effectively reduce heavy menstrual bleeding but its use has been limited because of its recommended short term use (6 months or less) and side effects. Gestrinone is similar to danazol but is a twice per week dose. GnRH agonist have a very limited role in treatment of DUB.

c. *Surgical treatment*

The decision to perform surgery for treatment of DUB will depend on:

i. Failure of medical therapy
ii. For bleeding resulting in hemodynamic instability
iii. For patients who do not wish future fertility and requests surgery.

Surgical options include Dilatation and Curettage (D and C), endometrial ablation, hysterectomy and trans cervical resection of endometrium.

i. *Dilatation and curettage:* The surgical approach of D&C is usually reserved for cases of significant uterine bleeding not responding to medical treatment. D&C can be done in conjunction with hysteroscopy for direct visualization of the uterine cavity to diagnose possible underlying pathology to exclude malignancy in peri menopausal women. D&C can stop acute bleeding and can no longer considered as curative treatment for DUB.

ii. *Endometrial ablation:* Endometrial ablation is usually performed when the women wants to keep her uterus but not willing for future fertility or when the woman is unable to tolerate major surgery. The principle of endometrial ablation is to destroy the basal layers of the endometrium, preventing the regeneration of the endometrium. This results in complete amenorrhea in approximately 50% of women or reduced bleeding in approximately 90% of women with menorrhagia, but it is not 100% effective. First generation techniques include roller ball diathermy or resection, laser ablation and second generation technique include microwave ablation.

iii. *Hysterectomy:* Hysterectomy results in definitive and permanent cure of DUB. Hysterectomy is considered in perimeno-pausal women when medical treatment fails. There are three types of hysterec-tomy—laparoscopically assisted, vaginal and abdominal. Laparoscopic hysterec-tomy has less morbidity and rapid recovery following the procedure.

EXERCISES

Answer the following questions

1. What is dysfunctional uterine bleeding?
2. What causes dysfunctional uterine bleeding?
3. How does dysfunctional uterine bleeding often present?
4. What basic tests can be done in a case of dysfunctional uterine bleeding?
5. How dysfunctional uterine bleeding is treated?
6. How do you manage if bleeding is heavy?

Explain or justify the following statements

1. All DUB are AUB but all AUB are not DUB
2. Dysfunctional uterine bleeding is diagnosis of exclusion of other causes.

Write short notes on

1. Medical treatment of DUB
2. Pathophysiology of DUB

Fill in the blanks with appropriate word/s

1. In anovulatory DUB ———— is the first line drug treatment.
2. DUB is most common in ———— and ———— age group.

Questions for practical (Read the case summary at the beginning of the topic before answering the questions)

1. What is menorrhagia?
2. What are the common causes of puberty menorrhagia?
3. What should be immediate measures to stop bleeding?
4. How she should be investigated?
5. How she should be treated?

Bibliography

1. Casablanka Y. Management of dysfunctional uterine bleeding Obstet Gynecol Clin N Am 35 2008: 219–234.
2. Farrel E. Dysfunctional uterine bleeding Australian Family Physician Vol. 33, No. 11, November 2004.
3. Pinkerton JV. Dysfunctional uterine bleeding Merck Manual Jan 2010, Johnson BA.
4. Walden SM. Primary care management of dysfunctional uterine bleeding **JAAPA** Vol. 19, No. 2 February 2006.

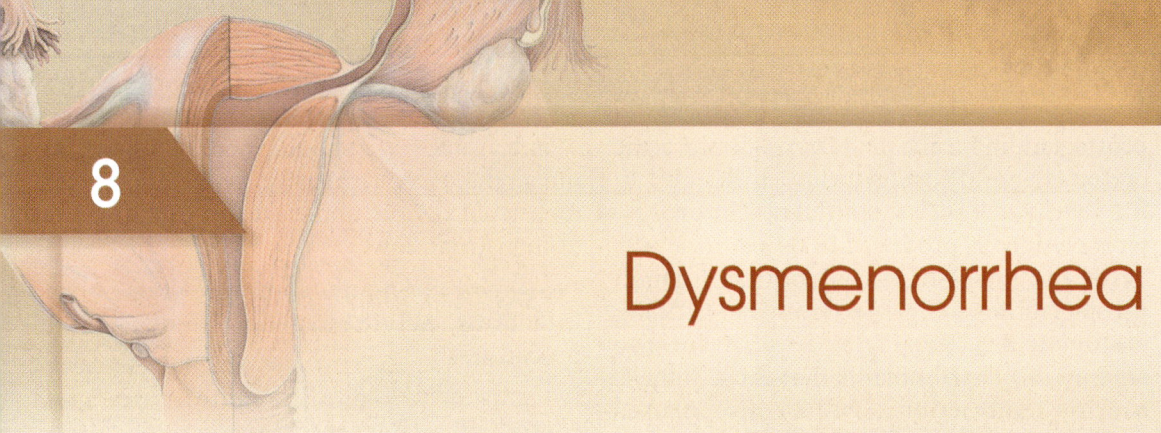

8

Dysmenorrhea

A 16-year-old girl has presented to outpatient department (OPD) with complain of lower abdominal cramping pain during menstruation. Her menarche was at 13 years of age and her initial periods for one year were painless. She also complains of nausea and vomiting for first 2 days of menstruation. All her symptoms subside from 3rd day of mens onwards. She was unable to attend school during her last period. Her general and abdominal findings are within normal limit. How she should be treated?

In this chapter we will learn:

- What is dysmenorrhea
- What are the different types of dysmenorrhea
- What causes dysmenorrhea
- How to differentiate among different types of dysmenorrhea
- Its clinical presentation, investigations and treatment

Introduction

Dysmenorrhea is defined as painful menstruation that prevents a woman from performing normal activities. Dysmenorrhea itself is not a life-threatening condition but is found to have a profound impact on daily activities and may result in missing work or school, inability to participate in sports and other activities. It is considered as leading cause of school absence in adolescent girls and a common problem in women of reproductive age. The prevalence of dysmenorrhea to be between 45 and 95% among reproductive age women.

menorrhea (also known as spasmodic dysmenorrhea) is defined as painful menstrual cramps in the absence of any identifiable pelvic pathology that could account for it. This is the most common problem in adolescent girls and is characterized by cramping pain in pelvic region at the onset of menstruation.

In secondary dysmenorrhea (also known as congestive dysmenorrhea), the painful menstruation is accompanied by identifiable pelvic pathology that accounts for the pain. Such a classification allows practical differentiation in the management approach, which is based on the causal mechanism.

Classification

Dysmenorrhea is classified as primary or secondary dysmenorrhea. Primary dys-

Etiology

Current evidence suggests primary dysmenorrhea which is caused by excess prostaglandin F 2 alfa (PGF2α) produced in the endometrium. Prostaglandin production in the uterus is under the influence of progesterone which is produced in ovulatory cycle. With the onset of menstruation formed prostaglandins are released from the shedding endometrium. Prostaglandins are intense smooth muscle stimulants that cause intense uterine contractions. PGF2α also causes contractions in smooth muscle elsewhere in body resulting in nausea, vomiting and diarrhea. In addition to increase in prostaglandins from endometrial shedding, necrosis of endometrial cells provides increased substrate arachidonic acid from cell walls for prostaglandin synthesis. Prostaglandin E2 (PGE2), a potent vasodilator and platelet anti aggregator, has been implicated as cause of primary menorrhagia. Multiple other factors like behavioral and psychologic factors, cervical stenosis or narrowing, increased vasopressin release, increased uterine activity have been implicated in the cause of primary dysmenorrhea.

Secondary dysmenorrhea is caused by structural abnormalities or disease processes that occur outside the uterus, or within the uterine wall or within the uterine cavity. Common causes of secondary dysmenorrhea include endometriosis, adenomyosis, PID, uterine leiomyoma and adhesions (*see* Table 8.1).

Clinical Presentation

History

History of present illness: History should include an assessment of the onset, duration, type, and severity of pain. Clinicians should also ask about the age at which symptoms began, factors that relieve or worsen pain, degree of disruption of daily life, and presence of pelvic pain unrelated to menses. Presence of accompanying symptoms such as cyclic nausea, vomiting, bloating, diarrhea, and fatigue should also be enquired.

Menstrual history should include the age at menarche, cycle regularity, cycle length, last menstrual period, and duration and amount of menstrual flow.

Past history: Enquire about previous pelvic infections, pelvic surgeries, injuries, and procedures.

Sexual history should include effect of contraceptives on pain, dyspareunia and prior or current history of sexual abuse.

Family history should include Endometriosis

Physical Examination

Pelvic examination focuses on detecting causes of secondary dysmenorrhea. Women with primary dysmenorrhea usually have normal findings on examination and pelvic examination is not usually indicated in young women. In sexually active women the vagina, vulva, and cervix are inspected for lesions and for masses protruding through the external cervical os. Pelvic structures are palpated to check for polyp or fibroid, uterine masses, adnexal masses, thickening of the rectovaginal septum, induration of the cul-de-sac, and nodularity of the uterosacral ligament.

Diagnosis of Primary Dysmenorrhea

Primary dysmenorrhea usually occurs 6–12 months of menarche, once ovulatory cycles have been established. Pain is usually lower abdominal and cramping in nature. Pain may radiate to the back and to the inner thigh. It usually lasts from 8 to 72 hours and accompanies menstrual flow or precedes it by only a few hours. The pain is associated with other systemic symptoms such as nausea, vomiting, diarrhea, fatigue and headache. Physical examination reveals no abnormality and clinical investigations fail to reveal any underlying pathology.

Diagnosis of Secondary Dysmenorrhea

By contrast, secondary dysmenorrhea usually occurs years after the onset of menarche and

Table 8.1: Causes of secondary dysmenorrhea		
Intrauterine	*Extrauterine*	*Non-gynecological*
Adenomyosis	Endometriosis	Psychosomatic disorders
Leiomyoma	PID	Irritable bowel syndrome
IUD	Adhesions	Inflammatory bowel disease
Congenital mullerian anomaly	Ovarian cyst or tumor	
Cervical stenosis	Pelvic congestion syndrome	
Uterine polyp		

may arise as a new symptom when the woman is in her 30s or 40s of age. The pain is not consistently related to menstruation alone, and may occur throughout the luteal phase of the menstrual cycle. It may also worsen as menses progresses rather than being confined to the first 24 to 48 hours of menstruation. Accompanying symptoms such as an irregular bleeding pattern, heavy periods, vaginal discharge, and dyspareunia can be suggestive of underlying pathology. Physical examination will reveal underlying pelvic pathology which can be confirmed by relevant investigations. Possible causes of secondary dysmenorrhea are mentioned in Table 8.1. Table 8.2 shows the differences between primary and secondary dysmenorrhea.

Clinical pearl: The diagnosis of secondary dysmenorrhea should be considered when symptoms appear after many years of painless menses.

Investigations

When the history and clinical examinations are suggestive of primary dysmenorrhea, further investigations are not required. Diagnosis is made based on clinical findings.

However, further investigations may be necessary in the presence of nonspecific symptoms, abnormal clinical findings, treatment failure of primary dysmenorrhea, or suspicion of secondary dysmenorrhea, or when the diagnosis is in doubt.

Further investigations may include the following:
Ultrasonography: Uterine leiomyoma, adnexal pathology, endometriomas, and intrauterine contraceptive devices are best assessed with ultrasonography. Transvaginal ultrasound is preferable as it offers better resolution.

WBC, ESR, CRP: An elevated WBC count along with a high ESR and CRP can be

Table 8.2: Differences between primary and secondary dysmenorrhea		
Characteristics	*Primary dysmenorrhea*	*Secondary dysmenorrhea*
Age	Onset soon after menarche	Usually in elderly, onset years after pain free menses (typically after 25 yrs)
Cycle	Before/during mens	Starts much before onset of menstruation
Pattern	Similar in each period	Increases with time
Associated symptoms	PMS, nausea, vomiting, bloating	Menorrhagia, infertility, dyspareunia
Part history	Nil	Exposure to STI, past surgery, IUCD
Pelvic examination	Normal	Tenderness, adnexal mass, fixed retroverted uterus Cervical tenderness
Ultrasonography	Normal	Pelvic pathology usually present
NSAID	Usually relieves the pain	Minimal improvement, if any
COC	Usually relieves the pain	Minimal improvement, if any

evidence of an acute or chronic inflammatory disease.

Cervical culture to exclude sexually transmitted diseases particularly Chlamidya and gonorrhea.

Laparoscopy: Helps in the diagnosis of endometriosis, adhesions, and pelvic inflammatory disease and at the same time can offer treatment.

Hysteroscopy: May be indicated to evaluate intrauterine pathology if the sonographic findings are unclear.

MRI/CT of abdomen and pelvis may be done when ultrasonography results are equivocal.

Clinical pearl: Laboratory testing or imaging is not required to make a diagnosis of primary dysmenorrhea.

Treatment

Treatment of primary dysmenorrhea: The treatment of primary dysmenorrhea aims to relieve pain or symptoms. There are three approaches to the management of primary dysmenorrhea:

- Pharmacological
- Non-pharmacological
- Surgical

General consideration: The overall approach to management should include skillful manipulation of the psychologic and behavioral factors and the specific pharmacotherapy. Careful assessment of the proportion contributed by the psychologic or reactive component of the pain in dysmenorrhea in each of the patients is essential to appropriate therapy or a combination of therapies. Explanation and reassurance will go a long way in curing the patient.

a. Pharmacological

Non-steroidal antiinflammatory drugs (NSAID): NSAIDs are the first line choice for treatment of primary dysmenorrhea. It is unclear which NSAIDs are superior in terms of efficacy and side effects. Drugs that are used:

First choice:
- Propionic acid: Ibuprofen 400–800 mg per oral 6 hrly. Naproxen 250–500 mg PO 6 hrly
- Fenamates: Mefenamic acids—250–500 mg PO 6 hrly
- Acetic acids: Indomethacin 25–50 mg PO 8 hrly

The second choice include:
- *Pyrazolones:* Phynylbutazone has bone marrow toxicity
- *Oxicams:* Pyroxicams

Generally therapy is started with mefenamic acid 250–500 mg 6 hrly. If pain is not relieved with the first agent after two or more cycles at maximum recommended dose, then a second agent may be added.

Combined oral contraceptive pills: These are second line treatment if birth control is not desired. The combined oral contraceptive pill inhibits ovulation and leads to thinning of endometrium. This will result in less prostaglandin synthesis with lower level of menstrual fluid volume and thus relief of dysmenorrhea in 90% of women. Monophasic and triphasic COC pills are equally effective.

Other therapies: Other therapies for dysmenorrhea have been proposed, but most are not well studied. These include thiamine, vitamin E, omega-3 fatty acids, magnesium, various herbal medicines, transdermal nitroglycerin, calcium-channel blockers, beta-adrenergic agonists, antileukotrienes.

b. Non-pharmacological Treatment

Transcutaneous electrical nerve stimulation (TENS): TENS involves use of electrodes to stimulate the skin at various frequencies and intensities in an attempt to diminish pain sensation. High frequency TENS provides effective pain relief when compared with placebo but not better than ibuprofen. High frequency TENS may be considered as a supplementary treatment in women unable to tolerate medication.

Topical heat: Low level topical heat therapy was as effective as ibuprofen for the treatment of dysmenorrhea. Faster improvement in pain relief was noted when heat therapy was combined with ibuprofen compared with ibuprofen alone.

Other therapies: There is limited evidences to support the use acupuncture or spinal nerve stimulation for treatment of dysmenorrhea.

Surgical Therapy

Laparoscopy: In women who do not obtain adequate pain relief with NSAIDs and OCPs, the likelihood of pelvic pathology such as endometriosis is high and laparoscopy may be considered. However, the risks of laparoscopic documentation must be weighed against the predicted advantages of having a diagnosis of endometriosis when the symptoms are controlled without surgery.

Cervical dilatation: Cervical dilatation as a primary method of treatment for primary dysmenorrhea is not warranted. However, dilatation of the cervix should be undertaken when laparoscopies are performed. This surgical manipulation does relieve primary dysmenorrhea temporarily, although with a progressive return of the symptoms.

Presacral neurectomy (PSN): Presacral neurectomy involves the total transection of presacral nerves lying within the boundaries of the interiliac triangle. Presacral neurectomy is rarely indicated for treatment of most forms of primary dysmenorrhea. Use of this procedure should be extremely limited and reserved for patients with chronic pelvic pain when other methods of pain relief have failed.

Laparoscopic uterosacral nerve ablation (LUNA): Resection of uterosacral ligaments achieve in theory a more complete uterine denervation than pre-sacral neurectomy. However, laparoscopic utero sacral nerve resection has not been shown to reduce dysmenorrhea and not advocated as mainstream treatment option.

Treatment of Secondary Dysmenorrhea

Women wearing the intrauterine device should be treated with nonsteroidal anti-inflammatory drugs for their intrauterine device-induced dysmenorrhea and the medication should be given continuously throughout the duration of the menstrual flow.

Treatment for most of the other causes of secondary dysmenorrhea should be directed to the specific underlying condition. Surgery has a greater role to play in the treatment of most forms of secondary dysmenorrhea and is usually more definitive. Nonsteroidal anti-inflammatory drugs may be given only as a temporary measure to obtain some relief while waiting for surgery. In endometriosis patients, specific hormonal therapy (i.e. danazol, gonadotropin releasing hormone agonist, progestins, and oral contraceptives) could also be employed to obtain adequate relief.

EXERCISES

Answer the following questions

1. What is dysmenorrhea?
2. What are the two main categories of dysmenorrhea?
3. Describe the typical pattern of pain in primary dysmenorrhea?
4. What is the mechanism for development of primary dysmenorrhea?
5. How do you approach a patient of dysmenorrhea?
6. What are the causes of secondary dysmenorrhea?
7. How do you treat primary and secondary dysmenorrhea?
8. Differentiate primary and secondary dysmenorrhea.

Write short notes on

1. Role of prostaglandins in dysmenorrhea
2. Diagnosis of primary dysmenorrhea

Explain or justify the following statements

1. Classification of dysmenorrhea allows practical differentiation in the management of dysmenorrhea
2. Non-surgical treatment is the main form of treatment in primary dysmenorrhea.
3. Surgical treatment is often required in secondary dysmenorrhea

Fill in the blanks

1. Three uterine causes of secondary dysmenorrhea are _____ , _____ , and _____ .
2. _____ are first line choice for treatment of primary dysmenorrhea.

Questions for practical (Read the case summary at the beginning of the topic before answering the questions)

1. What type of dysmenorrhea she is having?
2. Why she suffers from nausea and vomiting during mens?
3. What are the points in favor of diagnosis?
4. When she should be investigated?
5. What are the treatment options for her?
6. How do you choose appropriate NSAIDs to relieve her symptoms?

Bibliography

1. Dawood, Y, *Glob. libr. women's med.*, (ISSN: 1756-2228) 2008; DOI 10.3843/GLOWM.10009.
2. French L. Dysmenorrhea Am Fam Physician 2005;71:285–91, 292.
3. Pinkerton JAV. Dysmenorrhea Merck Manual 2010.
4. Reddish L. Dysmenorrhea **Australian Family Physician,** Vol. 35, No. 11, November 2006.
5. SOGC Clinical Practice Guideline. Primary Dysmenorrhea Consensus Guideline no. 169, 2005.
6. Tu F et al. Dysmenorrhea Contemporary Issues International Association for the Study of Pain, 2007.

9

Premenstrual Syndrome

A 31-year-old nulliparous woman has presented with recurrent symptoms of fatigue, abdominal bloating, breast tenderness, increased appetite, irritability and headache that have occurred for many years, predominantly 1-week before the start of menses. The symptoms had improved when she was on oral contraceptives following her marriage three years ago. Recently these symptoms have become more troublesome, interfering with her relationship with husband and her ability to perform optimally at work as school teacher. Physical examination reveals normal findings with normal breast and pelvic examination. How she should be managed?

In this chapter we will learn:
- What is premenstrual syndrome (PMS) and how it differs from premenstrual symptoms and premenstrual dysphoric disorders (PMDD)
- How PMS and PMDD are diagnosed and treated

Definition

Premenstrual syndrome (PMS) is a cyclical luteal phase (the time period between ovulation and onset of menstruation) condition characterized by physical, psychological, and behavioral changes of sufficient severity to result in deterioration of interpersonal relationships and normal activity. Premenstrual dysphoric disorder (PMDD) is considered a severe form of PMS.

Classification

Premenstrual symptoms: Up to 75% of women with regular menses describe a few symptoms during the luteal phase but may not interfere with day to day activity, and thus may not meet the criteria for premenstrual syndrome (PMS) or PMDD.

Premenstrual syndrome: Clinically significant cluster of premenstrual symptoms produce premenstrual syndrome (PMS), with the most common physical symptom being abdominal bloating, followed by breast tenderness and headaches.

Premenstrual dysphoric disorder (PMDD): PMDD is less common than PMS. If the mental symptoms predominate, are very severe, and are associated with impairment, then the patient is classified as having premenstrual dysphoric disorder (PMDD) which may be viewed as a severe subtype of PMS. The DSM-IV requires at least 1 affective symptom, such as anger or irritability, with psychiatric conditions excluded (see below).

Etiopathology: The etiology of premenstrual syndrome remains unknown and may be complex and multifactorial. PMS and PMDD are conditions that occur in women with regular menses. Cyclicity and physiologic hormonal variations of estrogen and progesterone make an impact on central neurotransmitters which seem to be the basis of the condition. Serotonin and GABA are the neurotransmitter which are mostly involved along with beta endorphins. Autonomic system may also play a role.

Diagnostic approach: While premenstrual symptoms are common among most women, a diagnosis of PMS or of PMDD is less common.

History

Age: PMS affects women in all ages from adolescence till menopause. Women in their fourth decade of life tend to be affected most severely.

Symptoms: Common symptoms are abdominal bloating, breast tenderness, and headaches. More than 100 symptoms of PMS have been reported in literature, many of which are shown in Table 9.1. A careful history should be taken to assess the cyclicity of symptoms and their adverse effect on the patient's work, school, family life, and interpersonal relationships. A prospective diary of at least 2 cycles is recommended, particularly for a diagnosis of the severe variant of PMS, PMDD.

Physical examination: There are no physical examination findings specific to PMS or PMDD.

Investigations

There are no standard laboratory tests for PMS or PMDD. Tests may be conducted to rule out other disorders, such as thyroid function tests if thyroid dysfunction is suspected, and FSH or LH levels if menopause or perimenopause is a differential diagnosis.

Diagnosis of PMS

One distressing symptom from a list of physical or behavioral symptoms is required for an ICD-10 (International statistical classification of diseases and related health problems—revision 10) diagnosis of PMS. Symptoms may include the following:

- Feeling sad, hopeless, or self-deprecating
- Tension, anxiety, mood liability, fearfulness, or persistent irritability
- Anger
- Decreased interest in usual activities
- Difficulty in concentrating
- Feeling fatigued
- Changes in appetite
- Hypersomnia or insomnia
- Feeling overwhelmed or out of control
- Other physical symptoms such as headaches, breast tenderness, or swelling, joint or muscle pain, bloating or weight gain.

Diagnosis of PMDD

DSM IV criteria for diagnosis of PMDD requires 5 of 11 symptoms during the leuteal

Table 9.1: Common premenstrual symptoms	
Psychological symptoms	*Somatic symptoms*
Irritability, labile mood or depressed mood, anger, oversensitivity, social withdrawal, insomnia, difficulty in concentrating, subjective memory difficulties, anxiety, subjective sense of feeling overwhelmed or out of control	Abdominal bloating, food craving, breast tenderness, headaches, fatigue, gastrointestinal upset, muscle stiffness, joint pain, generalized aches, appetite changes, acne, edema

phase. At least one symptom must be among the first four listed:

- Depressed mood
- Significant anxiety
- Affective lability
- Persistent anger or irritability
- Decreased interest in usual activities
- Concentration difficulty
- Lethargy
- Change in eating habits
- Insomnia or hypersomnia
- Sense of being overwhelmed
- Other physical symptoms such as headache, breast tenderness, bloating or weight gain.

The symptoms severely interfere with usual activities and relationship. Symptoms should not be associated with another psychiatric disorder. Evidence must be recorded in a diary for at least 2 symptomatic menstrual cycles.

Clinical pearl: PMS differs from other menstrual cycle symptoms because symptoms: (i) tend to increase in severity as the cycle progresses (ii) are relieved when menstrual flow begins or shortly after (iii) are present for at least two consecutive menstrual cycles

Treatment

The aim of treatment is to provide relief of symptoms during leuteal phase and to improve quality of life.

1. General measures
2. Pharmacotherapy

1. *General measures:* Non-pharmacologic therapy can be offered for patients with mild PMS. Treatment begins with adequate rest and sleep and regular exercise. Regular exercise may help alleviate bloating as well as irritability, anxiety, and insomnia. Dietary changes—increasing protein, decreasing sugar, and taking vitamin B complex (especially pyridoxine, a form of vitamin B_6) or Mg supplements—may help. Calcium supplementation 1200 mg in divided doses has been shown to reduce PMS. Fluid retention may be relieved by reducing Na

intake and taking a diuretic (e.g. hydrochloro-thiazide or spironolactone).

2. *Pharmacotherapy:* Two primary approaches are used when symptoms are not relieved by lifestyle modification only. (i) Hormonal manipulation to suppress fluctuation of hormonal level in leuteal phase (ii) Non hormonal pharmacotherapy to regulate neurotransmitters in brain

i. *Hormonal treatment:* For some women, hormonal treatment is effective. Options include:

1. Oral contraceptives
2. Progesterone by vaginal suppository (200 to 400 mg once/day)
3. An oral progestin (e.g. micronized proges-terone 100 mg at bedtime) for 10 to 12 days before menses
4. A long-acting progestin (e.g. Depot medroxy progesterone 150 mg IM every 3 mo)
5. Rarely, for very severe or refractory symptoms, a gonadotropin-releasing hormone agonist (e.g. Leuprolide depot 3.75 mg IM, goserelin 3.6 mg sc q mo) with low-dose estrogen/progestin (e.g. estradiol 0.5 mg once/day plus micronized progesterone 100 mg at bedtime) is given to minimize cyclic fluctuations. Spiro-nolactone, bromocriptine, and monoamine oxidase inhibitors are not useful.

ii. *Nonhormonal pharmacotherapy* to regulate neurotransmitters include selective serotonin reuptake inhibitor (SSRIs) and anxiolytics. SSRIs (e.g. fluoxetine 20 mg po once/day) may be used to reduce anxiety, irritability, and other emotional symptoms, particularly if stress cannot be avoided. SSRIs are effective in relieving symptoms of PMDD. Anxiolytics such as alprazolam may be indicated as second-line therapy for refractory behavioral symptoms.

Other therapies: Evening primrose oil is a popular self-treatment, but trials are of poor quality. NSAIDs such as Mefenamic acid are effective at relieving pain.

Clinical pearl: Good, level I evidence supports using calcium carbonate and selective serotonin reuptake inhibitors.

Less conclusive evidence suggests some relief with aerobic exercise, high-complex carbohydrate diets, stress reduction, spironolactone for swelling, magnesium, nonsteroidal anti-inflammatory drugs, hormone treatment, evening primrose oil, oral contraceptives, and vitamins B_6 and E.

Keywords: ICD 10—ICD-10 is the 10th revision of the International Statistical Classification of Diseases   and Related Health Problems (ICD), a medical classification list by the World Health Organization (WHO).

DSM: The Diagnostic and Statistical Manual of Mental Disorders (DSM), published by the American Psychiatric Association. It offers a common language and standard criteria for the classification of mental disorders.

EXERCISES

Answer the following questions

1. What is PMS?
2. When during menstrual cycle does PMS occur?
3. In which age group is it common?
4. Name the symptoms of PMS.
5. What are the criteria for diagnosis of PMS and PMDD?
6. How do you clinically evaluate PMS?
7. What is the treatment of PMS?

Write short notes on

1. Premenstrual symptoms
2. Premenstrual syndrome

Explain or justify the following statements

1. Presence of premenstrual symptoms is not adequate enough to diagnose premenstrual syndrome
2. PMDD is a subtype of severe form of PMS

Fill in the blanks with appropriate word/s

1. Three common premenstrual symptoms are _____ , _____ , and _____ .
2. Premenstrual syndrome typically occurs in _____ phase of menstruation.
3. Neurotransmitters that are involved for development of PMS are _____ and _____ .

Questions for practical (Read the case summary at the beginning of chapter before answering the questions)

1. Identify the premenstrual symptoms present in this patient.
2. Is she suffering from PMS or PMDD?
3. What are the treatment options for her?

Bibliography

1. Douglas A. Premenstrual syndrome. Evidence based treatment in family practice, Can Fam Physician 2002;48:1789–1797.
2. Kwan I, Onwude J. Premenstrual syndrome. Am *Physician.* 2008, Jan 1;77(1):82–84.
3. Marriam Z. Premenstrual syndrome—a review. Journal of Pharmaceutical Sciences and Research, 2012.
4. Pinkerton JV. Premenstrual Syndrome Merk Manual 2010

10

Primary Amenorrhea

A 16-year-old teenage girl has not started menstruation yet, while her elder has started her first period at age 13. Physical exam shows breast development at Tanner stage 2, external genitalia at Tanner stage 1. Examination shows no other abnormalities. How will you investigate this patient?

In this chapter we will learn:
- Definition of primary amenorrhea
- Causes of primary amenorrhea
- Diagnostic approach to a patient with primary amenorrhea
- Investigations
- Treatment

Definition

Primary amenorrhea is defined as absence of menstruation by 16 years of age in the presence of normal secondary sex character development or by 14 years of age where there is no visible secondary sex character development. Thus if a patient aged 15 years comes for consultation because she has not menstruated is not necessarily abnormal since the normal range of the age of menarche is 10–16 years. However, if the patient has no sign of secondary sexual development, this is abnormal and demands further investigation.

Fact sheet: Historical treatment of primary amenorrhea often consisted of ammonia injections into the vagina, as the intense pain was thought to stimulate normal menstrual cycles. Although not practiced today, this treatment frequently showed positive results.

CAUSES OF PRIMARY AMENORRHEA

We divide the causes of primary amenorrhea based upon development of secondary sex characters as secondary sex character is most evident to clinician and clinician can reach to a diagnosis from immediate examination of patient. However, we must remember that whichever way we classify causes of primary amenorrhea, there will be always an overlap of condition from one compartment to another.

A. *Secondary sexual development is good apart from amenorrhea* (Presence of breast development indicates production of estrogen at one point of time): The causes are:
   a. Anatomic defects of outflow tract
   b. Resistant ovary syndrome
   c. Androgen insensitivity syndrome

d. Some women with constitutional delay in puberty

Now let us further divide the causes—anatomic defects of outflow tract may be due to:

a. Imperforate hymen
b. Transverse vaginal septum
c. Müllerian agenesis: Agenesis of the vagina, cervix, or uterus

B. *If secondary sex character development is poor or absent* (absent breast development indicates lack of estrogen production), the causes can be
   a. Hypothalamic/pituitary abnormality (central)
   b. Gonadal or ovarian abnormality (peripheral)
   c. Constitutional delay in appearance of pubertal changes.

Let us further divide the causes:

- *Hypothalamic causes:* Kallmann syndrome, Anorexia nervosa, use of psychotropic medications
- *Pituitary causes:* Hyperprolactinemia, pituitary tumor, cranioparyngioma, empty sella syndrome, pituitary infarct, hemachromatoses, and sarcoidosis
- *Gonadal/ovarian abnormality:* Turner's syndrome, Mosaic turner, pure gonadal dysgenesis, mixed gonadal dysgenesis, ovarian failure

- *If secondary sexual development is heterosexual,* the diagnosis may be (production of estrogen and excess testosterone)
   a. Congenital adrenal hyperplasia
   b. Adrenal tumor
   c. Masculinizing ovarian tumor
   d. One of the forms of XY female
   e. Cushing's syndrome.

Clinical pearl: The common causes of primary amenorrhea seen in gynecological practice are (i) Constitutional delay in puberty, (ii) Turner syndrome and (iii) Müllerian agenesis

Diagnostic Approach to a Patient with Primary Amenorrhea

General considerations:

- Assessment of the adolescent patient requires a sensitive approach. Clinicians need to consider the young age and emotional maturity of the patient when examining the adolescent.
- History and physical examinations frequently direct the clinician towards a working diagnosis; however, ancillary studies are often necessary.
- An absence of any breast development or pubertal growth spurt by age 13–14 years in girls is distinctly abnormal and requires investigation.
- Breast development, pubertal growth spurt, and adrenarche are delayed or absent in girls with hypothalamic pituitary failure. In case of isolated ovarian failure, adrenarche occurs normally, while estrogen-dependent breast development and the pubertal growth spurt are absent or delayed.
- Most systemic disorders may be diagnosed with laboratory tests assessing neuro-endocrine and ovarian function, and the majority of structural abnormalities are identified through pelvic examination or imaging studies.

History

Complaint

- A history of cyclic pelvic pain in association with primary amenorrhea suggests the possibility of a congenital outflow tract abnormality such as imperforate hymen or agenesis of the vagina, cervix.
- Associated galactorrhea, headaches, or reduced peripheral vision could be a sign of intracranial tumor such as prolactinoma.
- An impaired sense of smell in association with primary amenorrhea and failure of normal pubertal development may be related to isolated gonadotropin deficiency,

as is observed in persons with Kallmann syndrome.

Medical History

- *Chronic systemic illness* may present with fatigue, malaise, anorexia, and weight loss.
- Dieting with excessive restriction of energy intake, especially fat restriction, may lead to amenorrhea and associated bone loss.

Family History

A history of familial delayed puberty, in addition to onset of menarche in the patient's mother and female siblings, should be elicited.

Past History

- History of a traumatic head injury or infection: A remote history may be elicited from the patient or parents.
- Prior history of chemotherapy or radiation therapy may be associated with ovarian failure.

Physical Examination

General Examination

- The patient's weight and height should be measured. Shortened height may suggest a chromosomal abnormality like Turner's syndrome.
- Assess overall nutritional status and general health and seek evidence for chronic disease or cachexia.
- Examine the skin for evidence of androgen excess, such as hirsutism and acne. Acanthosis nigricans may be present in association with androgen excess related to insulin resistance.
- Large pituitary tumors can cause visual-field defects by impinging on the optic tract.
- Assess the state of breast development by using Tanner stages. Also examine the breasts for galactorrhea.

- Associated anomalies such as webbed neck and cubitus valgus, and absent breast development will suggest Turner's syndrome.
- Examine for the presence of axillary and pubic hair. These are a marker of adrenal and ovarian androgen secretion. Pubic and axillary hairs are absent in androgen insensitivity syndrome.

Pelvic Examination

- Most structural anomalies are identified during pelvic examination. The hymen must be assessed first. A blind vaginal pouch (Fig. 10.1) will be noted in patients with Müllerian agenesis, transverse vaginal septum, or androgen insensitivity syndrome (the latter along with inguinal hernias). The uterine cervix should be noted on examination. Internal examinations are not always possible and the clinician may need to proceed with imaging options or an examination under anaesthesia.
- Measuring the clitoris is an effective method for determining the degree of androgen effect. The clitoral index can be determined by measuring the glans of clitoris in the anteroposterior and transverse diameter. A clitoral index greater than 35 mm^2 is evidence of increased androgen effect. A clitoral index greater than 100 mm^2 is evidence of virilization.

Investigations

All patients with primary amenorrhea, regardless of physical examination findings, should have preliminary laboratory studies which include FSH, oestradiol, TSH, and prolactin. Based on these results, other investigations are done:

- *Follicle-stimulating hormone* (FSH) along with oestradiol levels, help to determine if amenorrhea is due to gonadal failure, hypothalamic dysfunction, or systemic or functional causes. Low serum estradiol levels along with elevated FSH are suggestive of primary ovarian failure and low FSH suggests suppressed hypothalamic function.

- *Serum prolactin:* Elevated levels of circulating prolactin (hyperprolactinemia), whether idiopathic or due to a pituitary adenoma, result in hypogonadotrophic hypogonadism. For persistently elevated levels, neuroimaging is indicated to rule out intracranial neoplasm.

- *Thyroid-stimulating hormone (TSH)* is indicated to rule out (primary) hypothyroidism. Mild or sub-clinical hypothyroidism is unlikely to result in primary amenorrhea. It is proposed that elevated thyrotrophin-releasing hormone (TRH) stimulates prolactin secretion from the pituitary, suppressing FSH production.

- *Serum androgens:* Done for signs of hyperandrogenism. Levels such as dehydroepiandrosterone sulphate (DHEAS) and free testosterone will be elevated in patients with polycystic ovary syndrome, but might be significantly higher in patients with androgen-producing tumors.

Other Tests

- Pelvic ultrasonography may identify congenital abnormalities of the uterus, cervix, and vagina, or absence of these organs. However, a report of absence of uterus on ultrasonography does not always mean that the patient does not have a uterus. In primary amenorrhea in association with estrogen deficient states, the uterine fundus may be underdeveloped and may not be readily visible at the time of ultrasonography to less experienced examiners. Pelvic ultrasonography may be helpful in determining ovarian morphology as well.

- *Karyotype* helps to identify patients with androgen insensitivity syndrome, or gonadal dysgenesis.

- MRI is the most effective tool for characterizing specific structural abnormalities and may prevent the need for surgical diagnosis. On MRI, müllerian agenesis (Mayer-Rokitansky-Küster-Hauser syndrome) or asymmetrical fusion defects of the müllerian system (unicornuate uterus) can be identified as well as renal anomalies, which can occur in up to 30% of these patients.

- If prolactin levels are significantly elevated, cranial MRI is indicated to rule out pituitary adenoma.

SECONDARY SEXUAL DEVELOPMENT IS GOOD APART FROM AMENORRHEA

The conditions to be considered here are:

- Congenital and anatomical abnormalities (imperforate hymen, transverse vaginal septum, vaginal agenesis, uterine agenesis with vaginal dysgenesis, Mayer-Rokitansky-Küster-Hauser syndrome)
- Resistant ovary syndrome
- Androgen insensitivity syndrome

Congenital and Anatomical Abnormalities of Vagina and Uterus

When pubertal changes occur at the appropriate age and secondary sexual characteristics have developed normally but menses have not appeared, primary consideration should be given to the genital tract as the site of the problem. For unknown reasons, in some genetic females the müllerian ducts or the urogenital sinus do not develop or develop abnormally. In such girls, the external genitalia are normal, but the fallopian tubes, uterus, and upper third of the vagina are abnormal.

Cryptomenorrhea

Cryptomenorrhea also known as hematocolpos (collection of blood inside vagina), is a condition where menstruation occurs but menstrual blood does not come out due to an obstruction of the outflow tract. Specifically the endometrium is shed, but a congenital obstruction such as a vaginal septum or imperforated hymen or absence of vagina or cervix retains the menstrual flow. The patient usually presents at the age of puberty when the commencement of menstruation blood gets collected in the vagina and gives rise to cyclic abdominal pain.

Symptoms

Adolescent girls usually present with cyclic lower abdominal pain and primary amenorrhea. Patient may also present in emergency with acute retention of urine.

Signs

- *Abdominal examination:* A swelling is felt on palpation.
- *On vulval inspection:* A tense, bulging, bluish membrane is seen, this finding varies according to the thickness of the obstructing membrane. It may be absent in patients with complete or partial vaginal agenesis.
- On rectal examination: A large bulging mass is felt.

Complications

1. Hematometra (collection of blood in the uterine cavity)
2. Hematosalpinx (collection of blood in fallopian tubes)
3. Endometriosis

Treatment

Imperforate hymen is treated with cruciate incision over the bulging membrane and excising the margins of cut edges. The retained blood drains out over next few days. A thicker transverse vaginal septum can be treated with excision of transverse septum with re-anastomosis of upper and lower vagina. A blind vagina will require a partial or complete vaginoplasty. Hematosalpinx may require laparotomy or laparoscopy for removal and reconstruction of affected tube.

MAYER-ROKITANSKY-KÜSTER-HAUSER (MRKH) SYNDROME

This condition is caused by agenesis or partial agenesis of the müllerian duct system. It is characterized by congenital agenesis of the uterus and upper two-thirds of the vagina in women showing normal development of the secondary sexual characteristics and a normal 46, XX karyotype. There are two forms of MRKH. One is associated with the absence of just the vagina and uterus (Fig. 10.1), while the other affects additional parts of the body, too. Of those suffering from the latter form, 40% will have kidney abnormalities (15% of these individuals will be born with only one kidney), 10% will have hearing problems, and 10–12% will have skeletal abnormalities.

Diagnosis

1. Normal female appearance
2. Normal external genitalia (i.e. vulva)
3. Absence of vaginal canal
4. Absent or rudimentary uterus on per rectal examination
5. Normal functioning female ovaries evident from normal breast development

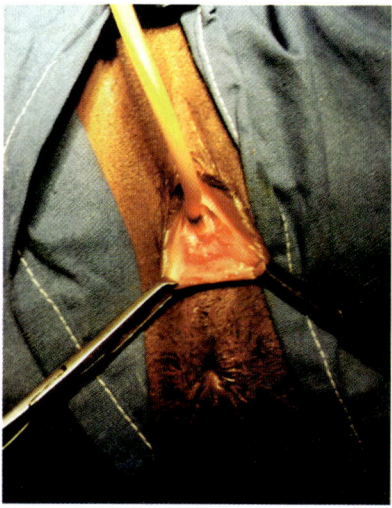

Fig. 10.1: Absence of vaginal canal in a case of MRKH syndrome

Investigations

1. Ultrasound pelvis and kidneys—absence of uterus with presence of ovaries
2. Chromosome analysis
3. IVU and X-ray spine

Treatment

The treatment is directed for capacity of sexual intercourse, and genital appearance by creation of neovagina. Menstrual function can not be achieved, however, with assisted reproductive techniques, women with Mayer-Rokitansky-Küster-Hauser syndrome can become pregnant by having oocytes harvested, fertilized, and implanted in a surrogate.

Treatment options for creation of vaginal canal (neovagina) are:

- *Frank technique or perineal dilation:* In this treatment, the patient presses a small dilator against the skin or the small vagina for 15–20 minutes a day. Progressively larger dilators are used to expand and lengthen the vagina.
- *McIndoe technique:* In this technique, using a blunt dissection, a space is created between the urethra and rectum (Fig. 10.2). After covering a cylindrical mould with the skin graft or amnion, is placed into the potential space.
- *Williams vaginoplasty:* Williams vaginoplasty uses a vulval flap to make a vaginal tube.
- *Intestinal neovagina:* This technique uses an isolated segment of bowel for vagina
- *Vecchietti technique:* This utilizes an acrylic olive shape apparatus that is applied under tension (via threads that are brought up through the abdominal wall via incision in the abdomen) against the vaginal dimple and thus exerts continuous progressive pressure through the potential neovaginal space and the abdominal wall.
- *Davydov procedure:* Utilizes the patients own peritoneum as the new vaginal canal.

Resistant Ovary Syndrome

It is also called Savage syndrome. It is due to a functional defect in the gonadotrophin receptors on the ovarian follicles and so the ovaries are resistant to endogenous FSH and exogenous gonadotrophin stimulation as well. The patient may present with primary or secondary amenorrhea. Diagnosis requires that the patient has a normal 46,XX karyotype, normal secondary sexual characteristics, elevated plasma FSH and LH—in the menopausal range—and that normal, multiple follicles are seen on ovarian biopsy.

Androgen Insensitivity Syndrome (AIS)

Androgen insensitivity syndrome occurs when patients are resistant to testosterone. These 46, XY women have been found to have mutations in their androgen receptor genes that render their androgen receptors nonfunctional. Despite normal testes development and normal male testosterone production, they are unable to convert the testosterone signal into the end organ events of masculinization of the external genitalia in utero or at puberty. At puberty, their androgens are converted to estrogens with normal breast development. It is an X linked

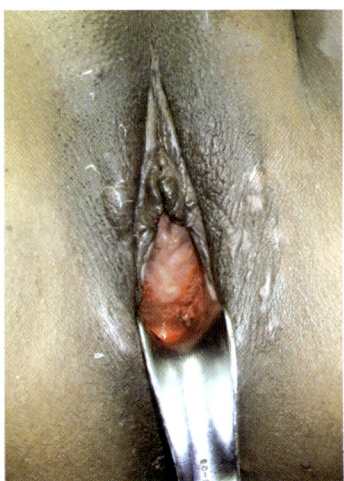

Fig. 10.2: Neovagina is created by McIndoe vaginoplasty of the same patient of Fig. 10.1

disease. Patients appear as phenotypically normal females. The testes, located internally and sometimes in the labia or inguinal area, do make müllerian-inhibiting hormone, so all müllerian structures, fallopian tubes, uterus, and upper third of the vagina are absent. The syndrome is divided into two main categories (i) Complete AIS and (ii) Incomplete AIS.

Clinical Features

A patient with complete AIS appears to be female but has no uterus with small blind vaginal pouch and has very little axillary and pubic hair. At puberty, female secondary sex characteristics (such as breasts) develop, but menstruation and fertility do not.

Persons with incomplete AIS may have both male and female physical characteristics. Many have partial closing of the outer vaginal lips, an enlarged clitoris, and a short vagina.

Investigations

Tests used to diagnose this condition may include:

1. Blood tests to check levels of testosterone, luteinizing hormone (LH), and follicle-stimulating hormone (FSH)
2. Karyotyping
3. Pelvic ultrasound

Treatment

Unusually located testicular tissue may not be removed until a child completes puberty and growth is complete. At this time, the testis may be removed because they can develop malignancy like any undescended testicle. Estrogen replacement is prescribed after puberty. Treatment and gender assignment can be a very complex issue, and must be individualized with great care.

SECONDARY SEXUAL DEVELOPMENT IS ABSENT/POOR APART FROM AMENORRHEA

The conditions to be considered here are:
1. Hypothalamic amenorrhea
2. Pituitary amenorrhea
3. Ovarian causes of amenorrhea
4. Constitutional delay in puberty.

Hypothalamic Amenorrhea

Hypothalamic dysfunction results in decreased or inhibited GnRH secretion, which affects the pulsatile release of LH and FSH.

A common cause of amenorrhea is functional hypothalamic amenorrhea. It is characterized by abnormal hypothalamic GnRH secretion, decreased gonadotropin pulsations, low or normal LH concentrations, absent LH surges, abnormal follicular development, and low serum estradiol. Serum FSH concentrations are usually in the normal range, with high FSH to LH ratio. This can be caused by eating disorders, exercise, or high levels of prolonged physical or mental stress. This can also include major psychiatric disorders such as depression.

Congenital GnRH deficiency leads to low gonadotropin levels. When this occurs with anosmia, it is diagnosed as Kallmann syndrome. Kallmann syndrome may be associated with midline facial defect, renal agenesis, and neurologic deficiency. Most often, it occurs as X-linked recessive disorder. Autosomal dominant and autosomal recessive inheritances are possible but less common.

Anorexia nervosa is a serious psychiatric disease with severe medical complications including primary amenorrhea (15%), osteopenia (52%), and osteoporosis (35%).

Functional causes of amenorrhea include severe chronic disease, rapid weight loss, malnutrition, depression or other psychiatric disorders, recreational drug abuse, and psychotropic drug use.

Pituitary Amenorrhea

A deficiency in FSH and LH may be a result of GnRH receptor gene mutations. Mutations in the FSH beta gene have been associated with amenorrhea. These women have low

FSH and estradiol levels and high LH levels. Primary amenorrhea caused by hyperprolactinemia is a rare condition characterized by the onset of thelarche and pubarche at appropriate ages but arrest of pubertal development before menarche. Hyperprolactinemia is associated with suppression of the GnRH from the hypothalamus and subsequent inhibition of LH and FSH, suppressed gonadal function and galactorrhea. Prolactinomas are the most common cause of persistent hyperprolactinemia, accounting for 40–50% of pituitary tumors.

Pituitary tumors may suppress gonadotropin secretion such as in Cushing disease or hypothalamic tumors, craniopharyngioma, or germinoma. Brain injury or cranial irradiation may also result in amenorrhea. Other pituitary causes include empty sella syndrome, pituitary infarct, hemachromatoses, and sarcoidosis.

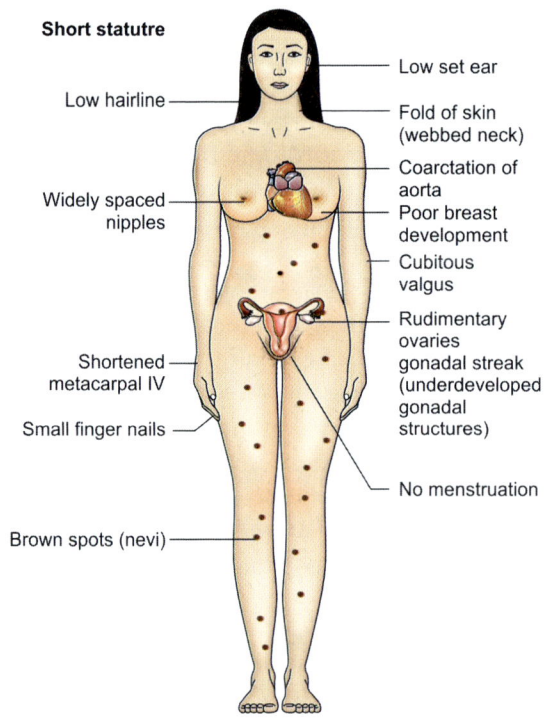

Short statutre

Low hairline

Widely spaced nipples

Shortened metacarpal IV

Small finger nails

Brown spots (nevi)

Low set ear

Fold of skin (webbed neck)

Coarctation of aorta

Poor breast development

Cubitous valgus

Rudimentary ovaries gonadal streak (underdeveloped gonadal structures)

No menstruation

Fig. 10.3: Clinical phenotypic findings in Turner's syndrome

Treatment

Treatment depends on its cause. Estrogen replacement therapy will stimulate maturation and development of the secondary sexual characteristics. When pregnancy is desired, ovulation can be induced by gonadotropin therapy or, in hyperprolactinemic states, by bromocriptine.

Ovarian Causes of Primary Amenorrhea

In many patients with primary amenorrhea, the cause is failure of gonadal differentiation or inappropriate gonadal function during early fetal and neonatal development. Gonadal dysgenesis most commonly occurs in Turner syndrome (45, X). The following are the clinical conditions in this category.

Turner's Syndrome (Gonadal dysgenesis)

Turner's syndrome encompasses several conditions of which monosomy X (absence of an entire sex chromosome) is most common. Other sex chromosome karyotypes that has been described are 45, X/46, XX and 45, X/ 46, XY.

Clinical Features

Approximately 95% of individuals with Turner's syndrome have both short stature and feature of ovarian failure upon clinical examination (Fig. 10.3).

Common features of Turner's syndrome include:

1. Short stature
2. Amenorrhea
3. Poor breast development
4. Broad chest (*shield chest*) and widely spaced nipples
5. Low hairline
6. Low-set ears
7. Rudimentary ovaries—gonadal streak (underdeveloped gonadal structures that later become fibrosed)
8. Increased weight, obesity
9. Shortened metacarpal IV

10. Webbed neck from cystic hygroma in infancy
11. Cubitous valgus
12. Coarctation of arorta
13. Bicuspid aortic valve
14. Horseshoe kidney
15. Nonverbal Learning Disability (problems with math, social skills and spatial relations)

Turner's syndrome manifests itself differently in each female affected by the condition, and no two individuals will share the same features.

Investigations

1. A standard Karyotype is required for diagnosis of Turner's syndrome, and will exclude mosaicism. Diagnosis is confirmed by the presence of a 45,X cell line or a cell line with deletion of the short arm of the X chromosome
2. Both LH and FSH are elevated and in menopausal range.
3. Because of the high prevalence of hypothyroidism in Turner's syndrome, obtain thyroid function tests at diagnosis.
4. At diagnosis, perform ultrasonography of the kidneys and renal collecting system.
5. Perform echocardiography of the heart and aorta.

Treatment

The treatment is directed towards increasing final height and induction of secondary sexual development and menarche. Growth hormone supplementation: Growth hormone supplementation should be started at the age of 4 or at the time of diagnosis of the disorder, whichever is earlier. It is now known that after 3–7 years of treatment, patients may be able to gain a height of about 8–10 cm. No side effects have been documented.

- **Estrogen therapy:** Estrogen is used to induce breast development and other features of puberty. Estrogen is usually started at age 12–15 years. Treatment can be started with continuous low-dose estrogens at 12 years. These can be cycled in a 3 weeks on, 1 week off regimen after 6–18 months; progestin can be added later. Patients should be maintained on estrogen-progesterone treatment to maintain their secondary sexual development and to protect their bones from osteoporosis until at least the usual age of menopause (50 years).
- Current assisted reproductive technology may allow women to become pregnant with donated oocytes.

Pure Gonadal Dysgenesis

This term is used to distinguish sexually immature girls who appear normal and who are taller than 150 cm from those with typical Turner's syndrome. It encompasses a more heterogeneous group of patients, with different etiologies implicated in ovarian failure. Many of these patients have a 46,XX or 46, XY karyotype. Patients with a normal chromosomal component tend to be tall, because the epiphyses stay open in the absence of ovarian steroids. The gonads are similar to the rudimentary streak gonad seen in Turner's syndrome. The distinction between the two is clinically important, because patients with pure gonadal dysgenesis have a higher incidence of presence of a Y chromosome. The syndrome also occurs more frequently in siblings than does classic Turner's syndrome.

XY Gonadal Dysgenesis (Swyer's Syndrome)

Affected persons have an XY chromosomal component, but phenotypically they are feminine, with normal female internal and external genitalia and streak ovaries. Because of the high frequency of malignant degeneration, persons with XY forms of gonadal dysgenesis should undergo prophylactic excision of the rudimentary gonads.

Mixed Gonadal Dysgenesis

This term refers to the rare anomaly of asymmetrical gonadal development, with a germ cell tumor or testis on one side and a streak or no gonad on the other side. Such persons usually are mosaics with X/XY karyotypes. They have anomalous external genitalia and exhibit virilization at or after puberty. The Y-containing gonad should be removed as soon as possible.

Constitutional Delay in Puberty

Puberty can be delayed in otherwise healthy girl. Constitutional delay of puberty refers to a common condition for which patients will go through puberty but at a time that is late from the normal time limit.

A number of these patients often have a family history of delayed puberty. Other causes of delayed puberty includes chronic systemic illness, e.g. chronic renal failure, malnutrition, prolonged high level of physical exertion, e.g. from being an athlete. A complete medical history, review of systems, growth pattern, and physical examination will reveal most of the systemic diseases and conditions capable of arresting development or delaying puberty.

Since bone maturation is a good indicator of overall physical maturation, an X-ray of the hand to assess bone age usually reveals whether the girl has reached a stage of physical maturation at which puberty should be occurring. Visible secondary sexual development usually begins when girls achieve a bone age of 10.5 to 11 years. Menstruation should start if the bone age is more than 14.5 years. Constitutional delay of growth and puberty is indistinguishable from that associated with hypothalamic or pituitary failure. Determination of the serum levels of TSH, T4, FSH, LH and prolactin is usually indicated, and a GnRH stimulation test will be useful. MRI scanning of the brain and pituitary gland is indicated if an abnormality of the hypothalamic-pituitary axis is suspected. Since not every adolescent with chromosomal abnormalities will have the classic clinical features, a chromosome analysis should be considered, especially in short girls with delayed puberty.

Treatment

If a girl is healthy, reassurance and prediction based on the bone age can be provided. No other intervention is usually necessary. In more extreme cases of delay, or cases where the delay is more extremely distressing to the adolescent girl, a low dose of estrogen for a few months may bring the first reassuring changes of normal puberty.

If the delay is due to systemic disease or undernutrition, the therapeutic intervention is likely to focus mainly on those conditions.

SECONDARY SEXUAL DEVELOPMENT IS HETEROSEXUAL

The conditions to be considered here are:
a. Congenital adrenal hyperplasia
b. Adrenal tumor
c. Masculinizing ovarian tumor
d. One of the forms of XY female
e. Cushing syndrome

Congenital adrenal hyperplasia (CAH): This condition usually presents at birth posing difficulty in gender allotment but if this does not happen, the problem may present at puberty with clitoral enlargement. It is an autosomal disorder results from enzyme deficiency in the synthesis of cortisol, most commonly being 21-hydroxylase deficiency. 21-hydroxylase deficiency leads to inadequate production of cortisol which in turn leads to excess production of ACTH. As a result there is increased production of cortisol precusur 17-hydroxy progesterone which gets converted to androgens. The elevated level of androgens results into varying degree of musculinization. The vagina is always present. Internal genitalia are normal. The labia may be fused or lower two-thirds of vagina are severely stenosed.

Clitoral enlargement during puberty may be the first sign of elevated androgen level in body. The clinician must look for androgenic tumors arising from ovary and adrenal gland. Estimation of 17-hydroxy progesterone and ACTH will help to diagnose CAH. MRI, CT scan, ultrasound can be judiciously used if androgenic tumors are suspected.

Treatment consists of administration of cortisol in appropriate doses in consultation of endocrinologist. Some reconstruction of external genitalia will be required such as clitoral reduction or division of fused labia.

Other causes: Incomplete androgen insensitivity syndrome (XY female) may present with female phenotype and genital ambiguity. Other possibilities which must be considered are presence or an ovarian masculinizing tumor, an adrenal adenoma or carcinoma or a pituitary lesion giving rise to the features of Cushing's syndrome.

Keywords

Mayer-Rokitansky-Küster-Hauser syndrome: This condition is characterized by müllerian agenesis resulting in absence of uterus and fallopian tubes and absence of upper portion of the vagina . It is the second most common cause of primary amenorrhea after gonadal failure (such as from Turner syndrome). The condition is named after August Franz Joseph Karl Mayer, Karl Freiherr von Rokitansky, Hermann Küster and G A Hauser.

Turner's syndrome: In 1938, Henry Turner first described Turner syndrome, which is one of the most common chromosomal abnormalities characterized by missing or incomplete X chromosome.

EXERCISES

1. Answer the following questions

- What is primary amenorrhea?
- How are the causes of primary amenorrhea categorized?
- Enumerate the causes of primary amenorrhea.
- What are the common causes of primary amenorrhea?

- What history should be covered when dealing with a case of primary amenorrhea?
- What are the important aspects of examination when you are dealing with a case of primary amenorrhea?
- What investigations are to be undertaken?
- How do you investigate and treat a girl with suspected müllerian agenesis?
- How do you investigate and treat a girl with suspected Turner's syndrome?
- How do you investigate and treat a case of constitutional delay in puberty?

2. Write short notes on

- Cryptomenorrhea
- Imperforate hymen
- MRKH syndrome
- Turner's syndrome
- Androgen insensitivity syndrome.

3. Explain or justify the following statement(s)

Cause of primary amenorrhea can be determined easily by clinical examination and few investigations.

4. Fill in the blanks

- Apart from müllerian anomaly, MRKH syndrome may be associated with _____, _____, _____ anomaly.
- In Turner syndrome, the karyotype is _____ .
- Resistant ovary syndrome is due to absence of _____ in ovarian follicle.
- Androgen insensitivity syndrome occurs due to _____ defect.

5. Questions for practical (Read the case summary at the beginning of chapter before answering the questions)

- What are the probable causes of amenorrhea in this girl?
- Name the investigations you consider for her.
- How she should be treated if she is diagnosed as a case of constitutional delay in puberty?

Bibliography

1. Bondel R, Foster MB, Dave K. Disorders of puberty Am Fam Physician. 1999 Jul 1;60(1):209–218.
2. Frank G Constitutional Delay of Growth and Puberty The Endocrinologist, Vol. 13, Number 4, August 2003, 341.
3. Master Hunter T, Heimal DL. Amenorrhea: Evaluation and Treatment Am Fam Physician 2006;73:1374–82, 1387.
4. Paul R. Gindoff Raphael Jewelewicz Amenorrhea Global Library of Medicine.
5. Reindollar RH, Davis J. A Abnormalities of Female Pubertal Development Endotext.
6. Sybert VP, McCauley E. Turner's Syndrome N Engl J Med 2004;351:1227–38.
7. Warne LG. Complete androgen insensitivity syndrome Department of Endocrinology and Diabetes Royal Children's Hospital Flemington Road Parkville, Victoria 3052, Australia 1997.

11

Secondary Amenorrhea

A 16-year-old girl presents for evaluation of amenorrhea. Her menarche was at the age of 12 years. Since she started running for exercise and sport at the age of 14 years, her menstrual periods have become lighter and less frequent. Her last menstrual period was 6 months ago. She has lost 2.5 kg over the past 3 months and reports a 2-week history of right foot pain. She typically runs 10 km per day, at least five times per week. On physical examination, her body-mass index is 19. How should her problem be evaluated and managed?

In this chapter we will learn:
- Definition of amenorrhea and secondary amenorrhea
- Pathophysiology of secondary amenorrhea
- Causes of secondary amenorrhea
- Diagnosis—Symptoms and Signs
- Investigations
- Approach to a patient with secondary amenorrhea
- Treatment

Introduction

Amenorrhea means absence of menstruation or suppression of menstruation. Amenorrhea is a symptom and not a disease and it has a variety of causes. Amenorrhea may be physiological, it may be primary (a patient who has never menstruated) or secondary (a patient who previously had normal menstrual function). A normal uterus with outflow tract and physiologically coordinated function of hypothalamopituitary ovarian axis is required for menstruation to occur. Any interruption in this relation will result in amenorrhea. Although many of the investigations of primary and secondary amenorrhea are similar, in most, probable diagnosis differ. Most congenital anomalies involving genetic aberrations and gross developmental anomalies of either the ovarian or müllerian structures present as primary amenorrhea. Secondary amenorrhea is more likely to result from acquired disease, is generally more amenable to treatment, and has a much better prognosis, at least for the restoration of fertility. The laboratory aspects of reproductive endocrinology have developed tremendously in last few years. Many of the sophisticated tests, however, are extremely expensive and do not add much of practical diagnostic value. It is therefore important to choose tests carefully, using only those essential for correct diagnosis and rational treatment.

> **Fact sheet:** The term, amenorrhea is derived from Greek: a = negative, men = month, rhoia = flow. Derived adjectives are **amenorrhoeal** and **amenorrhoeic**. The opposite is the normal menstrual period (eumenorrhea).

PHYSIOLOGICAL AMENORRHEA

Amenorrhea is normal before puberty, during pregnancy and lactation, and after the menopause. In any event, when amenorrhea is present in a woman of childbearing age, pregnancy must first be ruled out. In most cases, a routine pregnancy test in conjunction with a pelvic examination is sufficient to confirm or exclude pregnancy.

SECONDARY AMENORRHEA

Definition

Secondary amenorrhea is defined as the absence of menses for more than 3 cycle intervals, or 6 consecutive months, in a previously menstruating woman. It does not include physiological causes of amenorrhoea namely, pregnancy, lactation and menopause. The incidence of secondary amenorrhea is around 3% in the general population .

Pathophysiology

Regular and predictable menstrual cycles occur if the ovarian hormones estradiol and progesterone are secreted in an orderly fashion in response to stimulation by the hypothalamus and pituitary. Circulating estradiol stimulates growth of the endometrium. Progesterone, produced by the corpus luteum formed after ovulation, transforms proliferating endometrium into secretory endometrium. If pregnancy does not occur, this secretory endometrium breaks down and sheds during the ensuing menstrual period.

Amenorrhea occurs if the hypothalamus and pituitary fail to provide appropriate gonadotropin stimulation to the ovary, thereby resulting in inadequate production of estradiol and/or failure of ovulation and progesterone production. Amenorrhea can also occur if the ovaries fail to produce adequate amounts of estradiol despite normal and appropriate gonadotropin stimulation by the hypothalamus and pituitary. In some cases, the hypothalamus, pituitary, and ovaries all may be functioning normally, yet amenorrhea occurs because of uterine abnormalities such as adhesions in the endometrial cavity, or due to destruction of endometrium.

Causes

a. Uterine Causes

1. *Intrauterine adhesions (Asherman syndrome):* This results from acquired scarring of the endometrium, usually following procedures such as dilatation and excessive curettage for elective abortion or treatment of postpartum hemorrhage .This abnormality prevents the normal build up and shedding of the endometrium leading to scant or absent menses.

2. Endometrial destruction may be due to tuberculous endometritis, radiation.

b. Ovarian Causes

1. Premature ovarian failure or primary ovarian insufficiency
2. Polycystic ovary syndrome
3. Turner's syndrome—mosaic variety
4. Autoimmune oophoritis
5. Radiation or chemotherapy (iatrogenic premature ovarian failure)
6. Galactosemia
7. Androgen producing ovarian tumor.

c. Pituitary Causes

1. *Prolactinoma:* This is the most common pituitary etiology and accounts for almost

20% of cases of secondary amenorrhea. Elevated prolactin levels may suppress GnRH secretion, leading to low gonadotropin and low estradiol levels.

2. Other pituitary tumors (Cushing disease, acromegaly)
3. Postpartum pituitary necrosis (Sheehan's syndrome)
4. Autoimmune hypophysitis
5. Pituitary radiation
6. Neurosarcoidosis
7. Hemochromatosis
8. Pituitary apoplexy
9. Panhypopituitarism (secondary to trauma, after pituitary surgery or radiation, or idiopathic)

d. Hypothalamic Causes

1. Tumors such as craniopharyngioma or teratoma
2. Infiltrative disorder such as sarcoidosis, Langerhans cell histiocytosis, lymphoma

e. Functional Causes

1. Anorexia/bulimia
2. Extreme obesity
3. Chronic disease
4. Weight loss
5. Malnutrition
6. Depression or other psychiatric disorders
7. Recreational drug abuse
8. Psychotropic drug use
9. Prescription medications (opiates, antiepileptics)
10. Excessive exercise
11. Severe stress or severe illness
12. Idiopathic

Diagnosis

Symptoms

History of present illness

- History should include duration of amenorrhea, history of irregular menstrual cycle may be associated with conditions like polycystic ovary syndrome.

- Headache or visual field changes are suggestive of a central nervous system tumor.
- Chronic systemic illness may present with fatigue, malaise, anorexia, or weight loss.
- Symptoms of vaginal dryness, hot flashes, night sweats, or disordered sleep may be a sign of primary ovarian insufficiency or premature ovarian failure
- Galactorrhea suggests hyperprolactinaemia, which is commonly associated with secondary amenorrhea.

Past obstetric history

- A history of hemorrhage after childbirth can lead to failure of regular menses to return. This may be an indication of postpartum pituitary necrosis (Sheehan's syndrome). Failure of lactation is an even earlier sign. Detecting this condition early is important because of the possible development of associated central adrenal insufficiency, a potentially fatal condition.
- Postpartum endometritis, dilatation and curettage, or other intrauterine infection can result in Asherman's syndrome (obliterative endometrial process resulting in amenorrhea.

Personal history

Poor nutritional status due to systemic illness, an eating disorder, and/or low body fat may result in hypothalamic dysfunction. An inquiry into a patient's health status, eating habits, and body image is necessary. Emotional stress can also impair hypothalamic function, resulting in hypogonadotrophic hypogonadism. Extreme athleticism, especially with low BMI, may result in a similar phenomenon.

Past medical history

- A remote history of a traumatic head injury or infection may be elicited.
- A complete medication history is important. Oral contraceptives, long-acting progestogens, androgens, antipsychotic

medications, and chronic opioid use can induce amenorrhea. The type of medication may help to identify a treated disorder that is the cause of amenorrhea.

Signs

General examination

- The patient's weight and height should be measured. Low BMI may suggest an eating disorder or the athletic triad (amenorrhea, osteoporosis, eating disorders). BMI is generally > 30 in women with polycystic ovary syndrome.
- Skin examination may show acanthosis nigricans, acne, and hirsutism (polycystic ovary syndrome, *see* Chapter 12) or purple striae (Cushing's syndrome). Presence of male pattern baldness, deepening of voice, acne, hirsutism, cliteromegaly suggests hyperandrogenemia. These patterns may vary based on ancestry. If symptoms are slowly progressive, polycystic ovary syndrome or non-classic congenital adrenal hyperplasia is possible. If acute and progressive, the patient may suffer from an androgen-producing tumor (ovarian or adrenal).

Systemic Examination

- Large pituitary tumors can cause visual-field defects by giving pressure on the optic tract. In some cases, these visual-field defects can be detected by simple visual field testing.
- Examine the breasts for galactorrhea. In some cases, breast discharge can be expressed, yet the condition is not true galactorrhea. If the discharge is indeed milk, this can be confirmed by finding fat globules in the fluid using low-power microscopy.
- An abdominal examination may reveal unexpected findings that are indirectly related to the loss of menstrual regularity (e.g. discovery of hepatosplenomegaly,

which may lead to detection of a chronic systemic disease).

Pelvic Examination

- Measuring the clitoris is an effective method for determining the degree of androgen effect. The clitoral index can be determined by measuring the glans of the clitoris in the anteroposterior and transverse diameter. A clitoral index greater than 35 mm² is evidence of increased androgen effect. A clitoral index greater than 100 mm² is evidence of virilization.
- On speculum and bimanual exam thin and pale vaginal mucosa with absent rugae is evidence of estrogen deficiency The uterine cervix should be noted on examination. Ovarian enlargement may be found in cases of androgen producing ovarian tumors, autoimmune oophoritis, 17-hydroxylase deficiency, or 17, 20-desmolase deficiency.

Investigations

- *Urine for pregnancy test:* This is the first test performed in any patient of reproductive age presenting with secondary amenorrhoea.
- *Serum gonadotrophins (serum FSH and LH):* After ruling out pregnancy, this is the next test ordered. Measuring serum gonadotrophins (follicle stimulating hormone, luteinizing hormone) will help to distinguish between a hypothalamic-pituitary or primary ovarian cause of amenorrhea.

Low gonadotrophin concentrations indicate a hypothalamic cause for amenorrhea, which is often associated with stress or excessive exercise or weight loss with or without an eating disorder. In cases associated with weight change or excessive exercise, serum gonadotrophins may be normal, and a thorough history may give important clues.

Raised gonadotrophins concentrations indicate premature ovarian failure in a woman within the premenopausal age range. Follicle stimulating hormone concentration of > 30 IU/l (normal range 5–30 IU/l) in a woman under 40 with secondary amenorrhea indicates ovarian failure and affects 1% of women.

> **Clinical pearls**
> - Pregnancy needs to be excluded in women presenting with secondary amenorrhea
> - When gonadotrophins are of low value, the problem is at the higher centers (hypothalamus and pituitary) and when gnadotrophins are high, the problem is at the ovary/follicle (no estrogen = no negative feedback)

- Serum oestradiol: Low levels are suggestive of either primary ovarian failure (along with elevated FSH) or suppressed hypothalamic function (low FSH). Oestradiol concentration will be low or undetectable in cases of hypothalamic amenorrhea or premature ovarian failure and can be low in hyperprolactinemia. Assessment of endogenous oestradiol is not necessary for diagnosis, as levels can fluctuate significantly even in cases of premature ovarian failure, but oestradiol concentration is important in the management of amenorrhea. Oestrogen replacement to prevent long term hypoestrogenic complications and for control of symptoms should be considered. Oestradiol can also be low in the early follicular phase of a normal menstrual cycle.

A more accurate assessment of endogenous oestradiol concentrations is a progestogen challenge. If a vaginal bleed has not occurred after a short course of a progestogen this indicates either an uterine cause or that the patient is hypoestrogenic.

- *Serum prolactin:* Elevated levels of circulating prolactin (hyperprolactinaemia), whether idiopathic or due to a pituitary adenoma, result in hypogonadotrophic hypogonadism. For persistently elevated levels, neuroimaging is indicated to rule out intracranial neoplasm. Prolactin may be above normal (> 29 ngm/ml in a normal, non-pregnant woman) during stressful events, in primary hypothyroidism, and as a result of taking certain classes of drugs (phenothiazines, domperidone, metoclopramide). Mild or moderate hyperprolactinemia needs confirmation with a second specimen, and macroprolactinemia needs exclusion. Concentrations above 100 ngm/ml may indicate a prolactin secreting pituitary adenoma; such patients should be referred for further investigation and pituitary imaging.

- *Thyroid-stimulating hormone (TSH)* is indicated to rule out (primary) hypothyroidism. Mild or sub-clinical hypothyroidism probably will not result in menstrual irregularities. It is proposed that elevated thyrotrophin-releasing hormone (TRH) stimulates prolactin secretion from the pituitary, suppressing FSH production. Suppressed TSH suggests hyperthyroidism, which may cause oligomenorrhea.

- Serum androgens are measured for signs of hyperandrogenism. Levels of androgens such as dehydroepiandrosterone sulphate (DHEAS) and free testosterone will be elevated in patients with polycystic ovary syndrome, but might be significantly higher in patients with androgen-producing tumors.

- Transabdominal or transvaginal ultrasound confirms normal anatomy, and may obviate the need for progestogen challenge. Transvaginal is the preferred modality, if possible, to evaluate endometrial thickness.

- Progestogen challenge test has been traditionally used to evaluate a functional outflow tract that has been adequately primed by normal levels of circulating estrogen. A course of medroxyprogesterone acetate, 10 mg/day orally for 7 to 10 days, or an intramuscular injection of 100 mg progesterone in oil is given. Occurrence of bleeding within 2 weeks indicates activity along the HPO axis,

Table 11.1: Dosage schedule of progestogen and estrogen progestogen challenge test		
Drugs	*Dosing*	*Duration*
Progestogen challenge test		
Medroxy progesterone acetate	10 mg orally once per day	7–10 daya
Estrogen progestogen challenge test		
Estradiol valerate	2 mg orally daily	21 days
Followed by Medroxy progesterone acetate	10 mg orally once per day	Day 16–Day 25

estrogen production, a responsive endo-metrium, and a normal outflow tract. The diagnosis is probably anovulation. Patients who fail to bleed after progestin should be challenged with estrogens and progestin (Table 11.1). Failure to bleed after this maneuver suggests that the endometrium is unresponsive, and further studies should be undertaken to detect endometrial pathology (Asherman's syndrome or endometrial destruction). If withdrawal bleeding occurs, the uterus is normal and able to respond to the hormonal challenge, and the defect is along the HPO axis. Determination of gonadotropin and prolactin levels will help establish a diagnosis.

- If prolactin levels are significantly elevated, cranial MRI is indicated to rule out pituitary adenoma.
- Bone density measurement may be indicated in selected patients such as those with chronic hypo-oestrogenaemia.
- Asherman's syndrome may be diagnosed by transvaginal ultrasound (shows lack of a developed endometrial stripe); however, sonohysterography or hysterosalpingo-graphy are typical first tests used to assess the patient. Hysteroscopy remains the gold standard for diagnosis.
- A karyotyping helps to diagnose patients <30 years with premature ovarian failure.

Approach to Patient with Secondary Amenorrhea

The following simple strategy for investigating amenorrhea, which requires a limited number of tests and in most instances leads to a diagnosis, **is appropriate for patients whose initial examination is negative.** Figure 11.1 provides a diagram of the steps in this strategy.

Treatment

The treatment of secondary amenorrhea depends on the etiology as well as the desire of the patient, such as a desire to have regular menstruation, to become pregnant or to treat hirsutism.

Medical Treatment

- Dopamine agonists such as bromocriptine, cabergolin are effective in treating hyperprolactinemia. In most cases, this treatment restores normal ovarian endocrine function and ovulation.
- Hypothyroidism should be treated with thyroid replacement.
- Gonadotropin therapy or the use of pulsatile GnRH therapy may be required to induce ovulation in patients with infertility whose underlying pathology cannot be reversed.
- Estrogen replacement—In conditions leading to estrogen deficiency (premature ovarian failure/hypogonadotrophic hypo-gonadism), hormone replacement therapy is required to maintain bone density (*see* Chapter 31), and it may have other possible health benefits in patients whose underlying pathology cannot be reversed to restore normal endocrine function.
- Treatment of PCOS—Women with PCOS should be treated with combined oral

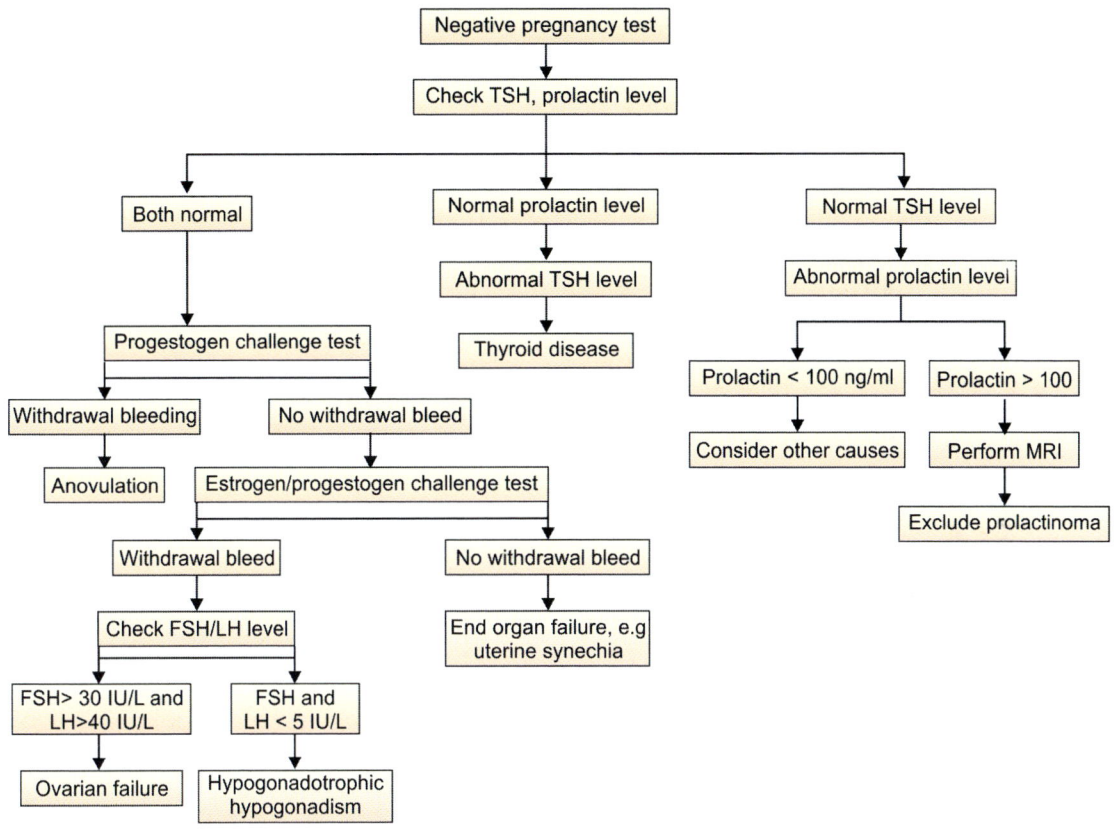

Fig. 11.1: Diagnostic scheme for evaluating secondary amenorrhea

contraceptive pills or cyclic progesterone therapy. Insulin sensitizing agents such as metformin is indicated in those with insulin resistance. Hyperandogenism due to PCOS may be treated with oral contraceptives and/or spironolactone (*see* Chapter 12).

- Women with late onset congenital adrenal hyperplasia may be treated with cortico-steroids to partially block ACTH stimulation of adrenal function and thereby decrease overproduction of adrenal androgen.

- *Contraceptive induced:* Stop contraception if this is what the patient wants. Discuss how long it will take for periods to return, and discuss other methods of contraception with them if they do not want to become pregnant.

Surgical Treatment

Some pituitary and hypothalamic tumors may require surgery and, in some cases, radiation therapy. Asherman syndrome requires hysteroscopic lysis of the intrauterine adhesions.

Consultations

In some complex cases referral to a specialist is required.

- *General medicine specialist:* In certain cases in which an underlying chronic disease process is present, the expertise of a physician may be needed.

- *Medical endocrinologist:* Referral to an endocrinologist is required in following situations—in cases of pituitary/hypothalamic tumor, central hypothyroidism, central adrenal insufficiency, in cases of hyperthyroidism or Cushing syndrome.

- *Geneticist:* With hereditary causes of secondary amenorrhea, such as galacto-semia, a geneticist's opinion can be helpful for the extended family and in counseling patients regarding the disorder.
- *Psychiatrist:* Cases of major depression, anorexia nervosa, bulimia nervosa, or other major psychiatric disorders require consultation with a psychiatrist.
- *Nutritionist:* In many cases, exercise-induced amenorrhea is due to an imbalance in energy intake and expenditure. Nutritional counseling to increase energy intake without reducing exercise is a means of reversing the underlying pathology. Women who are underweight or who appear to have nutritional deficiencies should receive nutritional counseling and can be referred to a multidisciplinary team specializing in eating disorders.

Diet

In some cases, nutritional deficiencies induced by dieting and exercise can cause amenorrhea even in the absence of a psychiatric disorder. Strict fat restriction often plays a role. Frequently, simply explaining the need to balance energy expenditure with energy intake resolves the problem. In this situation, nutritional counseling may be all that is required.

Activity

More than 8 hours of vigorous exercise a week may cause amenorrhea. As noted above, in some cases, this resolves with appropriate adjustment of the diet.

Clinical pearls
- The absence of menstruation for longer than six months in a woman with a previous regular menstrual cycle always requires a thorough history and further investigations

- The most common causes of secondary amenorrhoea encountered in routine practice are polycystic ovary syndrome, hypothalamic amenorrhoea, hyperpro-lactinaemia, and premature ovarian failure
- Initial evaluation of amenorrhoea—including history, physical examination and progestogen challenge test with few investigations —should identify the underlying defect in most cases
- Referral to secondary care should be considered in cases of secondary amenorrhoea where the diagnosis or management is not clear after initial investigation, as well as when the patient has concerns about fertility.

Keywords
Pure gonadal dysgenesis: A form of gonadal dysgenesis (underdeveloped and dysfunctioning ovaries) associated with female 46,XX genotype and female internal and external phenotype

Galactosemia is a rare metabolic disorder that affects galactose metabolism leading to accumulation of toxic levels of galactose 1 phosphate in various tissues. Classic galactosemia results in hepatosplenomegaly, cirrhosis, renal failure, cataracts, brain damage, and ovarian failure.

Autoimmune hypophysitis results from autoimmune destruction of pituitary gland resulting in below normal production of one or more pituitary hormones.

EXERCISES

Answer the following questions

1. What is amenorrhea?
2. What are the two types of amenorrhea?
3. How secondary amenorrhea differs from primary amenorrhea?
4. What is secondary amenorrhea?
5. What is most common cause of secondary amenorrhea?
6. What are the common causes of secondary amenorrhea?
7. What history should be covered when dealing with a case of secondary amenorrhea?
8. What are the important aspects of examination when you are dealing with a case of secondary amenorrhea?
9. What investigations are to be undertaken?

10. What is the procedure for progestogen challenge test?

11. What are the possible etiologic factors for lack of estrogen production?

12. What are the normal values of FSH?

13. What are the abnormal values of FSH and their significance?

14. How is secondary amenorrhea treated if fertility is not desired?

15. How is secondary amenorrhea treated if fertility is desired?

16. Is surgery indicated for treatment of secondary amenorrhea ?

Write short notes on

1. Uterine causes of secondary amenorrhea
2. Progestogen challenge test

Explain or justify the following statement

Pregnancy test is the initial investigation in women with secondary amenorrhea

Fill in the blanks

1. Physiological causes of amenorrhea are

_____ , _____ , _____ .

2. Skin examination in patient with secondary amenorrhea may reveal _____ , _____ , _____ .

3. Drugs used for hyperprolactinemia are

_____ , _____ .

4. More than _____ hours of vigorous exercise may lead to amenorrhea.

Questions for practical (read the case summary at the beginning of chapter before answering the questions)

1. What are the probable causes of amenorrhea in this patient?
2. How would you approach this patient to find out cause of amenorrhea?
3. How would you treat her?

Bibliography

1. Cheung J, Shaw RA. Case of secondary amenorrhea BMJ 2009;338:b2282.
2. Current evaluation of amenorrhea. The Practice Committee of the American Society of reproduc-tive Medicine Fertil Steril 2008:90; S 219–225.
3. Dickerson EH, Raghunath AS , Atkin SL. Initial investigation of amenorrhoea BMJ.
4. Disorders of menstruation by Paul B Marshburn, Bradley Hurst.
5. Gindoff PR , Jewelewicz R. Amenorrhea GLOWM
6. Master-Hunter T, Heiman DL. Amenorrhea – evaluation and treatment *Am Fam Physician.* 2006 Apr 15;73(8):1374–1382.
7. Popat V, Cowan BD. Secondary amenorrhea Medscape.

12

Polycystic Ovary Syndrome

An 18-year-old girl comes to genecology OPD with complaints of excessive facial hair growth for the past 3 years. The hair is worse on her chin, but is on other parts of her body as well (see Figs 12.1 to 12.3). She had menarche at age 13, and has irregular menses. Her last menstrual period was 3 months ago and lasted about 2 weeks. Her physical examination is unremarkable except acanthosis nigricans over nape of the neck (see Fig. 12.4). Her BMI is 28. What is your provisional diagnosis?

In this chapter we will learn:
• What is polycystic ovary syndrome and why it occurs
• Clinical presentation of PCOS
• Investigations and management of women with PCOS

Definition

It is a clinical syndrome characterized by mild obesity, irregular menses or amenorrhea, and signs of androgen excess (e.g., hirsutism, acne). Polycystic ovary syndrome occurs in 5 to 10% of women.

Pathophysiology

The precise mechanism by which polycystic ovary syndrome (PCOS) occurs has not been established. Some investigators explain it as primarily an intrinsic ovarian problem (excess ovarian production of androgens), others as adrenal (excess adrenal production of androgens), and again others as hypothalamic-pituitary dysfunction (exaggerated gonado-tropin releasing hormone pulsatility resulting in hypersecretion of luteinising hormone). Current studies suggest that excess androgen production may induce polycystic ovarian morphology and perpetuate the endocrine disruption of this disorder. Theca cell is the primary source for androgen production in this disorder. Increased androgen production may also contribute to inappropriate gonadotropin secretion in PCOS. In addition to increased LH secretion, the theca cell also exhibits increased responsiveness to LH stimulation. There is clear evidence to suggest a major role of insulin resistance and hyperinsulinemia in PCOS. As to whether insulin resistance constitutes a primary mechanism has yet to be established.

Symptoms and Signs

Symptoms typically begin during puberty and worsen with time. The typical symptoms are mild obesity, hirsutism, and irregular menses

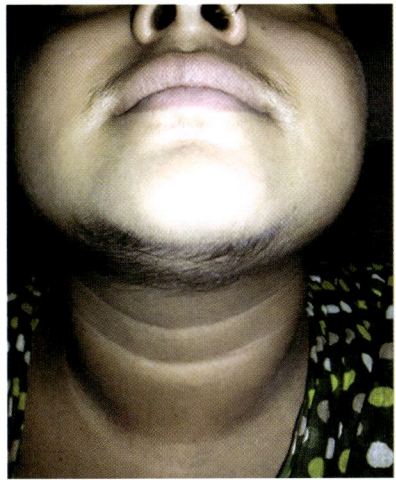

Fig. 12.1: Hairs over the chin and upper lips

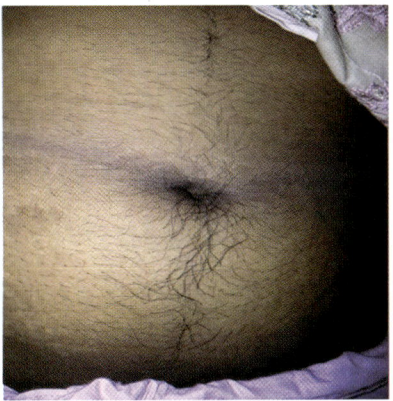

Fig. 12.2: Hairs on the abdomen

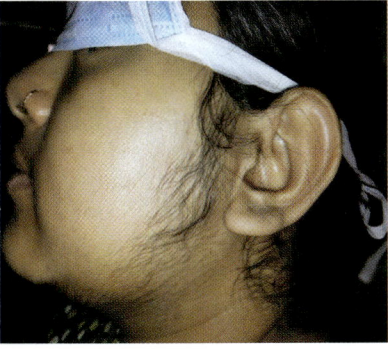

Fig. 12.3: Hairs over the side of face

or amenorrhea (Table 12.1). In most cases hirsutism occurs on the face and chin, although dark pigmented hair may occur over other regions such as the lower abdomen, chest, back, and extremities (Figs 12.1 to 12.3). Some women have other signs of virilization, such as acne and temporal balding. Areas of thickened, darkened skin (acanthosis nigricans) may appear in the axillae, on the nape of the neck, and in skin folds (Fig. 12.4); the cause is high insulin levels due to insulin resistance. When found in conjunction with hyperandrogenism, the condition is termed HAIR-AN (hyperandrogenic-insulin resistant-acanthosis nigricans) syndrome.

Diagnosis

The diagnosis requires at least 2 of the following 3 criteria (Table 12.2 for details) provided other causes for hyperandrogenism that mimic PCOS (e.g. congenital adrenal hyperplasia, Cushing syndrome, androgen secreting tumors) are excluded:

- Ovulatory dysfunction causing menstrual irregularity

Table 12.1: Clinical features that may be observed in women with PCOS

Reproductive
- Menstrual cycle disturbances resulting from anovulation (oligomenorrhea, amenorrhea, dysfunctional uterine bleeding)
- Obesity
- Infertility
- Hyperandogenisation (hirsutism or acne or androgen dependent alopecia)
- Acanthosis nigricans
- Recurrent spontaneous abortion
- Endometrial hyperplasia or cancer

Metabolic
- Impaired glucose intolerance
- Type 2 diabetes mellitus
- Gestational diabetes
- Dyslipidemia
- Cardiovascular disease

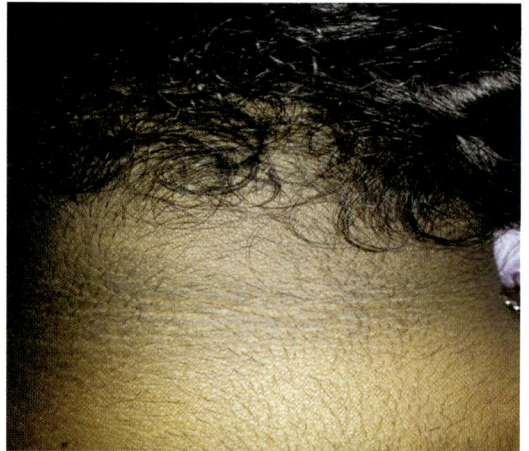

Fig. 12.4: Acanthosis nigricans (areas of thickened darkened skin) on back of neck

- Clinical or biochemical evidence of hyperandrogenism
- Polycystic ovaries on ultrasound, 12 or more follicles per ovary, usually occurring in the periphery and resembling a string of pearls.

Investigations

Tables 12.2 and 12.3 *outline* the general approach to standard investigations.

Which tests to perform in order to help confirm the diagnosis of PCOS and exclude other hyper androgenic disorders (congenital adrenal hyperplasia, Cushing syndrome and androgen secreting tumors) that mimic the

PCOS phenotype depends on clinical presentation and discretion of the clinician.

Clinical pearl: PCOS affects 5–10 % of reproductive aged women and is characterized by chronic anovulation, hyperandrogenism and polycystic ovaries.

Differential Diagnosis

Differential diagnosis of PCOS include:
1. Nonclassical CAH
2. Adrenal tumor, ovarian tumor, pituitary tumor, androgen secreting tumor
3. Cushing's disease or syndrome
4. Androgenic drugs
5. Hyperprolactinemia
6. Acromegaly

Treatment

PCOS is a chronic condition, there is no cure. Treatment depends upon clinical presentation of patient. Therapy is directed on either improvement of fertility or treatment of symptoms such as menstrual irregularities or hirsutism. In general following are treatment modalities:
1. Intermittent progestins or oral contraceptives for oligomenorrhea / amenorrhea
2. Infertility treatments in women who desire pregnancy
3. Management of hirsutism.

Table 12. 2: The Rotterdam Consensus Group criteria for the definition of PCOS

The diagnosis of PCOS requires at least two of the following three criteria:
1. Oligo-ovulation and/or anovulation
2. Clinical and/or biochemical signs of hyperandogenism. Clinical hyperandrogenism includes hirsutism, acne, or androgenic alopecia. Biochemical hyperandrogenism (or hyperandrogenaemia) includes a raised level of circulating androgens such as total testosterone, free testosterone or free androgen index (FAI), or dehydroepiandrosterone sulphate (DHEAS)
3. Polycystic ovaries on ultrasound (defined as the presence of 12 or more follicles in either ovary measuring 2–9 mm in diameter, and/or increased ovarian volume greater than 10 mL). If a follicle >10 mm in diameter is present, the scan should be repeated at a time of ovarian quiescence in order to calculate the ovarian volume other causes for hyperandrogenism that mimic PCOS (e.g. congenital adrenal hyperplasia, Cushing syndrome, androgen secreting tumors) should be excluded

Table 12. 3: Suggested routine testing for PCOS

- Pelvic ultrasound (preferably transvaginal for best imaging)
  i. Endometrial thickness (to exclude endometrial pathology including endometrial hyperplasia)
  ii. Ovaries (presence of polycystic ovaries, exclude ovarian androgen producing tumors)
- Urinary pregnancy test if amenorrhea (exclude pregnancy, the commonest cause of secondary amenorrhea)
- Hormone assays (time for days 2–5 of cycle if oligomenorrhea)
  1. FSH, LH (LH:FSH ratio 3:1), E2 ($\uparrow$) (raised LH in up to 50% of patients, exclude other causes of anovulation such as hypogonadotropic hypogonadism or premature ovarian failure)
  2. Thyroid function tests (exclude hypothyroidism, another cause of anovulation)
  3. Prolactin (exclude hyperprolactinaemia, another cause of anovulation, with the caveat that some PCOS patients may have prolactin levels slightly above normal)
  4. 17 α hydroxyprogesterone (exclude congenital adrenal hyperplasia)
  5. Androgens (DHEAS[a], total testosterone ($\uparrow$), SHBG[b] ($\downarrow$) FAI[c] to possibly help confirm PCOS and exclude androgen producing tumours)
- Metabolic screening
  1. 2 hour 75 g OGTT if BMI > 28 kg/m^2 (exclude IGT and type 2 diabetes mellitus)
  2. Fasting lipids (exclude dyslipidemia such as total cholesterol, LDL cholesterol, triglycerides, HDL cholesterol)

[a]dehydroepiandrosterone sulphate, [b]sex hormone binding globulin, [c]free androgen index

i. Presenting with Menstrual Irregularities-Oligomenorrhea/Amenorrhea Alone

- These women are anovulatory and chronic anovulation may lead to dysfunctional bleeding, endometrial hyperplasia and endometrial cancer. Therefore, treatments that induce ovulation (e.g., weight loss or metformin) or provide progesterone exposure (oral contraceptive pills or cyclic progesterone) should be given to these women.
- Weight loss is the preferred treatment for overweight or obese women. Oral contraceptive pills or metformin is used if ineffective or if weight is normal. Cyclic progestin is used in refractory cases (Table 12.4).

ii. Presenting with Infertility where Fertility is Desired

- The first-line and safest measure to restore ovulation is weight loss (in overweight or obese patients). Weight loss alone (even as little as 5 to 7%) may restore ovulation in up to 80% of overweight or obese patients (possibly by reducing hyperinsulinemia and thus hyperandrogenism).

- If weight loss is unsuccessful, metformin may be added. Metformin can restore ovulation/menses to the point where conception is possible. However, 6 to 9 months may be needed for the full effect.
- If these measures do not result in pregnancy, clomiphene should be given in Table 12.4. It is first line if weight is normal.
- If these measures fail, injectable treatments such as gonadotropins should be given.
- In the most difficult cases, in vitro fertilization or laparoscopic ovarian drilling is performed. In clomiphene-resistant women with PCOS, laparoscopic ovarian drilling results in ovulation and pregnancy in most women.

iii. Presenting with Hirsutism or Hyperandrogenic Features Alone (Not desirous of fertility)

- Weight loss should be encouraged, but is less efficacious for androgenic symptoms.
- At any stage of therapy for hirsutism, mechanical or local hair removal is a useful adjunct to remove hairs that do not respond

to medical therapy. There are many nonpharmacologic treatment options, including electrolysis, waxing, bleaching, plucking, depilatory creams (a form of hair removal that dissolves the hair), thermolysis (use of heat), and laser therapy. Topical eflornithine cream ameliorates hirsutism in many patients.

- If hyperandrogenic symptoms are mild, an antiandrogen or oral contraceptive pill as monotherapy may be efficacious as initial treatment. If monotherapy is to be used, the decision is tailored to the patient's needs, with a particular focus on adverse effects.

- Antiandrogens are indicated if hirsutism is significant. Antiandrogens are androgen receptor blockers (spironolactone, cypro-terone, flutamide) or 5α reductase inhibitors (finasteride). Antiandrogens should be used for at least 6 months before judging efficacy. The maximal effect on hirsutism may take 9 to 12 months (compared with the effect on acne, which usually responds within 2 months). Acne is more responsive to therapy while alopecia is less responsive. Adding metformin might improve results to monotherapy or dual therapy.

Clinical pearls
- The Rotterdam Consensus Group recommend that PCOS be defined when at least two of the following features are present (after exclusion of other etiologies): oligo- or an-ovulation, clinical and/or biochemical hyperandrogenism, or polycystic ovaries.
- Women with PCOS are at increased risk of developing impaired glucose in tolerance, type 2 diabetes mellitus and possibly CVD.
- Lifestyle intervention with attention to diet and exercise is first line treatment in overweight or glucose intolerant women with PCOS.

Keywords
Stein Leventhal Syndrome—Stein, Irving Freiler (1887-1976), and Leventhal, Michael Leo (1901-1971), American gynecologists. Stein and Leventhal published the first description of polycystic ovary syndrome in 1935.PCOS is also known as Stein Leventhal Syndrome . Hirsutism—is the excessive hairiness on women in those parts of the body where terminal hair does not normally occur or is minimal—for example, a beard or chest hair. It refers to a male pattern of body hair (androgenic hair) Virilization—the presence of male secondary sexual characteristics in a female.
Free androgen index (FAI) is a ratio used to determine abnormal androgen status. The ratio is the total testosterone level divided by the sex hormone binding globulin (SHBG) level, and then multiplying by a constant, usually 100. FAI has no units. FAI = Total testosterone/SHBG × 100

Table 12.4: Medical treatment options in PCOS

Drugs	Dosage	Benefits
Oral contraceptives	21 day/month	Restore menstrual cyclicity Suppression of hyperandrogenism Prevent endometrial hyperplasia
Medroxy progesterone acetate	10 mg daily for 10 days	Restore menstrual cyclicity
Micronised progesterone	400 mg daily for 10 days	Restore menstrual cyclicity
Spironolactone	50–200 mg daily	Suppression of hyperandrogenism
Metformin	500–850 mg three times daily	Restore menstrual cyclicity Suppression of hyperandrogenism, facilitate ovulation, facilitate weight loss, reduce hyperinsulinemia
Clomiphene citrate	50–150 mg for five days	Facilitate ovulation, restore menstrual cyclicity, prevent endometrial hyperplasia

EXERCISES

Answer the following questions

1. What is polycystic ovary syndrome?
2. How many women have polycystic ovary syndrome?
3. What causes PCOS?
4. What are the differential diagnoses of PCOS?
5. What investigations should be undertaken to confirm diagnosis?
6. Are there any long term consequences of PCOS?
7. Outline the treatment of PCOS.

Write short notes on

1. Diagnosis of PCOS
2. Medical treatment in PCOS

Explain or justify the following statements

1. Weight reduction is first line treatment in obese PCOS
2. Treatment of PCOS depends upon clinical presentation

Fill in the blanks with appropriate word/s

1. Typical symptoms/signs of PCOS are _____ , _____ , _____ .
2. Metabolic features that may be present in PCOS are _____ and _____ .
3. In PCOS , LH level is _____ and SHBG level is _____ .

Questions for practical (read the case summary at the beginning of the topic before answering the questions)

1. What is your diagnosis?
2. What are the points favour of your diagnosis?
3. What is hirsutism?
4. Why she is having irregular menstruation?
4. What are the differential diagnoses?
5. How do you investigate her?
6. How do you treat her?

Bibliography

1. Aziz R, et al. POSITION STATEMENT: Criteria for Defining Polycystic Ovary Syndrome as a Predominantly Hyperandrogenic Syndrome: An Androgen Excess Society Guideline. The Journal of Clinical Endocrinology and Metabolism 91(11):4237–4245.
2. Balen AH, et al. Ultrasound assessment of the polycystic ovary: international consensus definitions. Human Reproduction Update, Vol.9, No.6 pp. 505±514, 2003.
3. Chang R, Kazer R. Polycystic ovary syndrome Glob. libr. women's med., (ISSN: 1756-2228) 2009; DOI 10.3843/GLOWM.10301
4. Chizen Dr. What says it's Polycystic ovarian syndrome? The Canadian Journal of Diagnosis/ September 2003; 77–83.
5. Costello MF. Polycystic ovary syndrome—a management update Australian Family Physician Vol. 34, No. 3, March 2005.
6. Glunz C. Polycystic ovarian syndrome.
7. Radosh L. Drug treatment in polycystic ovary syndrome Am Fam Physician. 2009;79(8):671–676.
8. Richardson MR. Current perspective in polycystic ovary syndrome Am Fam Physician 2003;68:697–704.
9. The Rotterdam ESHRE/ASRM-sponsored PCOS consensus workshop group. Revised 2003 consensus on diagnostic criteria and long term health risks related to polycystic ovary syndrome (PCOS). Hum Reprod 2004;19:41–7.
10. Zack P, Stephen E. Transcript of learning module Polycystic ovary syndrome: diagnosis and treatment Available online at http://learning. bmj.com/learning/search—?result.html? moduleId=10022955.

13

Reproductive Tract Infections

A 22-year-old sexually active woman presents with low-grade fever and non-specific lower abdominal pain. Examination reveals mild diffuse lower abdominal tenderness on deep palpation. She has cervical motion tenderness and a mucopurulent vaginal discharge on pelvic examination. How do you manage this patient?

In this chapter we will learn:
- Types of reproductive tract infections (RTI)
- Sites of RTI
- Endogenous infections of reproductive tract
- Iatrogenic infections of reproductive tract
- Sexually transmitted infections
- Syndromic management of sexually transmitted infections
- Pelvic inflammatory disease (PID)
- Specific sexually transmitted infections
- Prevention of RTI

Introduction

Reproductive tract infections (RTIs) refer to infection of female genital organs which include **vulva, vagina, cervix (lower genital tract) and uterus, fallopian tubes, ovaries (upper genital tract).** They can have serious consequences like infertility, ectopic pregnancy, chronic pelvic pain, abortion and increased risk of HIV. The morbidity associated with RTIs affects the quality of life of many individual women and consequently, of whole communities.

Fact sheet 1: The World Health Organization estimates that in each year there is over 333 million of new cases of curable sexually transmitted infections. 75–85% of these new cases because of the four main curable STIs (gonorrhea, chlamydial infection, syphilis and trichomoniasis) occur every year in developing countries.

TYPES OF INFECTION

Reproductive tract infections (RTIs) refer to three different types of infection which affect the reproductive tract:

1. *Endogenous infections* result from an overgrowth of organisms normally present in the vagina. Endogenous infections include bacterial vaginosis and candidiasis.

These infections can be easily treated and cured. They are probably the most common RTIs worldwide.

2. *Iatrogenic infections* occur when the cause of infection (a bacterium or other micro-organism) is introduced into the reproductive tract through a medical procedure such as menstrual regulation, induced abortion, the insertion of an IUD or during childbirth. This can happen if surgical instruments used during the procedure have not been properly sterilized, or if an infection that was already present in the lower reproductive tract is pushed through the cervix into the upper reproductive tract.

3. *Sexually transmitted infections (STIs)* are caused by viruses, bacteria, or parasitic microorganisms that are transmitted through sexual activity with an infected partner. About 30 different sexually transmitted infections have been identified, some of which are easily treatable, many of which are not. HIV is perhaps the most serious sexually transmitted infection as it eventually leads to death. STIs affect both men and women, and can also be transmitted from mothers to children during pregnancy and childbirth.

SITES OF REPRODUCTIVE TRACT INFECTIONS

Infections in the area of the vulva, vagina, or cervix are referred to as *lower* **reproductive tract infections.** Infections in the uterus, fallopian tubes, and ovaries are considered *upper* **reproductive tract infections** (Fig. 13.1).

An RTI which affects the external genital area and lower reproductive tract in women is frequently referred to as vulvovaginitis, or simply vaginitis, indicating that the vulva and/or vagina become inflamed and sometimes itchy or painful. Infection of the cervix (cervicitis) can be caused by a variety of pathogens, particularly sexually trans-mitted infections such as gonorrhea and chlamydia.

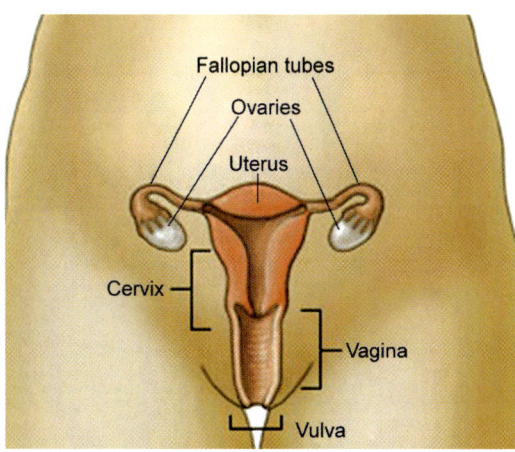

Fig. 13.1: Reproductive tract of woman

The migration of infections into the upper reproductive tract, including the uterus, fallopian tubes, and ovaries tends to be considerably more severe than infections in the lower reproductive tract. Upper reproductive tract infections are often a direct complication of lower reproductive tract infections, particularly sexually transmitted ones. Pelvic inflammatory disease (upper reproductive tract infection) for example, is one of the most serious consequences of gonorrhea or chlamydia.

ENDOGENOUS INFECTION OF THE REPRODUCTIVE TRACT

Endogenous reproductive tract infections result of overgrowth of organisms normally present in the vagina. When the normal balance of vaginal flora is disturbed, an overgrowth of organisms can occur. Candidiasis and bacterial vaginosis are the most common resulting infections. However, many studies show that even experienced clinicians cannot reliably distinguish between vaginal discharge caused by sexually transmitted or endogenous infections.

Candidiasis

Candidiasis (referred to as thrush, or a yeast infection) is caused by the fungus Candida.

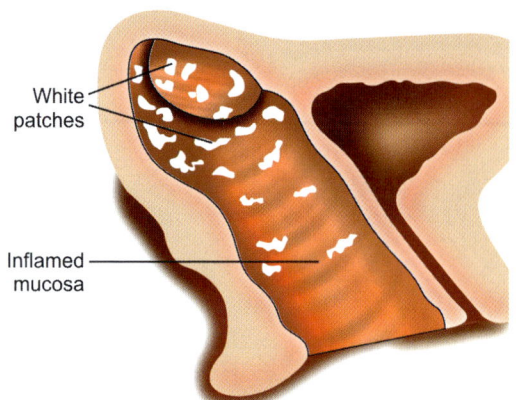

White patches

Inflamed mucosa

Fig. 13.2: Candida infection of vagina

This fungus is normally present in the mouth, gut and vagina, as are a number of other organisms. If the balance of microorganisms is disrupted, an overgrowth of fungus can occur. Some women appear to be naturally more prone to developing this type of infection for reasons that are not well understood. In addition, **recent use of antibiotics, oral contraceptives** that contain progesterone, or the presence of other conditions such as **diabetes, pregnancy, or immune suppression** (such as that caused by HIV) can also increase a woman's chances of developing candidiasis.

Symptoms

1. White, thick, curd-like discharge
2. Itching, soreness of the vulva and vaginal area (vaginitis)
3. Painful intercourse

Signs

1. White thick, curd-like discharge
2. Redness of vulva, vaginal, and cervical tissue.

Investigations

The diagnosis can be confirmed with any of the following tests:

1. A wet mount preparation (saline, 10% KOH) or Gram stain of vaginal discharge demonstrates yeasts, hyphae, or pseudo-hyphae (*see* Chapter 14 on vaginal discharge) or
2. A culture that yields a yeast species.

Treatment

Vaginal candidiasis is treated with antifungal medications. Several are available in the form of creams, suppositories and tablets that can be placed directly in the vagina.

Some Commonly Used Agents

Vaginal application

1. *Clotrimazole*

   1% cream 5 g in the vagina for 7–14 days, given twice a day, in the morning and evening

   100 mg vaginal tablet at night before sleep for 7 days

   Clotrimazole 100 mg vaginal tablet, two tablets (at bedtime) for 3 days

2. *Miconazole*

   2% cream 5 g in the vagina for 7 days

   100 mg vagina suppository, one suppository for 7 days

   200 mg vagina suppository, one suppository for 3 days

   1,200 mg vagina suppository, one suppository for 1 day

Oral Agent

Fluconazole 150 mg oral tablet, one tablet in single dose.

BACTERIAL VAGINOSIS

Bacterial vaginosis (BV) arises from an imbalance in the normal vaginal flora, and is not due to a single organism. The condition results in a loss of lactobacilli and increases the vaginal pH. This results in an increase in concentration of other organisms, especially anaerobic gram-negative rods. The major bacteria detected are *Gardnerella vaginalis*, Prevotella species, Porphyromonas species,

Bacteroides species, Peptostreptococcus species, *Mycoplasma hominis, Ureaplasma urealyticum,* and Mobiluncus species. The rise in pH also facilitates adherence of G. vaginalis to the exfoliating epithelial cells, thereby creating the "clue cells" that are diagnostic of the disorder (*see* Table 13.1). Thus, clue cells are vaginal epithelial cells studded with adherent coccobacilli that are best appreciated at the edge of the cell. Bacterial vaginosis is found more commonly among sexually active women although it is not clearly sexually transmitted and the treatment of male partners does not reduce recurrence (Fig. 13.3).

Diagnosis

Approximately 50 to 75 percent of women with BV are asymptomatic. Those with symptoms present with an **unpleasant, "fishy smelling" discharge** that is more noticeable after coitus. The discharge is **off-white, thin, and homogeneous.**

Dysuria and dyspareunia are rare, while pruritus, erythema, and vaginal inflammation (erythema, edema) are typically absent. BV can be associated with cervicitis (endocervical mucopurulent discharge or easily induced bleeding), with or without concomitant chlamydial or gonococcal infection. Because bacterial vaginosis is an imbalance in the proportion of bacteria normally present in the vagina, diagnosis is made on the basis of a set of criteria, rather than detection of a specific causal organism. Most typically, the Amsel criteria (listed in Table 13.1) are used.

Table 13.1: Amsel diagnostic criteria for bacterial vaginosis

A positive diagnosis is made if 3 of the following 4 criteria are present:
- Speculum examination reveals homogeneous discharge
- "Clue cells" are found on microscopy (> 20%)
- Vaginal pH > 4.5
- A "fishy" odor is produced when 10% Potassium Hydroxide is added to vaginal secretions

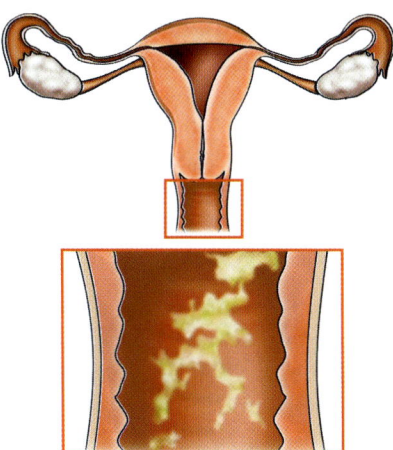

Bacterial vaginosis

Fig. 13.3: Homogenous discharge in bacterial vaginosis

Prevention

Vaginal douching should be avoided, as it can dry or cause imbalance in the vaginal environment and, hence, lead to bacterial vaginosis. The use of "drying" or "tightening" products can also cause imbalance and other harm.

Complications

In most cases, **BV causes no complications.** But there are some serious risks from BV including:

1. Increased chance of HIV infection.
2. Increased chance of complication during pregnancy such as preterm delivery.
3. Increased risk of developing an infection following surgical procedure such as hysterectomy.
4. Increased susceptibility to other STI such as herpes simplex virus, Chlamydia and gonorrhea.

Treatment

Two different antibiotics are recommended as treatment for BV: metronidazole or clindamycin. Oral medication may be more convenient, but causes more side effects.

Metronidazole: Metronidazole vaginal gel is one of the most effective treatments; it is applied inside the vagina at bedtime for five days. Metronidazole can also be taken in tablet form, 400 mg twice daily for seven days. The choice of pill versus vaginal gel depends upon the woman's preference. In general, there are fewer side effects with the vaginal treatment.

Clindamycin: Clindamycin is a cream that is inserted into the vagina at bedtime for seven days. A three day vaginal ovule are also available. Clindamycin cream should not be used with latex condoms due to the risk of condom breakage. Clindamycin can also be taken by mouth, 300 mg twice daily for seven days.

Sexual partners: It is not necessary to treat the sexual partner of a woman with BV. Treating the sexual partner does not improve the woman's symptoms or decrease the risk of the infection coming back.

Relapse and recurrent infection: Approximately 30 percent of women who initially improve after treatment have a recurrence of BV symptoms within three months, and more than 50 percent have a recurrence of symptoms within 12 months. It is not clear why this occurs, although it may be related to bacteria that were not completely treated or lack of a normal level of protective lactobacilli.

IATROGENIC INFECTION OF REPRODUCTIVE TRACT

Iatrogenic reproductive tract infections are a result of bacteria being introduced into the normally sterile environment of the upper reproductive tract through a medical procedure, such as the insertion of an IUD, an induced abortion, or during delivery. The causal bacteria originate either from improperly sterilized examination or medical instruments (such as vaginal specula) or from endogenous or sexually transmitted infections already present in the lower reproductive tract.

Why are they important: Because iatrogenic infections may affect the upper reproductive tract of women, they can result in extremely serious consequences. The uterus, endometrium, fallopian tubes, and ovaries can all be involved. Pelvic inflammatory disease (PID) may develop and cause severe abdominal pain, pelvic abscess, menstrual disturbances, ectopic pregnancy, spontaneous abortion, premature birth, and infertility.

Diagnosis and treatment: Many different bacteria can cause iatrogenic infection. Almost any infection already present in a woman's lower reproductive tract as well as sexually transmitted cervical infections, such as gonorrhea or chlamydia, can cause serious conditions when pushed into the sterile environment of the uterus. Bacteria on medical instruments can also introduce infection.

Depending on the specific nature of the condition, iatrogenic infections can often be treated successfully with antibiotics if they are diagnosed quickly. Unfortunately, many such infections receive attention only after they have caused irreparable damage, such as scarring or blockage of the fallopian tubes, or tissue damage. If a woman has recently undergone a transcervical procedure, the following symptoms may indicate the presence of an iatrogenic infection (Table 13.2).

Unsafe abortion: Although a variety of medical procedures can lead to the development of iatrogenic infections, unsafe abortion poses a particularly common risk. The vast majority of unsafe abortions take place in the developing world, and complications occur after 10–50% of them. Unsafe abortions are often sought if abortion is illegal, safe procedures are difficult to access or afford, or the woman is ashamed to seek care because she is young, unmarried, or the victim of sexual assault or oppression.

Table 13.2: Warning symptoms following gynecological procedures

- Pain in the pelvic region
- Sudden high fever
- Chills
- Menstrual disturbances
- Unusual vaginal discharge
- Pain during intercourse

Prevention of Iatrogenic Infections

- Minimizing the frequency and consequences of iatrogenic infections depends on improving the quality and accessibility of good medical services. Unlike STIs, which rely primarily on behavior change for their prevention, avoiding iatrogenic infections centers on maximizing access to good quality care, and in particular the technical competence of health care providers. It also requires resources and supportive public policy measures and encouragement of prompt health care seeking behavior by individuals.
- Medical institutions and health providers need adequate training and supervision to ensure that they carry out medical procedures with uncontaminated instruments and in a clean or sterile environment, as appropriate.
- Providers should be aware of the relationship between infections that may be already present and the risk of iatrogenic infection. For example, clients should be checked for endogenous or sexually transmitted infections before insertions of the IUD to avoid bacteria being pushed into the uterus. Alternatively, women selecting the IUD should be encouraged to choose a different form of contraception if they consider themselves at risk of exposure to an STI.
- Comprehensive reproductive health services should be made available, including the management of endogenous and sexually transmitted infections, to limit the risk factors for iatrogenic infection.

- The possibility of unsafe abortion should be reduced through the provision of good quality, affordable and accessible abortion services, within the limits of the law. Quality family planning services also reduce the prevalence of abortion.
- Women and their communities should be sensitized to the importance of seeking timely care for the symptoms of reproductive tract infection, and for the need to receive clinical care under safe and clean conditions.
- Women who have undergone transcervical procedures, such as IUD insertion, abortion, or surgically-assisted delivery, should be made aware of warning symptoms (Table 13.2) that could indicate subsequent infection and be told to seek immediate care if needed.

SEXUALLY TRANSMITTED INFECTIONS

Sexually transmitted infections (STIs) are those which are passed between people through sexual contact. Agents of infection include bacteria, viruses and other micro-organisms that can enter a person's urethra, vagina, mouth or anus. Some cause no symptoms at all, and some are easily treatable. Others result in severe long-term consequences and cannot be treated. HIV, the virus that causes AIDS, can lead to death.

Over 30 different organisms can be transmitted through sexual activity. They can cause symptoms and consequences including the following: genital ulcers, inflammation, pain, infertility, ectopic pregnancy, spontaneous abortion, fetal wastage and delivery, and neonatal blindness and infection. Sexually transmitted infections (STIs) are now recognized as a serious global threat to the health of populations.

Syndromic Management of Sexually Transmitted Infections

The World Health Organization (WHO) recommends that sexually transmitted infections (STIs) be managed at the first point of contact with the health services, using the Syndromic approach. STI syndromes are a way to group together infections which cause similar signs and symptoms. An STI syndrome is identified and then treated with combination therapy for all the common causes of the syndrome. Simple flowcharts have been developed to help health care workers to diagnose the syndrome and to treat the diseases within a particular syndrome (syndromic approach).

Syndromic approach focuses on common STIs like syphilis, gonorrhea, chlamydia, chancroid and trichomoniasis (*see* fact sheet 1) and is appropriate for primary health care settings as this approach does not require sophisticated laboratory tests and treatment can be provided by many different types of health care workers without a need of special skill. Thus people who are concerned that they may have an STI can get care right in their own community.

Syndromic approach is high quality STI care because it treats people who may have more than one STI infection with the most effective drugs available. Also, people with STIs are treated at the time of their first visit to a health care facility. Even if drugs cost more, treating in this way is less expensive in the long run because more people are cured the first time they come for care. Health care workers may notice that there is less emphasis placed on identifying the cause of a particular STI. This change can be difficult for those who have been trained to seek out and identify the cause of disease. Yet both health care workers and patients will be satisfied with the quality of care when they see that effective treatment is given more rapidly than is usually possible.

Treatment for multiple infections is built into the approach. Approximately 6 out of every 10 STI patients have two or more different infections at the same time. With the Syndromic Approach, multiple infections are considered from the beginning and patients are given effective drugs (Table 13.3).

An important part of the effort to control STIs is education about reducing the chances of future STI. **Patient education should be a standard for all types of STI care.**

The syndromic approach addresses this part of STI care by recognizing the valuable work of non-clinicians and the importance of working directly with people in the community. This is because health care workers who are comfortable talking with patients about sexual behaviour can obtain

Table 13.3: STIs using the syndromic approach (*Adapted from* World Health Organization guidelines)

	Syndrome	Treat for
Men	Urethral discharge	Gonorrhea and chlamydia
Women	Lower abdominal pain → →	Gonorrhea, chlamydia and other bacteria.
	Vaginal discharge → → →	Cervicitis—Gonorrhea and chlamydia Vaginitis—Trichomoniasis, bacterial and vaginosis candidiasis
Men and women	Genital ulcers	Syphilis, chancroid and genital herpes

Table 13.4: Advantages and disadvantages of syndromic management of STI

Advantages
- Highly sensitive when used to detect infection among symptomatic patients, does not miss mixed infections, which are common
- Treatment is given at first visit so delays in treatment are avoided and the patient is not lost to follow-up before treatment is initiated — this increases client satisfaction, and reduces further transmission and complications from untreated infections
- Provides opportunity and time for education and counselling
- Avoids expensive laboratory tests
- Can be implemented at primary care level because it is easy to use, does not require highly trained STI specialists
- Limits referral to specialist centres
- Problem-orientated (based on patient's symptoms)
- High rates of cure, provided that the effectiveness of the drugs selected is adequate and properly monitored
- The use of flowcharts standardises diagnosis, treatment, referral and reporting, allowing for improved surveillance and programme management.

Disadvantages
- Over-diagnosis and over-treatment that may result in increased drug costs, possible side-effects of multiple drugs, alterations in vaginal flora and potential for increased drug resistance
- Cannot be used to detect infections among asymptomatic individuals
- The syndromic approach for vaginal discharge is poorly predictive of the presence of cervical chlamydial and/or gonococcal infection
- Over-treatment of partners of women with vaginal discharge, most of whom do not have an STI, may lead to potentially serious social and physical consequences for the female index case
- Not easily accepted by doctors as thought of as inferior quality
- Does not address the issue of poor treatment-seeking behavior by symptomatic individuals

more complete and reliable information. They can use this information to help assess a patient's level of risk, help make a diagnosis and as the starting point for patient education.

Syndromic Management Protocol (Table 13.4)

The management of an individual STI case should always include the following steps:

- *Adopt a non-judgemental, caring and positive attitude.* Ensure privacy and ensure all information will be kept confidential.

- *Take a medical and sexual history* (include an assessment of the risk of exposure to an STI) and a history of drug allergies.

- *Perform a physical examination.* This should include a search for any signs of HIV disease, a bimanual digital examination in women to exclude cervical motion tenderness and a speculum examination. Feel and view the cervix. Carcinoma of the cervix must be excluded. Remember that one patient can have more than one STI syndrome.

- *Establish a diagnosis and provide treatment.* Identify one or more of the syndromes based on symptoms and signs and treat according to the appropriate protocol(s).

- *Do an RPR test for syphilis.* Ask the patient to return for the results and if positive, administer benzathine penicillin 2.4 MU IMI weekly for 3 weeks.

- *Promote VCT* (voluntary counseling and testing for HIV) since patients presenting with symptomatic STIs might be co-infected with HIV. Inform the patient that a negative HIV test result needs to be confirmed after 3 months.

- *Educate and counsel* the patient on how to prevent subsequent episodes of disease including risk reduction and on the importance of completing treatment.
- *Promote the use of condoms* and demonstrate how to use them.

Syndromic Management

Syndromic management for urethral discharge in men, and genital ulcers in men and women, has proved to be both valid and feasible. It has resulted in adequate treatment of large numbers of infected people, and is inexpensive, simple and very cost-effective. However, recent data have indicated that herpes simplex virus type 2 (HSV 2) is fast becoming the commonest cause of genital ulcer disease (GUD) in developing countries. This may negatively affect the treatment outcome of GUD if antiviral therapy is not appropriately instituted. A detailed discussion on these topics is out of scope of this chapter.

WHO's simplified generic tool includes flowcharts (Figs 13.4 and 13.5) for women with symptoms of vaginal discharge and/or lower abdominal pain. While the flowcharts for abdominal pain are quite satisfactory, those for vaginal discharge have limitations, particularly in the management of cervical (gonococcal and chlamydial) infections.

In general, but **especially in low-prevalence settings and in adolescent females, endogenous vaginitis rather than an STI is the main cause of vaginal discharge.**

Syndromic Management Protocol for Vaginal Discharge

A spontaneous complaint of abnormal vaginal discharge (in terms of quantity, colour or odour) is most commonly a result of a vaginal infection. It may in rare cases be caused by mucopurulent STI-related cervicitis. *T. vaginalis*, *C. albicans* and bacterial vaginosis (BV) are the commonest causes of vaginal infection. *N. gonorrheae* and *C. trachomatis* cause cervical infection. The clinical detection of cervical infection is difficult because a large proportion of women with gonococcal or chlamydial cervical infection is asymptomatic. The symptom of abnormal vaginal discharge is highly indicative of vaginal infection, but poorly predictive for cervical infection. Thus, all women presenting with vaginal discharge should receive treatment for trichomoniasis and BV (Table 13.5 and Fig. 13.4). Among women presenting with discharge, one can attempt to identify those with an increased likelihood of being infected with *N. gonorrheae* and/or *C. trachomatis*. To identify women at greater risk, therefore, of cervical infection, an assessment of a woman's risk status may be useful, especially when risk factors are adapted to the local situation.

Knowledge of the local prevalence of gonococcal and/or chlamydia in women presenting with vaginal discharge is important when making the decision to treat for cervical infection. The higher the prevalence, the stronger is the justification for treatment. Women with a positive risk assessment have a higher likelihood of cervical infection than those who are risk negative. Women with vaginal discharge and a positive risk assessment should, therefore, be offered treatment for gonococcal and chlamydia cervicitis (Table 13.6 and Fig. 13.4). Where resources permit, the use of laboratory tests to screen women with vaginal discharge should be considered. Such screening could be applied to all women with discharge or selectively to those with discharge and a positive risk assessment.

Protocol for Lower Abdominal Pain due to Pelvic Inflammatory Disease

All sexually active women presenting with lower abdominal pain should be carefully evaluated for the presence of salpingitis and/or endometritis—elements of pelvic inflammatory disease (PID). Pelvic inflammatory disease (PID) is an acute ascending infection of the upper female genital tract that is usually

Table 13.5: Treatment of vaginal infection (*Adapted from* World Health Organization guidelines)

Recommended syndromic treatment

Therapy for *T. vaginalis*	Therapy for BV	Therapy for *C. albicans*
1. Metronidazole 2 g orally, in a dose or single	1. Metronidazole 400 mg or 500 mg orally, twice daily for 7 days	1. Miconazole or clotrimazole 200 mg intravaginally, daily for 3 days OR
2. Tinidazole, 2 g orally, in a single dose		• Clotrimazole 500 mg intravaginally, as a single dose OR
Note. The reported cure rate in women ranges from 82 to 88% but may be increased to 95% if sexual partners are treated simultaneously.	**Note**	• Fluconazole 150 mg orally, as a single dose
	• Patients taking metronidazole should be cautioned not to consume alcohol while they are taking the drug and up to 24 hours after taking the last dose.	
Alternative regimen	**Alternative regimen**	**Alternative regimen**
Metronidazole 400 mg or 500 mg orally, twice daily for 7 days or tinidazole, 500 mg orally, twice daily for 5 days	• Metronidazole 2 g orally, as a single dose or	Nystatin 100 000 IU intravaginally, daily for 14 days
	• Clindamycin 2% vaginal cream, 5 g intravaginally, at bedtime for 7 days or	
	• Metronidazole 0.75% gel, 5 g intravaginally, twice daily for 5 days or	
	• Clindamycin 300 mg orally, twice daily for 7 days	

Table 13.6: Treatment of cervical infection (*Adapted from* World Health Organization guidelines)

Recommended syndromic treatment

Therapy for uncomplicated gonorrhea **PLUS**	Therapy for chlamydia
1. Ciprofloxacin 500 mg orally, as a single dose or	1. doxycycline 100 mg orally, twice daily for 7 days or
2. Ceftriaxone 125 mg by intramuscular injection, as a single dose or	2. azithromycin 1 g orally, in a single dose
3. Cefixime 400 mg orally, as a single dose or	**Alternatives**
4. Spectinomycin, 2 g by intramuscular injection, as a single dose	Amoxycillin
	Ofloxacin
	Erythromycin (if tetracycline is contraindicated)
	Tetracycline
Note	**Note**
• Ciprofloxacin is contraindicated in pregnancy, and is not recommended for use in children and adolescents.	• Doxycyline and other tetracyclines are contraindicated during pregnancy and lactation.
• There are variations in the anti-gonococcal activity of individual quinolones, and it is important to use only the most active	• Current evidence indicates that 1 g single-dose therapy of azithromycin is efficacious for chlamydial infection.
	• There is evidence that extending the duration of treatment beyond 7 days does not improve the cure rate in uncomplicated chlamydial infection.
	• Erythromycin should not be taken on an empty stomach

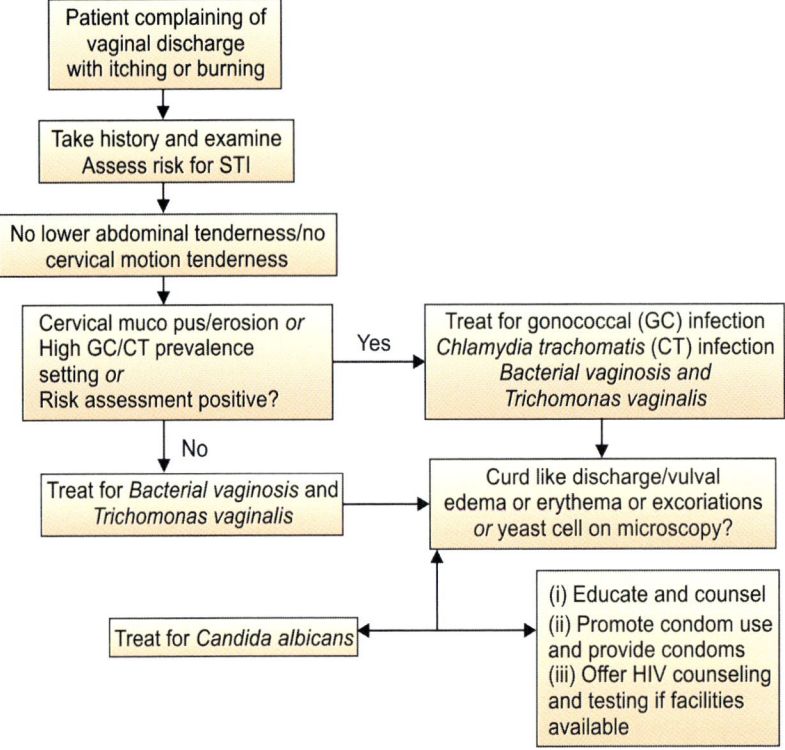

Fig. 13.4: Protocol for vaginal discharge (Flowchart for management of vaginal discharge (bimanual, speculum with or without microscopy) *Adapted from* World Health Organization guidelines)

caused by *Neisseria gonorrhoeae* or Chlamydia trachomatis which are sexually transmitted and less commonly by normal vaginal flora including streptococci, anaerobes and enteric Gram-negative rods. The infection usually begins in the cervix or vagina. PID includes endometritis, salpingitis, tubo-ovarian abscess, and pelvic peritonitis (upper genital tract infection).

Clinical Presentation

Presentation may vary widely. The most common presenting symptom is usually bilateral lower abdominal pain. Pain may be associated with dysuria, dyspareunia, or back pain or abnormal uterine bleeding (meno metrorrhagia). Symptoms of lower genital tract infection such as abnormal vaginal odor,

itching, bleeding, or discharge may also be present. Nausea, vomiting, fever or other constitutional symptoms may be present. In some instances, symptoms are mild or even absent.

General examination: The patient's temperature may be elevated [oral temperature over 38.3°C (101°F) increases specificity of diagnosis] but is normal in many cases.

Perabdominal examination: Lower abdominal tenderness, a tender pelvic mass, and direct or rebound tenderness may also be present.

Pervaginal examination (bimanual examination): One or more of these are present on pelvic examination:

1. Cervical motion, uterine or adnexal tenderness.

2. Presence of abnormal cervical or vaginal mucopurulent discharge
3. A tender pelvic mass on palpation through fornices may also be present.

Routine bimanual and abdominal examination should be carried out on all women with a presumptive STI since some women with PID or endometritis will not complain of lower abdominal pain. In general, clinicians should err on the side of over-diagnosing and treating suspected cases.

Hospitalization of patients with acute PID should be seriously considered when:

- The diagnosis is uncertain
- Surgical emergencies such as appendicitis and ectopic pregnancy cannot be excluded
- A pelvic abscess is suspected
- Severe illness precludes management on an outpatient basis
- The patient is pregnant
- The patient is unable to follow or tolerate an outpatient regimen; or
- The patient has failed to respond to outpatient therapy.

Differential Diagnosis

1. *Ectopic pregnancy:* Lower abdominal pain, adnexal tenderness, and other symptoms of acute abdomen (nausea, vomiting, diarrhea) may be present. There may be history of amenorrhea of 6–8 weeks. May resemble severe case of PID. Positive pregnancy test will guide search for ectopic pregnancy: hCG hormone level is high in serum and urine. Ultrasound reveals an empty uterus and may show a mass in the fallopian tubes.

2. *Acute appendicitis*: Nausea and vomiting occurs in most patients with acute appendicitis. Cervical motion tenderness will occur in about 25% of women with appendicitis while this sign is usually present in all patients with PID. Laparoscopy confirms diagnosis.

3. Ovarian cyst complications (ruptured ovarian cyst, ovarian cyst torsion, hemorrhagic ovarian cyst)

Ruptured ovarian cyst: Rupture usually spontaneous, can follow history of trauma or sexual intercourse; mild chronic lower abdominal discomfort may suddenly intensify. On examination peritoneal signs (guarding, rebound tenderness, rigid abdomen) may be present in lower abdomen and pelvis; adnexal size unremarkable due to collapsed cyst.

Ovarian cyst torsion may present with sudden, acute, unilateral, lower quadrant abdominal pain, severe and colicky in nature; two-thirds of patients have nausea and vomiting. Low-grade fever usually correlates with necrosis; tender adnexal mass palpated in 90%; localized peritoneal irritation.

Hemorrhagic ovarian cyst presents with localized abdominal pain, nausea and vomiting. On examination florid septic or hypovolemic shock may be present; abdominal tenderness can signify overt peritonitis; pelvic mass may be palpated.

All the above mentioned conditions can be confirmed by Pelvic ultrasound and/or laparoscopy.

4. *Endometriosis:* Adnexal enlargement, cervical stenosis or lateral displacement of uterus; cyclic pain that is exacerbated by onset of menses and during the luteal phase; or dyspareunia. Cyclic pain is not a feature of PID. Transvaginal ultrasound may show ovarian endometrioma or evidence of deep pelvic endometriosis such as uterosacral ligament involvement. Laparoscopy confirms diagnosis by direct visualization of peritoneal implants with biopsy-confirmed endometrial glands or stroma outside of uterine cavity.

5. *Non-PID causes of vaginal discharge—Vulvovaginal symptoms:* Discharge, itching, burning, dyspareunia. Vulvovaginal symptoms may or may not present in PID

because upper genital tract infection may exist in the absence of symptoms of vaginitis. Vaginal discharge tested by wet mount or urethral swab identifies disease causative organism.

Investigations

Initial Evaluation

1. *WBC count:* Usually elevated
2. Elevated ESR and C reactive protein
3. Presence of abundant numbers of WBC on saline microscopy of vaginal secretions
4. Culture of vaginal secretion—positive gonococcal or chlamydia cultures (although negative cultures do not rule out PID).

When the diagnosis is questionable or the patient is not responding to therapy, further investigation is warranted. Several tests and procedures exist with varying costs and availability but no single laboratory test is diagnostic. However, in this context, normal results on serum WBC count, wet mount polymorphonuclear leukocytes and ESR effectively exclude upper genital tract infection.

Imaging and Invasive Tests

1. *Transvaginal ultrasound:* Transvaginal ultrasound is the primary imaging modality and may be normal in early stages or uncomplicated cases. Use of color Doppler can improve detection of subtle abnormalities of endometritis, salpingitis, and oophoritis. Classic signs are tubal wall thickness greater than 5 mm, incomplete septae within the tube, fluid in the cul-de-sac, and a cog-wheel appearance on the cross-section of the tubal view; may also see tubo-ovarian abscess.
2. *Laparoscopy:* Laparoscopy demonstrates visual evidence of salpingitis. Laparoscopy enables specimens to be taken from the fallopian tubes and pouch of Douglas, and is particularly useful in excluding alternative pathologies when there is

diagnostic doubt. It should not be used as a routine diagnostic tool, especially when symptoms are mild or vague.

3. *Endometrial biopsy:* Endometrial biopsy should not be used as a routine diagnostic test. It is indicated in women undergoing laparoscopy who do not have visual evidence of salpingitis.
4. *Pelvic CT scan:* Pelvic CT is indicated in patients with diffuse pelvic pain, peritonitis, or difficult or equivocal ultrasound. CT scan shows subtle changes in appearance of pelvic fascial floor planes, thickened uterosacral ligaments, inflammatory changes of the tubes and ovaries, abnormal fluid collection. In progressive disease, reactive inflammation of surrounding pelvic and abdominal structures may be seen.
5. *Pelvic MRI:* Pelvic MRI is considered superior to ultrasound at diagnosing PID when there is a tubo-ovarian abscess, pyosalpinx, fluid filled tube and/or enlarged polycystic ovaries with free intrapelvic fluid. However, both ultrasound and CT are more cost effective than MRI. Therefore, MRI is rarely used and plays only a complimentary problem-solving role.

Treatment

Empirical treatment of PID should be initiated at first consultation in sexually active young women and other women at risk of PID (Fig. 13.5). Due to serious health implications of untreated PID and lack of clear delineation of timing for invasive tests, clinicians usually start treatment in patients at risk who have lower abdominal tenderness, adnexal tenderness or pain on manipulation of the cervix. These physical findings are noted in over 90% of women with laparoscopically documented disease.

Many experts recommend that all patients with PID should be admitted to hospital for treatment (Table 13.7). As it is impossible to

Table 13.7: Outpatient therapy (*Adapted from* World Health Organization guidelines)

Recommended syndromic treatment
- Single-dose therapy for uncomplicated gonorrhoea (*see* Table 13.5) Single-dose ceftriaxone has been shown to be effective; other single-dose regimen have not been formally evaluated as treatments for PID)

PLUS
- Doxycycline 100 mg orally, twice daily, or tetracycline 500 mg orally, 4 times daily for 14 days

PLUS
- Metronidazole 400–500 mg orally, twice daily for 14 days

Note
- Patients taking metronidazole should be cautioned to avoid alcohol.
- Tetracyclines are contraindicated in pregnancy.

reach a precise microbiological diagnosist, the treatment regimen must be effective against a broad range of pathogens. The regimen recommended in Table 13.8 are based on this principle.

Adjuncts to Therapy: Removal of Intrauterine Device (IUD)

If PID should occur with an IUD in place, treat the PID using appropriate antibiotics. There is no evidence that removal of the IUD

Table 13.8: Inpatient therapy (*Adapted from* World Health Organization guidelines)

Recommended syndromic treatment options for PID
1. Ceftriaxone 250 mg by intramuscular injection, once daily
   PLUS
- Doxycycline 100 mg orally or by intravenous injection, twice daily, or tetracycline 500 mg orally 4 times daily
   PLUS
- Metronidazole 400–500 mg orally or by intravenous injection, twice daily, or chloramphenicol 500 mg orally or by intravenous injection, 4 times daily
2. Clindamycin, 900 mg by intravenous injection, every 8 hours
   PLUS
- Gentamicin 1.5 mg/kg by intravenous injection every 8 hours
3. Ciprofloxacin 500 mg orally, twice daily, or spectinomycin 1 g by intramuscular injection, 4 times daily
   PLUS
- Doxycycline 100 mg orally or by intravenous injection, twice daily, or tetracycline,500 mg orally, 4 times daily
   PLUS
- Metronidazole 400–500 mg orally or by intravenous injection, twice daily, or chloramphenicol 500 mg orally or by intravenous injection, 4 times daily

Note
- For all three regimen, therapy should be continued until at least two days after the patient has improved and should then be followed by either doxycycline 100 mg orally, twice daily for 14 days, or tetracycline 500 mg orally, 4 times daily, for 14 days.
- Patients taking metronidazole should be cautioned to avoid alcohol.
- Tetracyclines are contraindicated in pregnancy.

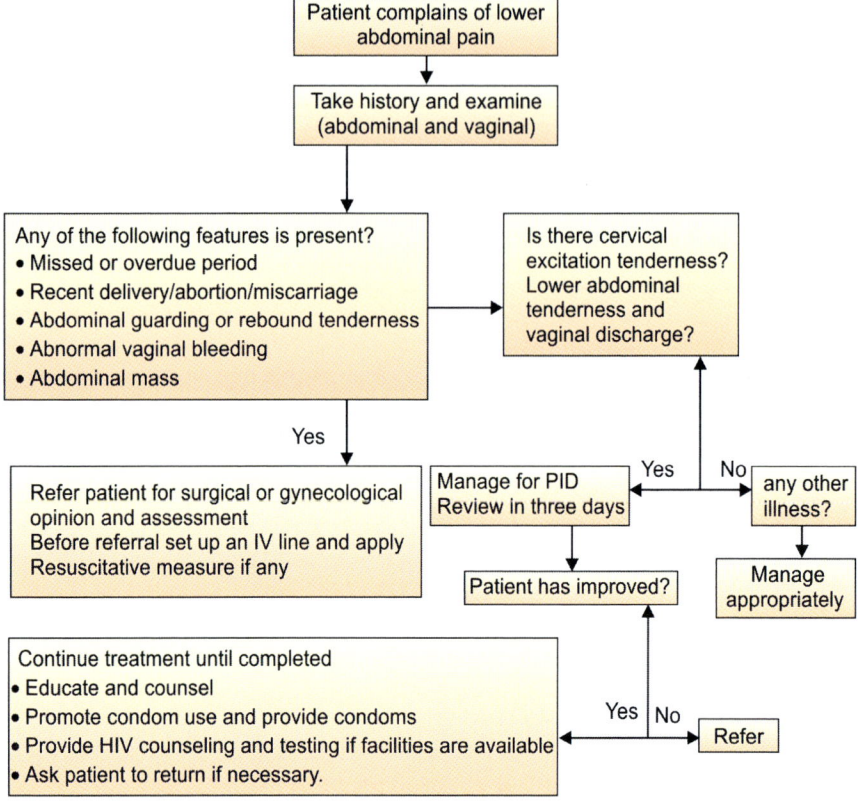

Fig. 13.5: Protocol for lower abdominal pain (Flowchart for management of lower abdominal pain *Adapted from* World Health Organization guidelines)

provides any additional benefit. Thus, if the individual should wish to continue its use, it need not be removed. If she does not want to keep the IUD, removal of the IUD is recommended after antimicrobial therapy has been commenced. When the IUD is removed, contraceptive counseling is necessary.

Follow-up

Outpatients with PID should be followed up after 72 hours and admitted if their condition has not improved.

Treatment of Sexual Partners

Men who have had sexual contact with a woman diagnosed with PID during the 60 days prior to her onset of symptoms should be evaluated and treated with regimens that are effective against chlamydia and gonorrhea. Women should be advised to avoid sexual intercourse until they and their partners have completed the treatment course. If adequate screening for gonorrhea and chlamydia in the sexual partner(s) is not possible, empiric therapy for gonorrhea and chlamydia should be prescribed.

Complications of PID

1. Tubo-ovarian abscess
2. Infertility
3. Chronic pelvic pain
4. Ectopic pregnancy
5. Fitz-Hugh-Curtis syndrome

Prognosis

Prognosis for complete recovery is good in patients treated within 3 days of symptom onset and who are able to complete the full course of therapy (cure rate 88–100%). The risks of tubal occlusion and infertility depend on severity of infection before treatment. Clinical improvement may not translate into improved fertility.

SPECIFIC SEXUALLY TRANSMITTED INFECTIONS

Trichomonas Vaginalis

Causative Organism

Trichomoniasis is caused by infection with a protozoan parasite called *Trichomonas vaginalis*. The parasite is passed from an infected person to an uninfected person during sexual intercourse.

Clinical Presentation

There may be no symptom or symptom can range from mild irritation to severe inflammation. Women with trichomoniasis may notice itching, burning, redness or soreness of the genitals, dysuria, or a thin discharge with an unusual smell that can be clear, white, yellowish, or greenish. The woman may have dyspareunia. Examination may reveal inflammation of cervix, vagina and urethra.

Diagnosis

Trichomoniasis is diagnosed by visually observing the trichomonads in vaginal discharge on wet mount microscopy (*see* Chapter 14, vaginal discharge).

Complications

Materno-fetal complications: premature rupture of membranes, preterm delivery, Low birth weight.

Treatment

See Table 13.6.

Gonococcal Infection

Causative Organism

Gonorrhea is a sexually transmitted infection caused by the *Neisseria gonorrhoeae* bacterium. *N. gonorrhoeae* infects the mucous membranes of the reproductive tract, including the cervix, uterus, and fallopian tubes in women, and the urethra in women and men. *N. gonorrhoeae* can also infect the mucous membranes of the mouth, throat, eyes, and anus.

Clinical Presentation

Most women with gonorrhea are asymptomatic. Even when a woman has symptoms, they are often so mild and nonspecific that they are mistaken for a bladder or vaginal infection. The initial symptoms in women include dysuria, increased vaginal discharge, or inter menstrual bleeding. Symptoms of rectal infection in both men and women may include discharge, anal itching, soreness, bleeding, or painful bowel movements.

Diagnosis

Urogenital gonorrhea can be diagnosed by testing urine, endocervical or vaginal specimens using nucleic acid amplification testing (NAAT). It can also be diagnosed using gonorrhea culture, which requires endocervical specimen. Gram stain of endocervical specimens is not sufficient to detect infection in most occasions.

Complications

Pelvic inflammatory disease, infertility, materno-fetal complications: premature rupture of membranes, premature delivery, potentially blinding neonatal conjunctivitis.

Treatment

Gonorrhea treatment is complicated by the ability of *N. gonorrhoeae* to develop resistance to antimicrobial therapies. Treatment options for uncomplicated gonorrhea are shown in Table 13.5. As the quinolone-resistant *N. gonorrhoeae* strains are now widely disseminated throughout the United States and the world, Centre for Disease Control (CDC) no longer recommend use of Ciprofloxacin as a treatment option.

Chlamydia Infection

Causative Organism

Chlamydia is a common sexually transmitted infection caused by the bacterium, *Chlamydia trachomatis*. Chlamydia can be transmitted during vaginal, anal, or oral sex. Chlamydia can also pass from mother to the baby during vaginal birth.

Clinical Presentation

Chlamydia is known as a "silent" disease because the majority of infected women have no symptoms. The bacteria initially infect the cervix and the urethra. Women who have symptoms might have an abnormal vaginal discharge or a burning sensation when urinating. If the infection spreads from the cervix to the fallopian tubes, some women still have no signs or symptoms; others have lower abdominal pain, low back pain, nausea, fever, pain during intercourse, or bleeding between menstrual periods (features of PID). Chlamydial infection of the cervix can spread to the rectum.

Women who have receptive anal intercourse may acquire chlamydial infection in the rectum, which can cause rectal pain, discharge, or bleeding. Chlamydia can also be found in the throats of women having oral sex with an infected partner.

Diagnosis

C. trachomatis urogenital infection in women can be diagnosed by testing urine or by collecting swab specimens from the endocervix or vagina. NAATs, cell culture, direct immunofluorescence, EIA, and nucleic acid hybridization tests are available for the detection of *C. trachomatis* on endocervical specimens.

Complications

Pelvic inflammatory disease, Peri-hepatitis, Chronic pelvic pain, infertility, ectopic pregnancy and neonatal complications: Conjunctivitis, pneumonia

Treatment

Chlamydia can be easily treated and cured with antibiotics. A single dose of azithromycin or a week of doxycycline (twice daily) is the most commonly used treatments (Table 13.5). HIV-positive women with chlamydia should receive the same treatment as those who are HIV negative.

Syphilis

Causative Organism

Syphilis is a systemic sexually transmitted infection caused by the bacterium *Treponema pallidum*. Syphilis is transmitted from person to person by direct contact with a syphilitic sore, known as a chancre. Transmission of syphilis occurs during vaginal, anal, or oral sex. Pregnant women with the disease can transmit it to the fetus.

Clinical Presentation

Primary: Painless ulcers at site of inoculation (genital area, rectum, mouth)

Secondary: 4–8 weeks after ulcers, generalized lesions on skin and mucous membranes fever, malaise

Latent: No symptoms/signs: Tertiary syphilis will develop in about 1/3 of untreated cases and has numerous systemic manifestations.

Diagnosis

The definitive method for diagnosing syphilis is visualizing the spirochete via darkfield microscopy. This technique is rarely performed today because it is a technologically difficult method. Diagnoses are thus more commonly made using blood tests. There are two types of blood tests available for syphilis: (1) nontreponemal tests and (2) treponemal tests.

Nontreponemal tests (e.g., VDRL and RPR) are simple, inexpensive, and are often used for screening. Treponemal tests (e.g., FTA-ABS, TP-PA, various EIAs, and chemiluminescence immunoassays) detect antibodies that are specific for syphilis. Persons with a reactive nontreponemal test should receive a treponemal test to confirm a syphilis diagnosis. This sequence of testing (nontreponemal, then treponemal test) is considered the "classical" testing algorithm.

Treatment

A single intramuscular injection of long acting Benzathine penicillin G (2.4 million units administered intramuscularly) will cure a woman who has primary, secondary or early latent syphilis. Three doses of long acting Benzathine penicillin G (2.4 million units administered intramuscularly) at weekly intervals is recommended for individuals with late latent syphilis or latent syphilis of unknown duration. Treatment will kill the treponema and prevent further damage, but it will not repair damage already done.

Complication

Late complications: Neurological problems that can lead to paralysis and blindness cardiovascular disease. Severe lesions in skin, mucous membranes, bones and viscera. Materno-fetal complications: Stillbirth, congenital syphilis.

Genital Herpes

Causative Organism

Genital herpes is a sexually transmitted infection caused by the herpes simplex viruses type 1 (HSV-1) or type 2 (HSV-2). Infections are transmitted through contact with lesions, mucosal surfaces, genital secretions, or oral secretions. HSV-1 and HSV-2 can also be shed from skin that looks normal.

Clinical Presentation

Most individuals infected with HSV-1 or HSV-2 are asymptomatic, or have very mild symptoms that go unnoticed or are mistaken for another skin condition. When symptoms do occur, they typically appear as one or more vesicles on or around vulva, vagina, rectum or mouth. The average incubation period after exposure is 4 days (range, 2 to 12). Recurrent episodes are common particularly in first year of onfection.

Diagnosis

Numerous herpes diagnostic tests are available. Direct (or virologic) tests such as PCR, test for viral DNA or RNA and allow for more rapid and accurate results. Indirect (or serologic) tests are blood tests that detect antibodies to the herpes virus. Several ELISA-based serologic tests are available commercially. Viral culture is currently the reference standard for diagnosing genital herpes.

Treatment

There is no cure for herpes. Antiviral medications can, however, prevent or shorten outbreaks during the period of time the person takes the medication. Treatment regimen includes any of the following:

1. Acyclovir 400 mg orally three times daily for 7–10 days
2. Acyclovir 200 mg orally five times daily for 7–10 days
3. Famciclovir 250 mg orally three times daily for 7–10 days

Complications

Genital herpes causes painful genital ulcers in women that can be severe and persistent in HIV-infected persons. Both HSV-1 and HSV-2 can also cause rare but serious complications such as blindness, encephalitis, and aseptic meningitis. Development of extragenital lesions in the buttocks, groin, thigh, finger, and eye may occur during the course of infection. Can be transmitted to neonates resulting in infection and death of infant.

Human Papilloma Virus (HPV) Infection

Causative Organism

Genital human papilloma virus (also called HPV) is a common sexually transmitted infection (STI). There are more than 40 HPV types that can infect the genital areas of males and females. HPV is passed on through genital contact, most often during vaginal and anal and oral sex. Rarely, HPV can pass to the baby during delivery.

Clinical Presentation

In 90% of cases, the body's immune system clears HPV naturally within two years. But, sometimes, HPV infections are not cleared and can cause:

- Genital warts
- Rarely, warts in the throat—a condition called recurrent respiratory papillomatosis, or RRP. When this occurs in children it is called juvenile-onset RRP (JORRP).
- Cervical cancer and other, less common but serious cancers, including cancers of the vulva, vagina, anus, and oropharynx.

HPV Tests

HPV tests are available for women aged > 30 years undergoing cervical cancer screening. These HPV tests detect viral nucleic acid (i.e., DNA or RNA) or capsid protein. However, there is no general test for men or women to check one's overall "HPV status", nor is there an approved HPV test to find HPV on the genitals or in the mouth or throat.

Treatment

Treatment is directed to the macroscopic (i.e., genital warts) or pathologic (i.e, precancerous) lesions caused by infection. Subclinical genital HPV infection typically clears spontaneously, and therefore specific antiviral therapy is not recommended to eradicate HPV infection.

Prevention

Two HPV vaccines: A bivalent vaccine (Cervarix) containing HPV types 16 and 18 and a quadrivalent vaccine (Gardasil) vaccine containing HPV types 6, 11, 16, and 18. Both vaccines offer protection against the HPV types that cause 70% of cervical cancers (i.e., types 16 and 18), and the quadrivalent HPV vaccine also protects against the types that cause 90% of genital warts (i.e., types 6 and 11).

HIV Infection

HIV infection represents a spectrum of disease that can begin with a brief acute retroviral syndrome that typically transitions to a multiyear chronic and clinically latent illness. Without treatment, this illness eventually progresses to a symptomatic, life-threatening immunodeficiency disease known as AIDS. In untreated patients, the time between HIV infection and the development of AIDS varies, ranging from a few months to many years with an estimated median time of approximately 11 years.

Diagnosis

HIV infection can be diagnosed by serologic tests that detect antibodies against HIV-1 and HIV-2 and by virologic tests that can detect HIV antigens or ribonucleic acid (RNA). Antibody testing begins with a sensitive screening test (e.g., the conventional or rapid enzyme immunoassay [EIA]). Currently available serologic tests are both highly sensitive and specific and can detect all known subtypes of HIV-1. Most can also detect HIV-2. Positive screening tests for HIV antibody must be confirmed by a supplemental test before

Table 13.9: Three strategies of HIV prevention

Strategies	1. Reduce exposure	2. Reduce efficacy of transmission	3. Shorten duration of infectivity
Individual behavior	• Abstain from sex • Limit number of partners • Remain in mutually monogamous relationship	• Substitute safer sexual practices for risky sexual behavior • Use condoms	• Seek immediate treatment for infectious symptoms • Abstain from sex during treatment • Refer partners • Adhere to recommended therapy
Health policy	• Work to limit population prevalence of STIs • Target risk groups • Promote awareness of self-protection methods	• Promote safer sex through active, high-quality, gender sensitive information campaigns • Make condoms easily available (e.g. through social marketing)	• Provide accessible STI services (e.g. introduce syndromic management for symptomatic cases) • Encourage partner referral and treatment

the diagnosis of HIV infection can be established.

Management

Those persons who test positive for HIV should receive prevention counseling before leaving the testing site. Such persons should receive or be referred for a medical evaluation and, if indicated, be provided with behavioral and psychological services as determined by a thorough psychosocial evaluation, which can also be used to identify high-risk behaviors. A detailed discussion is out of scope of this chapter.

Prevention

To limit the morbidity and mortality associated with both STIs and HIV, prevention is crucial. Primary strategies for preventing the transmission of STIs are the same as those for HIV/AIDS.

Once contracted, however, many of the other sexually transmitted infections are curable whereas HIV is not. As a result, timely and appropriate management of other STIs can help curb the HIV pandemic.

There are three strategies of HIV prevention through STI management. They apply to both individual behavior and health policy strategy. These are shown in Table 13.9.

Prevention of Reproductive Tract Infections

The best strategy to limit the harmful effects of RTIs is to prevent new infections. Each RTI should be prevented by methods related to its transmission routes.

Endogenous infections are easier to diagnose and treat than to prevent (although avoiding vaginal douching is recommended as it has been shown to increase the occurrence of bacterial vaginosis). Their consequences can be reduced through good access to adequate health care facilities and prompt health care seeking behavior.

Iatrogenic infections can be prevented by proper sterilization of medical instruments, adherence to sterile protocols during examinations, and screening or treatment for pre-existing infections before transcervical medical procedures are conducted.

Sexually transmitted infections can be prevented by the avoidance of sexual activity or the adoption of "safer sex" strategies, including mutual monogamy, non-penetrative sex, and the correct and consistent use of barrier contraceptive methods, particularly latex male condoms.

The polyurethane vaginal sheath (female condom) is also considered to offer protection from STIs.

The following are important components of STI control measures undertaken by World Health Organization that are adopted by the countries in the South-East Asia:

- Information, education and communication strategies to improve awareness on STIs, STI treatment seeking behaviour and promote condom use.
- Integration of STI treatment services into primary healthcare
- Improved case management of STI
- Screening and presumptive treatment
- Targeted interventions to populations with high risk behavior
- STI surveillance including laboratory surveillance and data management.

EXERCISES

1. Answer the following questions

- What are reproductive tract infections?
- What are the different types of RTIs?
- What is endogenous RTIs and what are the common organisms involved?
- How candidiasis is diagnosed and treated?
- How bacterial vaginosis is diagnosed and treated?
- What is the effect of BV on pregnancy?
- What do you mean by iatrogenic infection of reproductive tracts?
- Why are they important?
- How do you prevent iatrogenic infection of reproductive tract?
- What do you mean by sexually transmitted infections?
- What are the consequences of STIs?
- What do you mean by syndromic management of STI?

- What are the characteristics of Syndromic approach?
- What are its advantages and dis advantages?
- Describe the syndromic management protocol for vaginal discharge?
- Describe the syndromic management protocol for lower abdominal pain?
- What is PID?
- What is the cause of PID?
- What are the most common infectious agents?
- What is the typical presentation of PID?
- How is diagnosis of PID confirmed?
- What is the goal of PID therapy?
- When is hospitalization is recommended for treatment of PID?
- Describe the specific treatment regimens commonly used for out patient treatment of PID?
- Describe inpatient treatment regimen for PID?
- What are its complications?
- How do you diagnose and treat trichomoniasis?
- How do you diagnose and treat gonococcal infection?
- What are the complications of chlamydia infection? How do investigate chlamydia infection and treat it?
- How do you diagnose and treat syphilis?
- How genital herpes is diagnosed and treated?
- How do you prevent HPV infection?
- How do you prevent HIV infection?

2. Write short notes on

- Amsel criteria to diagnose bacterial vaginosis
- Differential diagnosis of PID
- Prevention of RTI

3. Explain or justify the following statements

- Reproductive tract infections can have serious consequences in woman's life
- Syndromic approach is high quality STI care

4. Fill in the blanks with appropriate word/s

- Most common endogenous infections are _____ and _____ .
- Two risk factors for vaginal candidiasis are _____ and _____ .
- Two antibiotics recommended for bacterial vaginosis are _____ and _____ .
- During pregnancy bacterial vaginosis can lead to _____ .
- Four main curable STI are _____ , _____ , _____ , _____ .
- PID involves infection of _____ genital tract.
- Three complications of PID are _____ , _____ , and _____ .

5. Questions for practical (read the case summary in the beginning of chapter before answering the following questions)

- What is your provisional diagnosis and why?
- What are the differential diagnosis and why?
- If she is having PID, will you admit her in hospital?
- How do you treat her if she is having PID?

Bibliography

1. Bacterial vaginosis Sobel J D up to date 2011.
2. HIV/AIDS Prevention and Control. World Health Organization 2006.
3. Reproductive tract infection: an introductory overview. Population Council.
4. Sexually transmitted disease guidelines MMWR CDC 2010.
5. Sexually transmitted diseases Center for Disease Control and Prevention fact sheet.
6. Syndromic management of sexually transmitted diseases. A guide for decision makers, Health care workers and communicators World Health Organization Manila 1997.
7. Syndromic managemet of Sexually transmitted infections Altini L, Coetzee D 2005.

14

Vaginal Discharge

A 26-year-old married woman has noticed profuse vaginal discharge which has a offensive smell. She also has mild irritation over vulva and she has had some discomfort in passing urine. Her menstrual history is regular and most recent began 21 days before. There is no past history of sexually transmitted infection and her general health is good. Her vaginal speculum examination reveals greenish frothy discharge with redness of vaginal wall. What treatment you would provide to her?

In this chapter we will learn:
- Causes of vaginal discharge
- Differences between physiological and pathological vaginal discharge.
- Clinical presentation
- Diagnosis
- Treatment

Introduction

Vaginal discharge is a common presenting symptom seen in gynecological practice. Vaginal discharge may be physiological or pathological. Although abnormal vaginal discharge may result from sexually transmitted infections (STIs), vaginal discharge in most instances is not due to presence of an STI.

The term leucorrhoea, literally means, a white discharge. This is a very old term which should be restricted to excessive amount of normal vaginal discharge. The term is going out of fashion as it is very subjective and does not include pathological causes of vaginal discharge.

CAUSES OF VAGINAL DISCHARGE

Physiological Vaginal Discharge

Normal vaginal flora (lactobacilli) colonise the vaginal epithelium and may have a role in defense against infection. They maintain the normal vaginal acidic pH (*see* below). The quality and quantity of vaginal discharge may alter in the same woman in cycles and over time. Physiological vaginal discharge is a white or clear, non-offensive mucous like discharge that varies with the menstrual cycle.

Each woman has her own sense of normality and what is acceptable or excessive for her.

Composition of Physiological Vaginal Discharge

The normal physiological vaginal discharge is composed of:

1. Vulval secretions—From Bartholin's, sebaceous, sweat and apocrine glands.
2. Vaginal transudate—The vaginal wall is lined by stratified squamous epithelium, thus it has no secretory glands. Vaginal discharge is transudate from its cell walls. Maintenance of the normal environment of the vagina depends largely upon the levels of endogenous estrogen, an acidic PH and the presence of lactobacilli. These organisms produce hydrogen peroxide and lactic acid, which also helps to prevent other organisms to grow in the vagina. Microscopically, facultative aerobes and anaerobes remain in low concentration and the dominant organism is lactobacillus. Lactobacillus maintains the pH of vagina in a range of 3.5–4.5.
3. The cervix—The cervical secretions come from the numerous endocervical glands. The characteristic of discharge varies with the different times of the menstruation cycle. The discharge is thin and copious around ovulation and thick and scanty after that.
4. Uterine secretions from the endometrium.
5. Fallopian tubes secretions.

Amount of Physiological Vaginal Discharge

The amount of physiological vaginal discharge in the adult women is such that the introitus feels comfortably moistened, but it is not enough to leave more than an occasional stain on the under garments (1 to 4 ml per 24 hours). The physiological vaginal discharge is normally increased or noticeable in following situations:

1. *Ovulation:* During ovulation there is increased secretion from the cervix. The

Table 14.1: Characteristics of abnormal vaginal discharge

- Heavier than usual
- Thicker than usual
- Pus like
- White and clumpy (like cottage cheese)
- Grayish, greenish, yellowish, or blood-tinged
- Foul- or fishy-smelling
- Accompanied by itching, burning, a rash, or soreness

discharge may be blood stained on the day of ovulation.

2. *Pre-menstrual:* A few days before onset of menstruation, there is an increased secretion from all parts of genital tract.
3. *During pregnancy* there is increased vaginal and cervical discharge.
4. *Sex:* During sexual excitement there is an outpouring of Bartholin's secretions into the vulva.
5. When using estrogen progestogen contraceptive pills.

Physiological discharge may be sufficiently heavy to produce irritation but this does not always mean infection. If the amount of discharge has more in the recent past, specially, if there is accompanying irritation, infection is likely. A blood stained discharge is suspicious and needs investigations (*see* Table 14.1).

Pathological Vaginal Discharge

The causes of vaginal discharge are summarized in Tables 14.2 and 14. 3.

a. *Nonsexually transmitted infections causing vaginal discharge*—Bacterial vaginosis and vulvovaginal candidiasis are common; these conditions are thought to be caused by a disturbance of the normal vaginal flora. They are not sexually transmitted and the male partner does not need to be treated.
b. *Sexually transmitted infections causing vaginal discharge*—*Chlamydia trachomatis, Neisseria gonorrhea*, and *Trichomonas vaginalis* can

Table 14.2: Causes of vaginal discharge

Noninfective	Nonsexually transmitted infections	Sexually transmitted infections
Physiological	Bacterial vaginosis	Chlamydia trachomatis
Cervical ectopy	Candida infections	Neisseria gonorrhea
Foreign bodies, such as retained tampon	Postoperative infections, post abortal sepsis, puerperal sepsis	Trichomonas vaginalis
Vulval dermatitis		
Endocervical polyp, cervical cancer		

Table 14.3: Common causes of vaginal discharge in relation to age

During childhood	During child bearing age	During postmenopausal age
• An infection due to bacteria from the digestive tract • Chemicals in bubble baths or soaps • A foreign body, such as a piece of toilet paper or sometimes a toy	• Bacterial vaginosis • Candidiasis • Trichomonas vaginitis (trichomoniasis of the vagina), which is usually sexually transmitted • Other sexually transmitted infections such as gonorrhea, or chlamydial infection.	• Atrophic vaginitis • Cervical and endometrial cancer

present with vaginal discharge but may also be asymptomatic. These infections are associated with an increased risk of HIV transmission, especially in the developing world.

Fact sheet: Vulvovaginal candidiasis is a common infective cause of vaginal discharge that affects about 75% of women at some time during their reproductive life, with 40–50% having two or more episodes.

Clinical Presentation

The history should include:

1. Features of the discharge such as its timing, color, consistency, smell, and presence of itch (Table 14.4).

2. Pelvic pain and fever which is important features of pelvic inflammatory disease.

3. New or multiple sex partners to identify patients at high risk of a sexually transmitted infection

Table 14.4: Questions to ask women who complain of vaginal discharge

Discharge	Associated symptoms
Onset	Itching
Duration	Soreness
Amount	Dysuria
Color	Inter menstrual or post-coital bleeding
Blood staining	Lower abdominal pain
Consistency	Pelvic pain
Odor	Dyspareunia—superficial and deep
Previous episodes	

4. Contraceptive vaginal ring or IUD use
5. Douching.

The need for examination and investigations is usually determined on the basis of such a history. A vaginal examination using a speculum is often done routinely when a patient presents with vaginal discharge. The character of vaginal discharge may help to reach a diagnosis (*see* below). A bimanual examination is done to evaluate for pelvic mass or cervical motion tenderness.

Following findings are of help to reach a diagnosis:

1. *White curdy discharge* with vulval itching or soreness, erythema/vaginitis, fissuring suggestive of candida infection
2. *Thin, grey/white homogenous discharge* coating the vaginal walls, fishy/offensive odour, not generally sore suggestive of bacterial vaginosis
3. *Yellow, green frothy discharge with fishy/ offensive odor* + pruritus, vaginitis, dysuria suggestive of trichomoniaisis.
4. *Discharge has other appearance* consider other causes such as physiological, foreign body, STI, streptococcal, staphylococcal infections.

Clinical pearls

- A vaginal discharge may be accompanied by itching, redness, burning, and soreness and dysuria.
- Cause of vaginal discharge depends on age.
- Malodorous vaginal discharge is suspicious for the presence of the bacterial vaginosis and trichomoniasis
- Vaginal discharge with pruritus is suspicious for the presence of candidiasis and trichomoniasis.
- Any discharge that occurs in menopausal age requires prompt evaluation

---

Syndromic Management

World Health Organization recommends Syndromic management of vaginal discharge which is based on the patient's symptoms. Treatment is provided without or with few laboratory investigations. A flowchart is used to guide the healthcare provider to the most appropriate treatment for a given set of symptoms and signs in a woman with a specifically defined risk history (*see* Fig. 13.4 in Chapter 13—RTIs).

Investigations

When laboratory facilities are available, a woman with abnormal vaginal discharge should be investigated for gonorrhea, chlamydia, trichomoniasis, bacterial vaginosis, and candidiasis with samples taken from the vagina and endocervix (Box 14.1). After obtaining vaginal discharge, wet mount microscopy is performed by placing a small sample of discharge on 2 separate areas in a slide and adding normal saline to one and potassium hydroxide (10% KOH) to other area. KOH preparation results in better visualization of fungus and yeast elements by dissolving vaginal epithelial cells. Then, after placing cover slips on the slide, these are visualized with a microscope. If Amsel's criteria (*see* Table 13.1 in Chapter 13— Reproductive Tract infections) are met then the diagnosis is bacterial vaginosis or the wet mount reveals Trichomonads then diagnosis is trichomoniasis, and, if budding yeast and hyphae are found the diagnosis is candidiasis. Presence of WBCs without trichomonads or yeast in microscopy may suggest cervicitis or other inflammatory conditions. Patients who are at risk of sexually transmitted infection should be tested for gonococci and chlamydia infections.

Box 14.1

Triple swabs

- High vaginal swab to identify bacterial vaginosis, candida infection and *Trichomonas vaginalis*
- Endocervical swab in transport medium (charcoal or non-charcoal) to diagnose gonorrhea
- Endocervical swab for a chlamydial DNA amplification test to diagnose *Chlamydia trachomatis*

Treatment

The underlying condition is corrected or treated if possible. For example, bacterial vaginosis is treated with antibiotics. Or, if the discharge is accompanied by pelvic pain and/ or cervical motion tenderness, the patient should be treated for PID (*see* Chapter 13). Some general measures can help relieve symptoms, although they do not eliminate an infection.

General measures: The genital area should be kept clean as far as possible. Washing every day with a mild, unscented soap (such as glycerin soap) and rinsing and drying thoroughly are recommended. Changing underwear and bathing or showering once a day may help relieve symptoms. Improved hygiene is particularly useful if the cause is being incontinent or bedbound. Young girls should be taught good hygiene-to wipe from front to back, to wash their hands after bowel movements and urinating, and to avoid fingering the genital area.

Treatment of vaginal infections: The treatment of vaginal infections such as bacterial vaginosis, candidiasis, trichomoniasis, chlamydial and gonococcal infections, are described in detail in Chapter 13 on reproductive tract infections. An outline of treatment is mentioned in Box 14.2.

Box 14.2: Management of vaginal infections

Bacterial vaginosis

Metronidazole 400–500 mg twice daily for five to seven days, or Metronidazole 2 gm as single dose. Intra vaginal clindamycin cream (2%) once daily for seven days, or Intra vaginal metronidazole gel (0.75%) once daily for five days. The infection often recurs and acidic vaginal jelly may reduce relapse rates.
Partner notification not needed

Vulvovaginal candidiasis

Vaginal imidazole preparations (such as clotrimazole, econazole, miconazole-various preparations are available including single dose ones), or fluconazole 150 mg orally as single dose. Partner notification not needed

Chlamydia trachomatis

Doxycycline 100 mg twice daily for seven days (contraindicated in pregnancy), azithromycin 1 g orally in a single dose
Partner notification required

Gonorrhea

Cefixime 400 mg as a single oral dose or ceftriaxone 250 mg intramuscularly as a single dose
Partner notification required

Trichomonas vaginalis

Metronidazole 400–500 mg twice daily for five to seven days OR Metronidazole 2 g orally in a single dose
Partner notification required

Partner notification: Partner notification is considered when vaginal discharge is due to sexually transmitted infections such as Trichomoniasis, chlamydia infections, gonococcal infections. Partner notification of recent sexual contact is essential to prevent and treat sexually transmitted infections including HIV.

Clinical pearl
- Vaginal discharge is caused by non-sexually and sexually transmitted infections.
- Non-sexually transmitted infections may not need treatment, but sexually transmitted ones must be treated and partners notified.

Keywords
Douching: The word "douche" means to wash. Douching is washing or cleaning out the vagina with water or other fluids. Douching can change the delicate balance of vaginal flora and acidic pH of healthy vagina.

EXERCISES

1. Answer the following questions

- What are the characteristics of physiological vaginal discharge?
- What is the composition of physiological vaginal discharge?
- Name the conditions when physiological vaginal discharge increases in amount?
- When do you consider vaginal discharge is abnormal?
- What are the causes of abnormal vaginal discharge?
- How do you clinically examine a woman with abnormal vaginal discharge?
- Describe the syndromic management of abnormal vaginal discharge.
- How do you identify the different causative agents of vaginal discharge through laboratory investigations?
- Outline the treatment of vaginal discharge.

2. Write short notes on

- Wet mount microscopy of vaginal discharge
- Defense mechanism of vagina

3. Fill in the blanks with appropriate word/s

- The pH of vagina is _____ .
- Leucorrhoea is _____ .
- Sexually transmitted infections causing vaginal discharge are _____ , _____ , and _____ .
- White curdy discharge is seen with _____ infection.
- Green frothy discharge with offensive odor is seen with _____ infection.

4. Explain or justify the following statements

- Treatment of vaginal discharge depends on the cause.
- Likely causes of vaginal discharge depend on age.

5. Questions for practical (read the case summary in the beginning of chapter before answering the following questions)

- What is your diagnosis and why?
- What conditions you consider in differential diagnosis?
- What are the other causes of vaginal discharge in a sexually active woman?
- If laboratory facilities are available, how will you investigate her?
- How do you treat her?

Bibliography

1. Management and laboratpry diagnosis of abnormal vaginal discharge. Quick reference guide for primary care, British Infection Associa-tion 2011.
2. Mbilu NK. Essentials of obstetrics and gynecology for clinical officers and midwives volume 2 Writers club press 2002.
3. McMillan A. Sexually transmissible infections in clinical practice a problem based approach. Springer Verlag London 2009.
4. Mitchell H. Vaginal discharge causes , diagnosis and treatment BMJ Volume 328 29 2004.
5. Phelan ST, Chiang S. Obstetrics and Gynecology Hayes Barton Press 2003.
6. Spence D. Mekville C. Vaginal discharge BMJ 2007;335:1147–51.

15

Pruritus Vulvae and Other Vulval Lesions

A 25-years-old married woman has presented with 4 days history of itch in the vulvae and mild vaginal discharge. Her general health is good and she has not had similar symptoms before. Her last menstrual period is 10 days back and she uses combined oral contraceptive pill. Her husband also has had mild itch and redness of his penis, these symptoms usually developing few hours after most recent sexual activity 2 days back. What is your diagnosis?

In this chapter we will learn:
- Etiology of pruritus vulvae
- Clinical presentation
- Differential diagnosis
- Investigations
- Treatment
- Special considerations—Lichen sclerosus, Lichen planus, complications of pubic hair removal, chronic vulval pain, Bartholin's gland cyst and abscess

PRURITUS VULVAE

Introduction

Pruritus vulvae (vulvar itch) is an unpleasant sensation that provokes the urge to scratch vulva to obtain relief. It is itching and irritation of vulvae rather than soreness. Anogenital irritations are a common complaint encountered in gynecological practice and no age group is exempted. In this region pruritus is particularly distressing complaint because attempt to relieve it by scratching is socially unacceptable.

Etiology

Causes of pruritus vulvae include:

- Vulvovaginal candidiasis—Pruritus vulvae is the most common symptom in women with candidiasis and this diagnosis must be high on the list of probabilities.
- Dermatitis—most commonly exposure to irritants, e.g. soap, perfumes, creams, barrier contraceptives, urine. Less frequently, atopic dermatitis may occur in the vulval area. Scratching and rubbing may lead to chronic lichen simplex.
- Shaving, waxing and other methods of hair removal.
- Lichen sclerosus, lichen planus
- Pubic lice, thread worm, scabies
- Viral warts
- Atrophic vulvovaginitis

- Symptoms of more generalized skin lesions, e.g. psoriasis
- Premalignant, e.g. vulval intraepithelial neoplasia (VIN) and malignant conditions of vulva.

Clinical Presentation

Pruritus vulvae is not a diagnosis. It is a symptom of various disorders most of which are benign but sometimes malignant. The cause of pruritus vulvae varies across ages. In young patients infections are most common causes and in postmenopausal age group lichen sclerosus, lichen planus and intraepithelial neoplasia are more frequent than infections.

A thorough history of the mode of onset, duration, associated systemic illness, or change in materials of clothes, soap or powder, hair removal practice or any other vulval disease is asked for.

The clinical presentation of pruritus vulvae may be acute, chronic or recurrent. Acute pruritus vulvae is most frequently due to infections and chronic presentation is often due to inflammatory dermatoses (psoriasis, atopic dermatitis, lichen planus). Examination of vulva may reveal the location of pruritic lesion. If lesions are present in vaginal mucosa, infections are likely causes. Cutaneous lesions are usually related to inflammatory dermatoses. Vulvar intraepi-

thelial neoplasia may involve either the mucosa or the skin of vulva.

The pruritic lesions of the vulva are mainly red or white. The color of the lesion may help to reach to diagnosis (Table 15.1 and Fig. 15.1).

Differential Diagnosis

Pruritus vulvae must be differentiated from vulvodynia. Pruritus vulvae is almost always associated with abnormal visible findings, however in vulvodynia there is chronic vulval pain in absence of any obvious skin condition or infection. In pruritus vulvae scratching may induce excoriation of vulvar skin which may be source of burning pain. However, patient is aware that pain is the consequence of scratching and not the primary symptom.

Investigations

Investigations may include:

1. Bacteriological examination of vaginal secretions and scraping from the skin, if vaginal discharge is a complaint.
2. A full blood count
3. Blood sugar estimation and a glucose tolerance test if relevant
4. Biopsy from the skin of vulva

Clinical pearl: Vulval conditions often impact on sexual function and you may ask specifically, specially in sexually active women.

Table 15.1: Etiology of pruritus vulvae according to color of lesion		
Type of lesion	*Frequent conditions*	*Rarer conditions*
Red	Candidiasis	VIN
	Lichen simplex	Paget's disease
	Psoriasis	Herpes (pre ulcerative stage)
	Lichen planus	Trichomoniasis
		Contact dermatitis
		Tinea cruris
White lesions (leucoplakia)	Lichen sclerosus	VIN
	Lichen simplex	Paget's disease
Dark lesions	Pubic lice	VIN
		Fixed drug eruption

Treatment

Women tend to be very shy about pruritus and often delay treatment. Self medication often makes the condition worse. No treatment should be attempted without full examination of patient, as blind treatment may overlook a serious condition such as an early carcinoma. The help of a dermatologist may be sought in difficult cases. The treatment depends on identification of underlying cause.

Fungal infection should be treated with fungicides such as mycostatin or clotrimazole. Conventional oral antihistamines may help for symptomatic relief. Topical corticosteroid should be prescribed for women with contact dermatitis, lichen sclerosus, lichen planus and symptomatic psoriasis. In addition general advice may include information about soaps, shampoos and other products that may irritate or dry vulvar skin. Occlusive under wear and tight fitting clothes may cause irritation of vulvar area.

LICHEN SCLEROSUS
(LICHEN SCLEROSUS ET ATROPHICUS)

Clinical Presentation

Lichen sclerosus is an inflammatory skin disorder thought to be of autoimmune origin. Lichen sclerosus primarily affect vulval, perineal and perianal skin. Although it may occur in any women in any age, including prepubertal girls, it is most frequently seen in women aged over 50 years. Symptoms include itching, which is often severe and pain. On examination the skin may appear white, and thickened. Fissures and hemorrhages may be present. If the diagnosis is uncertain based on clinical appearance, biopsy may be necessary.

Treatment

Treatment with a topical steroid is not curative but reduces the symptoms to a tolerable limit. Initially a potent corticosteroid ointment, e.g. Clobetasol is used. However, once symptoms start to settle, less potent corticosteroid can

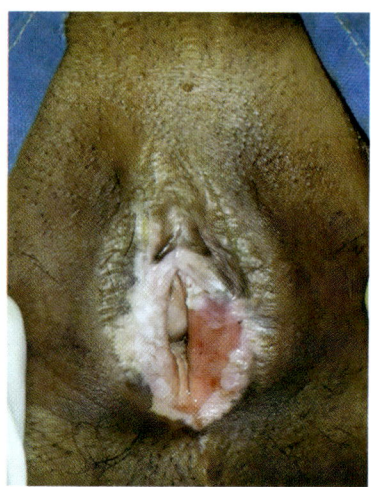

Fig. 15.1: Leucoplakia of vulva with ulceration

be prescribed or frequency of application of potent corticosteroid can be slowly reduced. Lichen sclerosus may be associated with scarring and distortion of genital anatomy. It is also associated with development of vulval intraepithelial neoplasia and invasive squamous cell carcinoma. So the vulval skin may be reviewed at least annually to detect malignancy early.

Lichen Planus

Lichen planus is also an inflammatory condition of autoimmune origin. However, it is less common and unlike lichen sclerosus, lichen planus may:
1. Affect other areas of the body
2. Involve vaginal mucosa
3. Rarely seen in children. Symptoms of lichen planus is similar to that lichen sclerosus, i.e. itching and pain. Scarring and distortion may occur and often more severe than lichern sclerosus. Diagnosis may be confirmed from biopsy.

Treatment is initially same as lichen sclerosus but can be challenging to control, and is more likely to require oral corticosteroids and immune suppressive medicines. Lichen planus is also associated with risk of development of vulval malignancies.

Complications of Pubic Hair Removal

There are many methods used for hair removal such as shaving, depilatory creams, electrical ipilation, waxing, electrolysis, light and laser devices. Complications may include infection, ingrown hairs and contact dermatitis. Most hair removal methods cause micro-trauma to the skin and allow introduction of bacteria from the skin or from items used in hair removal. Shaving or waxing of the pubic hair may cause irritation of the skin or folliculitis. An abscess may also develop and usually presents as isolated tender lump with surrounding folliculitis.

Folliculitis may resolve spontaneously with conservative treatment (warm compress, saline baths) although topical antibiotics may be required in some cases. If there is fever, or other systemic symptoms oral antibiotics should be prescribed. Treatment of an abscess will normally require incision and drainage and/or oral antibiotics depending on clinical presentation.

For ingrown hair, a warm compress can be held over affected area and then the hair lifted free of the skin with a sterile needle. If infections develop topical antibiotic may be required.

Chronic Vulval Pain

Chronic vulval pain affects all age groups; however, it is more common in women of reproductive age. It is frequently associated with sexual dysfunction.

Pain in the vulval area is classified according to whether it is:

- Due to specific disorder—vulval pain from infection, inflammation, neoplasia and neurologic causes.
- Without any evidence of specific disorder—burning discomfort of vulva in absence of specific lesion is described as vulvodynia. This may be localized to vestibule (vestibulodynia) and triggered by contact such as sexual intercourse. Sometimes it may be generalized and persistent when it is more likely to have a neuropathic origin.

A detailed history and physical examination is needed to make an accurate diagnosis of the cause of pain. Diagnosis of vulvodynia is made by exclusion of specific disorders. Treating any underlying lesion usually resolves the pain. Vulvodynia may be difficult to manage. Strategies include an assessment of pelvic floor, use of topical medicines (such as topical application of local anesthetic gels at night or before sexual intercourse) and oral medicines such as tricyclic antidepressants and gabapentin.

Bartholin's Gland Cyst and Abscess

If the duct from the Bartholin's gland becomes blocked a cyst may develop within the duct. Although such obstructions can result from gonococcal infection, other infections and trauma (mediolateral episiotomy, colpoperineorrhaphy) more commonly explain the occlusion. This produces a tense cystic lump, often 1–3 cm in size, which is usually asymptomatic and does not require treatment. During the acute infection, which may precede the actual cyst formation, an abscess often develops with symptoms of tenderness, swelling, and erythema. Incision and drainage bring almost immediate relief to the patient and can be performed under local anesthesia. Marsupialization is the procedure of choice for chronic or recurrent abscesses.

Keywords

Pruritus vulvae: Pruritus vulvae is an unpleasant vulvar sensation that provokes the urge to scratch to obtain relief.

Dermatitis: Some considers, dermatitis and eczema are synonyms, while others consider dermatitis implies an acute condition and eczema a chronic one. The two conditions are often classified together.

Psoriasis: Named for the Greek word psŏra meaning "itch", psoriasis is a chronic, non-contagious, autoimmune disease characterized by inflamed lesions covered with silvery-white scabs of dead skin.

Vulval intraepithelial neoplasia: The term denotes a squamous intraepithelial lesion of the vulva that shows dysplasia with varying degrees of atypia. The epithelial basement membrane is intact and the lesion is thus not invasive but has invasive potential.

Lichen sclerosus: Lichen sclerosus is a skin disease of unknown cause that results in white patches on the skin, which may cause scarring on and around genital skin.

Lichen planus: Lichen planus is a skin condition of unknown origin that produces small, shiny, flat-topped, itchy pink or purple raised spots on skin, genitalia and mouth, especially in middle-aged patients.

Lichen simplex: Lichen simplex chronicus (also known as "Neurodermatitis") is a skin disorder characterized by chronic itching and scratching resulting in thick, leathery, brownish skin.

Paget's disease: Paget's disease of the vulva, a rare disease, usually non-invasive intraepithelial (in the skin) adenocarcinoma, which may be a primary lesion or associated with adenocarcinoma originating from local organs such as the Bartholin's gland, the urethra, or the rectum and thus be secondary. Patients tend to be postmenopausal.

Vulvodynia: Vulvodynia is a term used to describe chronic vulval pain in absence of any obvious skin lesion.

Bartholin's gland: The Bartholin's glands are located on each side of the vaginal opening and produce mucous to assist with lubrication of the vagina.

EXERCISES

Answer the following questions

1. What are the causes of pruritus vulvae and which are common causes?
2. Which clinical characteristics will help you to find out cause of pruritus vulvae?
3. Which investigations you may consider to find out the cause of pruritus vulvae?
4. How do you treat a case of pruritus vulvae?
5. What is lichen sclerosus? How does it clinically present and treated?
6. What are the complications of pubic hair removal and how they are treated?
7. How Bartholin's abscess develops and treated?

Write short notes on

1. Vulvodynia
2. Lichen simplex
3. Chronic vulval pain

Fill in the blanks

1. Common white lesions of vulva associated with pruritus are _____ and _____ .
2. Commonest cause of pruritus vulvae is _____ .
3. Lichen sclerosus is treated with _____ ointment.
4. Lichen planus is differentiated from lichen sclerosus by _____ , _____ , and _____ .

Justify or explain the following statement (s)

1. Pruritus vulvae can be differentiated from vulvodynia by clinical examination.

Questions for practical (read the case summary at the beginning of the chapter before answering the following questions)

1. What is the most likely diagnosis?
2. Name the conditions where pruritus vulvae may be associated with vaginal discharge.
3. What treatment do you offer?
4. What conditions may predispose to acute vulvovaginal candidiasis?

Bibliography

1. Algorithmic diagnosis of signs and symptoms a cost effective approaches. R Doughlas Collins.
2. Hudson CN. Pruritus vulvae Gynecology in general practice British Medical Journal, 1971, 1, 656–657.
3. Pruritus by Laurence Misrey.
4. Textbook of Gynecology by Bhargaba.
5. Transmissible infections in clinical practice: a problem based approach. Alexander Mcmillan.
6. Vulvovaginal health in premenopausal women BPJ Isuue 41, 9–21.

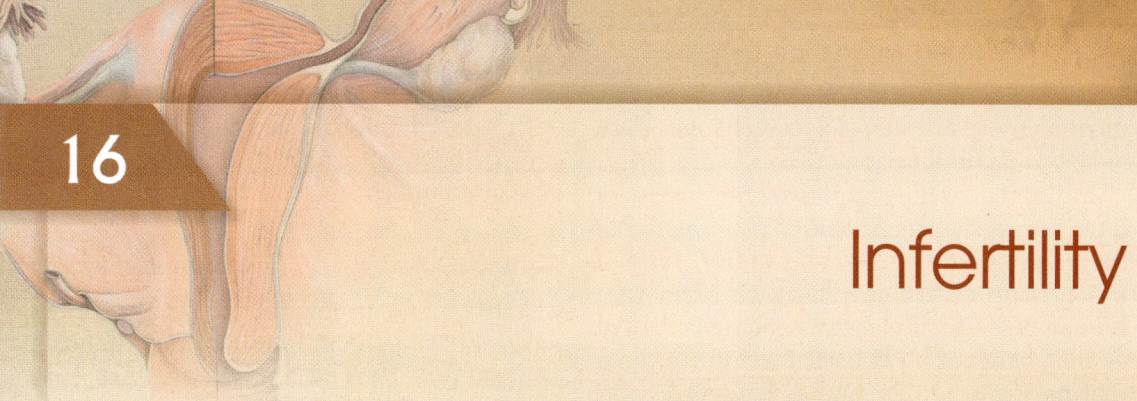

16

Infertility

A 30-year-old P 0+0 woman presents to gynecology outdoor with complaints of inability to conceive. She has been married for 3 years and stopped using contraception 2 years ago. Her menstrual cycles occur regularly every 28 days and are associated with moliminal symptoms (breast tenderness, bloating, and mood changes). She has no dysmenorrhea or dyspareunia. She has no significant medical history, has never had a sexually transmitted disease, and has never had surgery. Her husband is 35-year-old and has a history of hypertension controlled by beta-blockers. How the couple should be evaluated?

In this chapter we will learn:
- Definition, prevalence and causes of infertility
- Factors that are important in history and examination of infertile couple
- Basic and advanced investigations of infertile couple
- Benefits and limitations of different investigations used in infertile couple
- Management of infertile couple

Definition

Infertility is a common clinical problem. It affects 13 to 15% of couples worldwide. Infertility is defined as the failure to conceive after 1 year of regular unprotected intercourse. Sterility implies an intrinsic inability to achieve pregnancy, whereas infertility implies a decrease in the ability to conceive and is synonymous with subfertility. Infertility can be primary or secondary. Primary infertility applies to those who have never conceived, whereas secondary infertility designates those who have conceived at some time in the past. Fecundity is the probability of achieving a live birth in 1 menstrual cycle. Fecundability is expressed as the likelihood of conception per month of exposure. Fertility, as well as infertility, of a woman or couple is best perceived as fecundability, as few infertile patients are sterile.

Epidemiology

The prevalence of women diagnosed with infertility is approximately 13%, with a range from 7–28%, depending on the age of the woman. It has remained stable over the past 40 years; ethnicity or race appears to have little effect on prevalence. However, the incidence of primary infertility has increased, with a concurrent decrease in secondary infertility, most likely as a result of social changes such as delayed childbearing.

In normal fertile couples having frequent intercourse, the fecundability is estimated to be approximately 20–25%. Many, indeed most, couples are surprised to learn that human reproduction is not nearly as efficient as they believed. It is useful to inform them that normally fertile couples having regular intercourse will conceive at a rate of approximately 20% per month, that virtually all pregnancies result from intercourse occurring sometime within the 6-day interval ending on the day of ovulation, and that even when intercourse occurs on the very day of ovulation, the likelihood of achieving pregnancy is no greater than approximately 35%. Approximately 90% of couples with unprotected intercourse will conceive within 1 year (20% within 1 month, 50% within 3 months, and 75% within 9 months). Therefore, most couples should not be subjected to the rigors of an infertility work-up until they have tried to conceive for at least 1 year without success. Sterility affects 1–2% of couples.

> **Fact sheet**
> - Natural human fertility is low, and most couples have falsely high hopes of fertility treatments.
> - With more women pursuing careers and delaying childbearing, infertility is becoming an increasing problem in our society.

Etiology

Infertility can be due to either partner, or both. Overall, an etiology for infertility can be found in 90% of cases with an even distribution of male and female factors, including couples with multiple factors. In general:

- In about one-third of cases, infertility is due to a cause involving only the male partner.
- In another one-third of cases, infertility is due to causes involving both the male and female.
- In the remaining one-third of cases, infertility is due to a cause involving only the female.

In 10% of infertile couples, the etiology cannot be found and a diagnosis of unexplained infertility is made.

General Guidance on Evaluation of Infertility

Infertility is a problem that involves both partners. The consultation is incomplete if only the woman is evaluated. Anxiety is very common, and many couples seek consultation after a few months of unprotected intercourse. Diagnostic testing is unnecessary if the couple has not attempted to conceive for at least 1 year, unless the woman is 35 years old or older, or they have a history of male factor infertility, endometriosis, a tubal factor, pelvic inflammatory disease, or pelvic surgery. A brief explanation of the physiology of reproduction and reassurance are usually enough to lessen the anxiety of the couple.

Infertile couples are usually advised to start their investigations after 12 months of trying to conceive or after 6 months if the female partner is more than 35 years old or immediately if there is an obvious cause for their infertility or subfertility as mentioned before.

MALE INFERTILITY

Definition

The World Health Organization defines male factor infertility as the presence of ≥1 abnormalities in the semen analysis (*see* Table 16.1) or the presence of inadequate sexual or ejaculatory function.

Etiology

Male fertility requires normal sperm production and sperm transport, and adequate sexual performance. The causes of male factor infertility include abnormal spermatogenesis; abnormal sperm transport (reproductive tract anomalies or obstruction); inadequate sexual and ejaculatory functions; and impaired sperm motility.

Causes of Abnormal Spermatogenesis

1. Altered spermatogenesis is probably the most common reason for male infertility and is of unknown etiology (40–50%) in most cases.
2. Factors that alter spermatogenesis (30–40%) through low testosterone levels include obesity, endocrinopathies, and exposure to medicine (e.g., alkylating agents, anti-androgens, cimetidine, ketoconazole, spironolactone), radiation exposure or environmental toxins.
3. Other factors that have a direct deleterious effect on spermatogenesis include varicocele, increased scrotal heat, systemic diseases, smoking, and alcohol intake. Y chromosome deletions and other chromosomal anomalies, such as Klinefelter's syndrome (XXY), are less common causes. Testicular torsion and trauma, orchitis, including mumps orchitis and cryptorchidism can also affect sperm production.

Causes of Abnormal Sperm Transport (10–20%)

1. Ejaculatory duct obstruction may be congenital, such as congenital bilateral absence of vas deferens, or acquired secondary to epididymal or prostatic infections, vasectomy, or complications of surgical procedures (e.g., inguinal hernia repair or orchiopexy for testicular non-descent).
2. Prostatic surgery and some pharmaceuticals may be associated with retrograde ejaculation

Erectile and ejaculatory dysfunction may be associated with psychological factors, hypogonadism, spinal cord disease, and metabolic and vascular conditions such as diabetes.

Impaired sperm motility can be due to immotile cilia syndrome (Kartagener's syndrome) or in the presence of antisperm antibodies.

Evaluation of Male Partner

The main goal of evaluating male factor infertility is to find a correctable cause.

History

Most men with abnormal semen analysis are asymptomatic and have a normal physical examination and normal sexual function. A careful medical and surgical history including the duration of infertility, previous pregnancies, frequency of intercourse, previous treatments, and lifestyle identifies clues to the etiology of male infertility in less than half of the cases.

Key elements of history

Coital practices—infrequent coitus including impotence
Developmental history—cryptorchidism
Medical history (e.g., genetic disorders, chronic illness, genital trauma, orchitis), prior chemotherapy or radiation therapy
Medications (e.g., sulfasalazine, methotrexate, colchicine, cimetidine, spironolactone)
Potential sexually transmitted disease exposure, symptoms of genital inflammation (e.g., urethral discharge, dysuria)
Previous fertility
Recent high fever
Substance use—drug and alcohol abuse
Surgical history (e.g., previous genitourinary surgery)
Toxin exposure

Physical Examination

Physical examination should include the evaluation of secondary sexual characteristics, examination of the penis and spermatic cord, and evaluation of the testicular volume, consistency, and irregularity in the volume. Rectal examination may identify prostatic pathology.

Key elements in physical examination

Genital infection (e.g., discharge, prostate tenderness)
cryptorchidism
Hernia
Presence of vas deferens
Signs of androgen deficiency (e.g., increased body fat, decreased muscle mass, decreased facial and body hair, Tanner stage < 5, small testes)
Testicular mass
Varicocele

Investigations

The diagnosis of male infertility is based on semen analysis performed on 2 occasions 1 month apart.

The specimen is collected after the patient has abstained from any ejaculation at least 2 days (but not >7) through masturbation without any lubricants as they may contaminate the sample. An alternative to masturbation is the use of a semen collection device (a specialised condom kit made from non-toxic materials) during coitus.

WHO Reference Limit for Normal Semen Analysis

Semen analysis is a routine component of the laboratory evaluation of the infertile male. Key parameters assessed by the standard semen analysis include semen volume, total sperm number, sperm concentration, sperm motility, sperm vitality, and sperm morphology [World Health Organization (WHO), Department of Reproductive Health and Research, 2010]. The WHO has recently released revised guidelines for semen analysis, which establish the lower reference limits (Table 16.1). By WHO guidelines, semen samples should be collected after 2 to 7 days of sexual abstinence (WHO, Department of Reproductive Health and Research, 2010). Abstinence periods are important because sperm density increases by 25% for each day

of abstinence, up to four days. The semen specimen has to be analyzed in a laboratory about 30 minutes to one hour after collection. Additionally, at least two samples should be collected and analyzed over a period of several weeks to provide an adequate assessment of the patient's baseline spermatogenesis.

Terminology (WHO)

- Oligospermia is low semen volume.
- Oligozoospermia is low sperm count on semen analysis.
- Asthenozoospermia is decreased sperm motility.
- Teratozoospermia refers to abnormal sperm morphology.
- Azoospermia is absence of sperm in the semen. It can be obstructive or non-obstructive.
- Aspermia is absence of the ejaculate.

Clinical pearl: Semen analysis should be carried out in all cases, and if the result is abnormal it should be repeated.

Endocrine Evaluation

Assessment of FSH, LH, free and total testosterone, oestradiol, sex hormone-binding globulin, and prolactin levels is indicated in men with sperm counts < 10 million sperm/mL (Table 16.2). Low testosterone indicates

Table 16.1: Reference limit for normal semen analysis (WHO 2010)

Standard values for normal semen analysis	
Ejaculate volume	≥ 1.5 ml
pH-value	≥ 7.2
Sperm concentration	≥ 15 million sperms per ml
Total sperm count	≥ 39 million sperms
Motility	≥ 32% progressively moving spermatozoa, ≥ 40% motile sperms (progressive + non progressive)
Morphology	> 4% normal shape
Percentage of living sperms (vitality) (Eosin-test)	≥ 58%
Antisperm antibodies	
Mixed antiglobulin reaction (MAR)	< 50% sperms with particles attached
Leucocytes	< 1 million per ml

Table 16.2: Focused investigations for male partner

Basic investigation

1. Semen analysis (after 2–7 days of sexual abstinence): Interpreted for its volume, sperm count, motility, and morphology according to the WHO reference values (two analyses with 1 months apart at the same lab)

Advanced investigations

1. Hormonal assay: FSH, LH, testosterone, TSH and prolactin (for male with abnormal seminal analysis and suspected endocrine disorder)
2. Testicular biopsy: A fine-needle aspiration biopsy may required to differentiate between obstructive and non-obstructive azoospermia
3. Chromosomal karyotyping: For suspected genetic disorders as sex chromosomal aneuploidy, cystic fibrosis, and deletion of Y-chromosome
4. Post-coital test: No predictive value on the pregnancy rate (*see* below)
5. Anti-sperm antibodies (no evidence of effective treatment to improve fertility), and sperm function tests

hypogonadism. Increased LH and FSH in the presence of low testosterone are signs of testicular failure. Increased prolactin may be due to a pituitary tumour.

MRI of the brain is indicated to rule out pituitary or hypothalamic tumours or other disorders in the setting of hypogonadotrophic hypogonadism.

Testicular Biopsy

A testicular biopsy is performed to determine whether there is any evidence of sperm production. It is suggested for patients who may be candidates for IVF with intracyto-plasmic sperm injection who have evidence of obstruction of the reproductive tracts, or severe oligospermia or azoospermia.

Treatment Approach

The aim of treatment for male infertility is to achieve pregnancy and restore normal reproductive function for the man. However, there are many medical treatments which are empirical and remain of undemonstrated effectiveness.

Medical and Surgical Therapy

1. *Gonadotrophin or GnRH deficiencies:* Men with secondary hypogonadism, such as gonadotrophin deficiency or genetic conditions such as Kallmann's syndrome, can be treated with gonadotrophins or pulsatile GnRH.

2. *Hyperprolactinemia due to pituitary adenoma* can be treated with bromocriptine or cabergoline.

3. *Presence of antisperm antibodies:* Cortico-steroids are used in the presence of antisperm antibodies. However, there is no evidence that these are effective.

4. *Presence of varicocele and no other cause of infertility detected:* Varicocele is treated surgically with varicocelectomy or with embolization of the spermatic veins. Surgical treatment successfully eliminates 90% of varicoceles, but the effect on pregnancy rates is controversial.

5. *Unexplained male infertility:* For men with sperm counts of 10 to 20 million/ml and no endocrine disorder, clomiphene citrate (25 to 50 mg po once/day taken 25 days/mo for 3 to 4 mo) can be tried empirically. Clomiphene, an antiestrogen, may stimulate sperm production and increase sperm counts. However, whether it improves sperm motility or morphology is unclear, and it has not been proved to increase fertility. Supplementation with acetyl L-carnitine and antioxidants such as vitamins C or E are encouraged to enhance sperm maturation and function.

Assisted Reproductive Techniques (ART)

These techniques are recommended when medical/surgical intervention is ineffective, contraindicated, or unlikely to succeed.

The aim of ART is to facilitate oocyte fertilisation and to produce a pregnancy. ART includes insemination with or without controlled ovarian stimulation (COH) (However, according to definition of ART by WHO, IUI is not considered as ART). It also includes in vitro fertilization (IVF) with or without intracytoplasmic sperm injection (ICSI). Unlike conventional IVF, IVF with ICSI allows the sperm to bind and penetrate the zona pellucida of the oocyte. Thus, ICSI drastically improves the fertility prognosis of men who are severely oligospermic or asthenospermic (having decreased sperm motility).

Intrauterine Insemination

IUI is a technique by which a processed semen sample, washed to remove prostaglandins, leukocytes, and nonmotile sperm, is injected via catheter directly into the upper uterine cavity.

Indications

Intrauterine insemination (IUI) is recommended if:

1. The male partner presents with at least 10 million progressively motile sperm/ml in the ejaculate.
2. Normal deposition of semen cannot be achieved through intercourse, whether due to hypospadias, erectile dysfunction, or ejaculatory dysfunction.
3. Men with abnormal semen parameters can also benefit from IUI because the procedure allows sperm to bypass the cervical mucus, thus increasing the chances of conception.

The efficacy of IUI can be increased when combined with controlled ovarian hyperstimulation (COH) (*see* below). If antisperm antibodies are present, the ejaculate is collected directly into sterile sperm wash media in an effort to immediately dilute antibodies present in the seminal fluid. In the case of retrograde ejaculation, sperm can be retrieved from the urine.

If < 10 million progressively motile sperm/ml are present in the ejaculate or artificial insemination has failed, then the couple should be referred for IVF.

Intracytoplasmic sperm injection (ICSI): ICSI should be used for azoospermia or severe oligozoospermia (< 10 million sperm/ml). Some programs advocate ICSI for sperm penetration defects. In the case of azoospermia, sperm can be retrieved from the reproductive tract by testicular biopsy (testicular sperm extraction or TESE) or microsurgical epididymal sperm aspiration (MESA). MESA can only be used for obstructive azoospermia. Microsurgical testicular sperm aspiration (TESA) has also been studied in this regard, as has intrauterine insemination (IUI).

CONTROLLED OVARIAN HYPERSTIMULATION AND INTRAUTERINE INSEMINATION (COH-IUI)

After administering hCG, processed sperm were delivered into the intrauterine cavity and allowed to be propelled naturally to the site of the oocyte. Previous studies revealed that this transport occurred within two minutes.

Indications

Unexplained infertility was the initial indication for COH-IUI. This was later extended to include patients with male factor infertility as mentioned above and some patients with pelvic adhesions (but patent tubes).

Procedure

Beginning early in the menstrual cycle, gonadotropins are administered daily to patients. After approximately 5 days of therapy, ultrasound folliculograms and serum estradiol measurements are performed every 1 to 2 days to determine the dose and frequency of further gonadotropin administration. When three to four mature follicles are detected, human chorionic gonadotropin (hCG) is administered to trigger ovulation. Between 24 and 48 hours after hCG administration, an intrauterine insemination (IUI) is performed.

The sperm is prepared for IUI in a manner similar to that for IVF. After liquification, the ejaculate is diluted with a buffered media and centrifuged. The sperm is thus separated from the seminal plasma when the supernatant is discarded and the sperm-rich pellet is resuspended in media. Processing thereafter varies with the laboratory and sperm characteristics. The sperm suspension may be layered in a sephadex column (Percoll), recentrifuged with media, or allowed to "swim-up" into an overlying layer of media. These procedures are intended to remove non-motile sperm, debris, bacteria, and white cells before intrauterine insemination. They also remove 60–80% of the motile sperm. No technique has proved superior for pregnancy outcome.

Contraindications

Blocked fallopian tubes are a contraindication to COH-IUI because the tubes are required to pick up the oocytes from the ovary and facilitate the mechanical apposition of sperm and oocyte.

Outcome

Although pregnancy rates are to an extent dependent on motile sperm count, pregnancy rates of 10 to 18% per IUI cycle have been reported.

FEMALE INFERTILITY

Etiology

Female infertility has various etiologies including cervical/uterine abnormalities, tubal disease, ovulatory dysfunction, peritoneal factors and unexplained infertility. The most common etiology is ovarian dysfunction.

- *Ovulatory dysfunction (40%):* The causes of ovarian factor infertility are:
  i. Polycystic ovarian syndrome is the most common cause of eugonadotropic anovulation.
  ii. Endocrine disorders (hypothalamic/pituitary amenorrhea, hyperprolactinemia, thyroid disorders, adrenal disorders).
  iii. Premature ovarian failure
  iv. Aging and diminished ovarian reserve

- *Tubal factors (30%):* Tubal factor infertility may result from
  i. Pelvic inflammatory disease resulting in tubal blockage
  ii. Lower abdominal surgery leading to pelvic adhesions
  iii. Tubercular salpingitis
  iv. Previous tubal surgery
  v. Use of an intrauterine device (a rare cause of pelvic infection)
  vi. Any pelvic infection, including appendicitis and diverticulitis, can damage the fallopian tubes
  vii. Endometriosis.

- *Peritoneal factors and endometriosis (15%)*
Adnexal adhesions may result from pelvic inflammatory disease, previous pelvic surgery or endometriosis and may result in infertility. Either may distort pelvic anatomy and interfere with ovum capture or transport.

- *Uterine/cervical abnormalities (3–5%)*
  i. Congenital uterine anomaly
  ii. Submucosal or large intramural leiomyoma may impact implantation or cause tubal obstruction.
  iii. Asherman's syndrome (intrauterine adhesions).
  iv. Poor cervical mucous quantity/quality—Cervical mucus is critical to facilitate sperm entry into the uterus and to initiate

sperm capacitation, the final step in sperm maturation. During the peri-ovulatory period the mucus becomes abundant, thin, and stretchable. Cervical surgery or infection can disrupt the cervical glands and/or mucus production

- *Unexplained (10%)*
  - Unexplained infertility is defined as the failure to conceive after 2 years of regular sexual intercourse in the face of normal investigations (namely normal ovulation, normal semen analysis, patent fallopian tubes).
  - As couples go through the diagnostic and treatment pathways, an increasing number will acquire some form of diagnosis so that the proportion of couples with so-called unexplained infertility will decline.
  - The label of unexplained infertility recognizes that there are numerous candidate sites for abnormalities causing reduced fertility that cannot be recognized by standard diagnostic tests, but ultimately treatment may improve the chance of a pregnancy.

Evaluation of Female Partner

History Taking

Present history: The current problem/complaint, age, occupation, breast changes as milk-like discharges, excessive hair growth with or without acne on face and chest, hot flushes, eating disorders, any current associated medical illness as diabetes and/or hypertension, drug intake prescribed as non-steroidal anti-inflammatory drugs (NSAIDs), sex steroids and cytotoxic drugs or recreational as smoking, alcohol, and caffeine consumption.

Menstrual history: For age of menarche, cycle characteristics and any associated symptoms as painful menstruation or inter menstrual spotting and history of secondary amenorrhea. Menstrual history is the best evidence of normal ovulatory function. In a woman younger than 35 years of age, a history of a regular menstrual cycle is highly correlated with the presence of ovulation. This association is strengthened when menses are accompanied by monthly moliminal symptoms including breast tenderness, bloating, and/or mood changes. A long cycle is often associated with anovulation. In contrast, a short cycle may be associated with anovulation, inadequate follicular phase leading to poor endometrial development, or luteal phase deficiency.

Obstetric history: Previous pregnancies, if any, and its outcome, recurrent pregnancy loss, induced abortion, post-abortive infection or puerperal sepsis.

Contraceptive history: Previous use of any contraceptive method, particularly intra-uterine system, and any associated problems.

Sexual history: Coital frequency, timing in relation to the cycle, use of vaginal lubricant before, or vaginal douching after coitus, loss of libido, as well as, any associated problems as difficult or painful coitus.

Past history: Medical or surgical as pelvic infection, tuberculosis, ovarian cyst, appendicectomy, laparotomy, caesarean sections, and cervical conization.

Family history: For similar problem among the female members, consanguinity, diabetes mellitus, hypertension, twins delivery, breast cancer.

Examination

General examination: Vital signs (especially blood pressure), body height and weight (BMI = ratio between weight in kilograms and height in square meters) for over or under weights, secondary sexual characters, any excessive hairs with/without acne on face or chest, and acanthosis nigricans. Abnormal skin depigmentation as vitiligo may suggest an autoimmune systemic disease. Examination should include also the thyroid gland.

Breast examination: To evaluate its development and to exclude any pathology or presence of occult galactorrhea.

Chest examination: For lungs and heart.

Abdominal examination: For any abdominal mass, organomegaly, ascites, abdominal striae, and surgical scars.

Genital examination: Size and shape of clitoris, hymen, vaginal introitus, size, shape, surface, consistency, mobility and direction of uterus, any palpable adnexal mass, vaginal discharge, tenderness, uterosacral ligament thickening, and nodules in the cul-de-sac denoting either endometriosis or tuberculosis by per-vaginal (PV) examination.

Clinical pearl: For most couples, history and examination will not indicate a cause, and full infertility investigations will be needed.

The Infertility Evaluation

A basic infertility evaluation should include tests aimed at the 4 most important causes of infertility:

1. Abnormalities of semen
2. Ovulatory dysfunction
3. Abnormalities of the uterus and fallopian tubes
4. Reproductive aging.

When the medical histories and physical examination do not point clearly to a specific cause for infertility, the best approach is to begin with tests of semen analysis and ovulation and, deferring invasive diagnostic procedures in the female partner until those are completed (Tables 16.3 to 16.5).

Assessment of Ovulation

Available tests for ovulation are BBT (basal body temperature) monitoring, serum progesterone measurements, urinary luteinizing hormone (LH) monitoring (ovulation predictor kits), and serial transvaginal ultrasonography.

i. Basal Body Temperature (BBT) Monitoring

Basal body temperature has been traditionally used as a means of determining ovulation because progesterone production from the corpus luteum raises core body temperature by approximately 0.2°C (0.6°F) providing a "biphasic" pattern of temperature (body temperature taken each morning upon awakening, before arising, plotted on graph paper). Basal body temperature charting is a simple and inexpensive means of documenting ovulation. In ovulatory cycles, the first morning body temperature often increases from 97°F to 98°F (36.1°C to 36.6°C) to greater than 98°F as a woman's menstrual cycle progresses from the follicular phase to the luteal phase. The rise in temperature is generally noted two days after a surge in luteinizing hormone (LH) occurs. However, it is not a reliable test of ovulation and is cumbersome to undertake effectively. Since there are better assessments of ovulation its use has declined steadily in popularity in recent years.

ii. Serum Progesterone

Serum progesterone measurements are a simple and objective measure of ovulatory function, as long as they are appropriately timed. Levels generally remain < 1 ng/mL during the follicular phase, increase slightly at the time of ovulation, rise steadily thereafter to peak approximately one week after ovulation, and then decline progressively over the week preceding the onset of menses. Luteal-phase progesterone is a retrospective test of ovulation. Serum is assessed 7 days after the presumed day of ovulation, i.e. day 21 in a 28 day cycle (or 7 days before the presumed menstrual cycle). A progesterone value > 9.5 nanomol/L (> 3 nanogram/mL) is indicative of an ovulatory cycle. Some data suggest that a value < 31.8 nanomol/L (< 10 nanogram/mL) is associated with infertility.

Table 16.3: Focused investigations for female partner

Basic investigations

Hormonal assay: To predict ovulation and ovarian reserve. Mid-luteal serum progesterone level (7 days before the expected menstrual cycle). FSH (twice if female age > 35 years, on day 2–4 of the menstrual cycle). urinary luteinizing hormone using home prediction kit, and basal body temperature charting.

Transvaginal ultrasonography: to monitor natural ovulation, to detect any pelvic pathology as uterine or ovarian masses, abnormally-shaped or mal-directed uterus. No need for ultrasound scanning of endometrium Hysterosalpingography or Hysterosalpingo-contrast Sonography (HyCoSy): to evaluate shape of uterine cavity and patency of both fallopian tubes in low-risk women

Advanced investigations

Hormonal assay: Prolactin (if cycles are irregular with/without galactorrhoea or pituitary adenomas). Thyroid function tests (for women with symptoms of thyroid disease). Testosterone, SHBG, DHEA and DHEAS (for suspected cases with PCO syndrome)

Laparoscopy: For possible associated pelvic pathology or adhesions in cases with abnormal HSG findings, previous history of pelvic inflammatory disease or endometriosis

Hysteroscopy: For intrauterine space-occupying lesions detected on HSG as adhesions or polyp (no evidence linking it with enhanced fertility)

Chromosomal karyotyping: For suspected genetic disorders as Turner's syndrome.

Table 16.4: Changes in the basic infertility evaluation over time

	Traditional method	*Modern method(s)*
Semen quality	Semen analysis	Semen analysis
Ovulation	Serum progesterone concentration	Serum progesterone concentration
Fallopian tubes	Hysterosalpingography	Hysterosalpingography
Uterus	Hysterosalpingography	Hysterosalpingography/ sonohysterography
Cervical factor	Postcoital test	No longer recommended
Peritoneum	Diagnostic laparoscopy	Selective diagnostic laparoscopy
Ovarian reserve	Not previously evaluated	Serum AMH concentration

Table 16.5: Timing and coordination of infertility testing

Month 1	*Following 1st visit (barrier contraceptives recommended)*
Day 1	Initiate BBT
Day 3	Serum FSH
Days 7–11	HSG
Days 10–18	LH urine testing
Day 21 (or 1 week after LH surge)	Progesterone level
Days 25–28	Endometrial biopsy (dated to LH surge)
Days 1–28	Semen analysis
Month 2	
Days 12–14	PCT (or at LH surge) in selected cases
	Review test results, confirm diagnosis, and plan treatment or schedule other tests as indicated

iii. Ovulation Predictor Kits

Ovulation can be detected prospectively and accurately with urinary LH prediction kits. This utilises an enzyme-linked immunoassay against the beta sub-unit of LH. LH rises abruptly for approximately 18 hours before it peaks and ovulation typically occurs about 36 hours after the onset of the surge. Because the hormone needs to be conjugated before it is excreted, urinary LH will predict ovulation approximately 24 hours in advance. These tests are more accurate at predicting/demonstrating ovulation than basal body temperature charting. Additionally, this provides a prospective time of ovulation that also can be used to time intercourse.

Reliable use requires that testing be performed daily, usually beginning 2 to 3 days before the surge is expected, based on the overall length of the cycle. Although the test can be positive for more than one day, the first positive test best predicts the time of ovulation and further testing is unnecessary. Although early morning would seem the most logical time to test because urine typically is most concentrated then, results correlate best with the LH surge in serum when the test is performed during the late afternoon or evening (04:00 to 10:00 pm).

iv. Ultrasonography

Serial ultrasound can be used to document follicular growth and ovulation. Serial transvaginal ultrasonography can reveal the size and number of preovulatory follicles and provide the most accurate estimate of the time of ovulation. Serial ultrasonography can document progressive growth of the preovulatory follicle, followed by its collapse, the loss of distinct margins and an increase in internal echoes, and an increase in the volume of fluid in the cul-de-sac.

However, this is expensive and time prohibitive as an initial diagnostic tool. It is commonly used by clinicians to assess ovulation in patients who are receiving ovulation induction with exogenous gonadotropins.

Endometrial Biopsy

The endometrial biopsy may also be used to confirm ovulation and diagnose a luteal phase defect. It is usually performed late in the cycle, 2 to 3 days before expecting menstruation. The sample of endometrium is obtained with a curette from the anterior or lateral wall of the uterine fundus. The histological finding of secretory endometrium confirms ovulation. Luteal phase defect is a histologic diagnosis made when the endometrium lags more than 2 days behind the expected pattern at the time of endometrial biopsy (*see* below).

If ovulation is not confirmed then further diagnostic tests are indicated to establish the cause. These include assessment of FSH and LH (hypergonadotropic or hypogonadotropic hypogonadism), oestrogen levels, free testosterone (polycystic ovarian syndrome or other causes of hyper-androgenism), prolactin (pituitary tumor) with the possible addition of karyotype in the case of elevated gonadotrophins (Turner's syndrome), and other secondary investigations to find out a cause.

Assessment of Tubal Factors

The methods available for evaluating the fallopian tubes include traditional hysterosalpingography (HSG) and laparoscopic "chromotubation".

HSG

The most common test to evaluate reproductive anatomy is hysterosalpingography (HSG). This is the best first-line anatomical imaging test for the basic infertility workup because it evaluates both the uterus and the fallopian tubes. HSG is performed by injecting radio-opaque dye into the uterus and tubes and following the dye with fluoroscopy or radiography. Both water-soluble and oil-soluble contrasts are appropriate, depending on preference. Uterine abnormalities are outlined by the dye, and tubal obstruction is noted by the absence of free-spill into the peritoneal cavity. As a test of tubal patency, HSG is approximately 60% sensitive and 95% specific, meaning that when it suggests obstruction, the tubes are often truly patent, but when it demonstrates patency, the tubes are almost always truly open. The diagnosis of distal tubal obstruction generally is accurate, but apparent proximal tubal occlusions are often not real, representing artifacts of transient uterine contractions, so-called "tubal spasm", or catheter placement (with the tip lying near one tubal orifice). The HSG diagnosis of proximal tubal obstruction must, therefore, be confirmed, either by repeating the study, or by other methods such as chromotubation (Figs 16.1 and 16.2).

In addition to the diagnostic value of the HSG, the test may be therapeutic, i.e. pregnancy rates were increased in infertile women who underwent tubal flushing during HSG. A similar screening technique, hystero-salpingo-contrast sonography (HyCoSy), employs transvaginal ultrasound in combination with a reflective medium injected transcervically, giving a view of the endometrial cavity as well as an assessment of tubal integrity.

Laparoscopic "Chromotubation"

The alternative to HSG for the evaluation of tubal patency is laparoscopic "chromotu-bation". Laparoscopic chromotubation involves the introduction of a dilute solution of methylene blue or indigo carmine through the cervix during laparoscopy, and observing its movement through the fallopian tube. Tubal abnormalities such as agglutinated fimbria or adhesions (which restrict motion of the tubes) or peritubal cysts may suggest tubal disease that would not necessarily be detected on hysterosalpingogram. The diagnosis of endometriosis is usually based on laparoscopic findings.

Chlamydia Antibody Testing (CAT)

Chlamydia antibody testing (CAT) also has some clinical utility for the detection of tubal pathology. The CAT is based on the detection of immunoglobulin-G antibodies resulting from infection with *Chlamydia trachomatis*. Several European studies have suggested that the sensitivity of CAT for detection of tubal pathology approaches that of HSG and laparoscopic chromotubation. At least in theory, the CAT should help to identify women with tubal pathology who might

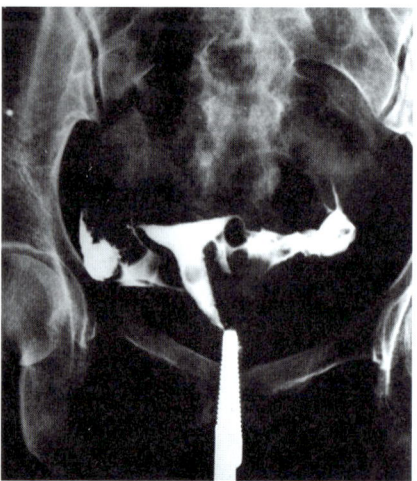

Fig. 16.1: Hysterosalpingogram showing normal uterine cavity with bilateral spillage of dye

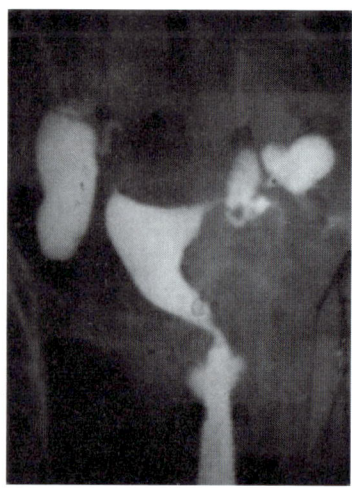

Fig. 16.2: Hysterosalpingogram showing bilateral tubal block with hydrosalpinx

benefit most from more specific tests, such as HSG or laparoscopic chromotubation. However, at present, the diagnostic accuracy of the CAT has not been established and the test is not used widely in clinical practice.

Assessment of Uterine Factors

Uterine factors include abnormalities of the uterine cavity and the disorder known as LPD, long regarded as a cause of both infertility and recurrent pregnancy loss.

Abnormalities of the Uterine Cavity

HSG: HSG has been, and remains, the most common test for evaluation of the uterine cavity. The test readily detects common developmental anomalies of the uterus, such as a septate or bicornuate uterus, although further clarification is required to reliably distinguish the two. HSG also detects other important acquired uterine abnormalities, including intrauterine adhesions, submucous myomas, and most, but not all, significant endometrial polyps. As a bonus, HSG provides useful information regarding tubal patency.

Ultrasonography: Transvaginal ultrasound scan (TVUS/s) will also allow an assessment of uterine structure (although this may require further clarification) including congenital abnormalities, the presence of fibroids and endometrial polyps. Sizeable hydrosalpinges indicating tubal pathology can also be detected. Thus TVUS/s will inform the decision for further detailed pelvic assessment. Additionally this allows the assessment of the ovaries, for evidence of follicular development, antral follicle count, polycystic appearance or the presence of significant cysts including endometriomas.

Saline-infusion sonography (SIS) can be used to follow up on intrauterine abnormalities seen on HSG or to evaluate the uterus when there is no suspicion regarding the fallopian tubes. Traditional ultrasonography is not sensitive enough to determine whether lesions are intracavitary, because the uterus is a potential space. Injecting saline into the uterus to provide a sonographic window within the endometrial cavity allows for better visualisation. The sensitivity and specificity of SIS have both been estimated to be 100% when surgery was used as a definitive test. The advent of 3-dimensional ultrasonography has improved the diagnostic capabilities of ultrasonography.

Hysteroscopy: Diagnostic hysteroscopy is the gold standard among methods for evaluating the uterine cavity, but generally offers few advantages over sonohysterography. Chief among these is that hysteroscopy has greater specificity than sonohysterography, because it distinguishes between endometrial polyps and submucous myomas, which sonohysterography often cannot, but that differentiation also is largely unimportant in the evaluation of infertile women because the finding of any mass lesion generally leads to operative hysteroscopy for excision.

MRI: Uterine abnormalities can also be visualised with MRI scanning (100% specificity and 80 to 100% sensitivity for the evaluation of pelvic anomalies). The production of images in multiple planes makes MRI an excellent preoperative assessment before reproductive gynaecological surgeries such as myomectomy or metroplasty.

Luteal Phase Defect (LPD)

LPD is a disorder classically characterized by a deficiency of corpus luteum progesterone production, in amount, duration, or both. The basic pathophysiological concept of LPD is that inadequate progesterone secretion causes delayed secretory endometrial maturation(out of phase by > 2 days). At least in theory, a severe delay predisposes to infertility caused by failed implantation, due to an unreceptive endometrium However, endometrial histologic dating is no longer recommended for the evaluation of infertility or recurrent early pregnancy loss. Endometrial histology does not reliably reflect the amount or duration of progesterone secretion, varies widely between individuals, between cycles within individuals, and among observers, and lacks the accuracy and precision required for a valid diagnostic test, primarily because it cannot discriminate fertile from infertile women.

Cervical Factors

Postcoital test (PCT): The post coitaltest is utilized to assess the adequacy of the cervical mucus and its interactions with sperm. After intercourse in the late follicular phase (day 12 of the cycle), the female partner is examined within 4 hours and a small amount of cervical mucus is obtained for assessment of spinnbarkeit (stretchability 8–10 cm) and microscopic examination of ferning and sperm motility (at least 5 motile sperm per high power field is considered normal).

However, routine PCT is no longer recommended, for several reasons. First, abnormalities of mucus or sperm-mucus interaction are rarely the primary cause of infertility, and the two most common causes of a "cervical factor" chronic cervicitis and cervical stenosis-can be identified by careful speculum examination. Second, the test is inconvenient and embarrassing for many women. Third, the PCT has no standardized methodology or interpretation and has poor reproducibility, even in specialty centers. Fourth, neither the results of the PCT nor treatment for an abnormal test have any measurable impact on outcomes. Lastly, results of the PCT seldom affect treatment, because contemporary treatments for unexplained infertility-IUI with or without ovarian stimulation and IVF-both "'treat'" any unrecognized cervical factor by bypassing the cervix altogether.

Nevertheless, at a minimum, information is gained about the adequacy of coital technique if a normal post-coital test is obtained. Therefore routine post-coital testing is unnecessary. It may be safely reserved for those few in whom results will clearly affect the treatment strategy.

Peritoneal Factors

Peritoneal factors relating to infertility include endometriosis and adnexal adhesions resulting from previous pelvic surgery or infection. Either may distort pelvic anatomy and interfere with ovum capture or transport. Diagnostic laparoscopy was long considered a routine and essential element of the infertility evaluation, primarily for detection of peritoneal factors that otherwise might escape detection, but the best available evidence indicates that routine diagnostic laparoscopy is neither justified nor cost effective.

Adnexal adhesions can adversely affect fertility without causing gross tubal obstruction, but women most likely to have such adhesions have risk factors, such as previous pelvic infection or a positive CAT, pelvic pain, other evidence of advanced endometriosis, or previous pelvic or adnexal surgery, including myomectomy or ovarian cystectomy in particular. Today, for all of the aforementioned reasons, diagnostic laparoscopy should be performed not routinely, but selectively, limited to those in whom it is most likely to yield findings that will influence the choice of treatment. Laparoscopy has a relatively high yield among women with signs, symptoms, or risk factors for peritoneal disease, and those with an abnormal HSG or transvaginal ultrasonography. In women without symptoms or risk factors having a normal HSG and ultrasonography, and perhaps also a negative CAT, laparoscopy has a very low yield and can be safely omitted.

Ovarian Reserve Tests

Age of the woman is considered as an important predictor of fertility. "Ovarian reserve" is the term used to describe the size and quality of the remaining supply of oocytes. The identification of diminished ovarian reserve is an increasingly important part of the initial infertility evaluation as patients present for diagnostic evaluation later in their reproductive lifespan. Ovarian reserve tests are aimed at identifying women having a "diminished ovarian reserve" (DOR), implying an advanced stage of follicular depletion that may result from normal aging, premature reproductive aging, or from previous ovarian trauma (surgery, radiation, chemotherapy).

There are three measures of ovarian reserve in common clinical use—the basal serum FSH concentration, the serum antimullerian hormone (AMH) concentration, and the "antral follicle count" (AFC) as determined by transvaginal ultrasonography.

The basal serum FSH concentration: As rising FSH levels are one of the earliest indications of reproductive aging in women, it's logical that the serum FSH concentration might be a useful ovarian reserve test, but because FSH levels vary widely across the cycle, the serum FSH concentration is best obtained during the early follicular phase (cycle day 2 to 4, usually on day 3) when concentrations generally are highest. With the assay systems currently in use, FSH levels >10 IU/L have relatively high specificity for predicting poor response to gonadotropins stimulation, but their sensitivity is rather low.

The serum antimüllerian hormone (AMH) concentration: AMH is produced by granulosa cells of preantral and small antral follicles. The serum AMH concentration has value as a measure of ovarian reserve because the number of small antral follicles correlates with the size of the remaining follicular pool; the AMH level falls progressively throughout reproductive life and becomes undetectable near the menopause.

A serum AMH level above 0.5 ng/mL is consistent with good ovarian reserve, while lower levels suggest the presence of a depleted ovarian follicle pool. Levels less than 0.15 ng/mL suggest the patient will have a poor response to IVF.

AMH can be measured anytime during the menstrual cycle and typically demonstrates minimal intercycle and intracycle variability.

Antral follicle count (AFC): Ultrasound examination can be used to determine the number of antral follicles in both ovaries (follicles measuring 2 to 10 mm in diameter). On transvaginal ultrasound, the presence of 4 to 10 antral follicles in early follicular phase (Cycle day 2–day 4) measuring between 2 and 10 mm in diameter suggests good ovarian reserve.

Unexplained Infertility

Unexplained infertility is a "diagnosis" of exclusion and applies when a systematic evaluation fails to identify a cause. The diagnosis requires, at a minimum, documented evidence of ovulatory function, normal semen quality, a normal uterine cavity, and bilateral tubal patency. Women with unexplained infertility also merit ovarian reserve testing to exclude DOR.

Clinical pearl: Most investigations to establish a cause of infertility are simple to undertake.

Treatment of Female Infertility

The treatment of infertility is directed at correcting any pathology and restoring reproductive function. The ultimate goal of treatment is to establish a healthy pregnancy that leads to a healthy live birth. Surgery is not usually performed as the first-line treatment for infertility unless there is a specific indication (other than infertility), for example, pelvic pain.

Clinical pearl: Duration of infertility and age of female partner are the most important factors when making a prognosis for treatment.

Treatment of Anovulation

Ovulation induction is the appropriate treatment for infertile patients who have dysfunction of the hypothalamic-pituitary-ovarian axis. The ovulation induction agents used include clomiphene citrate, hMG, hCG, recombinant FSH, and recombinant LH.

Clomiphene Citrate (CC)

Clomiphene citrate is considered a first-line treatment because of its low cost, relative ease of use, and minimal side effects. Clear indications for clomiphene citrate use include anovulation or oligo-ovulation due to hypo-thalamic pituitary dysfunction (women with PCOS, unexplained anovulation, hyper prolactinemia) and luteal phase defect. Clomiphene citrate has also been used in women with unexplained infertility, although limited data exist to justify such use.

Mechanism of action: Clomiphene citrate is nonsteroidal anti "estrogenic agent" which is recently reclassified as a selective estrogen receptor modulator. It competes for the estrogen receptor at the hypothalamus, pituitary, and ovarian levels. Because of the action at the estrogen-receptor level within the hypothalamus, CC alleviates the negative feedback effect exerted by endogenous estrogens. As a result, CC normalizes the GnRH release; therefore, the secretion of FSH and LH is capable of normalized follicular recruitment, selection, and development to reestablish the normal process of ovulation.

Dosage: The standard dose of CC is 50 mg PO od for 5 days, starting on the menstrual cycle day 3–5 or after progestin-induced bleeding. Ovulation usually occurs 5 to 10 days (mean 7 days) after the last day of clomiphene; if ovulation occurs, menses follows within 35 days of the induced bleeding episode. The daily dose can be increased by up to 50 mg every 2 cycles to a maximum of 200 mg/dose as needed to induce ovulation. Treatment is continued as needed for up to 4 ovulatory cycles. As an antiestrogen, CC requires that the patient have some circulating estrogen levels; otherwise, the patient will not respond to the treatment. The CC response is monitored by using pelvic ultrasonography, BBT chart or urinary monitoring of LH surge (day 12 onwards).

Success rate: Clomiphene successfully induces ovulation in 85% of women, although pregnancy rates are lower than 65%.

Side effects: Because of the antiestrogenic effect, CC may thicken the cervical mucus, creating an iatrogenic cervical factor that can be responsible for the lack of pregnancy in a patient who has otherwise ovulated. Other adverse effects associated with CC are hot flashes, scotomas, dryness of the vagina, headache, and rarely ovarian hyperstimu-lation.

Aromatase Inhibitors

Aromatase inhibitors (letrozole, anastrozole) inhibit the action of the enzyme aromatase, which converts androgens into estrogens by a process called aromatization. As a result, estrogen levels are dramatically reduced, releasing the hypothalamic-pituitary axis from its negative feedback. Aromatase inhibitors are not approved for ovulation induction due to the possibility of fetal toxicity and fetal malformations.

Gonadotropins

Human menopausal gonadotrophin (hMG) contains 75 U of FSH and 75 U of LH per mL, although the concentration may vary (ranges from FSH at 60–90 U and LH at 60–120 U). In the 1980s, a pure form of FSH became available that contains 75 U of FSH.

Indication of use: Gonadotropins are typically used as second-line treatment after selective oestrogen receptor modulation has failed. However, they may be first-line options for patients with hypothalamic amenorrhoea. For women with a non-functioning pituitary gland (e.g., with Kallman's syndrome).

Dosage: For all women with ovulatory dysfunction that does not respond to clomiphene, human gonadotropins (i.e., preparations that contain purified or recombinant follicle-stimulating hormone [FSH] and variable amounts of LH) can be used. Several IM and sc preparations with similar efficacy are available; they typically contain 75 IU of FSH activity with or without LH activity. They are usually given once/day, beginning on the 3rd to 5th day after induced or spontaneous bleeding; ideally, they stimulate maturation of 1 to 3 follicles, determined ultrasonographically, within 7 to 14 days. Ovulation is induced with human chorionic gonadotropin (hCG) 5,000 to 10,000 IU IM after follicle maturation; criteria for induction may vary, but typically, at least one follicle should be > 16 mm in diameter.

Success rate: When exogenous gonadotropins are used appropriately, > 95% of women treated with them ovulate, but the pregnancy rate is only 50 to 75%.

Side effects: Multiple adverse effects and complications may occur during the use of the gonadotropins, including:
1. Multiple pregnancy (24–33%)
2. Ectopic pregnancy (5–8%)
3. Miscarriages (15–21%)
4. Ovarian torsion and rupture
5. Ovarian hyperstimulation syndrome, which is the most severe. Ovarian hyperstimulation syndrome occurs in 10 to 20% of patients; ovaries can become massively enlarged, and intravascular fluid volume shifts into the peritoneal space, causing potentially life-threatening ascites and hypovolemia.

IVF is an appropriate second-line treatment option for anovulatory infertility when conception has not occurred within 6 to 12 ovulatory cycles, or where ovarian hyperstimulation has proved difficult to control.

Clinical pearl: Ovulation disorders often respond to simple treatments that can be safely initiated at primary care.

Treatment of Tubal Factor Infertility

Treatment depends on the type and degree of tubal dysfunction and various approaches are available. These include to less invasive techniques such as transcervical tubal cannulation and selective salpingography, and various microsurgical approaches. However, in vitro fertilization and embryo transfer (IVF-ET) is a viable alternative for all types of tubal dysfunction.

Proximal tubal occlusion: Treatment for proximal tubal occlusion include transcervical tubal cannulation, tubocornual anastomosis, and IVF-ET.

Transcervical tubal cannulation: Reversal of proximal tubal occlusion can be performed under fluoroscopic, or hysteroscopic guidance. Threading of an atraumatic guide wire through the catheter (tubal cannulation) allows for direct mechanical disruption of inspissated material.

Tubocornual anastomosis: With the microsurgical technique, the patent portions of the distal tube and the interstitial tube are reanastomosed using 10X to 20X magnification.

Distal tubal occlusion: Distal tubal disease is treated by IVF and surgical interventions, such as salpingostomy and fimbrioplasty.

Salpingostomy: Salpingostomy can be performed in the setting of adhesive disease, tubo-ovarian abscess, hydrosalpinx, and ectopic pregnancy. The overall pregnancy rate after salpingostomy is only 30% with one quarter of these being ectopic in nature.

Fimbrioplasty: Fimbrioplasty is the lysis of adhesions between fimbrial ends or dilatation of fimbrial phimosis, and thereby attempts to restore fimbrial function. With the use of microsurgical technique, the intrauterine pregnancy and ectopic rates are 59% and 6%, respectively.

Tubal reanastomosis: Female sterilization is the most commonly used method of contraception and woman may request conception following this procedure. Tubal reanastomosis for reversal of sterilization is feasible if adequate residual tube length remains; Sterilization reversal in younger patients has a high success rate and allows for multiple subsequent pregnancies.

In vitro fertilization and embryo transfer versus surgery: IVF-ET completely bypasses the tubal blockage, and offers an almost 30% delivery rate per cycle. As the pregnancy rates from IVF continue to improve, the value of surgical intervention (with increased surgical risk) has diminished. The exception to this may be tubal anastomosis after voluntary sterilisation. However IVF-ET success rates decrease with advancing age, is expensive, and not available to all infertility patients.

Treatment of Cervical Factors

Chronic cervicitis may be treated with antibiotics. Reduced secretion of cervical mucus due to destruction of the endocervical glands by previous cervical conization, freezing, or laser vaporization responds poorly to low-dose estrogen therapy. The easiest and most successful treatment is intrauterine insemination (IUI). Artificial insemination can be performed by depositing the sperm inside the endometrial cavity (intrauterine insemination).

Treatment of Uterine Factors

Until in vitro fertilization became available, a patient with congenital absence of the uterus and vagina (Rokitansky-Küster-Hauser syndrome) had no chance to have a biologic child. Today, it is feasible by using a surrogate mother or gestational carrier. Once patients desire to have children, they proceed with stimulation of the ovaries, oocyte aspiration, and in vitro fertilization, but the embryos are transferred to a gestational carrier (*see* in vitro fertilization).

Lieomyoma Treatment

In general, small and asymptomatic leiomyomas do not require treatment, but the patient should be periodically monitored. Leiomyomas should be treated if they are associated with abnormal uterine bleeding or if they are thought to be the cause of infertility. Uterine leiomyoma may be treated by myomectomy. Depending on the location of the leiomyoma, hysteroscopic or laparoscopic removal may be possible. Otherwise laparotomy is necessary.

Uterine Synechiae

Uterine synechiae are corrected using operative hysteroscopy. The surgery is performed during the early follicular phase. Once the synechiae have been resected, leaving an intrauterine balloon for 7 days is advisable to prevent a recurrence of adhesions. The patient should be prescribed high-dose estradiol (5 mg qd for 21 d) followed by medroxyprogesterone (10 mg for 10 d). A postoperative HSG should be performed 2 months later. In many instances, more than one hysteroscopy is required for total resection.

Endometrial Polyps

Endometrial polyps are removed through operative hysteroscopy associated with a dilatation and curettage, if necessary.

Uterine Anomalies

In uterine anomalies, most problems are related to preterm labor and pregnancy loss rather than infertility. Uterine anomalies such as septate uterus can be corrected through operative hysteroscopy. Ideally, the procedure should be performed during the early follicular phase and under laparoscopic surveillance to decrease the risk of uterine perforation.

Bicornuate uterus and septate uterus are treated with the Strassman metroplasty and the Jones metroplasty. The Strassman metroplasty consists of performing an incision at the fundus of the uterus between both cornual areas and closing the defect with an anteroposterior suture. The Jones metroplasty consists of resecting the septum using an anteroposterior wedge incision and closing the defect in the same direction .

Treatment of Peritoneal Factor, Infertility and Endometriosis

Treatment of Peritoneal Factors

Laparotomy is indicated in patients with severe pelvic adhesions that compromise the bowel, ovaries, and tubes, with obliteration of the cul-de-sac. The aim of the procedure is to correct what is necessary to allow the normal transport of the gametes; complete restoration of the anatomy is not intended. Lysis of adhesions should be meticulous, using hydrodissection and fine instruments. Blunt dissection should be avoided. Constant irrigation with Ringer lactate solution and heparin prevents fibrin formation. Meticulous hemostasis is imperative.

Fimbrial phimosis and periadnexal disease can be treated with laparoscopy. The pregnancy rate after salpingolysis is 50–60% during the first year after treatment. Fimbrioplasty for fimbria agglutination or phimosis without destruction of the cilial epithelium is equally successful. The incidence rate of ectopic pregnancy after surgery is in the range of 5%.

Endometriosis causing pain may be treated with surgical or medical therapy. Surgical extirpation of lesions and adhesions is successful in alleviating pain for endometriosis but is less effective in increasing fertility caused by endometriosis. Medical therapy does not have much effect on the adhesions associated with endometriosis and does not improve fertility in presence of pain. Similarly, endometriomas of the ovary are decreased in size by medical therapy but are rarely completely treated. In vitro fertilization is more effective than either surgery or medicine in increasing fertility caused by endometriosis

Treatment of Unexplained Infertility

Couples with unexplained infertility may conceive without therapy but it may take from 3 to 7 years. To decrease the waiting time, empiric therapy is instituted. Empiric therapy usually begins with parenteral gonadotropin therapy combined with intrauterine insemination. This combined therapy increases the cyclic fecundity over either alone in couples with unexplained infertility. After three or four unsuccessful cycles or alternatively, in vitro fertilization may be offered.

Assisted Reproductive Technology

World Health Organization (WHO, 2009) defines assisted reproductive technology (ART) as all treatments or procedures that include the in vitro handling of both human oocytes and sperm or of embryos for the purpose of establishing a pregnancy. This includes, but is not limited to, in vitro fertilization and embryo transfer, gamete intrafallopian transfer, zygote intrafallopian transfer, tubal embryo transfer, gamete and embryo cryopreservation, oocyte and embryo donation, and gestational surrogacy. ART does not include assisted insemination (artificial insemination) using sperm from either a woman's partner or a sperm donor.

The first successful human IVF attempt resulted in delivery of Louise Brown in England in the 1978 and is considered the beginning of a new era for the treatment of infertility. Since 1981, the understanding of the ovulatory process has been revolutionized and numerous technologies arose in the subsequent two decades: controlled ovarian hyperstimulation (COH-IUI), intracytoplasmic sperm injection (ICSI) and oocyte donation allowed pregnancy in couples without gametes. This section briefly describes the reproductive technologies available to infertile patients and referred to in treatment sections above in the chronological order of their introduction into the therapeutic armamentarium.

IVF indications have departed from the narrow scope of tubal infertility to other indications that were almost impossible to overcome, including infertility related to oligospermia and obstructive azoospermia.

IN VITRO FERTILIZATION (IVF) AND EMBRYO TRANSFER (ET)

In vitro fertilization (IVF) was first successfully performed by Patrick Steptoe, MD and Robert Edwards, PhD in a woman with tubal factor infertility.

Indications

Initially, IVF was indicated in patients with tubal factor infertility. The relatively high success rates have allowed extension to couples with endometriosis, drug-resistant polycystic ovarian disease, and unexplained infertility. Additionally, IVF can be used with donor oocytes to treat women with age-related ovarian dysfunction, ovarian failure or surgically removed ovaries. Combined with ICSI (*see* below) IVF can also be used to treat couples with sperm disorders and immunologic infertility.

Procedure

IVF consists of retrieving preovulatory oocytes from the ovary and fertilizing them with sperm in the laboratory, with subsequent embryo transfer (replacement) within the endometrial cavity. The following steps are required during an IVF cycle:

- Ovarian stimulation
- Follicular aspiration
- Oocyte classification
- Sperm preparation
- Oocyte insemination
- Embryo culture
- Embryo transfer

Ovarian Stimulation for IVF

IVF begins with ovulation induction. A variety of ovulation induction regimens are available. Most programs administer ovarian down regulation with a GnRH agonist in the luteal phase prior to the cycle of stimulation. Oral contraceptives are often added prior to down-regulation. After spontaneous ovarian activity is suppressed, folliculogenesis is stimulated with gonadotropins. The regimen used is particular to each program, but those that have been tested in clinical trials all seem to result in similar pregnancy and delivery rates. Choices are made based on cost, availability, route of administration, and familiarity of the physician with the regimen.

During ovulation induction, the ovaries are monitored for follicular growth by frequent transvaginal ultrasound examinations and serum estradiol concentrations. When clinical parameters suggest the presence of mature oocytes, human chorionic gonadotropin (hCG) is administered to mimic the LH surge and allow further progression of the oocytes through meiosis. Approximately 36 hours later, the patient undergoes a follicular aspiration.

Follicular Aspiration

Most aspirations are performed transvaginally with ultrasound direction. Conscious sedation is typically used. Concomitant identification of the oocyte by nearby laboratory technicians informs the physician to proceed with aspiration of each sequential follicle.

Oocyte Classification

The classification of the oocyte is a crucial step for success with IVF. The follicular fluid is scanned under either a dissecting microscope or an inverted microscope. The oocytes are graded according to the appearance of the corona-cumulus complex. The presence of a polar body (metaphase II stage) and/or germinal vesicle (prophase stage) is a determining factor for the preincubation time prior to the insemination.

Sperm Preparation and Oocyte Insemination

Between 4 and 6 hours after aspiration, the oocytes are mixed with 15,000–30,000 motile, previously prepared sperm. Human fertilization occurs in the next 18 hours.

Embryo Culture

The inseminated oocytes are incubated in an atmosphere of 5% carbon dioxide in air with 98% humidity. Ideally, the presence of 2 pronuclei and the extrusion of a second polar body are the criteria required to ascertain fertilization, which should occur approximately 18 hours after insemination. The fertilized oocytes (embryos) are transferred into growth media and placed in the incubator. No further evaluation is performed over the next 24 hours. A 4- to 8-cell stage pre-embryo is observed approximately 36–48 hours after insemination. A 10- to 16-cell embryo is observed after 48–72 hours. The morula or blastocyst stage is observed after 96–120 hours.

Embryo Transfer

Embryos are then transferred into the uterine cavity typically three or five days later. The American Society of Reproductive Medicine (ASRM) recommends determining the number of embryos to be transferred by patient criteria, with favorable prognosis patients generally receiving no more than 1–2 embryos, and poor prognosis patients of advanced maternal age receiving no more than 5 embryos.

Approximately 2 weeks later a pregnancy test is performed. Because aspiration removes granulosa cells which would otherwise produce the progesterone necessary for endometrial development, many programs support the luteal phase with exogenous progesterone supplementation.

Contraindications

IVF is contraindicated in women in whom pregnancy is contraindicated.

GAMETE INTRAFALLOPIAN TRANSFER (GIFT)

Gamete Intrafallopian Transfer (GIFT) is a procedure that begins in a therapeutic manner similar to IVF, however, when the oocytes are aspirated, they are mixed with sperm and immediately replaced in the patient's fallopian tubes. GIFT requires less laboratory services and expertise than does IVF, but does require the patient to incur the risks of general anesthesia and laparoscopy. With increasing training and availability of IVF laboratory personnel, GIFT is rarely utilized.

Indications

GIFT requires at least one normal, patent fallopian tube. Patients with unexplained infertility are those who benefit most by this procedure.

Contraindications

Patients with abnormal Fallopian tubes are not eligible for GIFT treatment. Any contraindication to pregnancy is a contraindication to GIFT.

INTRACYTOPLASMIC SPERM INJECTION (ICSI)

In the early 1990s the zona pellucida was incised (zona slitting) or treated with hyaluronic acid (zona drilling) to facilitate sperm transgression across it in cases of male factor infertility. Another technique injected sperm under the zona pellucida (sub zonal injection or SZI). Indeed, inadvertent penetration of the cytoplasm and injection of a sperm during a SZI procedure resulted in a pregnancy and became the best treatment of male factor infertility, intracytoplasmic Sperm Injection (ICSI).

Indications

ICSI is indicated for male factor infertility in which the count, motility, or strict morphology is low. The definite parameters will depend upon each program; in general, a sperm density $< 5 \times 10^6$, motility $<20\%$ and strict morphology $<5\%$ are indications. In addition, patients with antisperm antibodies may be best treated with ICSI. For 2008, ICSI also enabled men without sperm in their ejaculate to achieve a pregnancy. Sperm aspirated from the epididymis (MESA) and from the testicle (TESE) may be used for injection.

Procedure

Patients treated with ICSI undergo the same procedures as with IVF except that 5 hours after aspiration, one sperm is injected into each oocyte. The sperm is pretreated to remove it from the seminal plasma and placed in poly vinyl propylpyrrhidol (PVPP) which slows its movement and allows a single sperm to be aspirated into a glass micropipette. The tail of the sperm is frequently broken off to prevent migration from the cytoplasm after injection.

Contraindications

Contraindications to ICSI are those of IVF.

Outcomes of ART

A normal term pregnancy is the ultimate goal of IVF; thus, the pregnancy rate is the best indicator for evaluation of a program.

Success rates for fresh cycles are as follows:
- Overall pregnancy rate per initiated cycle— 35.0%
- Live birth rate per initiated cycle—28.6%
- Live births per oocyte retrieval—31.9%
- Live births per embryo transfer—35.7%

The incidence of miscarriage (spontaneous abortion 15.0%), stillbirths (0.5%), congenital malformation, or chromosome abnormality is similar to that of the general population. Ectopic pregnancy has been reported after IVF due to migration of the embryo through the cornual ostium. Ectopic pregnancy occurs in approximately 0.7% of cases. In some instances, ectopic pregnancy is associated with heterotopic pregnancy.

Keywords

Antisperm antibody: A man can make sperm antibodies when his sperm come into contact with his immune system. This can happen when the testicles are injured or after surgeries (such as a biopsy or vasectomy) or after prostate gland infection. The testicles normally keep the sperm away from the rest of the body and the immune system. The presence of these antibodies is detected by a test called mixed antiglobulin reaction (MAR). A woman can have an allergic reaction to her partner's semen and make sperm antibodies. This kind of immune response may affect fertility .

Sperm motility (progressive and nonprogressive): In evaluating motility, sperm are classified as non-motile, progressively motile or non-progressively motile. A progressively motile sperm swims forward in an essentially straight line, whereas a non-progressively motile sperm swims, but with an abnormal path, such as in circles.

Sperm vitality: Sperm may be alive, but not moving. A specialized staining technique using eosin is applied to determine the percentage of sperm alive. Eosin penetrates the cell membrane of dead cells, staining them effectively. The cell membrane of living cells however is impenetrable for eosin, leaving life cells unstained.

Sperm morphology: This describes the shape of the sperm and is a major aspect for assessing fertility. The sperm cell consists of a head, a midpiece and a tail. The sperm are examined under a microscope and must meet specific sets of criteria for several sperm characteristics in order to be considered normal.

EXERCISES

1. Answer the following questions

- Define infertility.
- What do you mean by primary and secondary infertility?
- What are sterility and fecundity?
- How common is infertility?
- What are the causes of infertility?

- When will you label a couple infertile and start investigations?
- How do you define male infertility?
- What are the causes of male infertility?
- What findings in the male history and physical examination suggest a male infertility factor?
- What is the basic investigation in male factor infertility?
- Describe the lower reference limit of semen analysis according to WHO?
- What do you mean by oligospermia, oligozoospermia, asthenozoospermia, teratozoospermia azoospermia and aspermia?
- Name some advanced investigations for male partner?
- What are the medical and surgical treatment options for male infertility?
- When do you consider IUI and ART for male factor infertility treatment?
- What are the causes of female infertility?
- What findings in female history suggest ovulatory factor infertility?
- What are the tests available for assessment of ovulation?
- What is the procedure for BBT?
- What are the methods available for evaluating tubal factor?
- What are the tests available for assessment of uterine factor?
- What abnormalities can be revealed with HSG?
- What do you mean by "Ovarian reserve"?
- What are the tests available to measure ovarian reserve?
- How anovulatory infertility is treated?
- Name the drugs used for ovulation induction?
- What are the indications for treatment with clomiphene citrate and how it is administered?
- What is the treatment of tubal factor infertility?

- How do treat uterine and peritoneal factor infertility?
- What is ART?
- Describe the role of ART in treatment of infertility.

2. Fill in the blanks with appropriate word/s

- Around 90% of couples with unprotected intercourse will conceive within _____ year.
- Semen analysis should be performed after _____ to _____ days of sexual abstinence.
- Most common cause of female infertility is _____ .
- A progesterone value _____ is indicative of an ovulatory cycle.
- Proximal tubal occlusion can be treated by _____ , or _____ , or IVF-ET

3. Explain or justify the following statements

- Age of the woman is considered as an important predictor of fertility.
- Unexplained infertility is a "diagnosis" of exclusion.

4. Write short notes on

- Controlled ovarian hyper stimulation and IUI
- Post coital test
- Intra cytoplasmic sperm injection (ICSI)

5. Questions for practical (read the case summary in the beginning of chapter before answering the following questions)

- When do you label a couple infertile?
- What are the basic investigations you advise to this couple?
- Is history suggestive of ovulation?
- How will you confirm ovulation?
- What should be the first test to evaluate male partner?
- If semen analysis report shows abnormality what will be your next step?
- What are the advanced investigations for male partner?

Bibliography

1. Adam H Balen, Anthony J. Rutherford Manage-ment of infertility BMJ | 22 SEPTEMBER 2007, VOLUME 335.

2. Carson SA, Mckenzie LJ. Evaluation of Infertility, Ovulation Induction and Assisted Reproduction Endogyn February 2010.

3. Choy,J. Ellsworth P. Overview of Current Approaches To the Evaluation and Management Of Male Infertility Urol Nurs. 2012;32(6):286–294.

4. D J Cahill, P G Wardle. Management of infertility BMJ Volume 325; 6 JULY 2002

5. Esteves S, Agarwal A. Impact of the New WHO Guidelines on Diagnosis and Practice of Male Infertility The Open Reproductive Science Journal, 2011;3:7–15.

6. Fritz AM. The Modern Infertility Evaluation Clinical Obstetrics and Gynecology Volume 55, Number 3, 692–705; 2012.

7. Infertility Evaluation and management ;Women's health and education

8. International Committee for Monitoring Assisted Reproductive Technology (ICMART) and the World Health Organization (WHO) revised glossary of ART terminology, 2009 Fertility and Sterility_ Vol. 92, No. 5, November 2009

9. Kamel MR. Management of infertlile couple : an evidence based protocol. Reproductive Biology and Endocrinology 2010, 8:21.

10. MILLER A J , BOYDEN J W, FREY K A Infertility American Family PhysicianVolume 75, Number 6, March 15, 2007.

11. Nirmupama Kakarla, Karen D. Bradshaw Evaluation and Management of the Infertile Couple Glob. libr. women's med., (ISSN: 1756-2228) 2008; DOI 10.3843/GLOWM.10321.

12. Pinar H. Kodaman, Aydin Arici and Emre Seli. Evidence-based diagnosis and management of tubal factor infertility Current Opinion in Obstetrics and Gynecology 2004, 16:221–229.

13. TB Hargreave, JA Mills. Investigating and managing infertility in general practice BMJ VOLUME 316 9 MAY 1998.

14. Vijayan P. Mashooq Spatial Divisions and Fertility in India International Journal of Population Research Volume 2012.

15. Wendy Kuohung, Mark D. Hornstein Evaluation of female infertility Up To Date February 2011.

17

Endometriosis

32-year-old nulliparous woman presents with a history of progressively worsening menstrual pain that is now causing her distress for most of the month. She finds no relief from ibuprofen and she misses 2–3 days of work each month. She is married for 6 months and her relationship with husband is affected by associated stress and pain during intercourse. On vaginal examination her uterus is of normal size and minimally tender. Recto vaginal examination reveals uterosacral nodularity and exquisite tenderness. What is your diagnosis?

In this chapter we will learn:
- What is endometriosis
- Why it occurs
- Pathophysiology
- Clinical presentation
- Differential diagnosis
- Investigations
- Treatment

Introduction

Endometriosis is defined as the presence of normal endometrial mucosa (glands and stroma) abnormally implanted in locations other than the uterus (outside the endometrium and myometrium). This endometrial tissue possesses the same steroid receptors as normal endometrium and is capable of responding to the normal cyclic hormonal changes. This results in microscopic internal bleeding, with the subsequent inflammatory response, neovascularization, and fibrosis formation. Resulted changes are responsible for the clinical consequences of this disease. Appearance during surgery varies from superficial blebs to infiltrating fibrosis. Direct visualization confirmed by histological examination remains essential for diagnosis.

Etiology

The exact cause and pathogenesis of endometriosis is not clear. Several theories (implantation theory following retrograde menstruation, metaplasia of coelomic epithelium, hematogenous or lymphatic spread, and direct transplantation of endometrial cells) exist that attempt to explain this disease, although none have been entirely proven.

- *Implantation theory following retrograde menstruation:* Early in the 20th century (1927), Samson proposed his implantation theory. The implantation theory proposes that endometrial tissue desquamated during menstruation passes through the fallopian tubes and once it reaches pelvic cavity, the tissue became implanted on peritoneal surfaces and grew into endometriotic lesions. This theory is simple, attractive, and easily explains why endometriosis is most commonly found on the peritoneal surfaces of the ovaries, cul-de-sac, and bladder and why lesions may develop in episiotomies and other incisions. However, this concept fails to explain the low rate of disease compared to such a common event (90% of menstruating women will manifest retrograde flow).

- *Immunologic dysfunction:* An altered immune response to the displaced endometrial tissue has been shown to play an important role as well. Studies have suggested that deficient cellular immunity results in an inability to recognize the presence of endometrial tissue in abnormal locations. Women with this disorder appear to exhibit increased humoral immune responsiveness and macrophage activation while showing diminished cell-mediated immunity with decreased T-cell and natural killer cell responsiveness. Humoral antibodies to endometrial tissue have also been found in sera of women with endometriosis.

- *Metaplasia:* Metaplasia, or the changing from one normal type of tissue to another normal type of tissue, is another theory. The endometrium and the peritoneum are derivatives of the same coelomic wall epithelium. Transformation of coelomic epithelium into endometrial-type glands in response to as yet unknown stimuli could explain endometriosis in unusual sites.

- *Remnant müllerian cells:* Another theory states that remnant müllerian cells may remain in the pelvic tissues during development of the müllerian system. Under situations of estrogen stimulation, they may be induced to differentiate into functioning endometrial glands and stroma.

- *Genetics:* Some women may have a genetic predisposition to endometriosis. Studies have shown that first-degree relatives of women with this disease are more likely to develop it as well. The search for an endometriosis gene is currently under way.

- *Vascular and lymphatic dissemination* suggested by presence of endometriosis in thoracic cavity.

Risk factors for endometriosis include the following:

- Inverse relationship to parity
- Family history of endometriosis
- Early age of menarche
- Short menstrual cycles (< 27 d)
- Long duration of menstrual flow (> 7 d)
- Heavy bleeding during menses
- Delayed childbearing
- Defects in the uterus or fallopian tubes

Fact sheet: It is generally acknowledged that an estimated 10% of all women during their reproductive years (from the onset of menstruation to menopause) are affected by endometriosis. This equates to 176 million women throughout the world, who have to deal with the symptoms of endometriosis during the prime years of their lives. Many remains undiagnosed and thereby not treated. Endometriosis is often labeled as "the missed disease".

Pathophysiology

Endometriosis is an estrogen-dependent disease and, thus, usually affects reproductive-aged women. Ectopic endometrial tissues are most commonly located in the dependent portions of the female pelvis (e.g., posterior and anterior cul-de-sac, uterosacral ligaments, tubes, ovaries), but any organ system is potentially at risk (Fig. 17.1). Transtubal dissemination is the most common route, although other routes, such as lymphatic and vascular channels, have been observed. This may explain how endometrial tissue can be found at distant, noncontiguous locations in the body.

The endometriotic implants are often functional causing pain during patient's menses. Over time, inflammation and scarring may ensue, which may distort the pelvic anatomy causing pain and infertility. As inflammation and scarring progresses patient's pain may be noted at any time during the cycle, not confined to menses.

There are three typical types of endometriotic lesions:

1. Superficial peritoneal and ovarian implants,
2. Endometriomas or chocolate cysts (ovarian cysts that are lined with endometrioid mucosa), and
3. Deep infiltrating endometriosis (complex nodules comprised of endometriotic tissue, adipose tissue, and fibromuscular tissue).

Iatrogenic deposition of endometrial tissue has been found in some cases following gynecologic procedures and cesarean sections (Fig. 17.2).

The ovary is the most common site for endometriosis. Lesions can vary in size from spots to large endometriomas. Endometriomas are cystic endometrial lesions contained within the ovary. The classic lesion is a chocolate cyst of the ovary that contains old blood that has undergone hemolysis. It has an appearance of smooth walled, brown cyst, may be unilocular but often multilocular when >3 cm in diameter. Laparoscopic visualization of ovarian endometriomas has a sensitivity and specificity of 97 and 95% respectively. Because of this ovarian biopsy is rarely required for diagnosis. The cyst may undergo rupture following rise in intra cystic pressure, spilling its contents within the peritoneal cavity. This can cause the severe abdominal pain typically associated with endometriosis exacerbations. The inflammatory response causes adhesions that further increase the morbidity of the disease.

Clinical Presentation

Women are usually nullipara and in reproductive age. There may be family history of endometriosis. The most common symptoms associated with endometriosis are pelvic pain, infertility, and abnormal uterine bleeding. Women usually present with regular, although short, menstrual cycles with

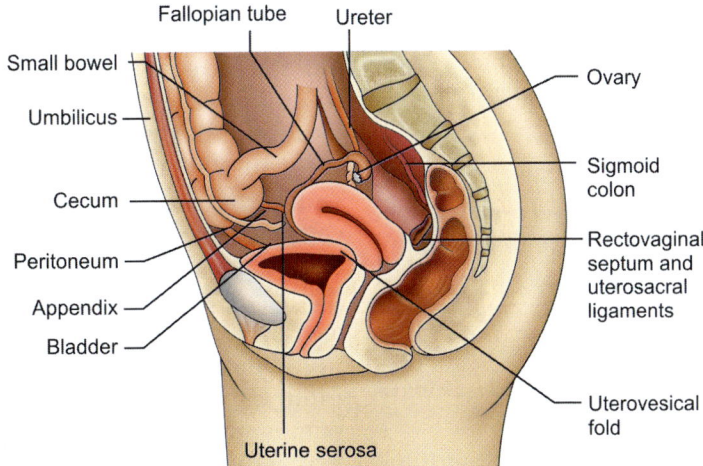

Fig. 17.1: Common locations of endometriosis within pelvis and abdomen (*Source:* New England Journal of Medicine 2001. Olive DL, Pritts EA. Treatment of Endometriosis. Vol. 345:267)

prolonged flow of 8 or more days. Onset of pain usually precedes flow by a few days and begins to resolve 1–2 days into the menses.

Occasionally women may present with endometriotic cyst of one or both ovaries. These masses can become quite painful, and patients with rupture present with an acute surgical abdomen.

Symptoms

Pain

Although pain is common, a significant number of women with endometriosis remain asymptomatic (approximately one-third). The most important point to remember is that the degree of visible endometriosis has no correlation with the degree of pain or other symptomatic impairment. However, pain does correlate with the depth of tissue infiltration, as pain is thought to be related to the degree of peritoneal inflammation rather than the volume of implants. Associated intrapelvic/intra-abdominal adhesions are also important determinants of the degree of pain experienced. Midline disease is generally believed to be more painful than lateral disease. In addition to pain, patients present with nonspecific symptoms of fatigue, generalized malaise, and sleep disturbances. Pain related to endometriosis may present as any of the following:

- Dysmenorrhea
- Dyspareunia (painful intercourse)
- Painful defecation (dyschezia)
- Lower back or abdominal pain
- Chronic pelvic pain (noncyclic abdominal or pelvic pain of at least 6 months duration)
- Painful micturition (dysuria)
- Inguinal pain
- Pain during exercise

Infertility

The next most common symptom is infertility. In women with moderate and severe endometriosis, there is adhesion of ovaries and fallopian tubes with adjacent structures resulting in decreased fertility rates. Interestingly, women with only minimal or mild disease may also have decreased fertility when compared to those without clinical evidence of endometriosis. In the absence of anatomic distortion of the pelvis, the mechanism of infertility associated with endometriosis implants alone is poorly understood. There are three other major theories that may explain the decreased monthly fecundity rates seen in women with endometriosis:

1. Increased incidence of luteinized unruptured ovarian follicle syndrome (trapped oocyte)
2. Increased peritoneal prostaglandin production or peritoneal macrophage activity (resulting in oocyte phagocytosis)
3. Non receptive endometrium (because of luteal phase dysfunction or other abnormalities).

Abnormal Uterine Bleeding

Abnormal uterine bleeding frequently has been associated with endometriosis. Abnormal uterine bleeding may be due to associated anovulation or coexisting pathology.

Other Symptoms

Uncommon symptoms are usually attributable to endometriosis involvement of atypical locations. In addition to bowel implants that can cause rectal bleeding or obstruction, endometriosis can be located in the bladder, causing suprapubic pain, frequency, urgency, dysuria, and hematuria. Ureteral involvement may cause upper urinary tract symptoms such as flank pain or backaches. Pulmonary involvement can result in pleuritic pain, pleural effusion, cough, hemoptysis, or pneumothorax. Cyclic headaches or seizures may indicate brain lesions. Sciatica has been reported from endometriosis in the retroperitoneal space.

Signs

Inspection

Endometriosis of the vagina, perineum, umbilicus, inguinal area, or surgical scars (*see* Fig. 17.2) may be visible as pigmented lesions that have cyclic pain and swelling.

Speculum Examination

Unfortunately, due to the diffuse and often varying nature of endometriotic lesions, the physical examination may not reveal any abnormality. Occasionally, bluish or red powder-burn lesions may be seen on the cervix or the posterior fornix of the vagina. These lesions may be tender or bleed with contact.

Bimanual Examination

Tender nodules may be palpable along the uterosacral ligaments, rectovaginal septum, or within the cul-de-sac, especially if the examination is performed just before menses. A fixed, retroverted uterus and thickened parametrial areas may indicate more advanced disease. Significant cystic formation may be detected as adnexal enlargement or tenderness. Because much disease is found in the dependent areas of the pelvis, a rectovaginal examination is particularly helpful in evaluating the posterior cul-de-sac structures.

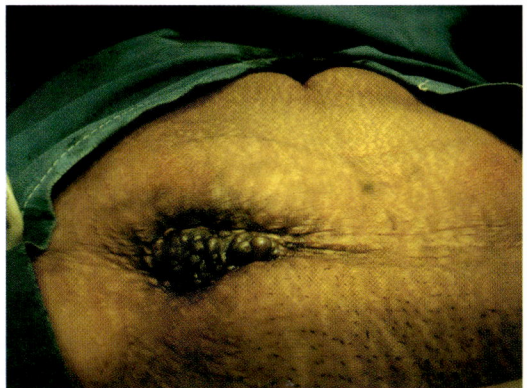

Fig. 17.2: Scar endometriosis—note the pigmented lesion over scar following previous caesarean section

Staging

At the time of laparoscopy, the extent of endometriosis lesions should be assessed to stage the disease. Surgically, endometriosis can be staged I-IV (Revised Classification of the American Society of Reproductive Medicine). The process is a complex point system that assesses lesions and adhesions in the pelvic organs. For the purpose of planning treatment, stages I and II can be combined as "early stage endometriosis" and Stage III and IV can be combined as "advanced endometriosis" (*see* below). However, it is important to note staging assesses physical disease only, not the level of pain or infertility. A patient with Stage I endometriosis may have little disease and severe pain, while a patient with Stage IV endometriosis may have severe disease and no pain or vice versa. In principle the various stages show these findings:

Stage I (Minimal)

Findings restricted to only superficial lesions and possibly a few filmy adhesions.

Stage II (Mild)

In addition, some deep lesions are present in the cul-de-sac.

Stage III (Moderate)

As above, plus presence of endometriomas on the ovary and more adhesions.

Stage IV (Severe)

As above, plus large endometriomas, extensive adhesions.

Differential Diagnosis

The differential diagnosis of endometriosis includes pelvic inflammatory disease, tubo-ovarian abscess, ectopic pregnancy, interstitial cystitis, adenomyosis, pelvic adhesions, uterine fibroids, chronic or acute endometritis, ovarian neoplasms, musculoskeletal disease, gastrointestinal neoplasms, appendicitis, and diverticular disease.

Investigations

Clinical suspicion of endometriosis usually is based on the history and physical examination. Confirmation of endometriosis, however, requires direct visualization and occasionally biopsy, if the surgeon is uncertain of the diagnosis. The initial clinical assessment identifies patients at risk for endometriosis who should undergo further evaluation by laboratory tests, diagnostic imaging, and laparoscopy.

1. Imaging Techniques

a. **Ultrasonography:** Ultrasound examination is the first line investigational tool for suspected endometriosis. It allows detection of ovarian cysts and other pelvic disorders such as uterine fibroids. The usefulness of ultrasonography in detecting focal implants is poor.

Endometriomas have several different ultrasonographic appearances. They usually appear as cystic masses with thick walls and scattered internal echoes. Some endometriomas contain septations, a combination of cystic and solid elements, or primarily solid components and may be indistinguishable from an ovarian abscess or neoplasm. The diagnostic accuracy can be improved by Doppler flow studies.

b. **Magnetic resonance imaging (MRI):** At present, magnetic resonance imaging is the best imaging for identifying endometriosis, and can identify implants as small as 3 mm in size. It can also differentiate benign from malignant lesions, with excellent sensitivity and specificity. Because of the large disparity in cost of an MRI versus a transvaginal ultrasound, physicians may resort to using an MRI in cases of ultrasonographically indeterminate pelvic masses.

2. Laparoscopy

Laparoscopy is the gold standard for the diagnosis of endometriosis. Endometriosis has wide variation in appearance. The classic lesions are blue-black or have a powder-burned appearance. However, the lesions can be red, white, or nonpigmented. Peritoneal defects and adhesions are also indicative of endometriosis. An advantage of surgical diagnosis of endometriosis at the time of laparoscopy is that therapeutic excision or ablation of endometriosis implant can occur at the same time of diagnostic surgery.

3. Histologic Features

Histologic demonstration of both endometrial glands and stroma in biopsy specimens obtained from outside the uterine cavity is required to make the diagnosis of endometriosis. Occasionally, the finding of fibrosis in combination with hemosiderin-laden macrophages is sufficient for a presumptive diagnosis.

4. Laboratory Tests

CA 125—Although serum level of cancer antigen 125 (CA 125) is elevated in moderate to severe endometriosis, its determination is not recommended as part of routine investigation. However, an undiagnosed pelvic mass may be evaluated with CA 125 level as a component of risk malignancy index.

Treatment

Treatment for endometriosis depends on symptom or clinical presentation of the patient. Most women with endometriosis typically present with one or more of the following three complaints:

1. Pelvic pain that interfere with daily activities

2. Infertility
3. A complex adnexal mass due to an ovarian cyst of ovary (endometrioma or chocolate cyst)

Treatment is either aimed at pain reduction, fertility restoration, or evaluating a mass, such as in the case of an endometrioma or chocolate cyst. Unfortunately, there are very few options for treatment of the patient who, both desires fertility and has pelvic pain. Sometimes pregnancy itself will relieve the pain of endometriosis.

There are general points which should be considered when treating a woman to decide which treatment option will be most suitable for her. These should include:

- The severity of the symptoms
- The type of symptoms
- The age of the patient
- The desire to get pregnant or not
- Length of treatment
- Coping with side-effects of drug treatment
- Cost

Endometriosis is an estrogen dependent lesion. The aim of some treatments is to reduce or stop the estrogen being produced in a woman's body, so that it does not continue to feed the endometriotic deposits. This is achieved by hormone drug therapy. This type of treatment is only successful for milder cases of endometriosis where the growths are relatively small and few in number. In more severe cases, treatment with surgery is usually needed to remove the endometriotic lesions. The options for treatment include:

- Observation with no medical intervention
- Medical treatment with NSAID or hormone medication
- Surgery
- Combined treatment

Observation with No Medical Intervention

This approach can be used for milder cases of endometriosis. Analgesics may be prescribed to help with any pain.

Medical Treatment

Medical treatment is indicated in patients with pain or dyspareunia, because no pharmacologic method appears to restore fertility.

Since endometriosis is a chronic disease, it would be most beneficial to use drugs that can be safely used long-term. Dysmenorrhea is one of the most common complaints in women with endometriosis, so many of the hormonal agents aim to cause amenorrhea. These treatments may also relieve deep dyspareunia, non-cyclic pelvic pain, and dyschezia. The drugs that can be used, include Oral contraceptives, progestins, danazol, gestrinone, medroxyprogesterone acetate, and GnRH agonists, aromatase inhibitors and are all supported by clinical trials showing approximately equal benefit . Their side-effect profiles and costs lead one agent to be preferred over another. However, once the agent is discontinued, the symptoms tend to recur.

NSAIDs (non steroidal anti-inflammatory drugs)

Historically, there has been a well-established role for prostaglandin inhibitors, such as ibuprofen, in the treatment of endometriosis-associated pain. However, recent evidences have not shown any benefit in placebo-controlled trials. Despite these evidences, prostaglandin inhibitors are relatively safe, have a tolerable side-effect profile, and can generally be taken on a long-term basis by most patients, so they remain part of the first-line therapy for the treatment of endo-metriosis-associated pain. However, their use is associated with undesirable and potentially severe gastrointestinal side-effects that may limit its use in every patient.

> *Clinical pearl:* A definitive diagnosis of endometriosis can only be made with surgery (laparoscopy/laparotomy). If there is sufficient clinical suspicion of endometriosis, it is reasonable to try empiric therapy with a single agent or a combination of agents.

Oral Contraceptive Pills

These agents have been the mainstay for treatment of pain associated with endometriosis. Oral contraceptive pills (OCPs) suppress LH and FSH and prevent ovulation. They also have direct effects on endometrial tissue, rendering it thin and compact. The decidualization of endometrial implants, coupled with reduced reflux related to lower menstrual volume, is the probable mechanism of pain relief with OCPs, making them comparable to other treatments in effect. Combination OCPs alleviate symptoms in about three quarters of patients. They can be taken continuously (with no placebos) or cyclically, with a week of placebo pills between cycles. The OCPs can be discontinued after six to 12 months or continued indefinitely, depending on such factors as patient satisfaction and the desirability of pregnancy.

Progestational Agents

Progestins are similar to combination OCPs in their effects on FSH, LH and endometrial tissue. They may be associated with more bothersome adverse effects than OCPs and, if a depot form [i.e., medroxyprogesterone suspension (Depo-Provera)] is used, return to fertility may be delayed. Nonetheless, progestins are effective in reducing the symptoms of endometriosis and progestins are much cheaper than either danazol or GnRH analogs. Progestins have been administered in numerous ways and include oral progestins (norethindrone/norethisterone, medroxyprogesterone, and levonorgestrel), depot medroxy progesterone acetate, a levonorgestrel releasing intrauterine device (IUD) and the newer selective progesterone receptor modulators (SPRMs).

The levonorgestrel releasing intrauterine device releases 20 μg/day and induces amenorrhea by causing the endometrium to become atrophic and inactive. It has been shown to improve dysmenorrhea, relieve deep dyspareunia and, as expected, reduce monthly blood loss. Reasons for discontinuation include irregular bleeding, pelvic pain, breast tenderness, and weight gain.

Danazol

Danazol has been highly effective in relieving the symptoms of endometriosis, but adverse effects may not permit its use. Danazol is a synthetic androgen (17α ethinyl testosterone) that inhibits leuteinizing hormone (LH) and follicle-stimulating hormone (FSH), and inhibits ovarian steroidogenesis resulting in a relatively hypo estrogenic state. Danazol occupies receptor sites on sex hormone binding globulin (SHBG) to increase serum free testosterone level and also binds directly to androgen and progesterone receptors. As a result a hyper androgenic, hypoestrogenic state is created resulting in endometrial atrophy and relieving pain from endometriosis. Adverse effects related to estrogen deficiency include headache, flushing, sweating and atrophic vaginitis. Androgenic side effects include acne, edema, hirsutism, deepening of the voice and weight gain. Danazol therapy should be started when the patient is menstruating. The initial dosage should be 800 mg per day, given in two divided oral doses, but this dosage can be titrated down as long as amenorrhea persists and pain symptoms are controlled. Patients with less severe symptoms may be given 200 to 400 mg per day, in two divided oral doses. Treatment duration is six months but can be extended to nine months in responsive patients with severe disease. The overall response rate is 84 to 92 percent, with beneficial effects lasting up to six months after treatment has stopped.

GnRH Agonists

These agents (e.g., leuprolide, gosarelin) inhibit the secretion of gonadotropin and are comparable to danazol in relieving pain. Like danazol, GnRH agonists are contraindicated in pregnancy and have hypoestrogenic side effects. In particular, they have been shown to produce a mild degree of bone loss, although this condition reverses after the medication is discontinued. Because of concerns about osteopenia, "add-back" therapy with low-dose estrogen has been recommended. The dosage of leuprolide is a single monthly 3.75 mg depot injection given intramuscularly. Gosarelin, in a dosage of 3.6 mg, is administered subcutaneously every 28 days. A nasal spray (nafarelin) is used twice daily. The response rate is similar to that with danazol; about 90 percent of patients experience pain relief. The pregnancy rate after the use of these agents is no different from that in untreated patients.

Aromatase inhibitors have recently become part of the armamentarium against endometriosis-associated pain. Aromatase is the enzyme responsible for the conversion of androgens into estrogens. Because endometriosis is an estrogen-dependent lesion and aromatase is responsible for estrogen production, aromatase inhibitors have therefore been employed to alleviate the painful symptoms caused by endometriosis. Combination therapy of an aromatase inhibitor with a progestin, oral contraceptive agent, or GnRH agonist is recommended in the treatment of endometriosis in premenopausal women because of their ovarian stimulatory properties in this population and to prevent pregnancy. Aromatase inhibitors have a tolerable side-effect profile and do not reduce bone mineral density. Table 17.1 summarizes the medical treatment schedule of endometriosis.

Surgery

Surgical treatment of endometriosis is based on two concepts:

1. Surgical treatment of endometriosis lesions can reduce the pain and may improve fertility associated with disease.
2. Surgical removal of both ovaries permanently stops 95% of the endogenous production of estrogen, which will cure the disease but cause surgical menopause.

Surgical treatment for endometriosis is usually indicated in one of the following situations:

- At the time of diagnosis for mild to moderate endometriosis with symptoms
- If medical treatment has not worked or contraindicated
- If infertility is a problem and associated factors like pain or pelvic mass is present
- If there is moderate to severe endometriosis involving bladder, bowel, ureter, pelvic nerves

Table 17.1: Medical treatment of endometriosis

Drug	Dosage	Adverse effects
Danazol	800 mg per day in 2 divided doses	Estrogen deficiency, androgenic side effects
Oral contraceptives	1 tablet per day (continuous or cyclic)	Headache, nausea, hypertension
Medroxyprogesterone suspension in Injection (Depo-Provera)	100 mg IM every 2 weeks for 2 months; then 200 mg IM every month for 4 months or 150 mg IM every 3 months	Weight gain, depression, irregular menses or amenorrhea
Medroxyprogesterone	5 to 20 mg orally per day	Same as with other oral progestins
Norethindrone acetate	5 mg per day orally for 2 weeks; then increase by 2.5 mg per day every 2 weeks up to 15 mg per day	Same as with other oral progestins
Leuprolide	3.75 mg IM every month for 6 months	Decrease in bone density, estrogen deficiency
Gosarelin	3.6 mg SC (in upper abdominal wall) every 28 days	Estrogen deficiency

- If the patient is having acute adnexal torsion or ovarian cyst rupture
- When endometriosis recurs

Surgery can either be conservative or radical. The aim of conservative surgery is to return the appearance of the pelvis to as normal as possible. This means destroying any endometriotic deposits, removing ovarian cysts, dividing adhesions and removing as little healthy tissue as possible.

Radical surgery means doing a hysterectomy with removal of both ovaries and is reserved for women with very severe symptoms, who have not responded to medical treatment or conservative operations.

Laparoscopic Surgery

Because primary method for diagnosis of endometriosis is laparocopy, surgical treatment at the time of diagnosis is an attractive option. The endometriosis spots are destroyed by diathermy, where an electric current is passed down a fine probe burning the lesion. Some surgeons use laser to evaporate the endometriosis. Fine adhesions can be cut using small scissors. Bleeding is usually minimal and having avoided an open operation means that the risk of subsequent adhesion development is reduced. Laparoscopic management also has the advantage of needing a minimal hospital stay, it is usually possible to go home the same or following day.

Where endometriosis is more advanced (stages III–IV), and in particular where there is more severe adhesions or an ovarian endometrioma, there is still the option of laparoscopic treatment. The aim of laparoscopy, as usual, is to restore anatomy back to normal.

Endometrioma resection—Ovarian endometriomas can be treated by drainage (to make a hole in the cyst wall, empty out the 'chocolate' collection of blood and diathermise the cyst base so all endometriotic deposits are destroyed.) or cystectomy (shelling out and removing the cyst from the underlying normal ovary tissue.). Laparoscopic cystectomy was found to yield better pain relief and pregnancy rates than drainage. Endometrioma on the ovary of any significant size (Approx. 2 cm +) must be removed surgically because hormonal treatment alone will not remove the full endometrioma cyst, which can progress to acute pain from the rupturing of the cyst and internal bleeding. Endometrioma is sometimes misdiagnosed as ovarian cysts.

Results of laparoscopic surgery—Surgical removal or destruction of endometriosis implants results in superior pain relief than diagnostic surgery where no implants are removed.

In women with stage I/II endometriosis, laparoscopic ablation of lesions may offer a small, but significant improvement in live birth rates.

In women with stage III/IV endometriosis, surgery is likely to be of benefit and is recommended by some authorities, but there are no randomized controlled trials to document efficacy and some studies show a negative effect of surgery on pregnancy rates.

Radical Surgery

Definitive surgery involves hysterectomy with bilateral salpingo-oophorectomy to induce menopause and ideally removal of all visible endometriotic nodule or lesions. This is indicated in:

1. Women who have significant pain and other symptoms despite conservative treatment and do not desire future pregnancy.
2. Women undergoing hysterectomy because of some other condition such as fibroid uterus.

Combined Treatment

This form of treatment involves combining surgery and drug therapy. An example is when Danazol is taken for 6 weeks prior to an operation to shrink the endometrial growths and ease the surgical removal. Following surgical removal of endometrial tissue, birth control pills may be prescribed that contain both estrogen and progesterone, to be taken continuously for up to nine months. This will induce a pseudo-pregnancy, with the aim to allow the body time to rest and heal.

Prognosis

As all form of current therapies offer relief but no cure, long term concerns are more guarded. The course of endometriosis is impossible to predict at present, and future treatment options should greatly be improved what can now be offered.

EXERCISES

1. Answer the following questions

- What exactly is endometriosis?
- What are the latest theories about the causes of endometriosis?
- How common is endometriosis?
- What are the common locations of endometriosis?
- What symptoms and signs does endometriosis produce?
- How does one diagnose endometriosis?
- What is the differential diagnosis?
- Does endometriosis cause infertility?
- What treatment options are available?
- Medical treatment is appropriate for which group of patients?
- What alternative therapy is available if medical treatment fails or not indicated?
- Who are the candidates of surgical interventions?
- What are the different surgical options in endometriosis?
- What is the definitive therapy of endometriosis?

2. Write short notes on

- Chocolate cyst (endometrioma) of ovary
- Staging of endometriosis

3. Explain or justify the following statements

- Retrograde menstruation is not the only cause of endometriosis
- Minimal endometriosis may cause infertility

4. Fill in the blanks

- Risk factors for endometriosis are _____, _____ , and _____ .
- Commonest site of endometriosis is _____ .
- Differential diagnosis of endometriosis include _____ , _____ , _____ .
- Drugs used for treatment of endometriosis are _____ , _____ , _____ .
- Best investigation to confirm the diagnosis of endometriosis is _____ .
- Chocolate cyst should be treated with _____ .

5. Questions for practical (read the case summary at the beginning of chapter before answering the questions)

- What is your diagnosis and why?
- What are the risk factors of endometriosis present in this patient?
- What are the causes of pain in endometriosis?
- How pain is related with severity of endometriosis?
- What are the differential diagnoses?
- Name the investigations you consider for this patent.
- Which investigation will confirm the diagnosis of endometriosis?
- How do you treat her?

Bibliography

1. Alford CE, Taylor RN, Decherny AH Endometriosis Endotext . com July 2010.
2. Blueprints Obstetrics and Gynecology.
3. Callaghan D. Endometriosis–an update Australian Family Physician Vol. 35, No. 11, November 2006.

4. Dunselman GAJ, et al. ESHRE guideline: management of women with endometriosis Human Reproduction, Vol.0, No.0 pp. 1-13, 2014

5. Endometriosis available at www.medstudents.com.br/ginob/ginob3.htm

6. Endometriosis available at www.mhprofessional.com/.../0071472576_chap10.pdf - United States

7. Endometriosis Diagnosis and management SOGC JOGC JUILLET 2010.

8. Endometriosis Up to Date

9. Investigation and management of endometriosis Green Top guideline no 24 2008.

10. Jenice Ryden, Paul D, Blumenthal Practical Gynecology: a guide for the primary care physician.

11. Mounsey AL, et al. Diagnosis and management of endometriosis Am Fam Physician 2006;74:594–600, 601–2.

12. Obstetrics and Gynecology by Mark Morgan

13. Obstetrics and gynecology the essential of clinical care.

14. Rajob V Gala, Alfa Omar Diallo. Endometriosis Patient encounters—the obstetric and gynecology workup.

15. Soder PR. Endometriosis Obstetrics and Gynecology.

16. Wellberry C. Diagnosis and Treatment of Endometriosis Am Fam Physician 1999 Oct 15;60(6):1753–1762.

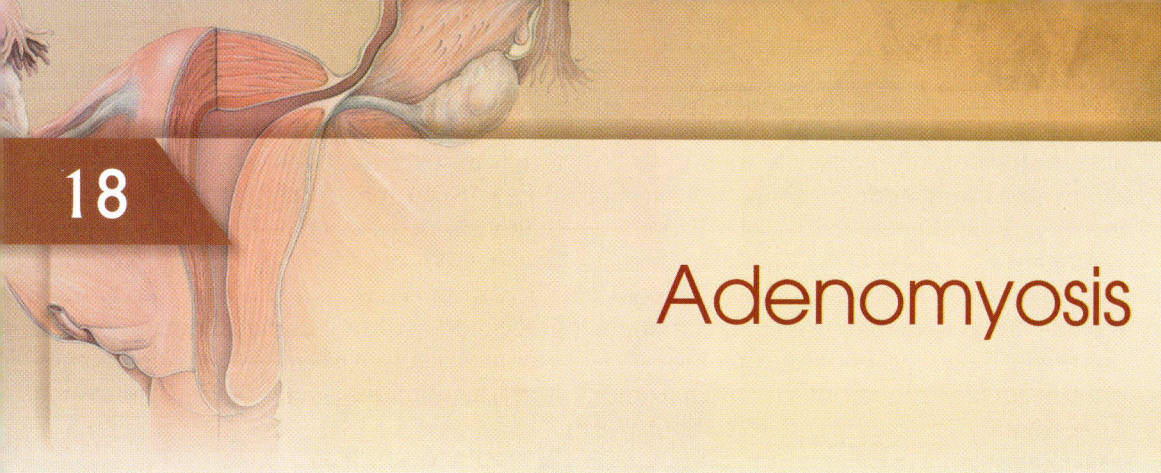

18

Adenomyosis

A 42-year-old P 4+0 woman has presented with excessive menstrual blood loss and progressive painful menstruation for last six months. She is moderately anemic. On pelvic examination, the uterus is enlarged to 12 weeks size pregnant uterus and the uterus is soft, globular and mildly tender without any mass felt through fornices. How will you investigate her?

In this chapter we will learn:
- What is adenomyosis
- Its pathophysiology
- Risk factors
- Clinical presentation
- Investigations
- Differential diagnosis
- Treatment

Introduction

Adenomyosis is perhaps the most infrequently investigated of all gynecological disorders. In this condition, endometrial glands and stroma are displaced within the uterine myometrium. The displaced endometrial tissue may be localized to a discrete mass termed as adenomyoma or be seen as diffusely scattered island of abnormal tissue throughout the myometrium (diffuse adenomyosis). The endometrial tissue is frequently (not always) surrounded by myometrium that has undergone hyperplasia and hypertrophy. Thus adenomyosis may be defined as the benign invasion of endometrium into the myometrium, producing a diffusely enlarged uterus which microscopically exhibits ectopic non-neoplastic, endometrial glands and stroma surrounded by the hypertrophic and hyperplastic myometrium. The term *adenomyosis* is derived from the terms *adeno-* (meaning gland), *myo-* (meaning – muscle), and *-osis* (meaning *condition*). Previously it was named as *endometriosis interna*. But adenomyosis is actually different from endometriosis and these two disease entities are found together in only 10% of the cases.

Pathophysiology

The precise etiology and the developmental events leading to adenomyosis is unknown. Two major theories exist for the origination of adenomyosis. One is de novo development from müllerian rests which is supported by observation of adenomyosis in müllerian remnants lacking endometrium. The second theory is that adenomyosis is derived from endometrium. All organs in human body that contains a cavity also possesses a submucous region with exception to uterus. It is thought that main function of submucous coat is to prevent inward growth of glands that lines these cavities. The disruption in continuity of basal layer and myometrium may occur during caesarean section and repeated delivery.

Gross Pathology

The uterus is uniformly enlarged (12 weeks of pregnant uterus size) and globular in shape. On cross-section, the haphazardly distributed hypertrophied muscular trabeculae is seen surrounding the foci of adenomyosis. Adenomyosis foci, on occasion, may contain brown staining old blood corresponding to hemolyzed blood and hemosiderin pigment deposits. The focally involved uterus with adenomyosis is termed as adenomyoma and often resembles appearance of uterine leiomyoma. Typically adenomyoma has poorly defined margins as they merge with surrounding normal myometrium. So adenomyoma can not be enucleated like leiomyoma (Fig. 18.1).

Microscopic Pathology

Histologically and by immunohistochemistry, both the endometrial glands and stroma in foci of adenomyosis resemble the basalis endometrium. Unlike endometriosis it seldom respond to hormonal stimuli, a phenomenon which explains why one sees occasionally hemorrhagic or reparative morphological events in foci of adenomyosis.

Risk Factors

Traditional belief is that adenomyosis is a disease of older parous women. However, this observation is influenced by diagnosis of adenomyosis in hysterectomy specimen. When radiologic criteria are used for diagnosis, disease can be found in all women irrespective of ages including adolescents. The other risk factors that have been associated with adenomyosis include prior uterine surgery (caesarean section, myomectomy), endometriosis and uterine leiomyoma.

Clinical Presentation

History: Around thirty percent of patients with adenomyosis are asymptomatic or have minor symptoms so that medical care is not asked for.

Age and parity: Symptomatic adenomyosis occurs most often in parous women between age 35 and 50.

Symptoms: The most frequent symptoms are menorrhagia, secondary dysmenorrhea and metrorrhagia. Occasionally dyspareunia may be an additional symptom. Patients typically present with increasingly heavy or prolonged menstruation (menorrhagia). The cause of menorrhagia may be due to:

1. Poor contractility of the adenomyotic uterus to stop menstrual blood loss
2. Altered prostaglandin synthesis
3. Associated anovulation and endometrial hyperplasia.

Patient may also complaint of progressive dysmenorrhea that may begin 1 week before onset of mens and last until cessation of menstruation. Other symptoms may

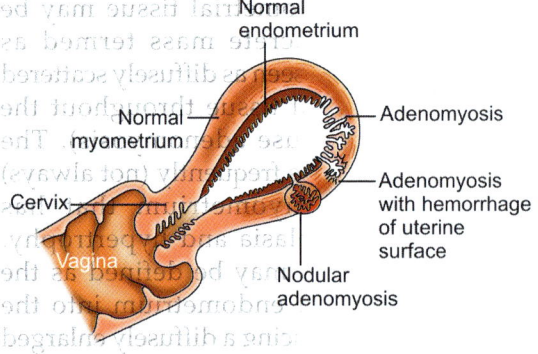

Fig. 18.1: Focal and diffuse adenomyosis

include pressure symptoms due to pressure on bladder or rectum by an enlarged uterus.

Signs

General examination may reveal varying degree of pallor due to menorrhagia.

Per abdominal examination—Uterus may be palpable

Pelvic examination may reveal an uniformly **enlarged globular uterus**. The uterus can be 2–3 times normal size but is usually < 14 cm. The consistency of the uterus is typically softer, and boggier than the firm, rubbery uterus containing uterine leiomyoma. The adenomyomatous uterus may be mildly tender just before and during mens but should have normal mobility and should not have any adnexal pathology.

Investigations

Pelvic Ultrasound

Ultrasound is usually the first and often the only imaging modality employed to investigate menorrhagia and dysmenorrhea. Unfortunately the sonographic features of adenomyosis are variable, and may be absent. Transabdominal ultrasound has limited diagnostic value. Trans vaginal ultrasonography has better accuracy to diagnose adenomyosis than transabdominal ultrasonography. The spectrum of findings includes (a) normal appearing uterus and (b) focal or diffuse bulkiness, typically of the posterior wall. When an adenomyoma is present, then appearances may closely mimic those of intrauterine leiomyoma, which may also co-exist.

Pelvic MRI

MRI is the modality of choice to diagnose and characterize adenomyosis, and has a very high diagnostic accuracy with a sensitivity of ~ 78–88% and a specificity of ~ 67–93%. However because of the cost, MRI may be prohibitive and ultrasonography may be the initial investigation.

Differential Diagnosis

The differential diagnosis includes disease processes resulting in uterine enlargement or menorrhagia or dysmenorrhoea. The conditions that are considered in differential diagnosis of adenomyosis are uterine leiomyoma, Polyps, endometrial hyperplasia, endometrial cancer, menstrual disorders, pregnancy and adnexal mass.

Clinical pearl: A definitive diagnosis of adenomyosis can only be made by histological examination of uterus.

Treatment

Hysterectomy

Hysterectomy is the most commonly employed treatment of adenomyosis as the results of medical treatment is often unsatisfactory. Although focal adenomyomas occasionally can be successfully removed, hysterectomy is the only treatment known to be highly (100%) effective.

Medical Treatment

The treatment of adenomyosis depends on severity of symptoms. At present medical therapy of adenomyosis can be attempted for symptomatic relief, especially in premeno-pausal women with mild symptoms and in women who wish to become pregnant. Nonsteroidal anti-inflammatory drugs, oral contraceptive pills, and menstrual suppression with progestins (oral, injectable or intra-uterine) or continuous combined oral contraceptives have found to be helpful. However, adenomyosis is less responsive to hormone therapy than endometriosis.

Other Treatments

Only a small number of women with adenomyosis have been treated with uterine artery embolization (UAE), and the results so far have been disappointing. According to a recent study, the progesterone-containing IUD (Mirena) can help with dysmenorrhea in about 70% of women. The IUD probably works because it slowly gives off progesterone directly to the lining cells in the uterus and in the uterine muscle wall.

Keywords

Adenomyosis: An extension of endometrial tissue into the uterine myometrium leading to menorrhagia, metrorrhagia and dysmenorrhoea. The uterus becomes soft and globular. The definitive treatment is hysterectomy.

Adenomyoma: A well circumscribed collection of endometrial tissue within the myometrium.

EXERCISES

1. Answer the following questions

- What is adenomyosis?
- How adenomyosis differs from endo-metriosis?
- How adenomyoma differs from leiomyoma?
- What are the risk factors of adenomyosis?
- Which investigations will help you to diagnose adenomyosis?
- What are its symptoms and signs?
- Name the conditions that may mimic presentation of adenomyosis?
- Which investigations are of help to diagnose adenomyosis?
- How do you treat adenomyosis?
- Who are the candidates of the medical treatment?
- How effective is medical treatment?

2. Write short notes on

- Adenomyoma
- Etiology of adenomyosis

3. Explain or justify the following statements

1. Adenomyosis is best diagnosed by histo-pathologial examination of hysterectomy specimen
2. Hysterectomy is the definitive treatment of adenomyosis.

4. Fill in the blanks with appropriate word/s

a. Typical symptoms of adenomyosis are _____ , _____ , and _____ .
b. In regard to parity adenomyosis is more common among _____ women.
c. _____ is the initial investigation in adenomyosis.
d. Differential diagnosis of adenomyosis includes _____ , _____ , and _____ .

5. Read the case summary at the beginning of the chapter before answering the questions

a. Identify the risk factors of adenomayosis present in this patient.
b. What are the differential diagnosis?
c. How do you investigate her.
d. What measures you take to correct anemia?
e. How you treat her menstrual abnormali-ties?

Bibliography

1. Adenomyosis Blueprints Obstetrics and Gynaecology.
2. Adenomyosis Obstetrics and Genecology The essential of clinical acre.
3. Benagiano GP, Brosen IE, Carrara S. Adenomyosis *Glob. libr. women's med., (ISSN: 1756-2228)* 2010; DOI 10.3843/GLOWM.104.
4. Delieger R, et al. Uterine adenomyosis in the infertility clinic Human Reproduction Update, Vol.9, No.2 pp. 139±147, 2003.
5. Ferencyzy A. Pathophysiology of adenomyosis Human reproduction update 1998 Vol 4 no 4 312-22.
6. Harris L Kohen Mimi C Berman Obstetrics and Genecology.
7. Paolo Vercellini. Chronic pelvic pain.
8. Sadhana Gupta A comprehensive text book of gynecology.
9. Wood C Surgical and medical treatment of adenomyosis, Human reproduction update 1998 Vol 4 no 4 323–336.

19

Chronic Pelvic Pain

A 35-year-old P 2+0 woman has presented with 3 years history of lower abdominal pain along with dyspareunia and dysuria. She has been seen by two physicians previously, tried an oral contraceptive pill and Ibuprofen and had laparoscopy twice to relieve her pain. Currently pain has become more severe in intensity so that she takes seven days off per month from her job. She was sexually abused by a close male relative at age of 16. She is otherwise in good health but having disturbed sleep and mildly depressed mood. Physical examination reveals diffuse lower abdominal tenderness. On bimanual examination she has tenderness on palpation through fornices in one side and tenderness on movement of cervix. How her case be managed?

In this chapter we will learn:
- Definition of chronic pelvic pain
- Causes of chronic pelvic pain
- Approach to diagnosis
- Management of chronic pelvic pain
- Sources of chronic pelvic pain

Introduction

Chronic pelvic pain in women is one of the most common and difficult problems encountered by gynecologist. Chronic pelvic pain accounts for about 1 in 10 out patient gynecology visits and is a common indication for laparoscopy. Chronic pelvic pain is defined as pain lasting for at least 6 months and localized at pelvis, the anterior wall at or below the umbilicus, lumbosacral back or buttocks, that is of sufficient severity to cause functional disability or lead to medical care. However, when pelvic pain is related to pregnancy or malignancy or who experience pain only around menstruation (dysmenorr-hea) or during sexual intercourse (dyspare-unia) are usually excluded from the chronic pelvic pain diagnosis.

Causes

Chronic pelvic pain may arise from any structure in or related to the pelvis, including the abdominal and pelvic walls and not uncommonly the cause of pain is multi-factorial. Furthermore, in some women no definitive diagnosis can be made. Table 19.1 provides a list of causes of chronic pelvic pain.

Table 19.1: Causes of chronic pelvic pain

Gynecological diseases: (1) Uterine causes—Adenomyosis, chronic endometritis, cervical stenosis, endometrial or cervical polyps leiomyoma, symptomatic pelvic relaxation (genital prolapse), intrauterine contraceptive device (2) Extrauterine pelvic causes—Endometriosis, adhesions, adnexal cysts, chlamydial salpingitis, endosalpingiosis, ovarian retention syndrome (trapped ovary syndrome) residual ovary syndrome (ovarian remnant syndrome), ovulatory pain, pelvic congestion syndrome, pelvic inflammatory disease, postoperative peritoneal cysts, residual accessory ovary, subacute salpingo-oophoritis, tuberculous salpingitis

Gastrointestinal diseases: Colitis, chronic constipation, diverticular disease, inflammatory bowel disease, irritable bowel disease, chronic intermittent bowel obstruction.

Genitourinary diseases: Chronic urinary tract infection, interstitial cystitis, radiation cystitis, recurrent cystitis, recurrent urethritis, urolithiasis, urethral curuncle.

Musculoskeletal disorders: Abdominal wall myofascial pain (trigger points), compression fracture of lumbar vertebrae, faulty or poor posture, fibromyalgia, mechanical low back pain, chronic coccygeal pain, muscular strains and sprains, pelvic floor myalgia (levator ani spasm), piriformis syndrome, rectus tendon strain, hernias (e.g. obturator, sciatic, inguinal, femoral, spigelian, perineal, umbilical)

Neurologic disorders: Neuralgia/cutaneous nerve entrapment (surgical scar in the lower part of the abdomen; usually iliohypogastric, ilioinguinal, genitofemoral, and lateral femoral cutaneous nerves), herpes zoster infection, degenerative joint disease, disk herniation, spondylosis, abdominal epilepsy, abdominal migraine, neoplasia of spinal cord or sacral nerve

Psychological and other disorders: Personality disorders, depression, sleep disorders, sexual and/or physical abuse

Diagnosis

Nowhere is the history more important than in assessing patients with chronic pelvic pain. A detailed history is important because of complex etiology and often the presence of multiple causes in same patient. It is crucial to get a detailed chronologic assessment of the problem. Perform a detailed review of systems, including reproductive, GI, musculo-skeletal, urologic, and neuropsychiatric. A thorough past history is also important to avoid repeating invasive and expensive procedures (Table 19.2).

Physical Examination

Physical examination should proceed slowly and gently because both the abdominal and pelvic part of examinations may be painful.

Abdominal examination may identify areas of tenderness, presence of masses or other anatomical findings that aid in the diagnosis. Palpation of outer pelvis and back may reveal trigger points that indicate a myofascial

component to the pain. Testing for Carnett's sign should be performed by placing a finger on the painful, tender area of the patient's abdomen and having the both legs off the table while lying in supine position (Fig. 19.1). A positive test occurs when pain increases during this maneuver. A positive test indicate that cause of pain is within the abdominal wall (myofascial pain, e.g. fibromyalgia). A visceral pain should not worsen during this maneuver.

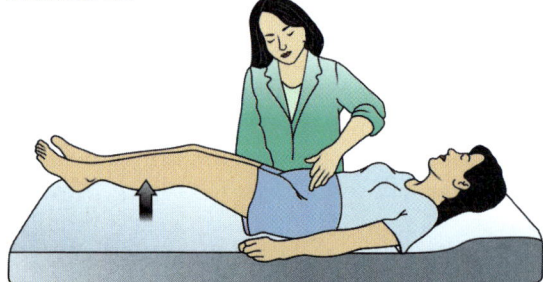

Fig. 19.1: Testing for Carnett's sign—The examiner places his/her finger on the tender area of patient's abdomen and asks the patient to raise both legs off the table. An increase in patient's pain during this maneuver is considered a positive test

Table 19.2: Key elements in history

History of pain: A detailed history of the pain is required including its character, location, radiation, duration, severity, aggravating and relieving factor, relation to menstrual cycle, bowel and urinary functions, physical activity, and its impact upon activities of daily living and personal relationship. Salient features of pain in relation to disease process are: (i) Pain that varies with the menstrual cycle is more likely to be adenomyosis or endometriosis, (ii) pain that worsens following sexual intercourse may be due to pelvic congestion syndrome, (iii) pain that worsens later in the day or with activity may represent fibromyalgia, (iv) bladder pain or irritative voiding symptoms may represent interstitial cystitis once bladder infection has been ruled out.

History specific to different systems: Gynecological—Excessive bleeding with menses suggests uterine leiomyomas or adenomyosis. Women with adenomyosis have higher levels of dysmenorrhea, pelvic pain, depression than women with uterine leiomyoma. History of previous surgery may suggest intra-abdominal or pelvic adhesions. Having multiple sexual partners is a risk factor for pelvic inflammatory disease.

Urologic: A detailed history to evaluate the urological system is important. Patients with interstitial cystitis report urgency and increased frequency of urination as the most distressing features.

Gastrointestinal: Presence of sigmoid adhesions are common in women with chronic pelvic pain and frequently are associated with GI symptoms.

Musculoskeletal: History of vaginal delivery with prolonged second-stage, episiotomies or tears may suggest pelvic floor relaxation disorder.

Neurologic: Constant burning pain is a common complaint in patients with pudendal neuralgia. Patients may report vulvodynia but usually not dyspareunia.

Psychologic: Obtain sufficient history to evaluate depression, anxiety disorder, somatization, physical or sexual abuse, drug abuse or dependence, and family problems, marital problems, or sexual problems. Sexual abuse occurring before age 15 years is associated with later development of chronic pelvic pain.

Pelvic examination should begin with single digit one handed examination. The patient should be checked for any nodule, masses, or point tenderness along the bladder or other musculoskeletal structures. Once single digit one handed examination is completed, a bimanual examination should be performed to check again for nodularity, tenderness, cervical motion tenderness, or lack of mobility of uterus.

Rectal examination may show rectal or posterior uterine masses, nodularity or pelvic floor point tenderness.

Clinical pearl: Thorough history taking that generates trust between physician and patient and a pain-focused physical examination should be part of complete evaluation of the patient with chronic pelvic pain.

Investigations

The investigations performed for women presenting with chronic pelvic pain will depend upon the history and physical examination findings. It is reasonable however, to support the use of following basic laboratory studies in all (or most) women presenting with chronic pelvic pain.

1. Complete blood count
2. Urine microscopic examination, culture and sensitivity
3. Endocervical swab for Chlamydia and culture and sensitivity.

Other selected investigations may include:
- *Ultrasound scan of pelvis (in particular trans vaginal ultrasonography)* when a mass is found in pelvis, ultrasonography is effective in evaluating pelvic masses (uterine or ovarian), in distinguishing solid and cystic masses. Doppler studies evaluate the vascular characteristics of the lesion.
- Laparoscopy is indicated in patients with chronic pelvic pain in whom a pelvic abnormality is suspected, the goal being to find and treat contributory conditions.

- *Magnetic resonance imaging (MRI):* MRI is useful noninvasive tool for diagnosing pelvic masses. It is useful in diagnosis of deep endometriosis, adenomyosis, endometriomas.

Treatment

Treatment should be directed at the underlying cause of chronic pelvic pain.

In patients for whom a specific diagnosis is not made, the empiric use of NSAIDs, oral contraceptives, and antibiotics, antispasmodics are indicated. Women who fail to respond to empiric therapy highly likely to have endometriosis, or adenomyosis and further diagnostic (laparoscopy) or therapeutic (GnRH) interventions should be directed toward the high likelihood of these diagnosis. A multidisciplinary approach (i.e. addressing social, dietary, environmental, psychological factors in addition to standard medication therapy) has been shown to improve outcome over medication therapy alone. Table 19.3 lists specific details regarding the most common medications used in treatment of chronic pelvic pain.

For pain that appears to be cyclic in nature, hormonal treatments (continuous or cyclic COC, progestins, GnRH agonists) should be considered, even if the cause is thought to be IBS, interstitial cystitis, pelvic congestion syndrome, because these conditions may also respond to hormonal therapy.

Although selective serotonin uptake inhibitors have not been shown to be effective for treatment of chronic pelvic pain, they may be used to treat concomitant depression.

Surgical Therapies

Among surgical therapies, only lysis of severe adhesions has been shown to benefit patients with chronic pelvic pain. Total abdominal hysterectomy showed some benefit in observational and cohort studies. Pre sacral neurectomy along with ablative therapy for endometriosis, has shown benefit in treatment of dysmenorrhea that is centrally located in pelvis but this finding can not be generalized to chronic pelvic pain.

Table 19.3: Common medications used for treatment of chronic pelvic pain

Treatment	Comment
NSAIDs	No study shows benefit for treatment of chronic pelvic pain
	Recommendation from experts /consensus opinion only
Combined oral contraceptive pill	Evidence supports use in patients with dysmenorrhea. No quality study show benefit in patient with chronic pelvic pain
Oral medroxy progesterone acetate 50 mg daily	Only medication with evidence showing some benefit in most patients with chronic pelvic pain
Depot medroxyprogesterone 150 mg IM every 3 months	Studies only show benefit in patients with chronic pelvic pain related with endometriosis
GnRH agonists (i.e. Goserelin)	Goserelin is effective for pelvic congestion syndrome and has longer duration of effect than medroxyprogesterone. Monitor patient for bone density loss.
LNG-IUS	One study supports benefit of patients with chronic pelvic pain related with endometriosis.
Danazol	Use for six months only; associated with high incidence of side effects.

Clinical pearl: Chronic pelvic pain cannot always be precisely diagnosed or cured, however, all women require reassurance that their pain can be managed and psychological support can be provided.

Sources of Chronic Pelvic Pain

Endometriosis

Although the data suggest an association between endometriosis and chronic pelvic pain, severity of endometriosis does not correlate with severity of pain. The pain is thought to be due to inflammation. Endometriosis associated CPP may be managed with an estrogen progestogen combination, a progestin alone, danazol, or a GnRH hormone agonist, with or without NSAIDs. Hysterectomy with bilateral salpingo-oophorectomy is generally regarded as most effective procedure for treatment of CPP associated with endometriosis.

Endosalpingiosis

It is the presence of ectopic fallopian tube like epithelium without stroma. The distribution and gross appearance of the lesions of endosalingiosis are the same as endometriosis.

Pelvic Inflammatory Disease (PID)

PID is a common condition that carries several long term sequelae, one of which is CPP. Although the pelvic adhesions are thought to be the cause of pain, the exact etiology remains unknown. A history of previous sexually transmitted infection, menstrual irregularity, dyspareunia, back ache, pelvic pain with fever is often obtained in women presenting with CPP due to PID. PID should also be considered as possible cause of CPP in women with late sequelae of PID (e.g. infertility, ectopic pregnancy), in women with adnexal tenderness/thickening (usually bilateral), cervical motion tenderness, or mucopurulent cervical discharge demonstrated on pelvic examination or in women whose endocervical swabs demonstrate an infective cause.

Appropriate antibiotics are recommended if PID is suspected.

Adhesions

Intraperitoneal adhesions are caused mainly by surgery and to a lesser extent by endometriosis and abdominal and pelvic inflammation or infection. It is thought that adhesions may be a cause of pain, particularly on organ distention or stretching. Dense vascular adhesions are likely to be cause of chronic pelvic pain, as dividing them appears to relieve pain. However adhesions may be asymptomatic.

Residual Ovarian Syndrome (ovarian remnant syndrome)

It is a condition in which a small amount of ovarian tissue is inadvertently left behind following oophorectomy which may become buried in adhesions. The treatment is removal of all ovarian tissue or ovarian function suppression using a GnRH agonist.

Trapped Ovarian Syndrome (ovarian retention syndrome)

This condition is characterised by recurrent pelvic pain or persistent pelvic mass after hysterectomy. In this condition a retained ovary following hysterectomy is buried in dense adhesions. The treatment is same as residual ovarian syndrome.

Pelvic Congestion Syndrome

Dilated pelvic vein have been observed in some women with chronic pelvic pain. Symptoms may include a dull aching pain as well as menstrual disturbances. Vulvar varicosities may be associated. Pelvic venography, Doppler ultrasonography, and MRI have been used to diagnose pelvic congestion syndrome. Treatment may include use of analgesic, ovulation suppression using oral contraceptive pills or continuous medroxyprogesterone in milder cases.

Hysterectomy as a management option of pelvic congestion syndrome has fallen out of favor. Ovarian vein ligation and percutaneous embolization of ovarian vein have been shown to be successful in relieving CPP.

Interstitial Cystitis

Interstitial cystitis (IC) is a clinical syndrome characterized by chronic urinary urgency and frequency, usually with suprapubic discomfort or pressure and usually relieved by urinating. In contrast to bacterial cystitis that results from an infection in the bladder, no infectious organism has been identified in women with interstitial cystitis. There may be breakages in the glycosaminoglycan layer of the bladder, exposing the underlying mucosa to the urine. Medical tests that help identify other conditions include a urine analysis, urine culture, cystoscopy, biopsy of the bladder wall. Medical management includes medication to protect the lining of bladder such as pentosan. Other medicine that are used includes antidepressant drugs, gabapentin, hydrodistenton at the time of cystoscopy can be very effective in properly selected cases.

Irritable Bowel Syndrome

Irritable bowel syndrome (IBS) is a symptom-based diagnosis characterized by chronic abdominal pain, discomfort, bloating, and alteration of bowel habits. IBS is a functional disorder and it has no known organic cause. Irritable bowel syndrome may represent the dys regulation of the enteric neural plexus potentially involving serotonin receptors. Treatment of IBS especially during exacerbation is centered along with excellent doctor patient relationship with drugs targeting the predominant symptoms.

EXERCISES

1. Answer the following questions

- Define chronic pelvic pain.
- Where is pelvic pain localized?

- What percentage of visits is for chronic pelvic pain?
- What are its causes?
- What are some common extrauterine gynecologic causes of chronic pelvic pain?
- What are some common uterine causes of chronic pelvic pain?
- How do you clinically evaluate a patient with chronic pelvic pain?
- What aspects of physical examination are important in evaluation of chronic pelvic pain?
- What laboratory studies are important for chronic pelvic pain?
- What imaging modalities are useful in the evaluation of chronic pelvic pain?
- How do you treat a case of chronic pelvic pain?
- What are the medical options for treatment of CPP?
- What are the surgical treatment options for CPP?

2. Write short notes on

- Carnett's sign
- Pelvic congestion syndrome

3. Fill in the blanks

- Pelvic pain related to _____ , _____ and _____ are usually excluded from definition of chronic pelvic pain.
- Only medication with evidence showing benefit in most women with CPP is _____.

4. Explain or Justify the following statement

- Thorough history and physical examination is essential in evaluation of CPP.

5. Questions for practical (read the case summary before answering the questions)

- What are the differential diagnoses?
- What laboratory investigations would you recommend to reach the diagnosis?
- How she should be treated if no specific diagnosis is made?

Bibliography

1. Consensus guideline for chronic pelvic pain J Obstet Gynecol Can 2005;27(8) 781–801.

2. Fraquhar C, Latthe P Chronic pelvic pain etiology and therapy Review in gynecological and perinatal practice 6;2006;177–184.

3. Guidelines on chronic pelvic pain European Association of Urology 2010.

4. Ortiz D Chronic pelvic pain in women American Family Physician vol 77 no 11;2008 1536–1542.

5. The initial management of chronic pelvic pain Royal College of Obstetricians and Gynecologists Guideline no 41 2005.

20

Uterine Leiomyoma (Fibroid, Myoma, Fibromyoma)

A 32-years-old woman, P 2+0 complains of an abdominal mass with excessive menstrual blood loss with irregular cycles. Her last menstrual period was 3 weeks ago and her previous period was 2 weeks prior to that. She had two normal deliveries and following her last childbirth she underwent bilateral tubal ligation. On general examination she was moderately anemic. A firm nodular mass is palpable in lower abdomen and estimated to be equivalent size of 20 weeks pregnancy. The mass is somewhat mobile side to side but up and down mobility is restricted. She is having no ascites. On pelvic examination the mass moves in continuity with cervix. What is the probable diagnosis?

In this chapter we will learn:
- Etiology and risk factors of uterine leiomyoma
- Classification of uterine leiomyoma
- Its pathology
- Degenerative changes
- Clinical presentation
- Differential diagnosis
- Investigations
- Treatment

Introduction

Uterine leiomyoma are also known as fibroids, myomas, and fibromyomas. Leiomyomas are well circumscribed, pseudo-encapsulated benign tumors composed of smooth muscles and fibrous connective tissues. Leiomyomas are most common uterine neoplasm as well as most common neoplasm found in female pelvis. They are present in 20–40% of women of 35 years of age or older. However, they often remain asymptomatic and do not require treatment. Leiomyomas may be single but most often they are multiple.

Etiology

The precise cause of leiomyomas remains unknown. Following are probable causes:

a. Cytogenetic studies suggest that leiomyomas take origin from single neoplastic smooth muscle cell; in other words they are monoclonal tumors resulting from somatic mutation. A number of chromosomal abnormalities have been identified (chromosomes 6, 7, 12, 14) suggesting a genetic role in pathogenesis of these tumors.

b. Hormones affect growth of leiomyoma. Evidence suggests that estrogen is promoter of growth of leiomyoma. Evidences are:

1. Leiomyomas are rarely found before puberty and stops growing after menopause.
2. New leiomyomas rarely develop after menopause.
3. Leiomyomas often grow rapidly during pregnancy
4. Gonadotropin releasing hormone agonists create a hypoestrogenic state and causes shrinkage of leiomyoma.

c. Local and paracrine factors such as blood supply and proximity of other tumors, may account in variation in tumor volume and rate of growth. In addition some peptide growth factors such as epidermal growth factor (EGF) may play an etiologic role and estrogen may exert its effects through EGF.

Risk Factors

Known risk factors for leiomyomas are black race, positive family history, nulliparity, and obesity. Uterine leiomyomas are thought to have an incidence in black women threefold that of white women. There is an association between nulliparity and the incidence of leiomyomas. The relative risk of leiomyomas decreases with an increasing number of term pregnancies. A woman with five term pregnancies has a 25% reduction in a risk for leiomyoma compared with a nulliparous woman.

Women weighing 70 kg or more have an almost threefold risk of developing leiomyomas compared with women weighing less than 50 kg. Obesity increases the risk of developing leiomyomas by 21% for each 10 kg weight gain.

Smoking, oral contraception use, and the use of depot medroxyprogesterone acetate, a progesterone derivative, have all been associated with protecting against the growth of leiomyoma.

Classification

Uterine leiomyomas are sometimes classified by where they grow in the uterus. However, these tumors may be found outside uterus including fallopian tube, vagina, round ligament, uterosacral ligament, vulva, ovary and gastrointestinal tract.

Figure 20.1 shows the different sites where leiomyoma may grow:

- Intramural leiomyomas are most common variety. These tumors arise within the myometrium and as they grow, they may move towards the uterine cavity or external surface of uterus. These tumors may produce symmetrical enlargement of uterus when they arise singly.

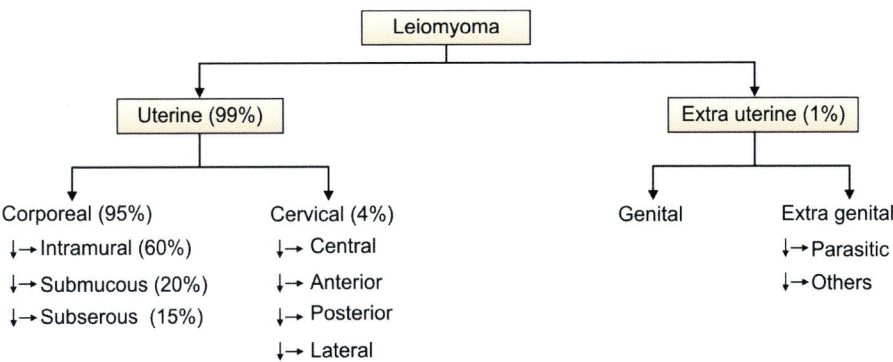

Fig. 20.1: Classification of leiomyomas

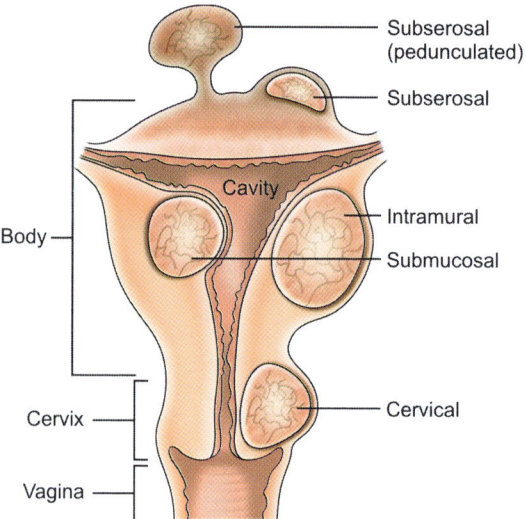

Fig. 20.2: Different types of uterine leiomyomas

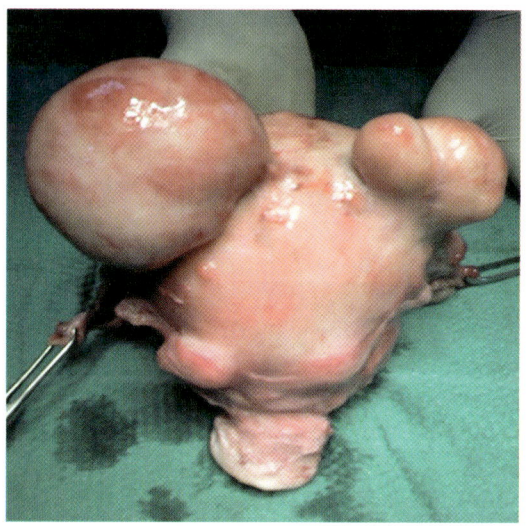

Fig. 20.3: Different types of uterine leiomyomas

- Submucosal leiomyomas are located beneath the endometrium and can grow into the uterine cavity. Pedunculated leiomyoma can protrude to or through the cervix. These tumors often produce abnormal uterine bleeding and known as uterine polyp.
- Subserosal leiomyomas are just beneath the serosal surface and grow towards peri-

toneal cavity, causing bulging over the peritoneal surface of uterus. These tumors may develop a pedicle and become pedunculated, and grow towards peritoneal cavity producing a large size without producing any symptom. When leiomyoma extends into the broad ligament they are known as intraligamentary leiomyoma. Pedunculated leiomyoma may rarely get attached with omentum or intestines and may develop a secondary blood supply. They may be detached from uterus and loose primary blood supply and the resulting structure known as parasitic leiomyoma (Figs 20.2 and 20.3).

Pathology

1. *Gross pathology:* Leiomyomas are pseudo-capsulated solid tumors well demarcated from surrounding myometrium. The pseudocapsule is not a true capsule but formed from the surrounding compressed myometrium and fibrous tissue on the surface of the tumor. Because the vasculature is located on the periphery, the central part of tumor is avascular and susceptible to degenerative changes. The tumors are smooth, solid and usually pinkish white depending on degree of vascularity. The cut surface typically has a fleshy, whorl like appearance (Figs 20.4 to 20.7).
2. *Microscopic pathology:* Leiomyomas are composed of groups and bundles of

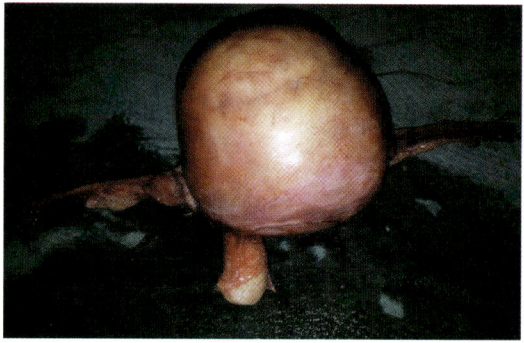

Fig. 20.4: Uterine leiomyoma arising out of body of the uterus

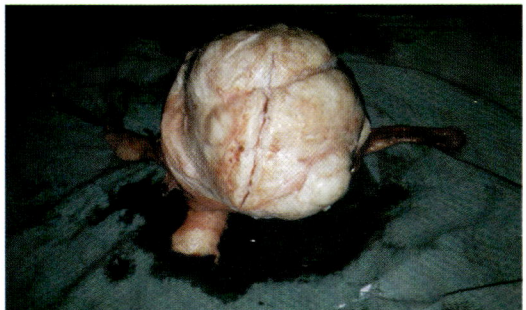

Fig. 20.5: Uterine wall is cut open, leiomyoma is shelled out, note the color of leiomyoma

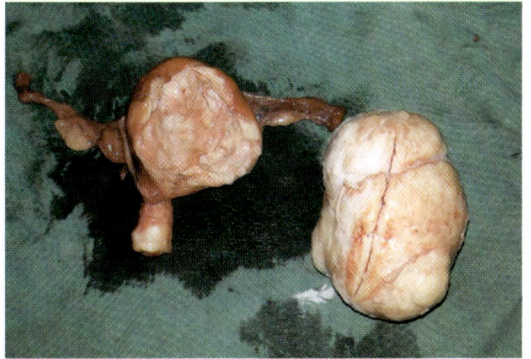

Fig. 20.6: Leiomyoma is separated from uterus, note the psuedocapsule

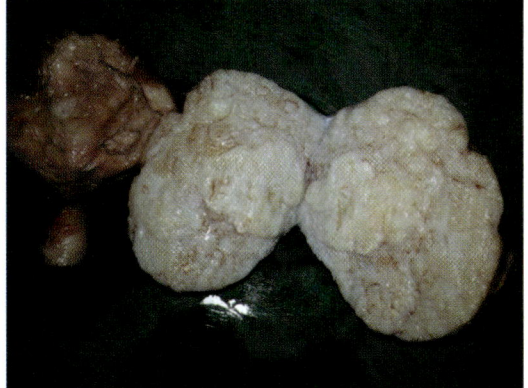

Fig. 20.7: Leiomyoma is divided to show cut surface - note the fleshy appearance

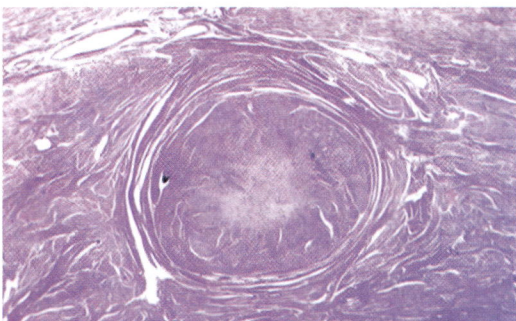

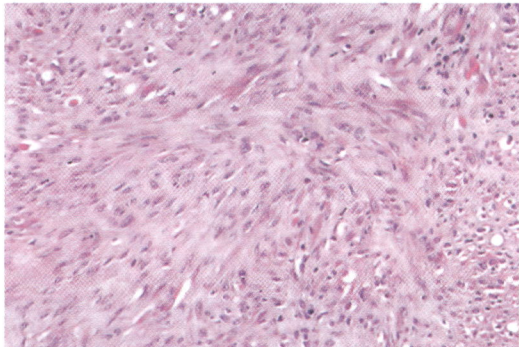

Figs 20.8 and 20.9: Low power and high power microscopic picture of uterine leiomyoma

smooth muscle fibers arranged in a twisted and whorled fashion. Microscopically, smooth muscle cell are arranged longitudinally or in cross section mixed with fibrous connective tissue. Vascular structures are few and mitoses are rare (Figs 20.8 and 20.9).

Secondary Changes

A variety of degenerative changes may occur in leiomyomas that alter the gross and microscopic appearance of the tumors. Most of these changes are of no clinical significance. These changes may be due to secondary to alteration in circulation (either arterial or venous) or postmenopausal atrophy or infection or may result from malignant transformation.

- **Hyaline degeneration:** This is most common degenerative change and present in almost every leiomyoma. The tumour becomes soft and there is loss of whorl appearance in cut section. Microscopically hyaline changes are seen in muscle and fibrous tissue.

- **Cystic degeneration:** This results from liquefaction of areas with hyaline changes

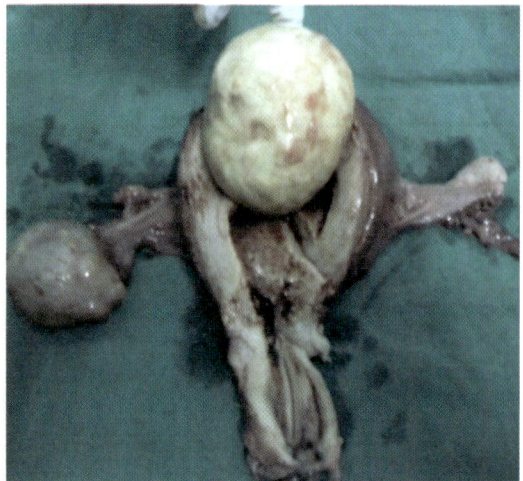

Fig. 20.10: Calcified leiomyoma in a postmenopausal uterus

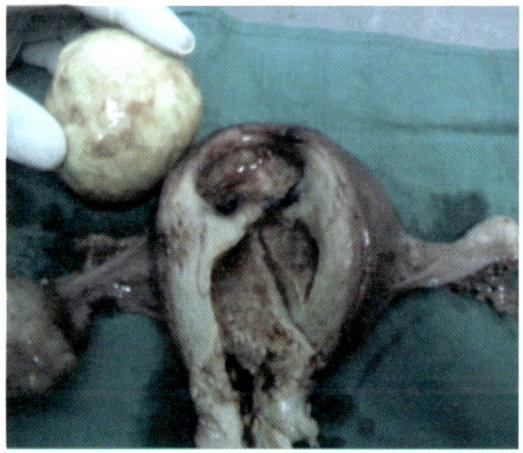

Fig. 20.11: Calcified leiomyoma—womb stone

following hyaline degeneration. Leiomyomas become soft with multiple cystic spaces and gives sponge like appearance.

- *Calcification:* There is deposition of calcium salt within tumour and commonly found in pedunculated subserous leiomyoma and in postmenopausal women. When calcium deposition occurs throughout the tumour, it becomes rocky hard and termed 'womb stone in old graveyards' (Figs 20.10 and 20.11).

- *Red degeneration:* This complication occurs in pregnancy especially in second trimester to puerperium. The tumor acutely becomes painful, tender and enlarged. The peripheral vessels are thrombosed and there are extravasation of blood which is responsible of red color of the tumor. The extravasated blood stretches the pseudo-capsule resulting in severe abdominal pain. The cut section of tumor has a raw beef appearance with a fishy odor from fatty acids. Apart from pain, patient can also have fever, vomiting and tachycardia. Blood examination shows peripheral leucocytosis and rise of ESR. The condition can be mistaken as torsion of pedunculated leiomyoma or other causes of acute abdomen in pregnancy. The condition is conservatively treated with bed rest, analgesics, sedatives and IV fluids. There is no place of surgery. Pregnancy usually proceeds uneventfully.

- *Fatty degeneration:* This is seen mostly in subserous leiomyoma. It is characterized by deposition of fat globules in muscle.

- *Infection:* A submucous tumor may become ulcerated in lower pole and get infected. Infection may also occur following abortion and delivery.

- *Malignant change:* Sarcomatous change is rare and only occurs in 0.5% of cases, mostly in postmenopausal women.

- *Pseudo-Meig's syndrome:* Pedunculated subserous leiomyoma may present with ascites by mechanical irritation of the peritoneum. If it is associated with right sided hydrothorax it is known as pseudo-Meig's syndrome.

Clinical Features

Although uterine leiomyomas are common, most are asymptomatic and require no treatment. Predominantly intramural or subserous leiomyomas are typically found as unsuspected pelvic masses at the time of ultrasound examination as an incidental finding.

The patients are usually between 30 and 50 years old. Leiomyomas are common in women with nulliparity or low parity.

The symptoms depend upon number, size and position of leiomyomas. The symptoms include abnormal uterine bleeding, abdominal pain or pressure, abdominal lump, infertility and pressure symptoms.

Menstrual Disorders

Menorrhagia

The most common presentation includes the development of progressively heavy menstrual blood loss that lasts longer than normal duration (menorrhagia defined as menstrual blood loss > 80 ml or menstruation persisting > 7 days or both). Submucous leiomyomas are most commonly associated with menorrhagia, however, intramural leiomyoma may present in similar manner if they become large enough to distort the endometrial cavity. The causes of menorrhagia are due to:

a. Increased endometrial surface area
b. Iincreased vascularity of uterus
c. Defective uterine contractions
d. Associated endometrial hyperplasia
e. Endometrial ulceration over a submucous leiomyoma
f. Uterine congestion due to compression of venous plexus within myometrium.

Metrorrhagia

Submucous pedunculated leiomyomas may cause metrorrhagia due to passive congestion, necrosis and ulceration of endometrium overlying leiomyoma.

Blood loss during menstruation may lead to chronic iron deficiency anemia, dizziness, weakness and fatigue, palpitation, dyspnoea.

Dysmenorrhea

Secondary dysmenorrhea is seen due to submucous and intramural leiomyoma. Dysmenorrhoea can also be correlated with coexisting endometriosis, adenomyosis and pelvic inflammatory disease (PID).

Pain

Leiomyomas are usually painless, however, pain may be due degeneration, torsion, infection or adhesion to other organs. Pain may be due to other coexisting pathology like endometriosis, PID.

Pressure Symptoms

Patient may present with pelvic pressure or feeling full in lower abdomen. Anterior leiomyomas may produce bladder irritability, frequency or retention of urine. Large broad ligament leiomyomas may cause hydro-nephrosis, hydroureter, and impairment of renal function because of pressure effect on ureter. Leiomyomas that fills the pelvis may lead to constipation, dyspareunia.

Abdominal Lump

Considerable number of patients may present with lump in lower abdomen with or without symptom.

Infertility

Uterine leiomyomas are associated with infertility in 5–10% cases. Leiomyomas, endometriosis, and infertility often coexists. The cause of infertility is not explainable in all cases but following are the possibilities.

1. Leiomyomas occurring near cornu of uterus may cause occlusion of fallopian tube, alteration of tubal functions, and motility. Multiple leiomyomas cause bilateral tubal block.
2. Submucosal leiomyomas may affect implantation and growth of embryo because of thin and poorly vascularised endometrium.
3. Leiomyomas may impair rhythmic uterine contractions that facilitate sperm motility through the uterus.

4. Cervical leiomymas can interfere with the movement of sperm to enter in uterine cavity.

Obstetrical Problems

Obstetrical complications that may be associated are recurrent pregnancy loss, preterm labor, malpresentation, increased caesarean section, postpartum hemorrhage, IUGR.

Signs

General Examination

The woman may be anemic.

Abdominal examination: An abdominal lump may be palpable arising out of pelvis with well defined margins, firm in consistency and nodular or smooth surface. The tumor is mobile side to side but up and down mobility is restricted. Side to side mobility, however may be restricted if it is very large or fixed due to adhesion or positioned in the broad ligament. The lump is non tender unless infected or malignant change. It is dull in percussion as the intestines lie behind and besides it.

Rapid growth in previously known leiomyoma should suggest the possibility of a sarcoma.

Pelvic examination: Vaginal findings vary according to size, number and position of leiomyoma. Small submucous leiomyoma may be missed during pelvic examination. Larger submucous leiomyoma cause symme-trical enlargement of uterus. Movement of the tumor per abdominally is transmitted to the cervix. The tumor is not felt separate from the uterus unless, it is pedunculated. In cervical leiomyoma the uterus is placed top on the low-lying tumor. The broad ligament and cervical leiomyomas displace the uterus from its position.

Small leiomyomas can only be felt by bimanual examination. The uterus is firm, uniformly enlarged with single leiomyoma but irregular with nodular surface in multiple leiomyoma.

In leimyomatous polyp, the lower pole is felt through open os. Chronic inversion should be ruled out.

Differential Diagnosis

- *Pregnant uterus:* The possibility of pregnancy should be kept in mind in all cases of uterine enlargement. A soft uterus due to cystic degeneration of leiomyoma should be distinguished from pregnant uterus by urine pregnancy test and ultrasonography.
- *Adenomyosis:* It shares the clinical feature of uterine leiomyoma and both cause infertility, dysmenorrhea, menorrhagia and enlarged uterus. Progressive severe dys-menorrhea and uterine tenderness favor diagnosis of adenomyosis. Adenomyosis tends to occur at younger age, rarely enlarges the uterus to more than 12–14 weeks pregnant uterus size and causes a regular than a nodular uterine enlargement. Ultrasound and MRI can confirm the diagnosis.

Table 20.1: Symptoms of uterine leiomyoma			
Menstrual symptoms	*Pressure symptoms*	*Pain*	*Reproductive symptoms*
Menorrhagia	Pelvic pressure	Acute infarct	Infertility
Metrorrhagia	Hydonephrosis, hydroureter	Dyspareunia	Recurrent abortion
Menometrorrhagia	Urinary frequency, retention	Coexisting pathology	Fetal malpresentation
Dysmenorrhea	Constipation		Preterm labor
			IUGR, increased caesarean section rate

- **Bicornuate uterus:** One horn of bicornuate uterus can be mistaken for leiomyoma. Hysterosalpingogram, ultrasound and hysteroscopy can help to confirm diagnosis.
- **Endometriosis and chocolate cyst:** Most common between 35 and 45 years of age. Pelvic pain is the presenting symptom. Physical activity and sexual intercourse will increase the pain. Infertility and menorrhagia can also occur. Chocolate cysts rarely exceed 12 cm diameter. The uterus is normal in size and adherent with pelvic mass. Nodularity of the uterosacral ligament is characteristic. Ultrasound and sometimes laparoscopy is required for correct diagnosis.
- **Old ectopic pregnancy:** The hematocele of old ectopic pregnancy may feel like leiomyoma and adherent to uterus. The history of amenorrhea, pregnancy test, ultrasound and laparoscopy will establish the diagnosis.
- **Tubo-ovarian mass (chronic pelvic inflammatory disease):** The uterus may be normal size but fixed. The mass will be tender and fixed in the pelvis.
- **Ovarian tumors:** Differentiating features are: (i) They are cystic or solid masses , paramedian, occur at any time of a woman's life. (ii) Ovarian tumors are usually not associated with menstrual symptoms. (iii) Bimanual examination reveals a normal sized uterus separate from the tumor. (iv) A groove can be felt between the tumor and uterus. (v) There is no movement of the cervix with movement of the tumor. Ultrasound examination helps to reach final diagnosis.
- **Endometrial carcinoma:** It is seen in elderly women, may be obese, diabetic and hypertensive. Common presenting symptom is abnormal uterine bleeding particularly menorrhagia. In 3% women over 40 years of age, leiomyomas may coexist with endometrial carcinoma.
- **Chronic inversion of uterus:** A submucous leiomyomatous polyp may be mistaken as chronic inversion of uterus. In case of uterine inversion, the leading part is uterine fundus and the mass can be reducible. The cervix is at normal position but the external os is not visible. It is not possible to insert an uterine sound. On bimanual examination body of uterus is not felt in its position.
- **Pelvic kidney:** It is not associated with menstrual abnormalities. It is retroperitoneal, fixed and firm and separate from the uterus. Ultrasound reveals absence of abdominal kidney and IVP will locate the kidney.
- **Carcinoma of fallopian tube:** It is a very rare malignancy in female genital tract. Occasionally presents with symptoms of several week of profuse, watery vaginal discharge.

Investigations

Ultrasonography: Pelvic ultrasonograhy is an adequate first line diagnostic modality in most cases of suspected leiomyomas. Transvaginal ultrasound is useful to know the utrine volume, number of leiomyomas and location in relation to endometrial cavity. Leiomyoma is seen as well defined rounded hypoechoic areas with cystic spaces if degeneration has occurred. Ultrasound also indentifies adenomyosis. It is also helpful in evaluation of adnexa and identifying hydronephrosis of kidney.

Sonohysterography or intrauterine infusion of sterile saline at the time of ultrasonography can indentify the presence of pedunculated submucous leiomyoma and endometrial polyp.

Hysteroscopy: It is very accurate in detecting submucous leiomyomas and helps in treatment planning for patients with menorrhagia due to leiomyoma. Hysteroscopy also recognizes a submucous polyp and also allows its excision under direct vision.

Hysterosalpingography is useful to indentify a submucous leiomyoma and to demonstrate tubal patency of fallopian tubes.

Table 20.2: Diagnostic imaging in uterine leiomyoma	
Diagnostic modality	*Advantages and disadvantages*
Transvaginal sonography	• Useful for detection of leiomyomas and following their growth • Not as accurate as MRI at determination of precise location and size of leiomyoma especially with larger uterus or with multiple leiomyomas
Sonohysterography	• Characterization of location and amount of endometrial cavity distortion caused by submucosal leiomyoma
Hysterosalpingography	• Evaluates the contour and patency of fallopian tubes • Does not evaluate the exact location of leiomyma
MRI	• Indentifies size and location of leiomyomas • Used before uterine artery embolization

MRI is very accurate and informative but very expensive, it is very useful in detecting the number, size, location of leiomyoma and signs of degeneration in complicated cases. It helps in differentiating adenomyosis from leiomyomas. MRI is safe in pregnancy (Table 20.2).

CT scan is not very useful in evaluating uterine leiomyoma because of its nonspecific diagnostic criteria.

Dilatation and curettage is required in perimenopausal women if endometrial malignancy is suspected.

IVP may be required in broad ligament leiomyoma to check anatomy of ureters and to exclude hydronephrosis. It also identifies a pelvic kidney.

Hemoglobin and hematocrit is obtained in cases of excessive menstrual bleeding to assess the degree of loss and adequacy of treatment.

Coagulation profile and bleeding time are ordered when history is suggestive of bleeding diathesis.

Treatment

If the leiomyoma is asymptomatic and the woman is not anemic no treatment is necessary. Treatment of uterine leiomyomas may involve one of the following approaches or a combination thereof: expectant management, medical management (GnRH analogues, progestational compounds, antiprogestins), surgical management (myomectomy or hysterectomy), uterine artery embolization, and other approaches, e.g., high frequency ultrasonography, laser treatment, cryotherapy, or thermoablation.

Expectant management: In asymptomatic leiomyoma, observation with periodic examination is appropriate. Bimanual examination should be performed every 3 to 6 months to determine the uterine size and the rate of tumor growth. After slow growth or stable uterine size has been confirmed, annual follow-up may be appropriate. Rapid growth—a change of 6 pregnancy weeks in size or more in 12 months observation or less is an indication for intervention. Follow-up with pelvic ultrasound is performed, if pelvic examination is inadequate as may occur in obesity.

Definitive treatment: When leiomyomas are associated with excessive or irregular menstrual bleeding, severe pelvic pain, infertility, pressure symptoms or recurrent pregnancy loss, treatment should be considered. Similarly when leiomyomas show evidence of postmenopausal or extremely rapid growth treatment should be initiated (Table 20.3). Choosing appropriate therapeutic options depends on many factors, including the woman's age, her desire for future fertility, the type and size of leiomyomas and the

Table 20.3: Indications for surgical management of uterine leiomyomas

- Abnormal uterine bleeding not responding to conservative treatments
- High level of suspicion of pelvic malignancy
- Growth after menopause
- Infertility when there is distortion of the endometrial cavity or tubal obstruction
- Recurrent pregnancy loss (with distortion of the endometrial cavity)
- Pain or pressure symptoms (that interfere withquality of life)
- Urinary tract symptoms (frequency and/or obstruction)
- Iron deficiency anemia secondary to chronic blood loss

specific symptoms experienced. Therapy for uterine leiomyomas must be individualized and may be nonsurgical or surgical.

Traditional Surgery

Hysterectomy: Hysterectomy has traditionally been the primary treatment for symptomatic leiomyoma. Leiomyomas are the most frequent nonmalignant indication for hysterectomy. Hysterectomy should be reserved for women who have completed childbearing and no longer wish to preserve the menstrual function of uterus. The surgery can be performed via the vaginal or abdominal route. In selected cases, the uterus may be removed with a laparoscopic approach.

Clinical pearl: The most common symptom of uterine leiomyoma is menorrhagia and most common cause of hysterectomy is uterine leiomyoma.

Myomectomy: Myomectomy is removal of single or multiple leiomyomas with preservation of the uterus. If fertility is a consideration and the patient has major symptoms, myomectomy is the procedure of choice. Myomectomy should be preceded by a hysterosalpingogram to determine the location and patency of the fallopian tubes and to screen for submucous myomas.

Abdominal myomectomy has been associated with more significant blood loss and higher morbidity than hysterectomy. However, with the recent improvements in surgical technique, the morbidity of myomectomy is now comparable with that of hysterectomy. A patient undergoing myomectomy should understand that the procedure is a treatment for leiomyoma, not a cure. There is a 15% recurrence rate of leiomyomas after myomectomy and a 10% reoperation rate (*see* Chapter 35).

New Surgical Interventions

Recent developments in surgical endoscopy have, in selected cases, allowed myomectomy to be performed with minimally invasive surgical procedures. These include hysteroscopic myomectomy, laparoscopic myomectomy, and laparoscopic myoma coagulation. These procedures offer several advantages, including shorter hospitalization, more rapid recovery, and cost savings per patient in hospital.

Hysteroscopic myomectomy: Hysteroscopic myomectomy is a potential treatment option in women with symptomatic submucosal or submucosal-intramural leiomyomas. In the case of a large submucosal leiomyoma with predominant intramural extension, two-step surgical hysteroscopy has been proposed. Laparoscopy can be performed simultaneously to reduce the possibility of uterine perforation. In women with leiomyoma-associated infertility, a postprocedural pregnancy rate of almost 60% has been reported. Menorrhagia or dysmenorrhea resolved in the majority of women after submucosal myomectomy was performed for menstrual abnormalities.

Laparoscopic myomectomy: Laparoscopic myomectomy is especially useful in cases of pedunculated subserosal leiomyomas. Relative contraindications are somewhat arbitrary; they include a leiomyoma larger than 7 cm in diameter, a leiomyoma adjacent to the uterine artery, or a leiomyoma near the tubal cornu if preservation of fertility is desired. Removal of the leiomyoma from the abdominal cavity is the most time-consuming part of this procedure, and the introduction of electromechanical morcellation may result in significant time savings. The late complications of uterine dehiscence or adhesion formation not that much reported.

Laparoscopic myoma coagulation: Laparoscopic myoma coagulation (myolysis) is accomplished with a neodymium:yttrium-aluminum-garnet (Nd: YAG) laser or bipolar needle electrodes, which may produce thermal injury resulting in protein denaturation, vascular destruction, and tumor degeneration. These effects lead to shrinkage of leiomyomas and symptomatic relief in many women. Laparoscopic myoma coagulation appears to be effective without regrowth of leiomyomas. This procedure may

be associated with significant adhesion formation; however, recent experience indicates that there is minimal postoperative adhesion formation when bipolar needle electrodes are used.

Medical Treatment

Gonadotropin-releasing hormone analogs: By inhibiting normal pituitary secretion of gonadotropins, GnRH analogs can induce a reversible hypoestrogenic state, resulting in amenorrhea and a reduction in the size of hormone-responsive leiomyomas. The maximum reduction is usually achieved with 12 weeks of GnRH analog treatment. However, after cessation of treatment, there is rapid re growth of the tumor (Table 20.4).

Short-term therapy may be used preoperatively in the following situations: hysterectomy, myomectomy in women with a large uterus (>600 cm^3), or new minimally

Table 20.4: Medical treatments of uterine leiomyomas		
Medication	*Advantages*	*Disadvantages*
GnRH analogue	Induce medical menopause thereby causing hypoestrogenic state and Shrinking of the leiomyoma	Expensive, many side effects (post-menopausal symptoms, osteoporosis) that limit use for > 6 months
		Usually used prior hysterectomy to shrink leiomyoma. Leiomyomas are grow rapidly when discontinued.
Selective estrogen Reuotake modulators (raloxifen, tamoxifen)	Act as estrogen antagonists in the uterus to decrease size of leiomyoma	No evidence yet to support routine use of these medications
Hormone therapy	Combined estrogen/progesterone May decrease endogenous estrogen level	No evidence to show effectiveness in limiting leiomyoma growth or improving symptoms
Mifepristone	Acts as a progesterone antagonist And may decrease size of leiomyoma	Small studies only. Require larger trial before clinical recommendation.
NSAIDs	Decrease prostaglandin levels	No evidence to show effectiveness in limiting leiomyoma growth or improving symptoms
Depot Medroxy progesterone	Induce endometrial atrophy possibly decrease serum estrogen level	Small uncontrolled studies show decreased menorrhagia in women with leiomyoma
Levonorgestrel Intrauterine system	May induce endometrial atrophy and decrease menstrual bleeding	May reduce menstrual blood loss but does not affect leiomyoma size (LNG IUS)

invasive procedures, including hysteroscopic myomectomy. Reduction of tumor size and vascularity secondary to a hypoestrogenic state may facilitate surgery and decrease intraoperative blood loss. In patients with anemia secondary to hypermenorrhea, GnRH analog therapy may allow recovery of normal hemoglobin levels before surgery, thus minimizing the need for transfusion or allowing autologous blood donation. Short-term GnRH analog therapy may also be indicated in perimenopausal women in whom permanent regression of leiomyomas may be expected after menopause.

There is not adequate evidence to support the use of nonsteroidal anti-inflammatory drugs (NSAID), hormonal therapy, raloxifen or Tamoxifen, or mifepristone, although some of these therapies show promise in decreasing the size of leiomyoma and improving the symptoms associated with leiomyoma (Table 20.4).

Uterine artery embolization: Uterine artery embolization is a promising new method of treating symptomatic leiomyomas. In this procedure, both uterine arteries are selectively catheterized from a femoral artery approach and subsequently embolized with polyvinyl alcohol particles or coils. Uterine artery embolization may result in shrinkage of the uterus and leiomyomas, along with relief of menorrhagia and symptoms due to local mass effect. As a percutaneous interventional technique, this procedure may offer the advantages of avoidance of surgical risks, potential preservation of fertility, and shorter hospitalization.

Clinical pearl: Uterine artery embolization and hysteroscopic myomectomy are 2 less invasive procedures that provide treatment options for women with leiomyoma who do not want hysterectomy.

EXERCISES

1. Answer the following questions

- What is leiomyoma?
- What causes leiomyomas?
- Which receptors are present in leiomyoma?
- What are the locations of leiomyomas?
- Which type is most symptomatic?
- What is the incidence of leiomyoma?
- What is the surgical impact of leiomyomas?
- What are the symptoms?
- Why do leiomyomas cause abnormal bleeding?
- Why do leiomyomas cause pain?
- What are the degenerative changes?
- Which degenerative change is most common?
- How do you treat red degeneration?
- When red degeneration is common?
- How leiomyomas are diagnosed?
- How do leiomyomas interfere with ability to achieve a term pregnancy?
- What surgical treatment available for leiomyomas?
- What are the indications of myomectomy?
- What are the indiacations of hysterectomy?

2. Fill in the blanks with appropriate word/s

- Most common neoplasm of uterus is _____ .
- Cytogenetic study suggests uterine leiomyoma takes origin from _____ .
- Three common risk factors of uterine leiomyoma are _____ , _____ and _____ .
- _____ type of leiomyomas are usually symptomless.
- Laparoscopic myoma coagulation (myolysis) is accomplished with _____ .

3. Explain or justify the following statements

- Growth of uterine leiomyomas depends on estrogenic stimulation.
- Several changes may occur in uterine leiomyoma.
- Different types of menstrual abnormality may be associated with leiomyomas.
- Uterine leiomyoma may cause infertility.
- Asymptomatic leiomyoma do not require treatment.

4. Write short notes on

- Types of uterine leiomyoma.
- Red degeneration

5. Questions for practical examination (read the case summary in the beginning of chapter before answering the following questions)

- What is your diagnosis?
- What are the points in favor of your diagnosis?
- What are the differential diagnoses?
- How do you differentiate uterine lump from ovarian lump?
- Why this woman is not having ovarian tumor?
- Why menorrhagia occurs in leiomyoma?
- How do you confirm your diagnosis?
- What other investigations you will do for her?
- How will you treat her?
- What is the role of GnRh analogue for treatment of this patient?

6. Questions for practical examination (look at the Figs 20.3 to 20.5 before answering following questions)

- Describe the specimens in each figure.
- How do you identify anterior and posterior surfaces of uterus.
- Name the operation that had been done in these cases.

- Looking at the specimen can you determine the age of the patient.
- Describe the clinical presentation of the patient from whom the specimen was obtained.

Bibliography

1. ACP Handbook of Women's Health.
2. Evans P, Brunsell S. Uterine Fibroid tumors - Diagnosis and treatment Am Fam Physician 2007;75:1503–8.
3. Flake GP, et al Etiology and pathogenesis of uterine leiomyoma - a review Environ Health Perspect 111:1037û1054 2003
4. Gynecology by Mark morgan
5. John Hopkins manual of obstetrics and gynecology
6. Lipscomb G. Uterine Artery Embolization and Minimally Invasive Techniques for Uterine Fibroids Glob. libr. women's med., (ISSN: 1756-2228) 2008; DOI 10.3843/GLOWM.10077.
7. Murase E, et al. Uterine Leiomyomas: Histopathologic Features, MR Imaging Findings, Differential Diagnosis, and Treatment
8. Neuwirth R, Moritz J. Leiomyomas of the Uterus Glob. libr. women's med., (ISSN: 1756-2228) 2008; DOI 0.3843/GLOWM.10007
9. Obsterics and gynecology, Charles RB Beckman
10. Obstetrics and gynecology by ST Phelan, S Chiang
11. Obstetrics and gynecology recall
12. Textbook of Gynecology—Sengupta
13. Wallach EE, et al. Uterine Myomas: An Overview of Development, Clinical Features, and Management Obstet Gynecol 2004;104:393–406.

21

Benign Ovarian Lesions

A 30-year-old P 2+0 woman presents to gynecology out patient department with a chief complaint of pelvic pain. The pain began about 3 weeks previously and is characterized as dull ache in the right lower abdomen. The pain is exacerbated by some movements and by sexual intercourse. She noted no change in intensity or character of pain with her last menses 2 weeks previously. Her past gynecological and medical histories are unremarkable. Previous surgeries include one caesarean delivery and an appendectomy. Physical examination reveals a well-nourished female in no acute distress who demonstrates mild tenderness on deep palpation of the right lower quadrant of her abdomen. On pelvic examination, palpation of the right adnexa elicits presence of a tense cystic mass separated from uterus with moderate tenderness. What is her provisional diagnosis?

In this chapter we will learn:
- Causes of different types of benign ovarian lesions
- Clinical presentation of benign ovarian lesions
- Investigations
- Differential diagnosis
- Complications of ovarian cysts
- Treatment

Introduction

An ovarian cyst is a sac filled with liquid or semi-liquid material arising in an ovary. Many ovarian tumors are cystic, but some cysts are not tumors. These cysts can develop in females at any stage of life, from the neonatal period to postmenopause. Most ovarian cysts, however, occur during reproductive period. Most are functional in nature and resolve with minimal treatment. The number of diagnoses of ovarian cysts has increased with the widespread use of ultrasonography. The discovery of an ovarian cyst causes considerable anxiety in women owing to fears of malignancy, but the vast majority of ovarian cysts are benign.

Etiology

Two-thirds of the ovarian lesions occur in women between the ages 20 and 44. These lesions can be grouped as given in Table 21.1.

1. Functional Cysts

Ovarian cysts arising in the course of ovarian function are called functional cysts and are

Table 21.1: Different types of benign ovarian lesions	
Functional ovarian cysts	Follicular cysts, corpus luteal cysts, theca-lutein cysts
Neoplastic cysts (benign)	Serous cyst adenoma, mucinos cust adenoma, benign cystic tearatoma (Dermoid cyst) fibroma, Brenner's tumor, adenofibroma, thecoma, mixed tumor
Inflammatory	Tubo-ovarian mass/abscess
Others	Chocolate cysts or endometriomas, poly cystic ovarian syndrome

always benign. They may be follicular and luteal, sometimes called theca-lutein cysts.

Follicular cysts: In the follicular phase, follicular cysts may result from a lack of physiologic release of the ovum due to excessive FSH stimulation or lack of the normal LH surge at midcycle just before ovulation. Hormonal stimulation causes these cysts to continue to grow. Follicular cysts are typically larger than 2.5 cm in diameter and manifest as pelvic discomfort and heaviness.

Corpus luteal cysts: In the absence of pregnancy, the lifespan of the corpus luteum is 14 days. If the ovum is fertilized, the corpus luteum continues to secrete progesterone for 5–9 weeks, until its eventual dissolution in 14 weeks' time, when the cyst undergoes central hemorrhage. Failure of dissolution to occur may result in a corpus luteal cyst, which is arbitrarily defined as a corpus luteum that grows to 3 cm in diameter. The cyst can cause dull, unilateral pelvic pain and may be complicated by rupture, which causes acute pain and possibly massive blood loss.

Theca-lutein cysts: Theca-lutein cysts are formed due to excessive stimulation from human chorionic gonadotropin (hCG). These cysts are predisposed to torsion, hemorrhage, and rupture. Theca-lutein cysts occur in presence of hydatidiform mole, multiple gestation, or exogenous ovarian hyperstimulation.

These cysts are usually bilateral and resolve spontaneously as the hCG level falls. Theca-lutein cysts may result in massive ovarian enlargement, a characteristic of the condition termed hyperreactio luteinalis.

2. Neoplastic Cysts

Neoplastic cysts arise via the inappropriate overgrowth of cells within the ovary and may be malignant or benign. Malignant neoplasms may arise from all ovarian cell types and tissues. The most frequent are those arising from the surface epithelium (mesothelium) and most of these are partially cystic lesions (*see* Chapter 24). The examples of benign neoplasm include serous cystadenoma, mucinous cystadenoma, adenofibroma, fibroma, thecoma, mature cystic teratoma (dermoid cyst), and Brenner's tumour. Although neoplastic cysts are tumours, all benign tumors are not cysts as some are solid tumors (*see* below).

Benign Epithelial Neoplastic Cysts (60% of benign ovarian tumors)

Serous cystadenoma
- Serous tumors are characterized by a proliferation of epithelium resembling that lining the fallopian tubes.
- The simple variety is mostly uniloculer and filled with clear yellowish flyid.
- The papillary variety develops papillary growths which may be so prolific that the cyst appears solid.
- Laminated calcified particles called psammoma bodies are often present in the walls of papillary serous cyst adenoma.
- They are most common in women aged between 40 and 50 years.

- About 15–25% are bilateral and about 20–25% are malignant.

Mucinous cystadenoma

- The most common large ovarian tumors which may become enormous(measuring up to 30 cm).
- Mucinous cysts are usually smooth-walled; compared with the serous variety, they rarely are associated with true papillae.
- They are filled with mucinous material and rupture may cause pseudomyxoma peritonei. They may be multilocular and the mucus-containing loculi appear blue through the tense capsules.
- They are most common in the 20–40 age group. About 5-10% are bilateral and around 5% will be malignant.

Benign Neoplastic Cystic Tumors of Germ Cell Origin

- They arise from primitive germ cells containing elements from all 3 embryonic germ layers, i.e., ectoderm, endoderm, and mesoderm.
- A benign mature teratoma (dermoid cyst) may contain well-differentiated tissue, e.g. hair, teeth, thyroid, bronchial, and central nervous system tissue (Figs 20.1 and 20.2).
- 20% are bilateral.

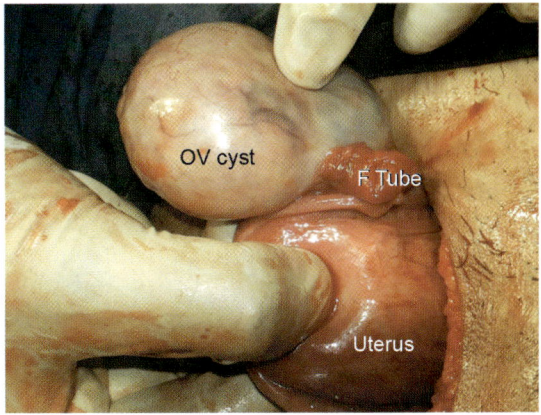

Fig. 21.1: Dermoid cyst of ovary at the time of operation

- They are most common in young women between age 20 and 40 years..
- A cystic teratoma is usually asymptomatic and is discovered incidentally on pelvic examination or on ultrasonography.
- During examination they are found close to anterior abdominal wall and quiet mobile, often migrating to upper quadrant during manipulation.
- Treatment is surgical removal of the cystic teratoma (ovarian cystectomy or ovariotomy) to confirm benign nature of the mass and to avoid complication like torsion or rupture.

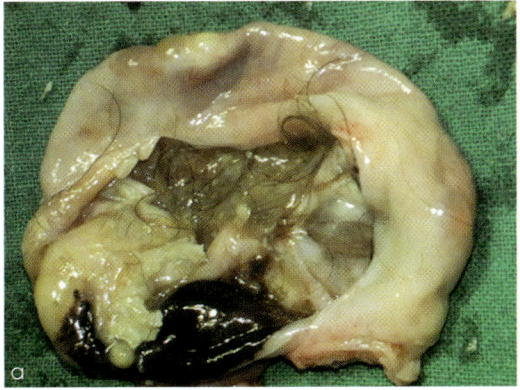
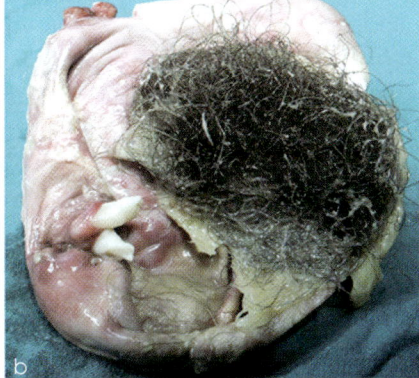

Fig. 21.2: and b: (a) Same cyst of Fig. 21.1 is cut open with presence of hairs (1 o' clock position) and **(b)** dermoid cyst is cut open with presence of hairs and teeth

- Most dermoid cysts are benign. Poorly differentiated, malignant teratomas are rare(< 2%).

Benign Neoplastic Solid Tumors

i. Fibroma (less than 1% is malignant); small, solid benign fibrous tissue tumours. The combination of benign ovarian fibroma with ascites and right plural effusion has been referred as Meig's syndrome.

ii. Thecoma (less than 1% are malignant).

iii. Adenofibroma.

iv. Brenner's tumour:
  - Rare ovarian tumors displaying benign, borderline or proliferative, and malignant variants.
  - Over 95% are benign and more than 90% are unilateral.
  - They may be associated with mucinous cystadenoma and cystic teratoma.

3. Endometriomas or Chocolate Cysts

Endometriomas are altered blood-filled cysts arising from the ectopic endometrium on the surface of the ovary. Usually these are bi-lateral, thick walled and adherent with uterus and other pelvic structures. The cysts are filled with a chocolate colored thick tenacious material. Endometriomas are associated with endometriosis, which causes a classic triad of painful and heavy periods and dyspareunia (*see* Chapter 17).

4. Polycystic Ovary Syndrome

In polycystic ovary syndrome, the ovary often contains multiple cystic follicles 2–5 mm in diameter as viewed on sonograms. The cysts themselves are never the main problem, and discussed in Chapter 12.

5. Tubo-ovarian Mass

Ovaries can be involved following inflamma-tion of fallopian tube as in PID or in ectopic pregnancy forming a tubo-ovarian mass or abscess.

Clinical Presentation

Age: Functional ovarian cysts occur at any age (including in utero), but are much more common in women of reproductive age. Most benign neoplastic cysts occur during the reproductive era but there is a wide age range and they may occur at any age.

Symptoms

- The majority of ovarian cysts are asymptomatic, with the cysts being discovered incidentally during ultrasono-graphy or routine pelvic examination. Some cysts, however, may be associated with a range of symptoms, sometimes severe.
- Pain or discomfort may occur in the lower abdomen. Torsion or rupture of cyst may lead to more severe abdominal pain, nausea, vomiting.
- Patient may complaint of abdominal swelling or a feeling of fullness or pressure.
- Patient may experience discomfort with intercourse, particularly deep penetration.
- There may be difficulty with having bowel movements, or there may be pressure leading to a desire to defecate.
- Frequency of micturition due to pressure on the bladder
- Irregularity of the menstrual cycle and abnormal vaginal bleeding may occur. Young children may present with precocious puberty and early onset of menarche.
- Endometriomas are associated with endometriosis, which causes a classic triad of painful and heavy periods and dyspareunia.

Physical Examination

General Examination

Usually there is no change in general examination findings unless the ovarian cysts undergo certain complications. Hemorrhage due to cyst rupture may lead to tachycardia and hypotension. Torsion of ovarian cysts may result in hyperpyrexia and tachycardia.

In huge mucinous cyst adenoma patient may have cachectic look because of protein loss.

Abdominal Examination

Inspection: Abdomen may be enlarged with a visible swelling arising out of the pelvis.

Palpation: A solid or cystic mass may be palpable in lower abdomen with well defined upper and lateral border but lower border cannot be reached. This indicates the mass is of pelvic origin. Surface is smooth and mass is freely mobile side to side but restricted mobility above down unless the pedicle is long.

Some complications of ovarian cysts, such as ovarian torsion, examination reveals moderate to severe unilateral or bilateral lower abdominal tenderness.

If hemorrhage or peritonitis ensues, the patient may present with a diffusely tender abdomen with rebound tenderness and guarding; in addition, a distended abdomen may be found on abdominal examination.

Percussion: Percussion note is dull on centre and resonant in the flanks (in ascites finding is reversed). Coexisting ascites is present in ovarian fibroma.

Pelvic examination: Bimanual examination reveals a round, solid or cystic mass, which is separate from the uterus. The cervix does not move with the movement of the mass. A groove may be felt between the lower pole of the mass and uterus.

Although normal ovaries may be palpable during the pelvic examination in thin, premenopausal patients, a palpable ovary should be considered abnormal in a postmenopausal woman. If a patient is obese, palpating cysts of any size may prove difficult.

Differential Diagnosis

Differential diagnosis varies according to the way in which a cyst presents, but there is considerable overlap. Torsion, is more likely to be confused with an inflammatory lesion. Any presentation of an ovarian cyst may be confused with:

1. Pregnancy
2. A distended bladder, which may contain up to 5 litres of urine
3. Pseudocysts
4. Hydrosalpinx
5. Uterine leiomyoma (fibroids)
6. A chronic ectopic pregnancy (hematocele)
7. A broad ligament cyst arising from the Wolffian ducts
8. An appendix mass, or a small-gut mass
9. Mesenteric cysts
10. An enlarged spleen with a long pedicle
11. Hydronephrosis

Investigations

Following investigations may be employed to confirm the diagnosis and to identify nature of ovarian lesion, i.e. benign or malignant (Table 21.2).

1. Ultrasonography

This is the primary imaging tool for a patient suspected of having an ovarian cyst. It can define morphologic characteristics of ovarian cysts.

- Simple cysts are unilocular and have a uniformly thin wall surrounding a single cavity that contains no internal echoes. These cysts have a very low chance of being malignant. Most commonly, they are functional follicular or luteal, or less commonly serous cystadenomas.
- Complex cysts may have more than 1 compartment (multilocular), thickening of the wall, projections (papulations) sticking into the lumen or on the surface, or abnormalities within the cyst contents. Malignant cysts usually fall within this

category, as well as many benign neoplastic cysts.

- Hemorrhagic cysts, endometriomas, and dermoids tend to have characteristic features ultrasonically that may help to differentiate them from malignant complex cysts.
- Ultrasound may not be able to differentiate hydrosalpinx, paraovarian, and tubal cysts from ovarian cysts.
- Transvaginal ultrasound can give detailed morphologic examination of pelvic structures. Although Transvaginal ultrasonography allows better resolution of the ovary, transabdominal ultrasound is better for large masses and allows assessment of other intra-abdominal structures such as the kidneys, liver, and ascites. It requires a full bladder.

Doppler flow studies: These studies can identify blood flow within a cyst wall and adjacent areas, including tumor surface, septa, solid parts within the tumor, and peritumorous ovarian stroma. Color flow dopler imaging helps to distinguish between benign and malignant cysts. The principle is that new vessels within tumors have lower resistance to blood flow because they lack developed smooth muscle in the walls. This can be quantitated into a resistive or pulsatility index. Thus neovascularization and low pulsatile index suggest increased blood flow in suspected malignant ovarian tumor.

2. CA-125

CA-125 is a protein expressed on the cell membrane of normal ovarian tissue and ovarian carcinomas. A serum level of less than 35 u/mL is considered normal. Post-menopausal women with elevations of CA-125 above the upper limit of normal (35 U/mL) and pre-menopausal women with markedly elevated values (>200 U/mL) warrant concern for malignancy. While CA125 is raised in 85% of epithelial ovarian carcinomas, overall it is raised in only 50% of stage 1 lesions confined to the ovary. It is also raised in some benign conditions (peritonitis, hemorrhage, cyst rupture, infection, as well as in menstruation, fibroids, and endometriosis), other malignancies, and 6% of normal patients. A raised CA 125 is most useful in conjunction with ultrasound in the assessment of a postmenopausal woman with an ovarian cyst.

Other tumor markers may be raised in neoplastic ovarian lesions. They include serum inhibin in granulosa cell tumors, alpha-fetoprotein in endodermal sinus tumor, LDH in dysgerminoma, and alpha-fetoprotein and beta-hCG in embryonal carcinoma.

3. MRI

MRI with gadolinium allows clearer evaluation of lesions indeterminate on ultrasound. It demonstrates better soft tissue contrast than CT scan, particularly for identifying fat and blood products and can give a better idea of the organ of origin of gynecologic masses. It is unnecessary in most cases.

4. CT scan

CT scanning is inferior to ultrasound and MRI for the definition of ovarian cysts and pelvic masses. It does, however, allow examination of the abdominal contents and retroperitoneum in cases of malignant ovarian disease.

At the present time the routine use of computed tomography and MRI for assessment of ovarian lesions does not improve the sensitivity or specificity obtained by transvaginal ultrasonography in the detection of ovarian malignancy.

5. Laparoscopy

Laparoscopy may be sometimes helpful in differentiating painful cystic masses from disturbed ectopic pregnancy.

6. Laparotomy

If the clinical and ancillary investigations fail to diagnose the mass, sometimes laparotomy may be justified to reach a diagnosis.

7. Histologic Findings

The definitive diagnosis of all ovarian cysts is made histologically. Each type has characteristic findings.

Complications of Ovarian Cysts

Ovarian Torsion
(Twisted ovarian cyst, axial rotation)

Ovarian torsion means the axial rotation of the ovarian vascular pedicle, causing

Clinical pearls

i. Benign ovarian neoplasms are more common than malignant tumors of the ovary at all age.
ii. The risks of malignant transformations increases with increasing age.
iii. The most important step in management is assessing the risk of malignancy.

obstruction to venous and, eventually, arterial flow that can lead to infarction. The pedicle of an ovarian cyst consists of:

1. The infundibulopelvic ligament and ovarian vessels
2. The ovarian ligament
3. A portion of the broad ligament
4. Frequently the fallopian tube.

Table 21. 2: Differentiation between benign and malignant ovarian tumors

Variables	Benign	Malignant
Age	Reproductive age	Post menopausal
Family history	-	Family history of ovarian cancer or breast cancer (BRCA-1- or BRCA-2- positive)
Symptoms	Asymptomatic	Dyspepsia, bloating, increased abdominal girth, weight loss
Physical examination	Mobile, smooth cystic mass	Fixed adnexal mass and ascites
USG findings	i. Unilocular cysts ii. Presence of solid components where the largest solid component <7 mm iii. Presence of acoustic shadowing iv. Smooth multilocular tumour with a largest diameter <100 mm v. No blood flow	i. Irregular solid tumour ii. Presence of ascites iii. At least four papillary structures iv. Irregular multilocular solid tumour with largest diameter ≥ 100 mm v. Very strong blood flow
CA-125	Not elevated	Postmenopausal ≥ 35 U/mL Premenopausal > 200 U/mL
Risk malignancy index (RMI)	< 200	> 200

Calculation of the RMI I

RMI I combines three presurgical features: Serum CA-125 (CA-125); menopausal status (M); and ultrasound score (U). The RMI is a product of the ultrasound scan score, the menopausal status and the serum CA-125 level (IU/ml) as follows: RMI = U x M x CA-125.

The ultrasound result is scored 1 point for each of the following characteristics: Multilocular cysts, solid areas, metastases, ascites and bilateral lesions. U = 0 (for an ultrasound score of 0), U = 1 (for an ultrasound score of 1), U = 3 (for an ultrasound score of 2–5).

The menopausal status is scored as 1 = premenopausal and 3 = postmenopausal.

Postmenopausal can be defined as women who have had no period for more than one year or women over the age of 50 who have had a hysterectomy.

Serum CA-125 is measured in IU/ml and can vary between zero to hundreds or even thousands of units.

Ovarian torsion is most common complication of ovarian cysts having an incidence of 12%. Ovarian cysts that are larger than 4 cm in diameter have been shown to have a torsion. Most torsion cases occur in premenopausal females of childbearing age. The most common ovarian mass associated with torsion is a dermoid cyst which is having a long pedicle. Mucinous cyst adenoma and parovarian cysts may undergo torsion because of free mobility. The etiology of torsion is unknown. It is suggested that, some vigorous or violent movement initiates the twist which causes venous occlusion and partial arterial compression. It initiates intermittent forcible arterial pulsation which further aggravates the axial rotation until it becomes complete (Fig. 21.3). The cyst may become tense and rupture or may be adherent with bowel loops. Ovarian torsion is more common on the right side owing to the sigmoid colon restricting the mobility of the left ovary.

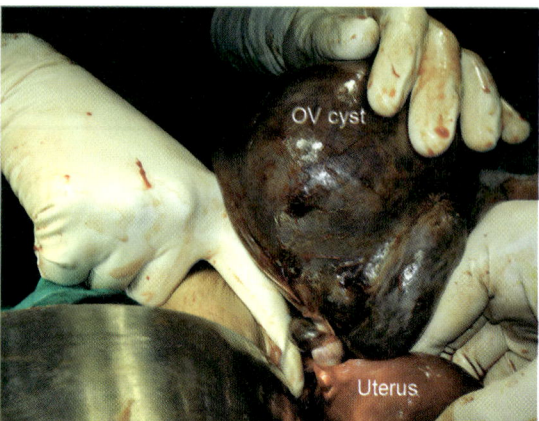

Fig. 21.3: Twisted ovarian cyst, note the torsion of the pedicle near the index finger of surgeon's right hand and color change of the cyst because of necrosis of ovarian tissue

Clinical Presentation

Symptoms: Sudden onset severe abdominal pain, nausea, vomiting.

Signs: Patient will be in agony, there will be tense, tender cystic lump with restricted mobility in lower abdomen arising from the pelvis. On pelvic examination tense cystic mass with restricted mobility will be felt separate from uterus.

Investigations: CT scanning and ultrasonography can assist with diagnosis. The absence of blood flow within an ovary can support the diagnosis of torsion.

Treatment: Ovarian torsion is surgical emergency and requires prompt surgical intervention. To suppress pain analgesic is given. Most early cases can be managed laparoscopically in young women. Laparoscopic "detorsion" with ovarian cystectomy and adnexal preservation is possible in premenopausal women when fertility and

ovarian function is desired. However, this type of treatment requires prompt diagnosis to avoid strangulation and necrosis of ovarian tissue having torsion. If strangulation and necrosis do occur, salpingo-oophorectomy should be done either via laparotomy or laparoscopy according to facility and expertise.

Rupture

Ovarian cyst rupture commonly occurs with corpus luteal cysts. They involve the right ovary in two-thirds of cases and usually occur on days 20–26 of the woman's menstrual cycle. Mittelschmerz is a form of physiologic cyst rupture. In pregnant women, hemorrhagic corpus luteal cysts are usually seen in the first trimester, with most resolving by 12 weeks' gestation. Hemorrhage and shock may occur and may present late in the symptomatology.

In ovarian cyst rupture, ultrasonography may demonstrate free fluid in the pouch of Douglas in 40% of cases. Cyst rupture and hemorrhage may be treated conservatively with observation if the patient is stable, with follow-up scanning in 6 weeks to confirm hemorrhage resolution. Laparotomy/Laparoscopy is indicated in hemodynamic compromise, possibility of torsion, no relief of symptoms within 48 hours, or increasing hemoperitoneum or falling hemoglobin concentration.

Infection

Infection of ovaraian cyst is infrequent and may occur in following situation:

1. Following acute salpingitis
2. During puerperium as part of ascending infection of upper genital tract
3. Following ovarian torsion.

Hemorrhage

Haemorrhage is more common for tumors of the right ovary. Immediate surgical intervention is indicated for a hemorrhagic cyst.

Psudomyxoma Peritonei

Pseudomyxoma peritonei is a condition caused by the production of abundant mucin by tumor cells, which fills the abdominal cavity (Fig. 21.4). It usually occurs with mucinous cyst adenoma of the ovary but also has been reported with mucocele of gall bladder, appendix and intestinal malignancy. The prognosis of this condition is bad as mesothelium of the peritoneum continues to

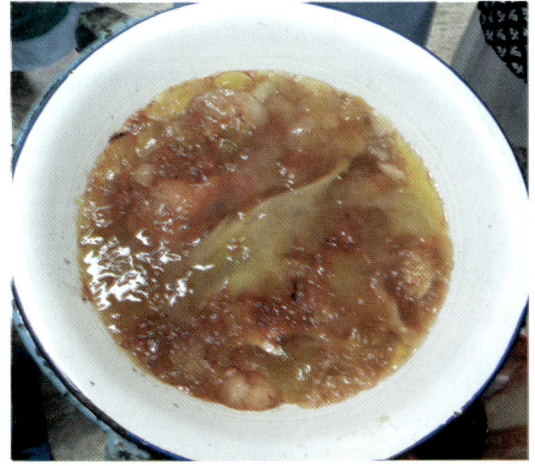

Fig. 21.4: Mucin like material in a case of pseudomyxoma peritonei

secrete mucinous material even after surgical removal of ovarian mass(debulking surgery). There is some largely anecdotal evidence in favor of intraperitoneal chemotherapy and radioisotope treatment.

Malignant Change

The potential of benign ovarian cystadenomas to become malignant has been postulated. Malignant change can occur in a small percentage of dermoid cysts and endometriomas.

Treatment

Medical Care

- Women in reproductive age with small (less than 5 cm diameter) simple ovarian cysts generally do not require follow-up, as these cysts are very likely to be physiological and almost always resolve within three menstrual cycle.

- In a postmenopausal patient, a persistent simple cyst less than 5 cm in dimension in the presence of a normal CA-125 may be followed with serial ultrasonography.

- Premenopausal women with asymptomatic simple cysts smaller than 10 cm on ultrasound in whom the CA-125 is within the normal range may be followed with a repeat ultrasound examination at 8–12 weeks (Fig. 21.6). Historically, oral contraceptive (OC) pills have been initiated while waiting for the repeat ultrasound. This was done to potentially suppress ovarian cyst formation secondary to gonadotropin suppression. OC pills may prevent the development of additional cysts, but the current literature shows OC pills are not effective in the resolution of the existing cyst.

Surgical Care

- Persistent simple ovarian cysts larger than 5–10 cm and complex ovarian cysts should be removed surgically (Fig. 21.6).

- A laparoscopic approach should be reserved for patients who have undergone thorough workup and are thought not to have malignant disease. Such patients include those considered to have a dermoid or endometrioma, those with functional or simple cysts that are causing symptoms and have not resolved with conservative management, and those presenting with acute symptoms.

In all cases, the cyst should be able to be removed intact.

- A laparotomy should be performed for patients thought to have a significant risk for malignant disease and also for patients with benign-appearing cysts that cannot be removed intact laparoscopically.

- Whether performing a laparoscopy or laparotomy, the aims are as follows:
  - Confirm the diagnosis of an ovarian cyst.
  - Assess whether the cyst appears malignant.
  - Take peritoneal washings for cytologic assessment.
  - Remove the entire cyst intact for pathologic analysis.
  - Assess the other ovary and other abdominal organs.

- *Ovarian cystectomy:* Excision of the cyst alone with conservation of the ovary (ovarian cystectomy) may be performed in patients who desire retention of their ovaries for future fertility or other reasons. Benign tumors like simple cystadenoma, endometrioma, dermoid, and functional cysts are treated by cystectomy in young women.

- *Ovariotomy:* Ovariotomy is usually done for a twisted ovarian cyst where the ovary has become gangrenous, large ovarian tumor where the ovarian tissue is compressed and destroyed, in older patients and in presence of suspicion of malignancy where conservation is not recommended. Some authors use the term oophorectomy as the synonym of ovariotomy.

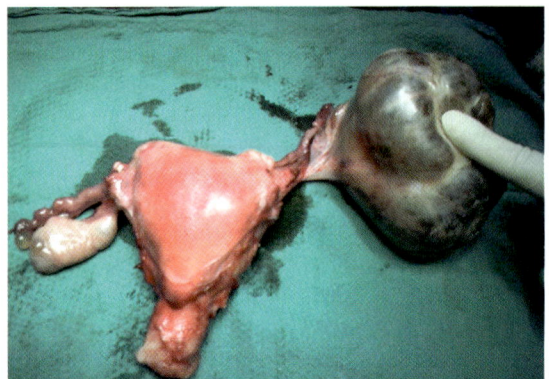

Fig. 21.5: Specimen showing large ovarian cyst, total hysterectomy with bilateral salpingo-oophorectomy was done

- Total hysterectomy with bilateral salpingo-oophorectomy (Fig. 21.5) is done in postmenopausal women, in perimenopausal women, and in premenopausal women over 35 years of age who have completed their family and who are considered at increased risk for subsequent development of ovarian carcinoma. These issues should be discussed with the patient preoperatively.

Clinical pearls

- The surgical treatment is indicated for benign ovarian neoplasms for their potential of malignancy and torsion.
- Surgical treatment may be conservative for benign tumors if future reproduction is desired.

Prognosis

- This is variable and depends on the type and size of ovarian lesion, associated complications and patient's age.
- Most small ovarian cysts in premenopausal women will resolve spontaneously.
- Ovarian torsion: If operated within six hours of onset of symptoms, tissue will usually remain viable.
- Prognosis of surgically removed cysts ultimately depends on the histology.

Figure 21.6 shows algorithm of ovarian cyst management.

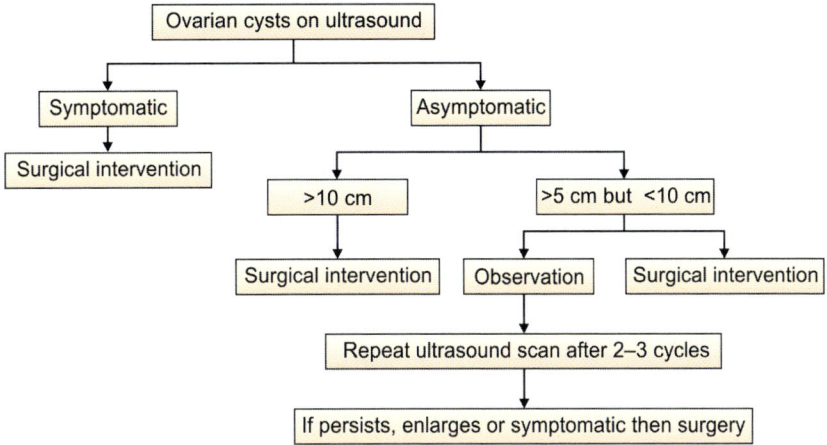

Fig. 21.6: Algorithm of ovarian cyst management

EXERCISES

Answer the following questions

1. Name the different types of benign ovarian lesions.
2. What are the nonneoplastic causes of ovarian cysts?
3. How functional ovarian cysts develop?
4. Differentiate serous cyst adenoma and mucinous cyst adenoma from clinico pathological aspect.
5. What is Meig's syndrome?
6. Describe the clinical presentation of benign ovarian cysts.
7. How clinical presentation of ovarian cyst differs from uterine leiomyoma?
8. Name the investigations for a patient with ovarian cyst.
9. How ultrasound appearances of simple and complex ovarian cysts differ?
10. How Doppler flow study helps to differentiate in benign and malignant cysts?
11. What is the normal value of CA-125?
12. Name some benign conditions where CA-125 may be raised?
13. Name some other tumor markers that may be raised in neoplastic ovarian lesions.
14. How do you differentiate benign and malignant ovarian cysts preoperatively?
15. What are the complications of ovarian cyst?
16. What do you mean by ovarian torsion?
17. Name the structures form the ovarian pedicle.
18. Name the common type of ovarian mass that are associated with torsion.
19. What is the mechanism of ovarian torsion?
20. Describe the clinical presentation of ovarian torsion.
21. How ovarian torsion is treated?
22. What is pseudomyxoma peritonei?
23. How it is treated?
24. Outline the treatment of benign ovarian lesions.
25. What do you mean by ovarian cystectomy? What are its indications?
26. What do you mean by ovariotomy? What are its indications?
27. When do you perform abdominal hysterectomy with bilateral salpingo - oophorectomy in management of ovarian cysts?

2. Fill in the blanks with appropriate word/s

1. Functional cysts are _____ , _____ , _____ .

2. Theca-lutein cysts are found in presence of _____ , _____ .

3. Psammoma bodies are present in _____ .

4. Pseudomyxoma peritonei may occur with _____ , _____ , _____ .

3. Explain or justify the following statements

1. Neoplastic cysts are tumors but all benign tumors are not cysts.

2. Benign ovarian cysts can be removed surgically either by laparotomy or laparoscopically.

4. Write short notes on

1. Dermoid cyst

2. Risk malignancy index

5. Questions for practical (read the case summary in the beginning of chapter before answering the following questions)

1. What is your diagnosis and why?

2. What are the differential diagnoses?

3. What is your primary imaging investigation?

4. What will be your preferred method, transabdominal or transvaginal sonography?

5. What other investigations you will consider for this patient and when?

6. How will you treat her if she is having a complex cyst?

6. Questions from specimens (look at the Figs 21.1, 21.2 and 21.5 before answering the following questions)

1. Describe the specimens.

2. Name the operations that has been done in Figs 21.2 and 21.5.

3. Name the type of ovarian cyst present in these specimens.

4. What was the age of the patient (from whom specimen was obtained) and why?

5. Describe the clinical presentation of the patients.

Bibliography

1. Evaluation of Ovarian Cysts Am Fam Physician. 2011 Aug 1;84(3):online.

2. Fleischer AC, et al. Ovarian Torsion, Medscape, Sep 2011.

3. Jackson WL. Ovarian cysts in the adolescents The Female Patient Vol 35 May 2010;31–34.

4. Key findings from the International Ovarian Tumor Analysis (IOTA) study: an approach to the optimal ultrasound based characterisation of adnexal pathology AJUM August 2012:15 (3);82–86.

5. Levine D, Brown DL, Anderotti RF, et al. Management of Asymptomatic Ovarian and Other Adnexal Cysts Imaged at US: Society of Radiologists in Ultrasound Consensus Conference Statement; Radiology: Volume 256: Number 3-September 2010;943–954.

6. Management of Suspected Ovarian Masses in Premenopausal Women Green-top Guideline No. 62 RCOG/BSGE Joint Guideline | November 2011.

7. Ovarian cysts in postmenopausal women RCOG guideline no 34 Review 2010.

22

Precancerous Lesions of Cervix—Cervical Intraepithelial Neoplasia (CIN)

A 37-year-old P 4+0 woman has attended gynecology outdoor with a Papanicolaou's smear report which is showing atypical squamous cells of undetermined significance (ASC-US). She reported having a long-standing monogamous sexual relationship. A general physical examination revealed no abnormalities. On pelvic examination, there were no vulvar, vaginal, or cervical lesions. How her report to be interpreted?

In this chapter we will learn:
- Cervical anatomy and role of HPV virus in development of cervical intraepithelial neoplasia (CIN)
- CIN and correlation of different terminology in relation with CIN
- Use of different screening methods for prevention of cervical cancer
- Diagnosis, prevention and treatment of CIN

Cervical Anatomy Review

- The cervix is the lower fibromuscular portion of the uterus. Ectocervix is the most readily visible portion of the cervix; endocervix is largely invisible and lies proximal to the external os.
- Ectocervix is covered by a pink stratified squamous epithelium, consisting of multiple layers of cells. The intermediate and superficial cell layers of the squamous epithelium contain glycogen. Colposcopically, the squamous epithelium of the cervix appears as a featureless, smooth, pale pink surface. Blood vessels lie below this layer and therefore are not visible or are seen only as a fine capillary network.
- Endocervix is lined by reddish columnar epithelium consisting of a single layer of cells. The columnar epithelium is characterized by infoldings or clefts and is commonly referred to as "glandular". During colposcopy the endocervix appears red and velvety due to the proximity of blood vessels beneath the one-cell-layer-thick epithelium.
- The location of squamocolumnar junction in relation to the external os varies depending upon age, menstrual status, and other factors such as pregnancy and oral contraceptive use. It everts outward onto the ectocervix during adolescence, pregnancy, and with use of combination hormonal contraceptives. It regresses into the endocervical canal with menopause and other low-estrogen states such as prolonged lactation and use of progestin-

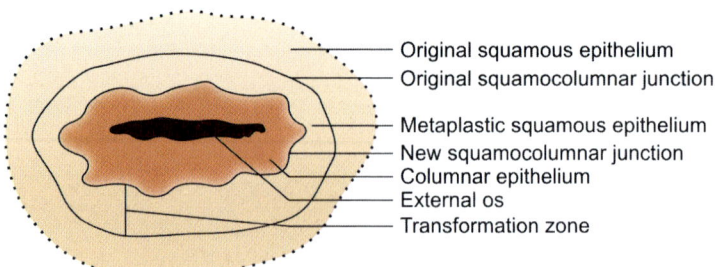

Original squamous epithelium
Original squamocolumnar junction

Metaplastic squamous epithelium
New squamocolumnar junction
Columnar epithelium
External os
Transformation zone

Fig. 22.1: A schematic diagram of the transformation zone

only contraceptives. Thus the original squamocolumnar junction is located on the ectocervix, far away from the external os. The metaplastic process mostly starts at the original squamocolumnar junction and proceeds centripetally towards the external os through the reproductive period to perimenopause. Thus, a new squamocolumnar junction is formed between the newly formed metaplastic squamous epithelium and the columnar epithelium remaining everted onto the ectocervix. As the woman passes from the reproductive to the perimenopausal age group, the location of the new squamocolumnar junction progressively moves on the ectocervix towards the external os (Fig. 22.1).

■ Squamous metaplasia [the conversion of one type of normal epithelium (columnar) into another, i.e. squamous] in the cervix refers to the physiological replacement of the everted columnar epithelium on the ectocervix by a newly formed squamous epithelium from the subcolumnar reserve cells. The rise in estrogen at puberty leads to glycogenation of the nonkeratinized squamous epithelium of the lower genital tract. Glycogen provides a carbohydrate source for lactobacilli, which dominate the normal vaginal flora in reproductive-aged women. The lactobacilli produce lactic acid, lowering the vaginal pH to less than 4.5. The exposure of the columnar epithelium to this low pH stimulates squamous metaplasia. Metaplasia is most active

during adolescence and pregnancy. This may explain why early age of sexual activity and first pregnancy are known risk factors for cervical cancer. Theoretically, cervical cells undergoing metaplasia are particularly vulnerable to the oncogenic effects of HPV and co-carcinogens.

■ The region of the cervix where squamous metaplasia occurs is referred to as the transformation zone. It corresponds to the area of cervix bound by the original squamocolumnar junction at the distal end and proximally by the the new squamocolumnar junction. Nearly all cervical neoplasia, both squamous and columnar, develops within the transformation zone, usually adjacent to the new SCJ. Identifying the transformation zone is of great importance in colposcopy (Fig. 22.1).

Human Papilloma Virus (HPV) and Carcinogenesis

■ The role of this virus in the genesis of cervical neoplasia is firmly established. Human papillomavirus is a nonenveloped DNA virus which infects epithelial cells exclusively. At least 100 HPV types have been identified; about 25 of these affect the male and female anogenital tract.

■ Clinically, HPV types are classified as high-risk (HR) or low-risk (LR) based upon their cervical cancer oncogenicity. Low-risk HPV types 6 and 11 cause nearly all genital warts and a minority of subclinical HPV infections. Low-risk HPV infections are rarely, if ever, oncogenic.

- In contrast, the HR HPV types include 16, 18, 31, 33, 35, 45, and 58 and account for approximately 99 percent of cervical cancer cases worldwide.

- Transmission of genital HPV usually requires sexual contact with the genital skin, mucous membranes, or body fluids of a partner with either warts or subclinical infection.

- In most women with an initial HPV infection, the infection clears spontaneously as a result of normal immunologic host defense mechanisms. In some women the virus may remain in the cell in a latent form in which a low number of about 100 copies of the viral genome are produced. This is termed a latent infection. Latent infections can be detected only by molecular techniques such as HPV DNA hybridization. Latent infection can also clears off spontaneously. In some individuals, however, for reasons that are not well understood, the latent papilloma virus begins to replicate independent of the host cell cycle, and large numbers of complete virions are produced. This is referred to as a productive viral infection. Productive infections have little or no malignant potential because eventual host cell death is required to complete the viral life cycle.

- Apart from productive infection, HPV infection may result in expression of neoplastic infection, causing preinvasive disease or malignancy. In neoplastic lesion, the circular HPV genome integrates linearly at random locations into a host chromosome and leaves the infected cell vulnerable to malignant transformation by loss of cell cycle control, cellular proliferation, and accumulation of DNA mutations. Neoplasia is the least common outcome of genital HPV infection.

- Infection with HPV is suspected by the appearance of clinical lesions and through the results of cytology, histology, and colposcopy, all of which are subjective and often inaccurate. Therefore, a definitive diagnosis can be made only by the direct detection of HPV DNA. This can be done histologically by in situ hybridization, by nucleic acid amplification via polymerase chain reaction (PCR), or by hybrid capture (HC) techniques. Currently, hybrid Capture 2 is the most common technique in clinical use. It is a chemiluminescent test that uses a mixture of RNA probes for the detection of 13 oncogenic HPV types.

Cervical Intraepithelial Neoplasia (CIN)

Invasive cervical cancers are usually preceded by a long phase of preinvasive disease. This is characterized microscopically as a spectrum of events progressing from cellular atypia to various grades of dysplasia or cervical intraepithelial neoplasia (CIN) before progression to invasive carcinoma. Thus **cervical intraepithelial neoplasia is defined as atypical proliferations of immature squamous epithelium that do not penetrate the basement membrane of the epithelium.** The correlation between the dysplasia/carcinoma in situ terminology and the various grades of CIN, as well as the Bethesda system are given in Table 22.1.

In cervical intraepithelial neoplasia (CIN), formerly called dysplasia, there is disordered growth and development of the epithelial lining of the cervix. There are various degrees of CIN. Mild dysplasia, or CIN I, is defined as disordered growth of the lower third of the epithelial lining. Abnormal maturation of the lower two-thirds of the lining is called moderate dysplasia, or CIN II. Severe dysplasia, CIN III, encompasses more than two-thirds of the epithelial thickness with carcinoma in situ (CIS) representing full-thickness dysmaturity (Fig. 22.2). **While histologically evaluated lesions are characterized using the CIN nomenclature, cytologic smears are classified according to the Bethesda system, which was revised in 2001.** Briefly, atypical squamous cells are

Table 22.1: Correlation between dysplasia/carcinoma in situ, cervical intraepithelial neoplasia (CIN) and the Bethesda terminology

Dysplasia terminology	Original CIN terminology	Modified CIN terminology	The Bethesda system
Normal	Normal	Normal	Within normal limits Benign cellular changes (infection or repair)
Atypia	Koilocytic atypia, flat condyloma, without epithelial changes	Low-grade CIN	ASCUS/ASC(H) LSIL
Mild dysplasia or mild dyskaryosis	CIN 1	Low-grade CIN	LSIL
Moderate dysplasia or moderate dyskaryosis	CIN 2	High-grade CIN	HSIL
Severe dysplasia or severe dyskaryosis	CIN 3	High-grade CIN	HSIL
Carcinoma in situ	CIN 3	High-grade CIN	HSIL
Invasive carcinoma	Invasive carcinoma	Invasive carcinoma	Invasive carcinoma

CIN—cervical intraepithelial neoplasia; ASC-US—atypical squamous cells of undetermined significance; ASC(H)—atypical squamous cells high grade lesion cannot be excluded; LSIL—low-grade squamous intraepithelial lesion; HSIL—high-grade squamous intraepithelial lesion

divided into those of undetermined significance (ASC-US) and those in which a high grade lesion cannot be excluded (ASC-H). Low-grade squamous intraepithelial lesion (LSIL) encompasses cytologic changes consistent with koilocytic atypia or CIN I. High-grade squamous intraepithelial lesion (HSIL) denotes the cytologic findings corresponding to CIN II and CIN III. **CIN may be suspected because of an abnormal**

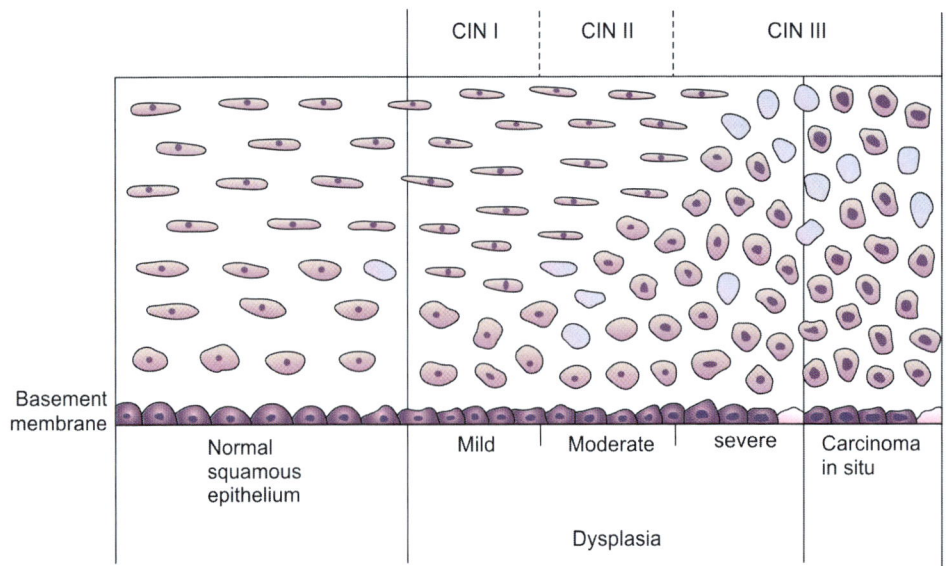

Fig. 22.2: Diagram of cervical epithelium showing various terminology used to characterize progressive degrees of cervical neoplasia. (*Source:* Modified from Richart RM: Can J Med Tech 38:177,1976; Canadian Society of Laboratory Technologists.)

Table 22.2: Approximate rates of spontaneous regression, persistence, and progression of CIN.

	CIN I	CIN II	CIN III
Regression to normal	60%	40%	30%
Persistence	30%	35%	48%
Progression to CIN	10%	20%	-
Progression to cancer	<1%	5%	22%

cytologic smear, but the diagnosis is established by cervical biopsy.

Natural history of CIN—Few CIN lesions have the potential to progress to frankly invasive cancer. Progressive potential increases with CIN grade. In addition to the grade of CIN, the course of a specific lesion is also influenced by a number of other factors, such as the patient's age, the inciting HPV type, the patient's immune competence, and smoking habits (*see* Chapter 23, Table 23.1). As summarized in Table 22.2, the majority of CIN I lesions will spontaneously regress without treatment. However, 9–16% of patients with untreated CIN I are diagnosed with CIN II/III over a 2 year follow up.

Clinical pearl: Progression of HPV infection to invasive cervical cancer on an average takes 15–20 years.

Clinical Findings

There are usually no symptoms or signs of CIN, and the diagnosis is most often based on biopsy findings following an abnormal routine cervical cytology smear. Because high-grade lesions probably are a transitional phase in the pathogenesis of many cervical cancers, early detection is extremely important. Many of these lesions, however, may turn white on application of 3–5% acetic acid, and may be iodine-negative on application of Lugol's iodine solution, as the CIN epithelium contains little or no glycogen.

Screening for Prevention of Cervical Cancer

After the introduction of cervical cytology for cervical cancer screening more than 50 years ago, multiple screening programs from all parts of the world have reported decreased rates of invasive cervical cancer and related deaths. Yet, even today, cervical cancer remains one of the leading causes of death for women in developing nations including India, where Papanicolaou smear screening programs are non existent. Cervical screening technologies include the following methods.

Conventional Pap Test

There are presently two cervical cytology techniques in use: conventional and liquid-based. The conventional Pap test is a smear of cells made directly from collection device to glass slide at the time of sampling.

Performing a Pap test: Pap tests should be scheduled in absence of menstruation. Patients should abstain from vaginal intercourse, douching, and use of vaginal tampons and medicinal or contraceptive cream preparations for a minimum of 24 to 48 hours before a test.

The woman is positioned on the table and a warmed Cusco's speculum is passed to expose the cervix. A glass slide should be labeled prior to undertaking the examination. The slide is marked in pencil with the woman's name, date-of-test and hospital number if known. A spatula is then used to scrape the whole squamo columnar junction (SCJ). If the external os is regular, the pointed end of a spatula can be passed into the canal and rotated twice by 360°. If the cervical os is stenosed, the brush end of a cytobrush should be used. This is common after surgery to the cervix for cervical abnormality or in postmenopausal women. The most commonly used spatula is the Ayers spatula with its elongated beak to go up the cervical canal. For traditional Pap smears, the endocervix and ectocervix should be sampled separately (spatula first, cytobrush last). The standard method for sampling the endocervix is with an endocervical brush, which enhances cell recovery. Insert the brush into the endocervical canal and rotate one-half to two full turns.

Transfer the cells onto a slide within 30 seconds. Both sides of the spatula should be drawn along the slide. If using a cytobrush, gently roll and twist the brush along the slide and mark the slide with a "C." The material on the slide must be spread thinly so that microscopic interpretation is possible. The glass slide is fixed immediately to prevent the cells drying in air either by immersing it in a jar of 95% ethyl alcohol and fixing for 15 minutes or by spraying with the fixative aerosol which dries rapidly, fixing the cells and nuclei. The slide can then go to the laboratory.

Liquid-based Testing

To decrease the false-negative rate of cervical cytology, attempts have been made to improve both specimen collection and quality and to reduce errors of interpretation. These techniques differ from the conventional method of Papanicolaou smear collection in several ways. Once the clinician obtains a scraping of the SCJ and transformation zone area of the ectocervix, the spatula and brush are dipped in a small bottle of fixative solution to elute the cells rather than being smeared on a glass slide. This bottle is then labeled and sent to the cytology laboratory rather than sending a slide. Collected cells in a liquid transport medium are subsequently processed to produce an even monolayer of cells on a glass slide.

Visual Inspection with Acetic Acid (VIA)

Simple visual inspection of the cervix after application of acetic acid has been effectively used in resource-poor settings for cervical cancer screening. Areas of cervical dysplasia turn white after application of acetic acid, and inspection of the cervix using handheld magnifying lenses can identify many CIN lesions. This technique, commonly referred to as VIA (visual inspection with acetic acid), has been effectively used in areas of Africa, India, and China. Nurses or even health care technicians can be trained to use the technique and do biopsies or refer women with suspicious lesions for more extensive evaluation. Although VIA is not as specific as cytology, it is almost as sensitive and does not require several visits or the considerable infrastructure needed by cytologic screening.

Human Papilloma Virus Testing

With the knowledge that significant cervical neoplasia is always associated with HPV infection, it has been suggested that HPV testing could be used to screen women for cervical neoplasia. The purpose of HPV testing is to detect the presence of high risk HPV types associated with cervical cancer. HPV testing is very sensitive. HPV testing could be used as a primary screening approach for women aged 30 years and over, with Pap tests reserved for women who test HPV positive. Screening women less than 30 years of age for HPV is not recommended, as with the high prevalence of HPV and low incidence of cervical cancer, the specificity of the test is low.

Initiation of Screening

In developed countries (USA) screening begins approximately 3 years after initiation of sexual activity or by age 21, whichever occurs first. Based on ACOG recommendations, cytology screening should be annual until age 30. After age 30, women at average risk for cervical cancer can be screened at 2- to 3-year intervals if three consecutive, annual negative Pap tests have been documented. Women at higher risk due to prior treatment for CIN II, CIN III, or cervical cancer, in utero DES exposure, or immunosuppressive illness or medications should receive at least annual screening. Specifically, HIV-infected women require a Pap test twice during the first year after diagnosis and annually thereafter (Centers for Disease Control and Prevention, 2002). Alternatively, women age 30 or older may undergo testing for HR HPV types as an adjunct to cervical cytology. If both tests are negative, rescreening should be no more frequent than every 3 years.

Discontinuation of Screening

Screening may be stopped at age 65 or 70 in women not at high risk for cervical cancer.

Fact sheet: There is no international consensus on the age at which to initiate and discontinue cervical cancer screening. Recommendations for age to start and stop screening and for screening interval vary from country to country and between professional organizations; they also have changed over time.

The 2001 Bethesda System

The Bethesda system for classification of abnormalities was developed to standardize nomenclature to minimize misunderstandings between cytologists and treating physicians, and was modified in 2001. Its components of epithelial cell abnormalities are shown in Table 22.3.

Clinical pearl: Cervical cytology results are not diagnostic of CIN or cancer; biopsy and histologic confirmation are required for diagnosis.

Epithelial Cell Abnormalities: Significance and Management

A cytology report is a medical consultation that interprets a screening test and is not a diagnosis. Thus, a final diagnosis is determined clinically, often with results from histologic evaluation. Pap tests are interpreted as either negative for intraepithelial lesion or malignancy, or consistent with one or more epithelial cell abnormalities.

Atypical Squamous Cells of Undetermined Significance

The most common cytologic abnormality is atypical squamous cells of undetermined significance (ASC-US), which indicates cells that are suggestive of, but do not fulfill the criteria for, SIL. Although an ASC-US result

Table 22.3: The 2001 Bethesda system: Epithelial cell abnormalities

Squamous cell

Atypical squamous cells (ASC) of undetermined significance (ASC-US); cannot exclude HSIL (ASC-H)

Low-grade squamous intraepithelial lesion (LSIL)
High-grade squamous intraepithelial lesion (HSIL)
Squamous cell carcinoma

Glandular cell

Atypical glandular cells (AGC)
Endocervical, endometrial, or not otherwise specified
Endocervical adenocarcinoma in situ (AIS)
Adenocarcinoma

often precedes the diagnosis of CIN II or III, this risk approximates only 5 percent and cancer is found in only 1 to 2 per thousand instances. Therefore, the evaluation of ASC-US should not be overly aggressive, particularly in adolescents who are at low risk of cervical cancer.

Atypical Squamous Cells, Cannot Exclude HSIL

Five to 10 percent of ASC is designated as atypical squamous cells, cannot exclude high grade (ASC-H). This describes cellular changes that do not fulfill criteria for HSIL cytology, but for which a high-grade lesion cannot be excluded. Histologic HSIL is found in upwards of 25 percent of these cases. This is higher than that seen with ASC-US, and therefore colposcopy is indicated for evaluation.

Low-grade Squamous Intraepithelial Lesion

This cytology result indicates the likely presence of HPV infection or low-grade neoplasia. Low-grade SIL encompasses the cytologic features of HPV infection and CIN I and carries a 15 to 30 percent risk of CIN II or III, similar to the ASC-US HPV-positive category. Therefore, colposcopy is indicated for most.

High-grade Squamous Intraepithelial Lesion and Glandular Abnormalities

High-grade SIL, all glandular epithelial cell abnormalities, and suspicion of carcinoma should all be evaluated by prompt colposcopic evaluation. High-grade SIL cytology encompasses features of CIN II and CIN III and carries a high risk of underlying histologic CIN II or CIN III (at least 70 percent), or invasive cancer (1 to 2%).

To address abnormal findings, evidence-based management guidelines have been developed and are summarized in Table 22.4 and Fig. 22.3. Alternative management strategies may be appropriate based on individual patient characteristics, available resources, and other clinical factors.

Diagnosis of CIN

As mentioned earlier, screening tests for CIN are imperfect, with limited sensitivity and specificity. The definitive diagnosis of CIN requires colposcopy and biopsy, with treatment based on histologic findings.

Colposcopy

A colposcope is a low-power, stereoscopic, binocular field microscope with a powerful light source used for magnified visual examination of the uterine cervix to help in the diagnosis of cervical neoplasia.

Objectives

- To visualise the cervix and vagina under magnification
- To identify squamocolumnar junction of the cervix
- To detect lesions suspicious for neoplasia
- To direct biopsy of lesions
- Monitor patients with a current or past history of lower genital tract neoplasia.

Table 22.4: Cervical cytology: Initial management of epithelial cell abnormalities

Epithelial cell abnormality	General recommendation	Special circumstances
ASC-US	Reflex HPV testing Repeat cytology at 12 months (if no HPV testing) colposcopy if HPV positive	Refer to colposcopy for recurrent abnormal cytology, or initial positive HPV DNA test; adolescents[b] managed with repeat annual cytology
LSIL	Colposcopy for non-adolescent women If co-testing shows HPV-negative LSIL, repeat co-testing at 1 year is preferred, but colposcopy is acceptable.	Adolescents managed with repeat annual cytology; HPV DNA test at 12 months or repeat cytology at 6 and 12 months are also acceptable for postmenopausal women
ASC-H, HSIL, squamous cell carcinoma	Colposcopy	
AGC, AIS, adenocarcinoma	Colposcopy, endocervical curettage[a] HPV DNA testing for AGC	Endometrial sampling is indicated if age >35 years, abnormal bleeding, chronic anovulation, or atypical endometrial cells specified

[a]Endocervical curettage and endometrial sampling are contraindicated in pregnancy.
[b]adolescents: age 13 to 20 years. AGC: atypical glandular cells; AIS: adenocarcinoma in situ; ASC-H: atypical squamous cells, cannot exclude high-grade squamous intraepithelial lesion; ASC-US: atypical squamous cells of undetermined significance; HPV: human papillomavirus; HSIL: high-grade squamous intraepithelial lesion; LSIL: low-grade squamous intraepithelial lesion (*Adapted from* 2012 ASCCP Consensus Guidelines)

Indications

- Abnormal cervical cytology
- Grossly visible genital tract lesions.

Procedure

The colposcopic examination begins with careful visual inspection of the vagina and cervix. The cervix is examined in a clockwise fashion, concentrating on the squamo-columnar junction, the border between squamous epithelium of the ectocervix, and the columnar epithelium of the endocervix, where most dysplasia appears to originate. If no obvious malignant lesions are noted, 3–5% acetic acid then is liberally applied to the cervix. This not only cleans the cervix, it also alters the reflectivity of superficial cells, accentuating atypia and highlighting vasculature. The cervix again is inspected, concentrating on the transformation zone, the area of metaplastic transition between the native squamous epithelium, which is red and smooth, and the columnar epithelium, which has a white, grape-like appearance after the application of acetic acid. Following application of 3–5 percent acetic acid to mucosal epithelium, the color or degree of whiteness obtained, rapidity and duration of acetowhitening, and sharpness of lesion borders are observed. Once inspection with white light has been completed, inspection is completed with a green filtered light, which enhances vascular patterns.

Abnormal findings indicative of CIN and carcinoma in situ (CIS) are those of:

1. Leukoplakia or hyperkeratosis, which is an area of white, thickened epithelium that is appreciated prior to the application of acetic acid and may indicate underlying neoplasia.
2. Acetowhite epithelium, which is epithelium that stains white after the application of acetic acid.
3. Mosaicism or punctation reflecting abnormal vascular patterns of the surface capillaries. As a general rule, capillary thickness and intercapillary distances correlate with the severity of the lesion and thus tend to be larger and coarser in higher-grade lesions.
4. High-grade lesions demonstrate a more persistent, duller shade of white, whereas low-grade lesions are translucent or bright white and fade quickly. Low-grade lesions characteristically have feathery margins, whereas high-grade lesions have straighter, sharper outlines. A lesion with an internal border, that is, a lesion within a lesion, is typically high-grade.
5. Atypical vessels with bizarre capillaries with so-called corkscrew, comma-shaped, or spaghetti-like configurations suggest early stromal invasion.

Biopsy

Ectocervical Biopsy

Under direct colposcopic visualization, suspicious lesions on the ectocervix are biopsied using a biopsy forceps. Generally, cervical biopsy does not require anesthesia. Extreme cases of bleeding are rare and can be controlled with vaginal packing.

Satisfactory Colposcopy

Within a neoplastic lesion, more severe disease tends to be at the proximal limit of the transformation zone. Thus, adequate visualization of the entire cervical SCJ and upper limits of all lesions defines whether a colposcopic examination is termed satisfactory or unsatisfactory. This determination can affect management. Therefore, with initially unsatisfactory colposcopy, an endocervical speculum may be used to dilate and fully visualize lesions that have extended cephalad into the endocervical canal.

Endocervical Curettage

For non-pregnant patients, endocervical curettage (ECC) is used to evaluate tissue within the endocervical canal not visualized by colposcopy. A normal ECC provides an added degree of assurance that a neoplastic endocervical lesion is not present. Endocervical curettage generally is indicated if:

- Atypical glandular cell cytology is evaluated
- Colposcopy is unsatisfactory, which is common in postmenopausal women
- Ablative treatment is planned. Endocervical curettage is performed by introducing an endocervical curette 1 to 2 cm into the cervical canal. The entire length and circumference of the canal is firmly curetted, carefully avoiding sampling of the ectocervix or lower uterine segment.

Prevention of CIN

Behavioral Interventions

Sexual abstinence, delaying onset of sexual activity, delayed child birth and limiting the number of sexual partners are useful strategies to avoid or limit genital HPV infection and its effects.

Condoms

Use of condoms is important for prevention of sexually transmitted infections (STIs) in general, but their efficacy specifically in preventing HPV transmission is less certain. Male condoms are more effective at preventing STIs transmitted through body fluids and across mucosal surfaces, and less so for STIs spread skin-to-skin, as is the case with HPV.

HPV Vaccine

Prophylactic vaccines have been found to prevent establishment of persistent infection and therefore, the development of cervical neoplasia. There are two types of vaccines:

- A recombinant quadrivalent vaccine against types 6, 11, 16, and 18 (Gardasil)
- A bivalent HPV vaccine against types 16 and 18 (Cervarix).

Both vaccines are administered in three intramuscular doses during a 6-month period, (0, 2, 6) and are extremely safe, effective and well tolerated. Protection provided by vaccination is nearly 100% when administered prior to initiation of sexual activity (girls aged 11–12 years). A history of previous sexual intercourse or HPV-related disease is not a contraindication to vaccine administration. Testing for HPV is not recommended prior to vaccination. However, it must be remembered that the current vaccines are effective only for preventing cancer and high-grade CIN related to HPV-16 or -18. Although these two viral types cause approximately 70% of all cervical cancer, several other viral types (31, 33, 45, and others) are responsible for almost a third of cervical cancer. In addition, women who have already been exposed to HPV-16 or -18 will not be protected by the vaccine.

Management of Histologic Diagnosis of CIN

- Patient management is based on the correlation of the results of the cervical cytology smear, findings at colposcopy and biopsy, and ECC results, as well as individual patient characteristics, such as pregnancy, HIV infection, and the likelihood of compliance with management recommendations.
- Since CIN typically occurs in women of childbearing age, the impact of the disease and its treatments on future fertility and pregnancy outcomes is an important consideration. Excisional therapy of CIN has been linked to preterm delivery.
- *Management of CIN falls into two general categories:* Observation and treatment. The objective of all treatment is surgical obliteration of the entire cervical transformation zone, including abnormal tissue. This may be done by use of ablation, that is, tissue destruction with cryosurgery or laser ablation, or by excision of tissue. Excisional modalities include laser conization, cold-knife conization, and

electrosurgical loop excision (Loop Electrosurgical Excision Procedure) (Table 22.5). All treatment modalities, particularly excisional procedures, are suspected of increasing the risk of adverse future reproductive outcomes, such as preterm delivery and premature rupture of membranes.

- In general, histologic CIN I can be observed indefinitely, especially in adolescents, or treated if it persists for at least 2 years. This is also the case for CIN II lesions in adolescents. However, CIN II in adult women and CIN III are treated by excision or ablation except in special circumstances. The "see and treat" approach in which loop excision is performed at initial colposcopy is an acceptable option for high-risk, adult patients who present with high-grade cytology and corresponding colposcopic abnormalities. In the case of unsatisfactory colposcopy and histologic CIN, a diagnostic excisional procedure is recommended to exclude the presence of occult high-grade CIN or invasive cancer (Fig. 22.3).

Modalities for the Treatment

Cryotherapy

In cryotherapy, an outdoor procedure not requiring anesthesia, nitrous oxide or carbon dioxide is used as the refrigerant for a supercooled probe. Using either carbon dioxide or nitrous oxide under pressure as the coolant, the cervical epithelium is frozen to a depth of 6 to 10 mm. The length of time for the freeze and the absolute temperature of the

Table 22.5: Techniques for treatment of squamous intraepithelial lesions

Ablative	Excisional
Cryosurgery	Laser excisional conization
Laser vaporization	Loop electrosurgical excision procedure (LEEP)
	Cold knife conization (CKC) (scalpel)
	Hysterectomy

probe will determine the depth of penetration and subsequent tissue loss. Tissue is sloughed off slowly, over a period of 10 to 14 days, as a watery discharge. The most widely accepted technique for cryotherapy is to freeze the cervix for 3 minutes after formation of an ice ball on the cervix, followed by a 5-minute thaw and a repeated 3-minute freeze. The advantages of cryotherapy include ease of use, low cost, widespread availability, and a low complication rate. Side effects include mild uterine cramping and a copious watery vaginal discharge for several weeks. Infection and cervical stenosis are rare.

Carbondioxide Laser

Carbon dioxide (CO_2) laser can be used either to ablate the transformation zone or as a tool for cone biopsies. The laser destroys tissue with a very narrow zone of injury around the treated tissue, and is therefore both precise and flexible. The tissue is vaporized to a depth of at least 7 mm to assure that the bases of the deepest glands are destroyed. Post treatment vaginal discharge may last 1–2 weeks, and bleeding that requires reexamination can occur in a small percentage of patients. The technique is expensive and requires significant training and attention to safety, as well as local or general anesthesia.

Loop Electrosurgical Excision Procedure (LEEP)

LEEP is the procedure of choice for treating CIN II and CIN III because of its ease of use, low cost, and provision of tissue for histologic evaluation. LEEP uses a small, fine, wire loop attached to an electrosurgical generator to excise the tissue of interest. Various sizes of wire loop are available. Following LEEP excision of the transformation zone, frequently an additional narrow endocervical specimen is removed to allow for histologic evaluation while avoiding excessive damage to the cervical stroma. Fulguration with a roller ball electrode is then used to achieve

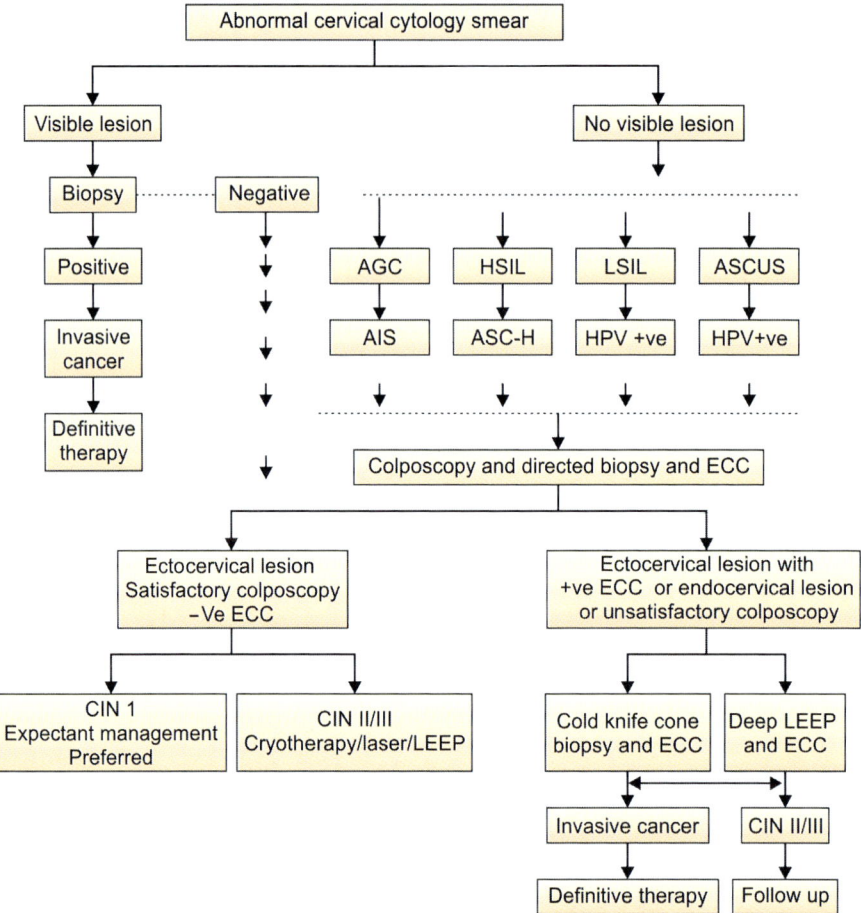

Fig. 22.3: Algorithm of management of the abnormal cytologic smear with visible or no visible cervical lesion

complete hemostasis in the excision bed. LEEP can be performed as an office procedure under local anesthesia. An insulated speculum to prevent conduction of electricity, a grounding pad, and a vacuum to remove the smoke are necessary. Complications are less frequent than with cold knife conization and include bleeding, infection, and cervical stenosis.

Cold Knife Conization

Cold knife conization of the cervix means the excision of a cone-shaped portion of the cervix using a scalpel. This technique can be individualized to accommodate the cervical anatomy and the size and shape of the lesion. For example, a wide, shallow cone specimen can be obtained from a young patient whose squamocolumnar junction is on the ectocervix. In an older patient, in whom the squamocolumnar junction tends to move more cephalad into the endocervical canal, a narrower, deeper cone is preferable. Endocervical curettage is performed after the conization to assess the remaining endocervical canal. Cervical cone biopsy is generally done in the operating room under local or general anesthesia. Complications include bleeding, infection, cervical stenosis, and cervical incompetence. The need to perform the procedure in the operating room and a higher complication rate are distinct disadvantages of cold knife conization.

However, it results in a specimen devoid of any thermal artifact that may complicate the histologic diagnosis and margin assessment seen with LEEP and laser conization. This becomes particularly important with suspected microinvasive carcinoma and adenocarcinoma in situ.

Hysterectomy

Hysterectomy is unacceptable as primary treatment for CIN I, II or III. However, there is still a limited role for hysterectomy such as in the scenario of repetitive CIN II/III that recurs despite less invasive treatments.

Keywords

Squamocolumner junctiom: The junction between the squamous and columnar epithelium on the cervix. Although it is found in the area of the external cervical os in most women during the reproductive years, it is a dynamic, ever-changing location.

Transformation zone: A colposcopic term for the area of cellular change that is observed adjacent to the squamocolumnar junction.

Cervical intraepithelial neoplasia (CIN): A cytologic and histologic classification of preinvasive cervical atypias or neoplastic changes. In general, CIN I = mild dysplasia, CIN II = moderate dysplasia, and CIN III = severe dysplasia/carcinoma in situ.

Cervical dysplasia: Dysplasia is a pathologic term to indicate noninvasive epithelial atypia that involves various degrees of the cervical epithelium. By convention, in mild dysplasia, the nuclear atypia, mitoses, and cellular irregularity involved the lower one third of the squamous epithelium. When the atypia involves the middle third, the diagnosis is moderate dysplasia; in severe dysplasia, the upper one third of the epithelial layer is involved. A full-thickness change is called carcinoma in situ.

The Bethesda system: Another classification system that was introduced in 1991 for grading cytologic abnormalities. It has also been used for histologic diagnoses. Low-grade squamous intraepithelial lesion (LSIL) = mild dysplasia/human papillomavirus changes. High-grade squamous intraepithelial lesion (HSIL) = moderate/severe dysplasia or carcinoma in situ.

HPV DNA testing: High risk HPV (hrHPV) DNA testing is a mainstay component of cervical cancer screening as the presence of hrHPV DNA is a necessary agent for the development of cervical cancer. Currently the use of hrHPV testing is approved in the following three scenarios: (1) Triage of patients having equivocal (ASC-US) Pap tests; (2) Use in conjunction with the Pap test in primary screening for women over the age of 30 years; (3) Use of HPV 16/18 testing for triage in women in the second scenario above who have positive hrHPV and negative Pap tests.

Koilocytic atypia: Koilocytosis or koilocytic atypia are terms used in histology and cytology to describe the presence of koilocytes in a specimen. A Koilocyte is a squamous epithelial cell that has undergone a number of structural changes, which occur as a result of infection of the cell by human papilloma virus. Koilocytes may have the following cellular changes (i) Nuclear enlargement (two to three times normal size), (ii) Irregularity of the nuclear membrane contour, (iii) A darker than normal staining pattern in the nucleus, known as hyperchromasia and (iv) A clear area around the nucleus, known as a perinuclear halo.

Carcinoma in situ: A histopathologic diagnosis involving severe epithelial atypia. In the cervix, the full thickness of the cervical epithelium is atypical, but the basement membrane remains intact. Despite the confusing name, the lesion is not a cancer. It does not metastasize.
LEEP or Loop electrosurgical excision procedure; also called a LLETZ (large loop excision of the transformation zone). A thin wire electrosurgical loop electrode of 1 to 2.5 cm in diameter is used to excise the transformation zone under local anesthesia.

EXERCISES

Answer the following questions

1. What is the significance of transformation zone in development of cervical neoplasia?
2. What is the role of HPV in genesis of cervical neoplasia?
3. What is CIN?
4. How do you correlate dysplasia, CIN and Bethesda terminology?
5. What is the natural course of CIN?
6. What are the different methods of screening for prevention of cervical cancer?
7. Name the different types of epithelial cell abnormalities detected during pap screening and what are their significance?

8. How epithelial cell abnormalities are managed?
9. How CIN is diagnosed?
10. What are the abnormal findings during colposcopy indicative of CIN?
11. How CIN is managed?
12. What are the different techniques of treatment of squamous intraepithelial lesions?

Write short notes on

1. Pap test
2. Colposcopy

Explain or justify the following statements

1. Terminology to express abnormal cervical cytology has changed over time.
2. Colposcopy plays an important role in management of abnormal cervical cytology report.
3. Hysterectomy is unacceptable as primary treatment of CIN.
4. HPV vaccination is not adequate enough to prevent cervical cancer.

Fill in the blanks with appropriate word/s

1. Ecto cervix is lined by _____ epithelium and endocervix is lined by _____ epithelium.
2. CIN lesions turn _____ on application of 3–5% acetic acid.
3. The glass slide with papsmear is fixed immediately with _____ .
4. The diagnosis of CIN requires _____ and _____ .

Bibliography

1. Apgar SB, Brotzman G. Mangement of cervical cytologic abnormalities Am Fam Physician 2004;70:1905–16.
2. Cervical cancer precursors and their management Rock, John A.; Jones, Howard W. TeLinde's Operative Gynecology, 10th Edition.
3. Cervical intraepithelial neoplasia, current obstetrics and gynecology Mc Grew Hill 2006.
4. Clinical practice guideline for general practitioners cervical screening the US Agency for International Development (USAID).
5. John W, Sellors R. Sankaranarayanan Colposcopy and Treatment of Cervical Intraepithelial Neoplasia: A Beginners' Manual International Agency for Research on Cancer, 2003 World Health Organization.
6. Mark Spitzerbarbara S. Apgar Gregory L. Brotzman. Management of Histologic Abnor-malities of the Cervix Am Fam Physician 2006;73:105–12.
7. Masad SL, Mark H Einstein, Warner K Huh, et al. 2012 Updated Consensus Guidelines for the Management of Abnormal Cervical Cancer Screening Tests and Cancer Precursors Obstet Gynecol 2013;121:829–46.
8. Preinvasive lesion of the lower genital tract Williams Gynecology McGrew Hill 2008
9. Programmatic Guidelines for Screening for Cancer of the cervix in Canada Society of Gynecologic Oncologists of Canada.
10. Vesco K, Whitlok EP, Eder M. Risk Factors and Other Epidemiologic Considerations for Cervical Cancer Screening: A Narrative Review for the US. Preventive Services Task Force Ann Intern Med. 2011;155:698–705.
11. Wright C T, Cox T, Masad S, et al 2001. Consensus Guidelines for the Management of Women with Cervical Intraepithelial Neoplasia Am J ObstetGynecol 2003;189:295–304.

23

Cervical Cancer

A 62-year-old woman has presented with bleeding per vagina for last few weeks. She is post-menopausal for last 12 years. On pelvic examination she has an exophytic mass arising out of the cervix. Biopsy from the mass shows moderately differentiated squamous cell carcinoma. How she should be managed?

In this chapter we will learn:
- Definition of cervical cancer
- Epidemiology
- Etiology
- Pathophysiology
- Primary prevention
- Clinical presentation
- Investigations
- Staging and prognosis
- Treatment
- Complications

Definition

Cervical cancer is a HPV virus induced malignancy of cervical mucosa.

Epidemiology

Cervical cancer is the second most common malignancy in women worldwide with an estimated 300,000 deaths annually. India has a high incidence of cervical carcinoma, representing the most frequent malignant neoplasm and cancer-related cause of death among women. In the year 2004, national estimate was 1,12,609 new cases cancer cervix, corresponding to an incidence of 26.1% new cases among all cases of cancer among women (Krishnan, 2005). The highest worldwide mortality rates from cervical cancer are reported in Romania (13.7 cases per 100,000 population) and the lowest in Finland (1.1 per 100,000).

HPV is the most important etiological factor. Incidence of cervical cancer correlates with early onset of sexual activity, multiple sexual partners, cigarette smoking, low socioeconomic status, poor nutrition, oral contraceptive use, and immunosuppression (Table 23.1). Effective screening with the Pap smear in developed countries has reduced the

Table 23.1: Risk factors for cervical neoplasia

- More than one sexual partner or have a male sexual partner who have had sex with more than one person
- First intercourse at an early age (younger than 18 years)
- Male sexual partner who has had a sexual partner with cervical cancer
- Smoking
- HIV infection
- STD infection
- Diethyl stilbesterol (DES) exposure
- Organ transplant (Specially kidney)
- Infrequent or absent pap screening test

incidence and mortality by 75% in the last 50 years.

Fact sheet: Cervical cancer disproportionately affects developing countries which have no screening system. According to WHO, in 2005, almost 2,60,000 women died of the disease , nearly 95% of them of developing countries , making cervical cancer one of the gravest threats to woman's life. In India, over 80% of the cervical cancer present at the fairly advanced stage and around 80,000 deaths are reported annually due to cervical cancer.

Etiology

HPV is the most important etiological factor, and is responsible for most (99.7%) tumours . HPV-16 and 18 are the 2 most common high-risk types detected in more than 70% of malignancies. Other high-risk types include 31, 33, 35, 39, 45, 51, 52, 56, 58, 59, 68, 73, and 82.The majority of the cervical cancers are caused by just four types of high risk HPV types: 16,18,31,45. In western population, peak infection incidence is in the late teens and early 20s, but in 80% of patients, the infection resolves within 12 to 18 months with a median duration of infection of roughly 8 months. Once infection resolves, the risk of cervical cancer returns to baseline. Cervical cancer in the absence of demonstrable HPV

infection does occur, but it is extremely rare, and HPV testing appears to be more sensitive than and superior to standard Pap smear screening (*see* Chapter 22).

Clinical pearl: The main risk factor for cervical cancer is Human papilloma virus infection which is a sexually transmitted infection

Pathophysiology

The HPV virus is cleared by the immune system in 93% patients by 3 years following infection. The incubation from latent infection to development of cancer is typically 15 years (Fig. 23.1). The oncoproteins E6 (which binds p53) and E7 (which interacts with retino-blastoma protein Rb), in conjunction with co-factors yet to be defined, drive CIN as a monoclonal proliferation (by loss of E2F cell cycle regulation) to invasive cancer. The research shows an annual rate of progression of high-grade squamous intraepithelial lesion to invasive cancer of 1.4%.

About 80 to 85% of all cervical cancers are squamous cell carcinoma; most of the rest are adenocarcinomas. Sarcomas and small cell neuroendocrine tumors are rare.

Spread of Cancer Cervix

Invasive cervical cancer usually spreads by direct extension into surrounding tissues or via the lymphatic to the pelvic and para-aortic lymph nodes. Hematogenous spread to lungs, liver and bone is possible but rare. Sites of spread by direct extension include cervical stroma, body of uterus, vagina and para-metrium. In later stage it spreads to urinary bladder and rectum causing urinary fistula. The lymphatic from cervix drain into parametrial group of lymph nodes. Then it goes into internal eliac, obturator and external eliac group of lymph nodes. Then the drainage goes to common eliac and para-aortic group of lymph nodes. Dissemination is mostly in this order.

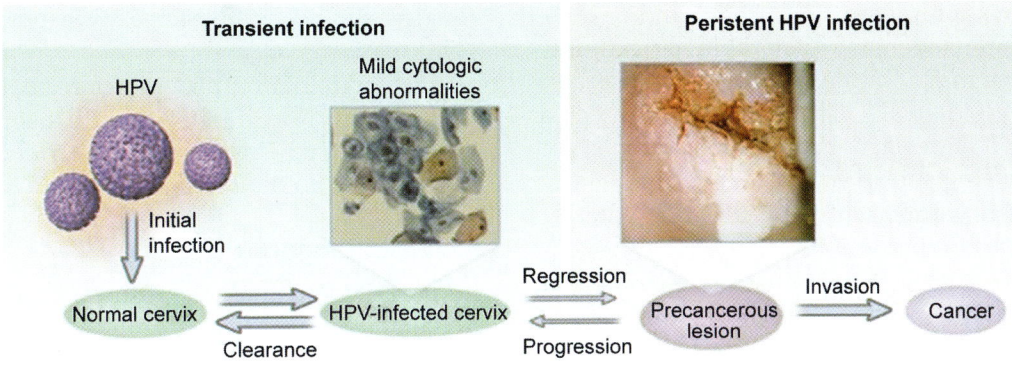

Fig. 23.1: Steps of cervical carcinogenesis (*Courtesy:* New England Journal of Medicine)

Primary Prevention

- As HPV is spread by skin-to-skin contact, safe sexual health and effective barrier contraception may play a role in primary prevention, although the issue is complex.
- Cervical cancer vaccine—Vaccines against HPV-16/18 could prevent more than 70% of cervical cancers. The recommend age for vaccination is 11 to 12 years for girls, but data support immunising as young as 9 years old or up to age 45. There are 3 IM injections at 0, 2, and 6 months. In HPV-naive patients, this vaccine proved to have 100% efficacy to prevent HPV-6-, 11-, 16-, and 18-related cervical, vaginal, and vulvar dysplasia and condyloma; longer-term outcomes regarding cervical cancer itself are not yet available. The immunogenicity data suggest a high level of persistent antibody titres 5 years after immunization. The vaccine is very safe, with typical adverse effects including pain, itching, irritation, erythema, and low-grade fever. Primary prevention in the low socioeconomic groups would be particularly useful given their increased risk, but advocacy for this often underserved population with poor access to health care has been challenging.

Secondary Prevention

See Chapter 22—screening for prevention of cervical cancer.

Clinical Presentation

CIN is usually asymptomatic. Early cervical cancer may be asymptomatic.

Early Symptoms

- Abnormal vaginal bleeding may take the form of post-coital bleeding, inter menstrual bleeding or postmenopausal bleeding.
- Serosanguinous discharge or yellowish vaginal discharge, at times foul smelling, may occur.

Clinical pearl: Suspect cancer cervix if the woman's age is 35 years or more and presents with abnormal vaginal discharge.

Late Symptoms

- Pelvic pain—Sciatic or back pain can be related to sidewall extension, hydro-nephrosis or metastasis.
- Bladder or rectal invasion by advanced stage disease may produce urinary or rectal symptoms (hematuria, urinary frequency, vaginal passage of urine or stool).
- Lower extremity swelling from occlusion of pelvic lymphtaics, or thrombosis of external eliac vein.

Signs

On general and systemic examination, advanced cervical cancer may present with anemia, plural effusion, ascites and or lower extremity edema. Unilateral lower extremity edema may indicate spread of the disease to pelvic side walls. Groin and supraclavicular lymph nodes may be indurated or enlarged, indicating spread of disease.

Most women with cervical cancer will have visible cervical lesion.

- On speculum examination, early lesions may be focally indurated or ulcerated or present as a slightly elevated and granular area that bleeds readily on contact (Fig. 23.2). It may resemble an ectropion or chronic cervicitis. More advanced tumors have several types of gross appearance: exophytic, endophytic, or infiltrative. Exophytic, lesion generally appears as a friable, bleeding, cauliflower like lesion in the portio vaginalis that characteristically bleeds on touch. In some cases tumor may arise from the endocervix and ecto cervix may appear normal .This is known as endophytic growth. In these cases, bimanual examination may reveal a firm indurated barrel shaped cervix. Infiltrative lesion produces enlargement, irregularity, and a firm consistency of the cervix and eventually of the adjacent parametria. The

vagina should be inspected for extension of disease.
- Rectal examination provides information regarding nodularity of uterosacral ligaments and helps to determine extension of disease into the parametrium.

Differential Diagnosis

The conditions that may mimic cervical carcinoma may include:

- *Cervicitis:* The cervix may be hypertrophied and bulbous in shape. Nabothian cysts may be visible. The infective organism may be nonspecific or Gonococci. The main complaint is usually mucopurulent vaginal discharge.
- Cervical polyp.
- Ulcers on the cervix—for example, syphilitic, tubercular or granuloma inguinale.
- Cervical ectropion .

Investigations

Investigations depend on abnormality seen on Pap smear in asymptomatic women. In symptomatic disease all patients require colposcopy and biopsy in the initial work-up. Further tests to stage the disease and check for complications are then carried out if indicated.

a. *Investigations for asymptomatic women* with abnormal pap smear -

Dysplasia: Following results are highly suggestive of malignancy or premalignancy, and should be investigated with colposcopy and biopsy

- LSIL (low-grade squamous intraepithelial lesion) also known as mild dysplasia,
- HSIL (high-grade squamous intraepithelial lesion) includes moderate dysplasia, carcinoma in situ, and cervical intraepithelial neoplasia (CIN) II and III
- Squamous cell carcinoma
- Adenocarcinoma in situ (ACIS)

For other types of abnormal pap smear report, investigations are mentioned in Table 22.3 in Chapter 22.

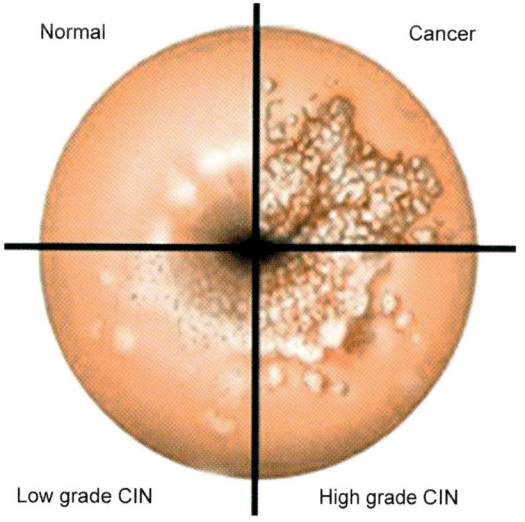

Normal   Cancer

Low grade CIN   High grade CIN

Fig. 23.2: Cervix viewed through speculum

b. *Investigations for symptomatic disease*

■ *Colposcopy and cervical biopsy.* Colposcopy may show abnormal vascularity, white change with acetic acid, or visible exophytic lesions. Biopsy establishes the diagnosis.

■ *Staging:* Staging of cervical carcinoma is clinical. Staging is traditionally based upon physical examination, colposcopy, and biopsy results, and the following limited studies are indicated: Chest X-ray, intravenous pyelogram (IVP), proctoscopy, cystoscopy, barium enema, and examination under anesthesia (Table 23.2).

■ *Subsequent investigations:* After diagnosis is established based on biopsy findings, and staging is done, full blood count (FBC), renal and liver function tests, are performed to screen for anemia due to bleeding, and kidney and liver involvement.

■ In developed countries, modern management uses advanced imaging [magnetic resonance imaging (MRI), positron emission tomography (PET)/computed tomography (CT)] to assist in planning treatment, although they are not permitted to be used in determining stage.

Staging and Prognosis

FIGO stages related to management and prognosis (Revised FIGO Staging 2009)

Stage I: Carcinoma confined to the cervix. Extension to the body of uterus is disregarded.

■ *IA:* Microinvasive carcinoma, strictly confined to the cervix. Can only be diagnosed by microscopy; it is not clinically visible (Fig. 23.3).

  • *Stage IA$_1$:* Stromal invasion no greater than 3.0 mm in depth and not more than 7.0 mm in horizontal spread. 5-year survival with optimal treatment: ~98%.

  • *Stage IA$_2$:* Stromal invasion of more than 3.0 mm but not more than 5.0 mm in

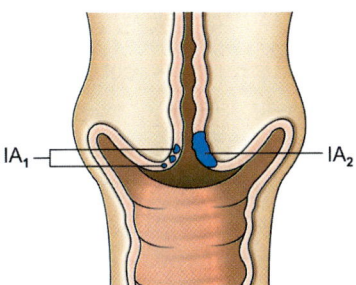

Fig. 23.3: Stage IA cervical cancer

Table 23.2: Investigations for staging and treatment for cervical cancer according to FIGO		
Mandatory for staging	*Supplementary for staging*	*Optional, for additional treatment, not for staging*
• Speculum, vaginal and rectal examination • Intravenous pyelogram (IVP) or • Abdominal ultrasound	Cystoscopy Proctoscopy Cone biopsy Endocervical curettage or smear Chest X-ray Skeletal X-ray or bone scan (If back pain)	Blood tests for haemogram and for HIV, syphilis CT scan of abdomen and pelvis MRI of pelvis

Occasionally a hysterectomy is performed for a reason unrelated to cervical disease and there is an incidental finding of cervical cancer. These cases cannot be clinically staged, but should be treated according to the characteristics reported by the pathologist

depth and with horizontal spread of 7.0 mm or less.

5-year survival with optimal treatment: ~95%.

- *IB:* Carcinoma strictly confined to the cervix and clinically visible; or a microscopic lesion greater than IA_2 (Fig. 23.4).
  - *IB_1:* Clinically visible lesion 4.0 cm or less in greatest dimension. 5-year survival with optimal treatment: ~85%.
  - *IB_2:* Clinically visible lesion more than 4.0 cm in greatest dimension. 5-year survival with optimal treatment: ~75%.

Stage II: Cervical carcinoma invades beyond the uterus, but not to the pelvic wall or to the lower one third of vagina Extension to the body of uterus is disregarded.

- *IIA:* Spread beyond the cervix, including upper two-thirds of the vagina, but not to tissues around the uterus (parametria) (Fig. 23.5). 5-year survival with optimal treatment: ~75%.
  - IIA_1 lesion—clinically visible lesion < 4 cm in greatest dimension
  - IIA_2 lesion—clinically visible lesion > 4 cm in greatest dimension
- *IIB:* Spread beyond the cervix, with parametrial invasion, but not as far as the pelvic wall or the lower third of the vagina (Fig. 23.6). 5-year survival with optimal treatment: ~65%.

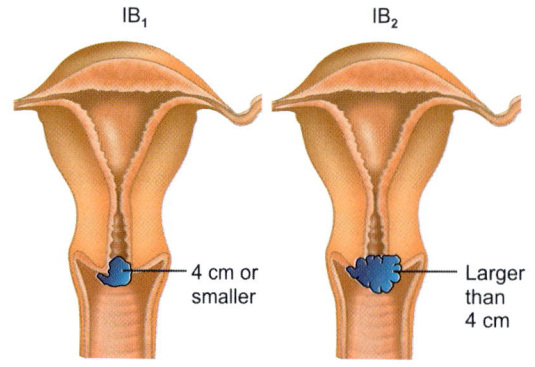

IB₁   IB₂

4 cm or smaller   Larger than 4 cm

Fig. 23.4: Stage IB cervical cancer

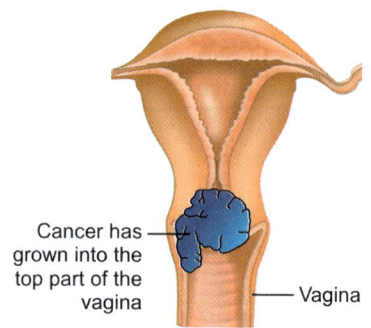

Cancer has grown into the top part of the vagina — Vagina

Fig. 23.5: Stage IIA cervical cancer

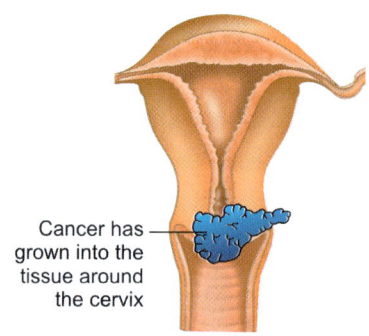

Cancer has grown into the tissue around the cervix

Fig. 23.6: Stage IIB cervical carcinoma

Stage III: Tumour extends to pelvic wall or involves lower third of the vagina, or causes hydronephrosis or non-functioning kidney.

- *IIIA:* Invasion of the lower third of the vagina, with no extension to the pelvic wall (Fig. 23.7). 5-year survival with optimal treatment: ~30%.
- *IIIB:* Extension to the pelvic wall, or hydronephrosis or nonfunctioning kidney (Fig. 23.8). 5-year survival with optimal treatment: ~30%.

Stage IV: Tumor has spread

- *IVA:* Spread to involve the mucosa of the bladder or rectum (Fig. 23.9). 5-year survival with optimal treatment: ~10%.
- *IVB:* Spread to distant organs, such as extrapelvic lymph nodes, kidneys, bones, lungs, liver and brain (Fig. 23. 10). 5-year survival with optimal treatment: <5%.

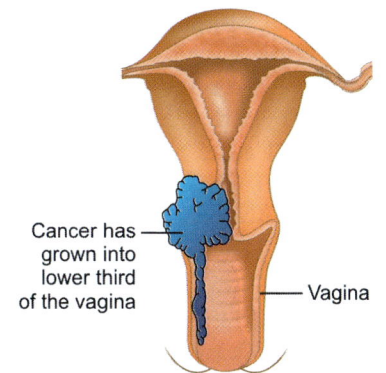

Cancer has grown into lower third of the vagina

Vagina

Fig. 23.7: Stage IIIA cervical carcinoma

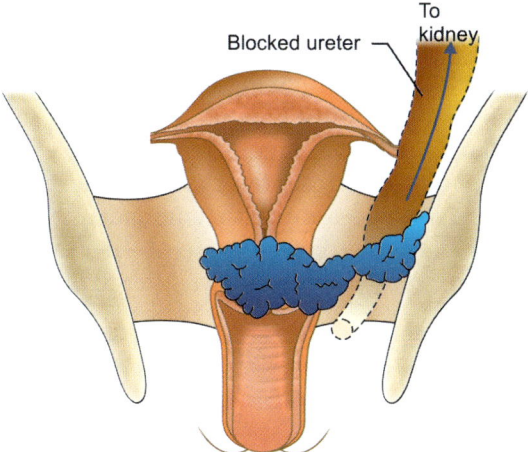

Blocked ureter

To kidney

Fig. 23.8: Stage IIIB cervical carcinoma

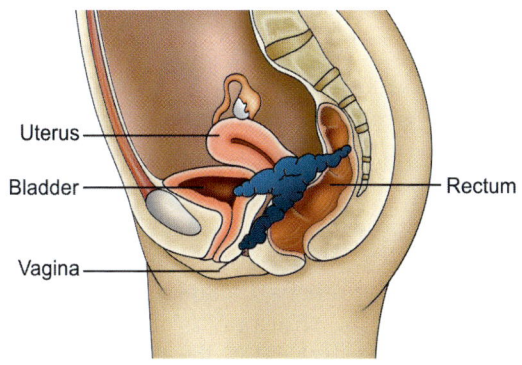

Uterus

Bladder

Rectum

Vagina

Fig. 23.9: Stage IVA cervical carcinoma

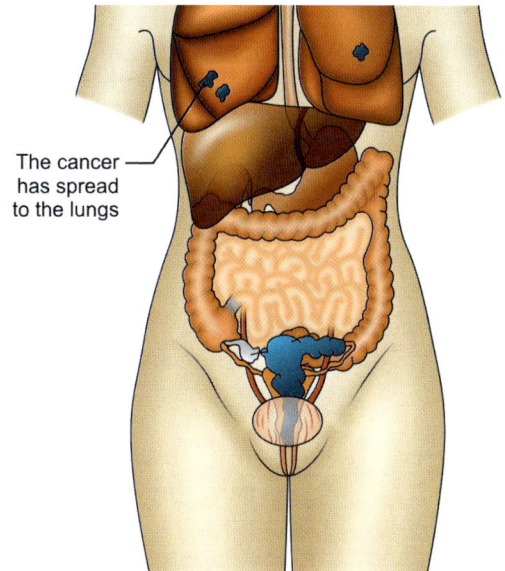

The cancer has spread to the lungs

Fig. 23.10: Stage IVB cervical carcinoma

Clinical pearl: Histological confirmation of cervical cancer and FIGO staging must be completed before proceeding to further investigations and treatment.

Treatment Approach

Preinvasive precancerous lesions may spontaneously regress, but untreated carcinoma of the cervix is uniformly fatal. The treatment of invasive cervical cancer is based on stage. Treatment plans are based on clinical acumen, local expertise and practice, and individualised discussion between the patient and physician. In specific circumstances, it may be appropriate to adjust treatment plans if there is a desire to preserve childbearing potential. Primary therapy may be surgery or radiotherapy or a combination of both. Chemotherapy is given concurrently with radiotherapy (chemoradiation). For early invasive cancer, surgery is the treatment of choice. In more advanced cases, radiation combined with chemotherapy is the current standard of care. Radiotherapy alone is not the standard of care for any subset of locally advanced or high-risk early stage cervical cancer at present.

Adenocarcinoma is associated with a worse prognosis at all stages, but there are no clear data that a more aggressive approach to this subtype results in a better outcome. For this reason, adenocarcinoma is treated using the same treatment principle based on stage as that used for other cancer types.

Stage IA_1 Disease

The treatment of choice for stage IA_1 disease is surgery. Total hysterectomy and conization are accepted procedures. Selected patients with stage IA_1 disease but no lymphovascular space invasion who desire to maintain fertility may undergo therapeutic conization with close follow-up, including cytology, colposcopy, and endocervical curettage.

Lymphadenectomy is not required for stage IA_1 disease as the risk of metastases is very small (1%). Subsequent care depends on margin involvement. If margins are positive, completion of hysterectomy or chemoradiation must be pursued. With negative margins, careful follow-up is adequate (Fig. 23.11).

Stage IA_2–IIA: Early Stage Disease

For patients with stage IA_2- IIA disease, there are 2 treatment options:
- Radical hysterectomy with bilateral pelvic lymphadenectomy
- Combined external beam radiation with brachytherapy and/or chemotherapy

Radical hysterectomy with lymphadenectomy is preferred to chemoradiation, especially for the following situations:
- Premenopausal women where ovarian function can be preserved
- An undiagnosed pelvic mass
- High risk of bowel toxicity on radiotherapy (very thin women, or existing adhesions due to pelvic inflammatory disease, endometriosis, inflammatory bowel disease)
- Difficulty complying with the radiotherapy schedule.

Age does not appear to be a significant contraindication to radical hysterectomy. Morbid obesity is a relative contraindication to surgery, and operative risk may need to be weighed against risks of alternative therapy (chemoradiation). Chemoradiation is second-line for those who have contraindications to surgery (Fig. 23.11).

After patients undergo radical hysterectomy, it is essential to evaluate the pathology to guide decisions on adjuvant therapy. If surgical pathology reveals a small tumour, minimal invasion, and no lymphovascular space invasion (LVSI), no further therapy is required and patients should be monitored for recurrence. If surgical pathology reveals positive nodes, involvement of parametrium, or positive margins, postoperative chemoradiation is required.

If patients have stage IA_2 to IB_1 disease and the patient desires preservation of fertility, radical trachelectomy with lymphadenectomy may be considered instead of radical hysterectomy for tumours smaller than 2 cm.

Clinical pearl: Fertility sparing surgery (conisation or radical trachelectomy (excision of the cervix)) is an option for women with early stage disease

Stage IIB–IVA: Locally Advanced Disease

Chemoradiotherapy is first-line therapy. For locally advanced cervical carcinoma (stages IIB, III, and IVA), radiation therapy was the treatment of choice for many years. However, the results from large, well-conducted, prospective randomized clinical trials have demonstrated a dramatic improvement in survival when chemotherapy is combined with radiation therapy. Radiotherapy alone is no longer indicated for any patient (Fig. 23.11).

- External beam radiation therapy shrinks the central tumor and treats regional lymph nodes. This therapy is followed by brachytherapy (local radioactive implants, usually using cesium) to the cervix, which

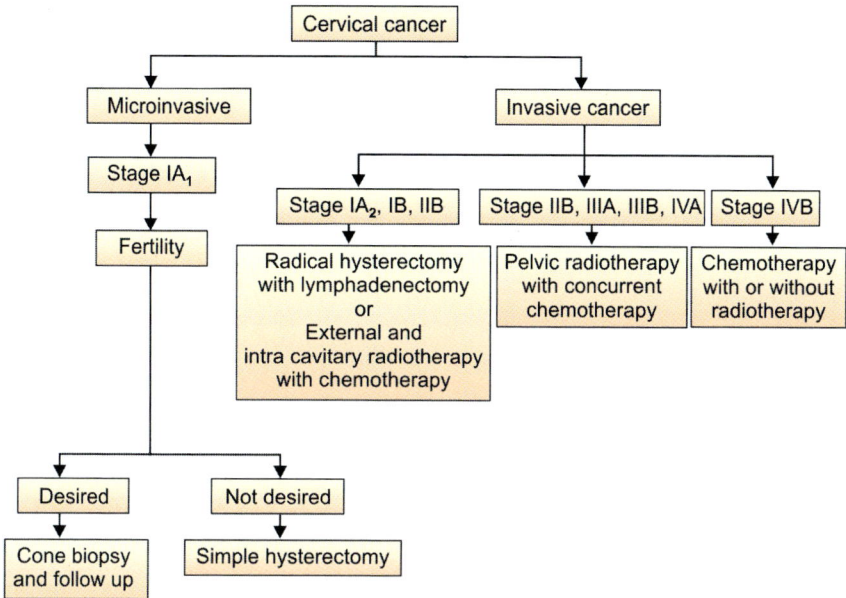

Fig. 23.11: Management of invasive cancer

destroys the central tumor. Radiation therapy may cause acute complications (e.g. radiation proctitis and cystitis) and, occasionally, late complications (e.g., vaginal stenosis, intestinal obstruction, rectovaginal and vesicovaginal fistula formation).

- Chemotherapy is usually given with radiation therapy, often to sensitize the tumor to radiation. Chemotherapeutic agents that are usually used are cisplatin alone, cisplatin + flurouracil or gemcitabine plus cisplatin.

Clinical pearl
- For locally advanced disease, chemo radiotherapy is significantly superior to radiotherapy alone.
- Chemo radiotherapy is the standard of care for locally advanced and early stage cancers with poor prognostic factors

Stage IVB: Metastatic Disease

Platinum-based dual-agent chemotherapy is first-line treatment. Cisplatin and topotecan is the only combination with a documented overall survival advantage (9.4 versus 6.5 months), but combination therapy with cisplatin and paclitaxel, or cisplatin and ifosfamide, is also associated with greater response rates than for any single agent. However, if dual agent chemotherapy is not tolerated single agent chemotherapy may be tried (Fig. 23.11).

As the response to chemotherapy is not always good and because of toxicity of chemotherapy, in some patient supportive care with no further chemotherapy is a reasonable alternate treatment option to consider. Best supportive care addresses physical, psychological, social, and spiritual issues. Common medical challenges include pain, nausea and vomiting, lymphoedema, obstruction (genitourinary and GI), and fistulae.

Complications

The complications of carcinoma of cervix include:
- Haemorrhage from the friable cervical growth will lead to anemia.
- Cachexia due to either poor nutrition or effect of carcinoma.

- Pyometra—collection of pus inside uterine cavity
- Vaginal fistula (urinary or fecal). These are common in stage IV disease.
- *Ureteric obstructions:* The ureters are immune to involved by malignant tissues but obstruction is due to fibrotic process surrounding ureters or inflammation of tissues surrounding ureters.
- Urinary tract infection—due to involvement of the bladder and ureteric obstruction.
- Infection of cervix

The cause of death in patient with carcinoma cervix includes:

- Uremia can lead to renal failure
- Cachexia
- Complications to treatment
- Metastasis to vital organs such as lungs, liver, brain.

Modalities of Treatment

Surgery

Curative surgery in cervical carcinoma aims to remove the primary tumor, with all its site of spread , in a single operation. The operation undertaken will depend on the clinical stage of the tumor and the findings of the surgeon when the operation is in progress. Palliative surgery is usually used to relieve distressing symptoms when radiotherapy has failed or caused complications, such as rectovaginal or vesicovaginal fistulae.

Surgical Procedures

The main surgical procedures are radical hysterectomy and pelvic lymphadenectomy, although simple hysterectomy and trachelectomy are indicated in specific cases.

Trachelectomy

Trachelectomy is the removal of the cervix. Radical trachelectomy includes removal of the parametria and upper vagina in addition to the cervix.

Simple Hysterectomy

Simple hysterectomy is the surgical removal of the entire uterus, including the cervix, either through an incision in the lower abdomen, or through the vagina. The tubes and ovaries are not routinely removed, but they may be, if they appear abnormal.

Radical Hysterectomy

Radical hysterectomy is the surgical removal of the uterus, cervix, and surrounding tissues (parametria), including 2 cm of the upper vagina (Fig. 23.12). The removal of as much cancer-free tissue from around the tumor as possible is associated with a much better cure rate. Ovaries are not routinely removed because cervical cancer rarely spreads to the ovaries. In a modified radical hysterectomy, less parametrium is removed than in standard radical hysterectomy. Recovery time is slightly longer than after simple hysterectomy.

Radiotherapy

Radiotherapy plays an important role in the treatment of most invasive cervical cancers. It is mainly used for cases with bulkier tumors (stages IB and IIA through to IVB) and those with extensive involvement of the lymph

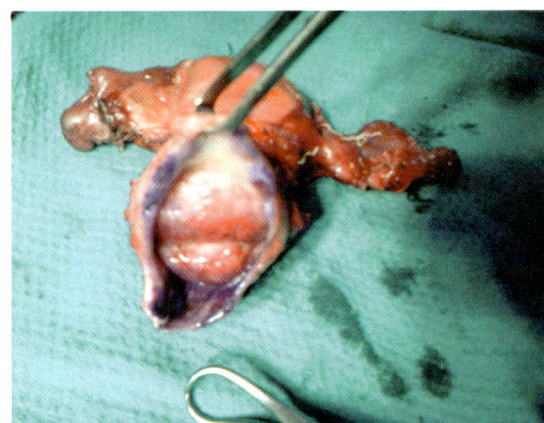

Fig. 23.12: A specimen of radical hysterectomy—note the ulcerative lesion over cervix and portion of vagina removed

nodes seen on laparotomy (without hysterectomy). It is also used to manage cancers in patients who are unable to tolerate general anesthesia. In addition to its curative role, radiation can also alleviate symptoms, especially bone pain and vaginal bleeding

How Radiotherapy Works

In radiotherapy, the tumour is treated with ionizing radiation. Radiation penetrates the body, damaging and destroying malignant cells. It also has a smaller effect on rapidly dividing normal cells in the skin, bladder and large bowel, which causes some of the reversible symptoms noted during and immediately after treatment.

Types of Radiotherapy

There are two broad groups of radiation treatment, which differ in terms of position of the source of radiation relative to the patient:

- Teletherapy, in which the source of radiation is distant from the patient
- Brachytherapy, in which small radioactive sources are placed in cavities within the body.

Curative treatments are based on a combination of pelvic teletherapy and intravaginal brachytherapy.

Teletherapy

Teletherapy is also called external beam radiation therapy (EBRT). The origin of the radiation is a shielded head, which has a small opening through which a beam of radiation can pass. The beam is aimed at the area of the cervix with cancer and the sites at risk of disease spread. Care must be taken to avoid the bladder and rectum, to protect their function. The treatment is administered in a specialist hospital, and takes place in an enclosed space (therapy bunker). No anaesthesia is needed because the patient feels no pain

Brachytherapy

In brachytherapy, the radiation source is in close contact with the tumour. The radiation sources are placed inside an applicator in the uterus and vaginal vault (intracavitary brachytherapy), the radiation is directed to the cancer on the cervix, uterus, upper vagina and tissue surrounding the cervix (parametria). Care is needed to avoid exposing the bladder and rectum to the radiation, in order to preserve their function as much as possible.

The dose rate is the speed of delivery of a radiation dose at a specified point. Intracavitary brachytherapy can be administered with a low dose rate (LDR), pulsed dose rate (PDR), medium dose rate (MDR) or high dose rate (HDR). The rate used determines the time the patient will be kept in isolation, as well as the total dose to be used, and the number of sessions the patient will have. The most commonly available brachytherapy devices are LDR and HDR, which have similar effectiveness.

Indications

Teletherapy is indicated when the entire area affected by the cancer cannot be removed by simple or radical hysterectomy. This means that most women with invasive cervical cancer without distant metastases (stages IB to IVA) should be treated with teletherapy. Brachytherapy is usually used in addition to teletherapy. Its use is mandatory if the intent is to cure cervical cancer. For stages IB_1 or lower, if surgery is not possible, brachytherapy can be used as the exclusive treatment.

Chemotherapy

National Cancer Institute (NCI) in US in 1999 identified a large survival advantage for the administration of concurrent chemotherapy with radiotherapy. The benefits of chemoradiotherapy over radiotherapy alone were further confirmed in a Cochrane meta-analysis. Weekly cisplatin during radiotherapy

Keywords

HPV: Human Papillomavirus, more commonly known as HPV, is a viral infection spread through skin to skin sexual contact (vaginal, anal, oral sex). HPV is a group of over 100 different viruses, with at least 30 strains known to cause different types of cancer.

Colposcopy: A colposcopy is a special way of looking at the cervix. Colposcope is a magnifying and photographic device that uses a light and a low-powered microscope to make the cervix appear much larger and thus used as an aid in the diagnostic examination of the vaginal and cervical epithelia.

Cone biopsy: A cone biopsy is an extensive form of cervical biopsy in which a cone-shaped wedge of tissue is removed from the cervix and examined under a microscope. A cone biopsy removes abnormal tissue that is high in the cervical canal. A small amount of normal tissue around the cone-shaped wedge of abnormal tissue is also removed so that a margin free of abnormal cells is left in the cervix.

Radical hysterectomy: Radical hysterectomy means the excision of the uterus en bloc with the parametrium and the upper one third to one- half of the vagina with the ovaries left or removed. The surgeon usually also performs a bilateral pelvic node dissection. Radical hysterectomy is performed as a primary therapy for (i) Stage 1A$_2$ - IIA cancer cervix (ii) Stage II adenocarcinoma of endometrium (iii) Upper vaginal carcinoma, uterine or cervical sarcomas and other rare malignancies confined to the area of cervix, uterus and/or upper vagina.

has been studied in more advanced stage rather than early stage disease; this approach would offer a more favorable toxicity profile compared with cisplatin and fluorouracil. However, many clinicians suspect that 2 drugs are better than 1.

EXERCISES

Answer the following

1. What is the incidence of cervical cancer?
2. What are its risk factors?
3. What HPV subtypes is highest risk for cervical cancer?
4. How does HPV induce malignancy?
5. What are the symptoms and signs of cervical cancer?
6. How is cervical cancer diagnosed?
7. What is the differential diagnosis?
8. How is cervical cancer staged?
9. What is micro invasive carcinoma?
10. How it is treated?
11. What procedures are used in staging of cervical cancer?
12. What are the histological types of cervical cancer? And their frequencies?
13. How does cervical carcinoma spread?
14. What are the treatment options?
15. What are the treatment options for stage 1A$_1$?
16. What is the treatment of stage 1A$_2$?
17. What is the treatment of stage 1B and stage II?
18. What is the treatment of stage IIB through IVA?
19. What are the complications of cervical carcinoma?
20. What are the common causes of death in cervical carcinoma?

Write short notes on

1. HPV Vaccine
2. Staging of cervical carcinoma
3. Brachytherapy

Explain or justify the following statements

1. Cervical cancer disproportionately affects developing countries
2. For locally advanced disease, chemo-radiotherapy is significantly superior to radiotherapy alone.
3. The treatment of cervical carcinoma is based on staging

Fill in the blanks with appropriate word(s)

1. Most commonly cervical cancer spread by _____ and _____.

2. Pelvic Lymph nodes that are involved in cervical carcinoma are _____ , _____ , _____ , _____ .

3. Investigations mandatory for staging of cervical carcinoma are _____ , _____ , or _____ .

4. Two main types of radiotherapy are _____ and _____ .

Questions for practical (Read the case summary at the beginning of chapter before answering the questions)

1. What will be your next step in management?

2. Name the investigations you will consider for her?

3. Which investigations are mandatory for staging?

4. If she is having an early stage disease how will you treat her?

5. Name the type of surgery which is done in early stage disease?

6. When will you consider radiotherapy following surgery?

7. If she is unfit for surgery, how do you treat her?

8. If she is having advanced stage disease (say Stage IIIB), how do you treat her?

9. What are the different types of radiotherapy?

10. Why chemoradiation is better than radiotherapy alone?

11. Which chemotherapeutic agent is used and why?

Questions from specimen (look at the Fig. 23.12 before answering the following questions)

1. Describe the specimen.

2. What are the structures removed in radical hysterectomy?

3. What was the indication of the operation?

4. How this patient (from whom the specimen was obtained) presented in hospital?

Bibliography

1. Bllomfield P. Management of cervical cancer Australian Family Physician Vol. 36, No. 3, March 2007.

2. Canavan TP Cervical cancer Am Fam Physician. 2000 Mar 1;61(5):1369–1376.

3. Comprehensive cervical cancer control: a guide to essential practice WHO Press, World Health Organization, 2006.

4. David M, et al. Cervical cancer Marke manual 2008.

5. Dinshaw, et al. Cancer Management Guidelines Members of Expert Sub? Committee on Guidelines for Management of Cancer of Cervix Uteri ICMR guideline 2010.

6. FIGO committee on gynecologic oncology. Revised FIGO staging for carcinoma of the vulva, cervix, and endometrium j.ijgo.2009.02.012

7. Management of cervical cancer A national clinical guideline Scottish Intercollegiate Guidelines Network 2008.

8. Moore D H Cervical cancer Obstet Gynecol 2006;107:1152–61.

9. Non ovarian cancer Clinical Care Options, LLC 2012.

10. Petignat P, et al. Diagnosis and managemet of cervical cancer BMJ. 2007 October 13; 335(7623): 765–768.

11. R Horvat. Quality assurance guidelines for pathology in cervical screening 2003.

24

Ovarian Malignancy

A 55-year-old postmenopausal woman presents with 3 months of progressive abdominal bloating and early satiety. On examination the abdomen is distended with dull to percussion and with minimal tenderness. A fluid thrill is present. On pelvic examination, a mass is palpable in the left adnexa extending down into the pouch of Douglas. What is your provisional diagnosis?

In this chapter we will learn:
- Epidemiology of ovarian malignancy
- Etiology
- Pathophysiology
- Classification
- Prevention
- Diagnosis
- Differential diagnosis
- Staging
- Treatment approach
- Prognosis

Introduction

Ovarian malignancy is a relatively uncommon gynecological cancer. In this condition there is malignant transformation of different parts of ovary (primary). In some cases ovarian cancer may be secondary following metatasis from a primary cancer from elsewhere in body. Primary lesions include epithelial ovarian carcinoma, germ cell tumors, sex cord stromal tumors, and other more rare types. Secondary metastasis to the ovaries are relatively frequent with most common being from the endometrium, breast, colon stomach and cervix. However, most (90%), ovarian cancers arise from the surface of ovary and classified as epithelial ovarian cancers. The primary focus of this chapter will be the epithelial ovarian subtype.

Epidemiology

Ovarian cancer is an important cause of morbidity and mortality, especially in the middle aged women. During the year 2002, it ranked third in frequency (4.1%) among all cancers in women, with an estimated 2, 04, 499 new cases occurring in the world (Parkin et al., 2005). In India, during the period 2004–2005, proportion of ovarian cancer varied from 1.7 to 8.7% of all female cancers (ranked 3rd or 4th) in various urban and rural population based registries operating under the network of the National Cancer Registry Programme (NCRP) of Indian Council of Medical Research.

The disease is more common in industrialized nations, with the exception of Japan. In the United States, females have a 1.4 to 2.5% (1 out of 40–60 women) lifetime chance of developing ovarian cancer.

Etiology

The exact etiology of ovarian cancer is not known. There are promising data that women who are having breast ovarian cancer gene 1 (BRCA1) and breast ovarian cancer gene 2 (BRCA2) are at risk of developing ovarian malignancy. Also, in patients with hereditary non-polyposis colon cancer (also known as Lynch II syndrome), mutations MSH2 and MLH1 can be associated with ovarian cancer.

Based on several epidemiological studies, there is good evidence that increased parity, use of oral contraceptive pills, tubectomy and hysterectomy reduce the risk of ovarian malignancy. Other factors such as lactation, age at menarche, age at menopause seem to have lesser effect on risk reduction. The effects of PCOS, infertility treatment, endometriosis on ovarian cancer the risks remain uncertain.

The incessant ovulation theory states that a woman's risk of developing ovarian cancer is related with number of ovulation occurring in her life. Ovulation results in disruption and repair of surface epithelium. An aberrant repair process is linked to origin of ovarian cancer. Thus the conditions where ovulation is suppressed such as multiparity, use of OC pill, lactation is having protective effects and vice versa (Table 24.1).

Pathophysiology

The majority of primary ovarian tumors derive from epithelial cells on the surface of the ovary, although they can also arise from

Table 24.1: Risk factors associated with ovarian cancer

Increased risk	Decreased risk
Delayed childbearing	Breastfeeding for 18 months or more
Early menarche	Early menopause
Estrogen replacement therapy for more than five years	Multiparity (risk decreases with each additional pregnancy)
Family history suggesting genetic predisposition	
Genetic syndromes	Hysterectomy*
High-fat diet	Late menarche
Late menopause	Low-fat diet
Low parity	Oral contraceptive use
	Tubal ligation*

*Hysterectomy and tubal ligation are likely associated with decreased risk of ovarian cancer because of decreased utero-ovarian blood flow, which limits local exposure to hormonal or potentially carcinogenic factors.

Fact sheet: Ovarian cancer is diagnosed in nearly a quarter of a million women globally each year. It is the eighth most common cancer in women and the seventh leading cause of cancer death among women, responsible for approximately 140,000 deaths each year. It has the highest mortality rate of all gynaecological cancers.

other cell types (germ cell tumors, sex cord-stromal tumors, and mixed cell type tumors).

The ovary develops from the genital ridge in the embryo. The genital ridge is composed of thickened coelomic epithelium, which is thought by some authors to have the potential for developing into ovarian-like tumors. This thickened coelomic epithelium forms the mesothelial (epithelial) covering of the ovary and gives rise to epithelial tumors. Epithelial cancer of the ovary derives from malignant transformation of the epithelium of the ovarian surface, which is contiguous with the peritoneal mesothelium. The germ cells originate in the primitive streak of the embryo and migrate to the gonad, where they proliferate into a component of the ovarian cortex. The mesenchyma of the medulla is the origin of the ovarian stromal cells. These three cell types are thought to give rise to the three types of malignant ovarian neoplasms: epithelial, germ cell, and stromal.

Spread of the Disease

Epithelial ovarian cancer does not typically invade into organ space parenchyma, but instead attaches to the surface of organs. Tumour cells implant along the lining of the peritoneal cavity (local advancement), bowel mesentery, and liver capsule, indicating metastatic disease. The most common method of metastatic spread is the exfoliation of ovarian cancer cells into the peritoneal fluid, resulting in the seeding of the pelvic/abdominal structures and lymphatic spread, with hematogenous spread being less common.

Exfoliated cancer cells follow the natural circulation of the peritoneal fluid, along the right paracolic gutter and sub-diaphragmatic space. Thus, the right liver edge and diaphragm peritoneum are common sites of tumour implantation. The omentum is also a common site of tumour implants (Figs 24.1 and 24.2). Thus, the initial spread pattern of ovarian cancer is by direct spread or

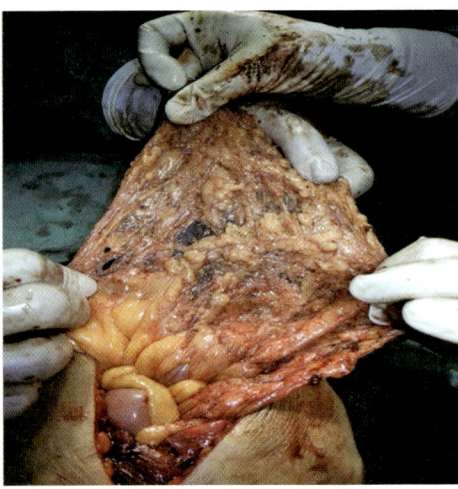

Fig. 24.2: Omental metastasis at the time of operation

lymphatic drainage. Haematogenous dissemination typically occurs late in the disease process.

Classification

Ovarian cancer types:

1. *Epithelial:* Derived from ovary surface cells; most common type (85–95%)

   Invasive carcinoma: Cystic and solid or solid neoplasm with stromal invasion by malignant epithelial elements

   - Serous cyst adenocarcinoma (most common)
   - Mucinous cyst adenocarcinoma (Figs 24.3 and 24.4)
   - Clear cell carcinoma
   - Transitional cell (Brenner's) carcinoma (rare)
   - Endometrioid carcinoma
   - Mixed epithelial carcinoma
   - Squamous cell carcinoma (very rare)
   - Undifferentiated carcinoma

2. *Germ cell:* Derived from egg-producing ovarian cells; rare (3 to 5%)
   - Dysgerminomas
   - Embryonal carcinomas
   - Endodermal sinus tumors
   - Choriocarcinomas

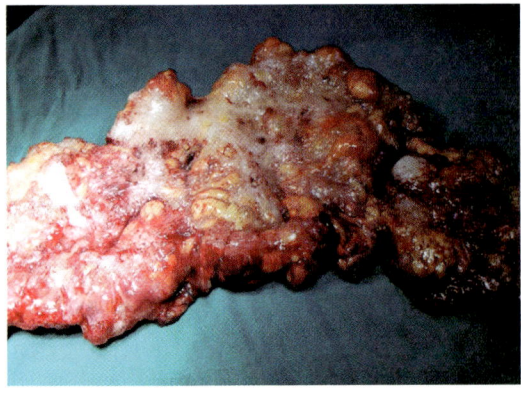

Fig. 24.1: Omental metastasis of ovarian cancer

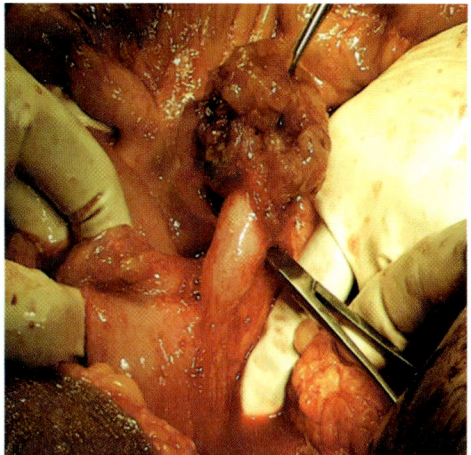

Fig. 24.3: Metastasis in appendix in a case of mucinous cyst adenocarcinoma

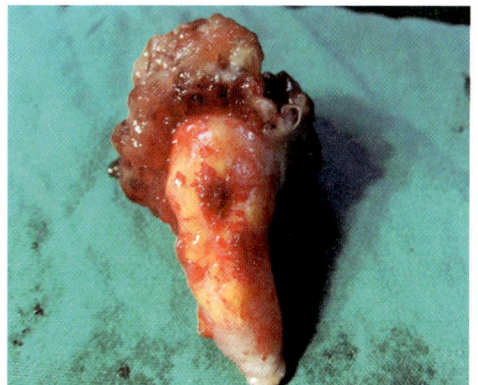

Fig. 24.4: Appendicectomy was done in same patient of Fig. 24.3

- Immature teratomas
- Polyembryoma

3. *Sex cord stromal:* Often produces steroid hormones; rare (5 to 8%)
- Granulosa cell tumour:
- Thecoma
- Sertoli-Leydig cell tumour:
- Sertoli cell tumour
- Leydig cell tumour
- Fibroma
- Fibrosarcoma
- Sclerosing stromal tumour

4. Secondary metastases to ovaries (5%) Krukenberg tumour—Breast cancer or the GI tract malignancy.

Prevention

In general, there are no true primary preventive measures for ovarian cancer. However the use of oral contraceptives for a period of 5 years is associated with a 50% decrease in the risk of ovarian cancer. Risk-reducing salpingo-oophorectomy is currently the most effective way to decrease the risk of ovarian cancer in high-risk patients with BRCA1 or BRCA2 mutations who have completed childbearing.

Screening

Asymptomatic Population

Screening of asymptomatic population is not indicated as the screening procedures results in high false-positive rates, leading to unnecessary surgery in asymptomatic women and the inability to diagnose early-stage disease.

High-risk Screening

There is limited evidence to support the effectiveness of screening high-risk women with family history of breast and/or ovarian cancer or hereditary nonpolyposis colorectal cancer; however, expert groups have recommended performing pelvic ultrasounds with concomitant CA-125 levels every 6 months (National Comprehensive Cancer Network [NCCN] practice guidelines). Currently, prophylactic bilateral salpingo-oophorectomy and oral contraceptives remain the only means of risk reduction in this population.

Clinical Presentation

Patient profile—Although ovarian malignancy may occur at any age group, in general, the prepubescent child and the postmenopausal woman are at greatest risk for a malignant ovarian neoplasm. The reproductive age woman is more likely to have a functional/benign ovarian cyst or endometrioma. Risk factors of ovarian malignancy may be present in history.

Symptoms

- Patients with early disease are typically asymptomatic; thus, a majority of patients (75%) present in advanced stages of the disease (stages 3 or 4).

- If symptoms are present, they are often vague and non-specific. Common symptoms are abdominal bloating, nausea and emesis, early satiety, dyspepsia, increased abdominal girth, abdominal cramping, a change in bowel habit, or weight loss suggestive of advanced disease.

- On occasion, patients with early-stage disease present with pelvic pain, however, most women with early-stage disease are asymptomatic.

- Abdominal distention may be due to the tumour, ascites or both. This is the most common symptom.

- Respiratory symptoms may result from the increased intra-abdominal pressure or transudation of fluid into the pleural cavity.

- Acute pain may result from torsion or rupture. Torsion is more often seen with benign tumours that are not adherent to tissues. The rupture is more likely to be a malignant tumour.

Signs

General examination: In early stage disease there may not be any change in general examination findings. In advanced stage, the patient may be cachectic. The supraclavicular and inguinal lymph nodes may be enlarged. Sister Mary Joseph's nodule refers to a metastatic implant in the umbilicus.

Chest examination: In stage IV disease, a pleural effusion can be detected as well.

Abdominal examination: On inspection, abdominal distention is one of the common findings. The presence of flank fullness indicates the presence of ascites or a large pelvic-abdominal mass. Recent eversion of the umbilicus in a patient with abdominal distention may result from an increase in intra-abdominal pressure secondary to ascites.

Palpation: A solid or cystic mass may be palpable in lower abdomen with well defined upper and lateral border but lower border cannot be reached. This indicates the mass is of pelvic origin. The mass is frequently firm, hard, and fixed with multiple nodularities. Small tumors may not be easily palpated in the presence of ascites. Presence of a fluid thrill indicates associated ascites.

Percussion: Percussion note is dull on centre and resonant in the flanks. Tympanitic percussion noted over the lateral abdomen is consistent with a large mass that displaces the bowel to the periphery. In contrast, a central tympanitic percussion note is suggestive of ascites.

Pelvic examination: A careful and thorough pelvic examination provides many helpful clues regarding the etiology of a pelvic mass. Fixed, bilateral masses and firm masses with nodularity are suggestive of, but not diagnostic of, an ovarian malignancy. Because no features seen on physical examination consistently distinguish malignant from benign neoplasms. Table 24.2 lists the characteristics of the mass that should be noted on pelvic examination.

Investigations

Initial investigations:

- *Pelvic ultrasound:* Presence of solid, complex, septated, multi-loculated mass with high blood flow suggests ovarian malignancy. Transvaginal pelvic ultrasound is the preferred method to evaluate a suspected ovarian mass, providing both qualitative and quantitative information

Table 24.2: Characteristics of a pelvic mass that should be noted on pelvic examination

Characteristics	Benign	Malignant
Mobility	Mobile	Fixed
Consistency	Cystic	Solid and firm
Cul-de-sac position	Unilateral	Bilateral
Cul-de-sac	Smooth	Nodular

valuable in management. Worrisome findings include bilateral masses, complex masses with thick septations or solid tumour nodules, and abnormal Doppler flow.

- CT scan is less sensitive than ultrasound in evaluation of pelvic organs; however, when upper abdominal disease is suspected, CT imaging of the abdomen and pelvis is more useful. CT/MRI scan of the abdomen and pelvis more accurately delineates the spread of disease showing peritoneal deposits, omental deposits, para-aortic node involvement and/or liver metastases, ureteric obstruction (rare in ovarian cancer).

- Serum CA-125 levels tend to be raised in >80% of women with advanced ovarian cancer; however, this test is not sufficiently sensitive or specific as a tool for preoperative diagnosis. Numerous non-cancerous conditions can cause an elevation of CA-125, such as uterine fibroids, endometriosis, pelvic inflammatory disease, and appendicitis. In post-menopausal women, an elevated CA-125 level is more predictive of malignancy, but it is by no means diagnostic. Postoperatively, the CA-125 level is useful in evaluating clinical response to chemotherapy and in detecting any relapse of ovarian cancer.

- *Chest X-ray:* Chest radiographs are routinely performed to look for malignant pleural effusions, which occur in 10% of patients, and metastatic pulmonary disease, which is very rare.

- Liver function tests to detect spread to the liver.

- Urea and electrolytes.
- Full blood count.

The latter two do not help in staging the disease but are important for preoperative assessment.

Other Investigations

- Barium enema examination may be helpful in patients with a left lower quadrant mass, blood in the stool, constipation, or anemia in whom a primary gastrointestinal tract malignancy must be ruled out. Barium enema examination is not very useful in predicting the need for colon resection.

- Mammography is necessary to rule out a possible metastatic or synchronous breast carcinoma.

Histopathology

When an ovarian mass is detected, biopsy is not routinely recommended as this can disseminate tumour cells in the peritoneal cavity. If transvaginal ultrasound demonstrates suspicious findings, surgery (laparotomy) is required for definitive diagnosis. An exploratory laparotomy is warranted for staging, histological diagnosis, and tumour debulking. Surgical staging guides further postoperative treatment primarily for early-stage disease (Table 24.4).

Staging

International Federation of Gynecology and Obstetrics (FIGO) Staging Guidelines

Stage characteristics:

- Stage I—tumor limited to 1 or both ovaries
  - Stage IA—tumor limited to 1 ovary; no ascites present; no surface involvement; no tumor rupture or spillage; negative peritoneal washings.
  - Stage IB—tumor limited to both ovaries; no ascites present; no surface involvement; no tumor rupture or spillage; negative peritoneal washings.

Table 24.3: Diagnostic imaging modalities to evaluate adnexal masses

Modality	Sensitivity*(%) Specificity*(%)	Use
Transvaginal ultrasonography	86/91	First-line detection and characterization of adnexal masses
Magnetic resonance imaging	91/88	Further delineation of indeterminate masses seen on ultrasonography
Computed tomography	90/75	Preoperative evaluation
Positron emission tomography	67/79	Treatment follow-up
		Evaluation of increased cancer antigen 125 in known ovarian cancer (e.g., recurrence) with nondetectable implants
		Detection of metastases in known ovarian cancer, in combination with computed tomography

*Sensitivities and specificities are for patients with a known pelvic mass.

Table 24.4: Differential diagnosis of adnexal masses

Benign ovarian tumor	Ovarian torsion
Cancer metastases	Pedunculated uterine fibroid
Endometrioma	Pelvic kidney
Endometriosis	Tubo-ovarian abscess

- Stage IC—tumor limited to 1 or both ovaries, with associated ascites, surface involvement, tumor rupture or spillage, or positive peritoneal washings.

Note: Lymph node dissection is recommended if disease appears to be confined to the ovaries or pelvis, for complete staging.

- Stage II—tumor involvement limited to the pelvis
  - Stage IIA—involvement of the uterus or fallopian tubes
  - Stage IIB—involvement of other pelvic organs or structures (e.g. bladder, rectum, pelvic side wall)
  - Stage IIC—involvement of other pelvic organs or structures (e.g., bladder, rectum, pelvic side wall); plus ascites, surface involvement, tumour rupture or spillage, or positive peritoneal washings

Note: Lymph node dissection is recommended if disease appears to be confined to the ovaries or pelvis, for complete staging.

- Stage III—tumor involvement of the upper abdomen or retroperitoneal lymph nodes:
  - Stage IIIA—microscopic upper abdominal disease
  - Stage IIIB—macroscopic upper abdominal disease; tumour deposits up to 2 cm
  - Stage IIIC—macroscopic upper abdominal disease; tumour deposits >2 cm in diameter; retroperitoneal lymph node involvement

Note: For stages IIIA and IIIB, tumour measurements should be made before debulking procedure, for staging purposes.

- Stage IV—pleural effusion; intraparenchymal liver or spleen involvement; distant metastases (e.g., lung, brain)
  - Pleural effusions must have positive cytology for stage IV disease
  - Surface involvement of the liver does not qualify as stage IV disease.

International Federation of Gynecology and Obstetrics Tumour Grades

Grade 1: < 5% solid tumor growth

Grade 2: > 5% solid tumor growth

Grade 3: > 50% solid tumor growth

Gynecological Oncology Group Classification Tumor Grades

Grade 1: Well differentiated

Grade 2: Moderately differentiated

Grade 3: Poorly differentiated

Note: The gynecological oncology group (GOG) grading system is based on tumor histology. Different guidelines are applied depending on whether the tumor is serous, endometrioid, mucinous, Brenner's, transitional cell, mixed, or small cell. Clear cell carcinomas are not graded according to the GOG.

Treatment Approach

The main two modalities of ovarian cancer management are surgery and chemotherapy. Management is based on the tumour stage (I to IV) and/or grade (1 to 3).

Surgery: Applicable in all stages of the disease, surgery plays an essential role in regards to establishing a diagnosis and determining the extent of disease (surgical staging). Furthermore, if necessary, surgery allows for the debulking of metastatic deposits at the time of surgical assessment and provides the necessary information for treatment and prognosis of the disease (Figs 24.5 to 24.9).

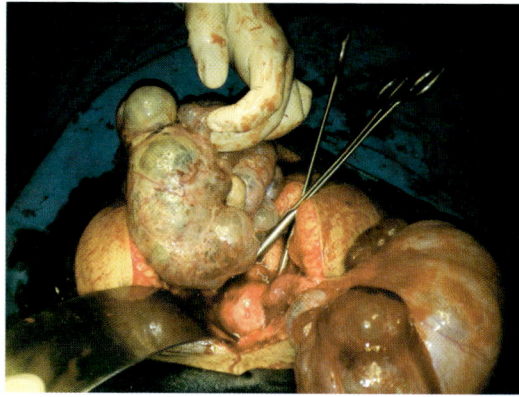

Fig. 24.6: Bilateral ovarian tumor at the time of laparotomy—note the rupture of capsule at places of left tumor mass

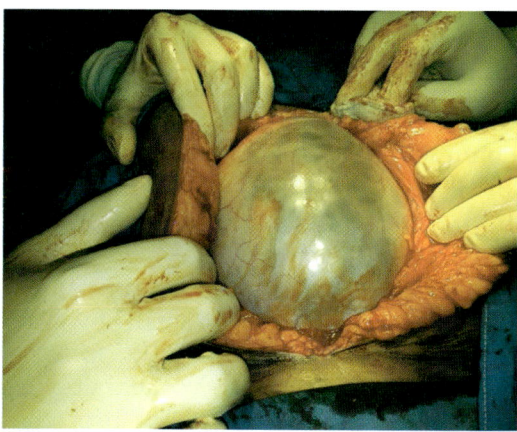

Fig. 24.7: Ovarian tumor at the time of laparotomy—note midline vertical incision

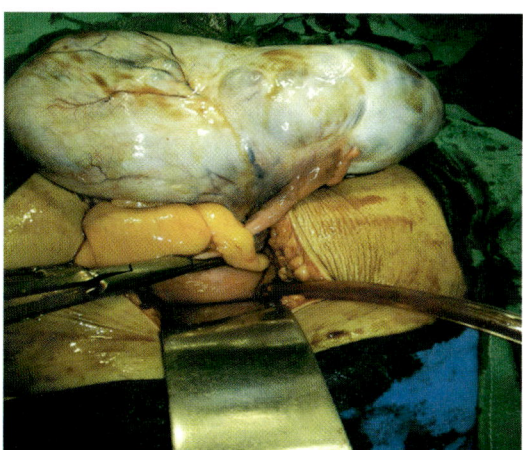

Fig. 24.5: A large ovarian tumor at the time of laparotomy

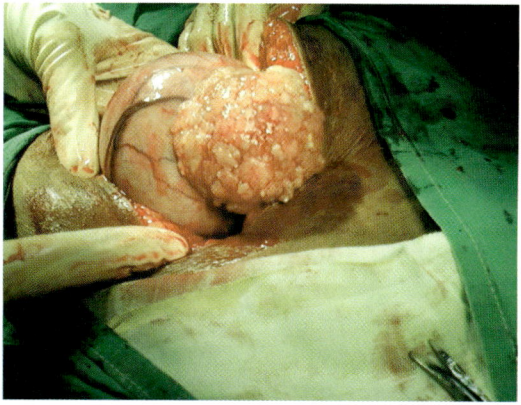

Fig. 24.8: Preresection operative findings of massive pelvic—abdominal tumor

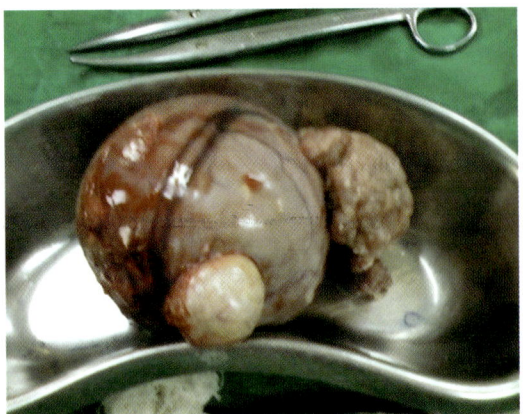

Fig. 24.9: Epithelial ovarian tumor

Surgical staging: The standard care for ovarian cancer includes surgical exploration for primary staging and for cytoreduction or debulking. If the disease appears to be confined to the pelvis (up to stage II), comprehensive surgical staging is indicated. The incision for surgery should be midline abdominal. Careful inspection and/or palpation of the abdominal contents should be performed, including all peritoneal surfaces, the liver, large and small bowel and mesentery, stomach, appendix, kidneys, spleen, retroperitoneal spaces, and all pelvic structures. The surgical staging procedure should include the following:

- Total abdominal hysterectomy, bilateral salpingo-oophorectomy
- Peritoneal cytology
- Multiple peritoneal biopsies
- Omentectomy
- Pelvic and para-aortic lymph node sampling.

When advanced disease is discovered at surgical exploration, a maximal surgical effort to debulk all tumour deposits is necessary. While the current accepted definition of optimal cytoreduction is less than 1 cm, the best outcomes occur in patients who have complete cytoreduction, or no macroscopic residual disease. Debunking or cytoreductive surgery can occasionally involve bowel resection, diaphragm stripping, and splenectomy. The morbidity of radical debulking procedures, however, is justified by the improvement in patient survival. [C Evidence] Patients who undergo "optimal" tumour debulking, where residual tumour nodules are ≤ 1 cm in diameter, experience improved survival compared to patients who have extensive residual disease at the completion of primary debulking surgery.

The majority of patients require adjuvant chemotherapy after surgical staging and debulking. Adjuvant chemotherapy is employed to eradicate any residual microscopic foci of cancer following complete or optimal cytoreduction.

Role of Chemotherapy

Chemotherapy plays an important role for the treatment of ovarian cancer. Unlike most other solid tumors, ovarian cancer has been shown to be exquisitely chemo-sensitive. As a result, chemotherapy, in combonation with surgical management, plays an essential role in the treatment of women with ovarian cancer. Initially (in 1970s), the use of single agents, such as melphalan, cyclophosphamide, thiotepa and chlorambucil, was advocated. In 1985, the application of platinum agents in ovarian cancer resulted in improved survival outcomes. In 1996, the introduction of paclitaxel in combination with platinum compounds resulted in further survival benefits. These studies established the use of a platinum agent and paclitaxel as the standard of care, which has remained the case. In 2006, the route of administration, intravenous versus intraperitoneal, of these two drugs was evaluated (in stage III disease), and results favored intraperitoneal chemotherapy for a select group of patients. In patients with stage III disease, who underwent optimal cytoreduction, intraperitoneal chemotherapy results in a 20% reduction of recurrence and 20–25% reduction in risk of death, with survival increasing from 8 to

16 months. However, the use of intraperitoneal chemotherapy is associated with a higher rate of toxicities.

Neoadjuvant Chemotherapy

Neoadjuvant therapy is administration of chemotherapy before the main treatment. When the ability to achieve optimal cyto-reduction is unlikely, the administration of neoadjuvant chemotherapy is recommended. The reasons for suboptimal results may be due to surgeon-dependent factors (e.g., level of experience, operative skill and philosophical approach), disease-dependent factors (e.g., extent and anatomic location of the disease), patient-dependent factors (e.g., medical comorbidities), or a combination of factors.

Clinical pearl: Surgery is the primary intervention in suspected ovarian cancer, both to obtain histological confirmation and stage as well as first line treatment.

Stages IA, IB, or Grade 1 or 2 Disease

Patients with early-stage low-risk disease (e.g., stage IA and stage IB) and favourable tumour characteristics (e.g., grade 1 or grade 2) do not require adjuvant chemo-therapy (Tables 24.5 and 24.6). However, these patients must have undergone appropriate surgical staging including omentectomy, lymph node dissection (pelvic and para-aortic), and staging biopsies.

Conservative surgery (fertility sparing surgery)—Fertility-sparing surgery (compre-hensive staging with preservation of the uterus and unaffected ovary) is considered in young patients who desire future childbearing potential. The selection of the appropriate candidates is critical and indicated in stages IA, IB, grade 1or 2 disease. Patients are typically not eligible for conservative surgery in grade 3 disease and when the disease is present outside the ovaries.

Stage IC to II or Grade 3 Disease

For patients with an early-stage ovarian cancer with a high risk of recurrence (stages IC, IIA, IIB, and IIC) or poor tumor charac-teristics (grade 3), adjuvant chemotherapy is warranted (Tables 24.5 and 24.6). Currently, paclitaxel and carboplatin is the combination regimen of choice [A Evidence].

Stage III (optimally debulked) or advanced

In most patients, the preferred approach is surgery followed by chemotherapy. For patients who are not surgical candidates, neoadjuvant chemotherapy should be considered. The goal of neoadjuvant chemo-therapy is to decrease the volume of disease present and allow time for optimization of the patient's underlying medical co-morbidities.

For patients with stage III disease who undergo optimal debulking surgery (no tumour nodule > 1 cm at the completion of surgery), intraperitoneal (IP) chemotherapy with carboplatin and paclitaxel is recom-mended (Table 24.6).

Stage IV Disease

Even for patients with stage IV disease, aggressive surgery may provide survival benefits. A recent ancillary study by the gynecologic oncology group demonstrated that the ability to achieve cytoreduction to less than 5 cm of residual disease results in a superior survival outcome when compared with greater than 5 cm residual disease. The use of radical procedures to achieve microscopic residual disease for this group of

Table 24.5: Gynecologic oncology group classifica-tion of early-stage epithelial ovarian carcinoma

Low-risk disease	High-Risk disease
Stage IA,IB; grade 1,2	Stage IA,IB; grade 3
	Stage IC
	Stage IIA, IIB, IIC, with no residual disease*

*Stage II patients with residual disease at the conclusion of primary cytoreductive surgery are classified as having advanced disease

Table 24.6: Postoperative treatment of ovarian cancer by stage and type

Stage and type	Treatment
Stage 1 A/ B grade 1 or 2	No postoperative therapy
Stage 1 A/B grade 3	6 courses of chemotherapy typically paclitaxel and carboplatin
Stage 1C	
Stage II A/B/C	
Stages III, IV	Six courses of chemotherapy with paclitaxel and carboplatin
	Consideration of intraperitoneal chemotherapy

patients has also been demonstrated, with median survival time greater than 3 years.

Sub-optimal Debulked Stage III or Stage IV (both advanced)

For patients who undergo sub-optimal debulking (extensive residual disease after primary surgery) for stage III, or for patients with stage IV disease, the current standard of care is treatment with paclitaxel and carboplatin for 6 to 8 cycles [A Evidence].

Prognosis

The 5 yr survival rates with treatment are as follows:

- *Stage I:* 70 to 100%
- *Stage II:* 50 to 70%
- *Stage III:* 20 to 50%
- *Stage IV:* 10 to 20%

Prognosis is worse when tumor grade is higher or when surgery cannot remove all visibly involved tissue; prognosis is best when the involved tissue can be reduced to < 1 cm in diameter. With stages III and IV, recurrence rate is about 70%.

EXERCISES

A. Answer the following questions

- How common is ovarian cancer?
- Why ovarian cancer is leading cause of mortality among women?
- How are the ovarian tumours categorized?
- Which ovarian malignancy is most common?

Keywords

BRCA gene: BRCA 1 and BRCA2 gene ate located on the long arm of chromosome 17 and 13 respectively. Germline mutations of these gene are responsible for hereditary ovarian cancers.

Hereditary breast and ovarian cancer syndrome (HBOC): A syndrome charecterized by multiple cases of early onset (< 50 years)breast and ovarian cancers.

Hereditary non polyposis colon cancer or Lynch type II syndrome: A syndrome characterized by early onset (<50 yrs) proximal colon cancer and associated with cancer of ovary and Endometrium.

Optimal debulking or cytoreduction: In advanced malignancy, where complete resection is not feasible, as much tumor as possible is removed (debulking surgery). The aim of debulking surgery is to leave behind no tumors larger than 1 cm. This is called optimally debulked. Patients whose tumors have been optimally debulked, have a better prognosis than those left with larger tumors after surgery.

- In which age group epithelial ovarian cancer more common?
- What is thought to be underlying hypothesis for development of epithelial ovarian cancer?
- Epithelial types include which histologic types?
- How does ovarian cancer spread?
- What is he role of screening for ovarian cancer?
- What are the common sign and symptoms of ovarian cancer?
- What is the initial investigation to evaluate a ovarian lesion?

- What are the radiographic tests should be considered in a patient with epithelial ovarian cancer (EOC)?
- Which tumour marker is often elevated in advanced stge EOC? What is its value?
- What is Gold stage standard in diagnosis of EOC?
- How is ovarian cancer staged?
- Describe the stages of ovarian cancer and their prognosis.
- Which lymph nodes are typically involved in advanced EOC?
- What is optimal treatment of advanced EOC?
- What is the most effective chemotherapy regimen?
- What are the most common side effects of chemotherapy?
- What are the poor prognostic factors?

B. Write short notes on

a. Incessant ovulation theory
b. Staging laparotomy for ovarian cancer
c. Neoadjuvant chemotherapy
d. CA 125

C. Justify/criticize or give reasons for following statements

a. Ovarian malignancy is often diagnosed in advanced stage
b. Surgery plays most important role in managing ovarian malignancy

D. Fill in the blanks with appropriate word/s

a. The three cell types that are thought to give rise to the three types of malignant ovarian neoplasms are _____ , _____ , and _____ .
b. The main two modalities of ovarian cancer management are _____ and _____ .
c. The incision for surgery of ovarian malignancy should be _____ abdominal.

d. Presence of microscopic upper abdominal disease is staged as stage _____ .

E. Questions for practical (read the case summary in the beginning of chapter before answering the following questions)

1. What is your provisional diagnosis and why?
2. What are the differential diagnoses for this patient?
3. How do you confirm your diagnosis?
4. How do you differentiate clinically between benign and malignant ovarian tumors?
5. What other investigations you consider for her?
6. How do you treat her?

Bibliography

1. Alleti G, Gallenberg MM, Cliby WA, et al. Current Management Strategies for Ovarian Cancer Mayo Clin Proc. 2007;82(6):751–770.
2. Bhoola S, Hoskins WJ. Diagnosis and management of epithelial ovarian cancer ACOG Vol 107 no 6: 1399–1410.
3. Epithelial ovarian cancer NCCN Clinical Practice Guidelines in Oncology for Epithelial Ovarian Cancer JNCCN 2011;9:82–113.
4. Epithelial ovarian cancer Scottish Intercollegiate Guidelines Net work 2003.
5. Hamilton W, Menon U. Easily missed Ovarian cancer BMJ 2009; 339:b4650.
6. Markman M. The Role of CA-125 in the Management of Ovarian Cancer The Oncologist February 1997 vol. 2 no. 16–9.
7. Olson SH. Symptoms of Ovarian Cancer VOL. 98, NO. 2, AUGUST 2001 0029-7844/01.
8. Ovarian cancer, American Cancer Society 2012.
9. Ovarian cancer—the recognition and initial management of ovarian cancer Nice clinical guideline 2011.
10. Roett M , Evans P. Ovarian Cancer - an overview Am Fam Physician. 2009;80(6):609–616.
11. Salani R, Backes FJ. Overview of Epithelial Ovarian Cancer and Updates in Management Strategies Medscape 2009.

25

Endometrial Carcinoma

A 63-year-old obese woman with history of treatment for diabetes and hypertension has presented with postmenopausal bleeding per vagina. She has onset of menopause 12 years ago. She is unmarried and her family history reveals her mother died of endometrial carcinoma. Bleeding is scanty but has persisted for more than 20 days. She has not used any hormone therapy in the past. On examination she is morbidly obese with BMI of 42 and pelvic examination reveals normal looking cervix with presence of vaginal bleeding. On bimanual examination uterus is enlarged to 8 weeks size of pregnant uterus and fornices are free. How she should be treated?

In this chapter we will learn:
- Etiology of endometrial carcinoma
- Its pathology
- Clinical presentation
- Investigations
- Staging
- Treatment
- Prognosis

Introduction

In developed countries, endometrial carcinoma is the most common gynecological cancer; however, in developing countries including India, it is much less common than carcinoma of the cervix. By definition, adenocarcinoma of the endometrium is an invasive disease, invading either the endometrial stroma or the underlying myometrium or the extrauterine tissues. Etiologically, endometrial carcinoma usually results from unopposed estrogen stimulation of the endometrium, although non-estrogen-related forms occur as well. The most common presentation of endometrial cancer is postmenopausal bleeding. A variety of diagnostic modalities are available to aid in the detection of the disease, each with its own strengths and limitations. Surgery, radiation, and chemotherapy play a role in treatment, depending on tumor stage and grade. At present, there are no recommendations for screening the general population.

Etiology

Endometrial cancer affects mainly postmenopausal women, particularly those aged 50 to 65. Major risk factors are:

1. Obesity
2. Diabetes
3. Hypertension

Other risk factors include:

- Unopposed estrogen. Unopposed estrogen (high circulating levels of estrogen with no or low levels of progesterone) may be associated with obesity, polycystic ovary syndrome, nulliparity, early menarche, late menopause, estrogen-producing tumors, anovulation (ovulatory dysfunction), and estrogen therapy without progesterone.
- Tamoxifen use for > 5 yrs
- Previous pelvic radiation therapy
- A personal or family history of breast or ovarian cancer
- Family history of hereditary nonpolyposis colorectal cancer or possibly, among 1st-degree relatives, endometrial cancer.

Heredity contributes to endometrial cancer in about 6% of cases, usually in families with hereditary nonpolyposis colorectal cancer (HNPCC) syndrome.

Clinical pearl
- Unopposed estrogen is a known risk factor for endometrial cancer.
- The benefit of tamoxifen use to pevent recurrence of breast cancer far outweighs the risk.

Pathology

Uterine cancer may develop from endometrial hyperplasia, which is associated with increased estrogen exposure. It may also develop from endometrial atrophy, which is not estrogen related. Endometrial adeno-carcinoma accounts for > 80% of endometrial cancers. They are also called the endometroid type because of its histologic similarity to the endometrium. Most tumors occur in the setting of unopposed estrogen stimulation, leading to endometrial hyperplasia. Previously, hyperplasia was thought to progress along a continuum that led to endometrial cancer. Recent studies show that although some hyperplasias do progress to

adenocarcinoma, others coexist with endometrial cancer. The probability of endometrial hyperplasia progressing to adenocarcinoma is greater in patients who have a higher degree of cytologic atypia, as described by the World Health Organization classification system. Simple hyperplasia without cellular atypia has a 1 percent probability of progressing to carcinoma if left untreated; with cellular atypia, the probability is 8 percent. Complex hyperplasia without cellular atypia has a 3 percent probability of progressing; with cellular atypia, the probability is 29 percent.

Other types include papillary serous, clear cell, squamous, mucinous carcinoma. These tumors manifest later in life, are typically diagnosed at a more advanced stage, and carry a poorer prognosis.

Spread: The cancer may spread from the surface of the uterine cavity to the cervical canal; through the myometrium to the serosa and into the peritoneal cavity; via the lumen of the fallopian tube to the ovary, broad ligament, and peritoneal surfaces; via the blood stream, leading to distant metastases; or via the lymphatics. The higher (more undifferentiated) the grade of the tumor, the greater the likelihood of deep myometrial invasion, pelvic or para-aortic lymph node metastases, or extrauterine spread.

Clinical Presentation

Endometrial adenocarcinoma occurs during the late reproductive and menopausal years. The patient may be nullipara. The history should include determination of risk factors (as mentioned earlier).

Symptoms

Because approximately 75% of women with endometrial cancer are postmenopausal, the most common symptom is postmenopausal bleeding. A vaginal discharge may occur weeks or months before postmenopausal bleeding.

Because 25% of endometrial cancers are in patients who are perimenopausal or premenopausal, symptoms suggestive of cancer may not be obvious. The idea that any type of bleeding during the perimenopausal period is probably due to menopause is a common misconception. This irregular bleeding is often ignored by the patient and even health care providers. Remember that the normal bleeding pattern during this time should become lighter and lighter and further and further apart. Heavy frequent menstrual periods or intermenstrual bleeding must be evaluated.

Signs

Physical examination should include calculation of the body mass index, detection of pallor, measurement of blood pressure. An abdominal examination will not reveal any abnormality in most women, however, in some women it may reveal a lower abdominal mass with hepatomegaly. The pelvic examination should include visual inspection to evaluate for any sources of bleeding (i.e., cervical, vaginal, rectal, urethral). The uterus and adnexa should be palpated for uterine size and position, as well as for any suspicious masses.

Clinical pearl
- Most patients (75%) with endometrial cancer present with postmenopausal bleeding; however, only 10% of women with postmenopausal bleeding have endometrial carcinoma.
- Endometrial cancer is usually detected in early stage due to an early symptom: postmenopausal bleeding

Investigations

An endometrial biopsy or curettage for histological examination is the only test that will definitely confirm the presence of endometrial cancer. However less than 10% of women with postmenopausal bleeding (PMB) subsequently turn out to have endometrial carcinoma. Therefore, it is reasonable to obtain a pelvic ultrasound as first step. Saline infusion sonography is an ultrasound method gaining popularity in some countries that may yield additional information. Discussion is ongoing about the optimal sequence and combination of procedures for evaluation. A variety of options exist, each with its own strengths and limitations.

Endometrial Biopsy

Traditionally, dilatation and curettage was the primary means of evaluating the endometrium. The development of newer sampling techniques, specifically the Pipelle device, has simplified this evaluation. The sensitivity of the Pipelle in detecting endometrial cancer has been calculated as high as 99 percent in postmenopausal women and 91 percent in premenopausal women. However, blind endometrial sampling techniques, such as the Pipelle, are most useful when the abnormality is global, rather than focal (i.e., endometrial polyp or focal hyperplasia). Further evaluation is warranted in the following circumstances: failure to obtain an adequate specimen; inconsistencies between biopsy and imaging; and persistence of symptoms despite a benign biopsy result.

Ultrasonography

Transvaginal and transabdominal ultrasonography of the uterus can be helpful when evaluating a patient with abnormal vaginal bleeding. In the premenopausal woman, ultrasonography may reveal a variety of structural abnormalities of the uterus and endometrium. In the postmenopausal woman, transvaginal ultrasonography has been used to assess endometrial thickness in an attempt to identify women who need further invasive testing (*see* Chapter 32—PMB)

Hysteroscopy

Hysteroscopy is direct endoscopic visualization of the endometrial cavity. A recent review indicates that hysteroscopy is highly accurate in diagnosing endometrial cancer and moderately accurate in diagnosing other endometrial conditions in women with abnormal bleeding.

Saline Infusion Sonography

In saline infusion sonography (also known as sonohysterography), sterile saline is instilled into the uterine cavity before ultrasound evaluation to allow for more precise visualization of the endometrial structures. Saline infusion sonography is often used as a second step in the evaluation of abnormal bleeding. It is particularly useful when ultrasonography suggests a focal lesion, when endometrial biopsy is non-diagnostic, or when abnormal bleeding persists despite normal initial workup.

Other laboratory tests: Once cancer is diagnosed, pretreatment evaluation includes Complete blood count (CBC), kidney and liver function tests, blood sugar, chest X-ray, and ECG. If an abdominal mass or hepatomegaly is detected during physical examination or if liver function tests are abnormal, pelvic and abdominal CT are also done to check for extrauterine or metastatic cancer.

Staging

The endometrial cancer is generally staged according to the International Federation of Gynecology and Obstetrics (FIGO) system. FIGO system has recommended surgical staging. In May 2009, a new FIGO staging system was published which is mentioned below.

Stage I—Tumor Limited to the Corpus Uteri

- IA no or less than 50% myometrial invasion
- IB ≥ 50% myometrial invasion (Fig. 25.1).

Stage II—Tumor invades Cervical Stroma, but does not Extend Beyond Uterus

Endocervical glandular involvement only should be considered as stage I and no longer stage II.

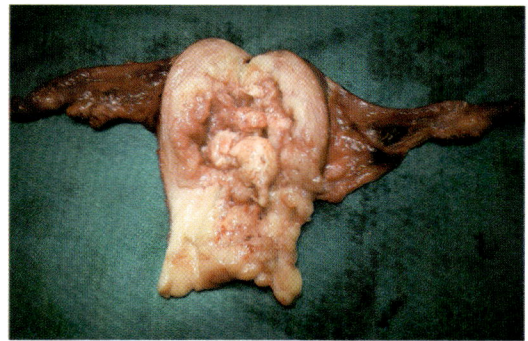

Fig. 25.1: Specimen showing endometrial carcinoma extending towards the cervix. Histopathology report confirmed more than 50% myometrial involvement and endocervical glandular involvement only - FIGO stage IB, grade 1

Stage III—Local or Regional Spread of the Tumor

- IIIA—tumor invades the serosa of the corpus uteri and/or adnexa, positive cytology has to be reported separately without changing the stage.
- IIIB—vaginal or parametrial involvement
- IIIC—metastasis to pelvic and or para aortic lymph nodes
- IIIC1—positive pelvic lymph nodes
- IIIC2—positive para-aortic lymph nodes with or without positive pelvic lymph nodes.

Stage IV—Tumor invades Bladder and/or Bowel Mucosa and/or Distant Metastasis

- IVA—tumor invades bladder and/or bowel mucosa
- IVB—distant metastasis including intra-abdominal metastasis and/or inguinal lymph nodes

Cases of carcinoma of the corpus should be classified (or graded) according to the degree of histologic differentiation. The histopathology and degree of differentiation is as follows:

- Class G1—nonsquamous or nonmorular solid growth pattern of 5% or less
- Class G2—nonsquamous or nonmorular solid growth pattern of 6–50%

- Class G3—nonsquamous or nonmorular solid growth pattern of more than 50%

All women with biopsy proven diagnosis of endometrial carcinoma will undergo surgical staging which includes:
- Exploratory laparotomy
- Total abdominal hysterectomy (TAH)
- Bilateral salpingo-oophorectomy (BSO)
- Peritoneal cytology
- Pelvic and para-aortic lymph adnenectomy

Clinical pearl

Diagnosis is confirmed at biopsy and histology and staging is confirmed at surgery (laparotomy).

Treatment

Once the diagnosis of endometrial cancer has been made, routine presurgical evaluation is performed. If the results are found to be normal, the patient is deemed a surgical candidate. Then, an exploratory laparotomy, total abdominal hysterectomy, bilateral salpingo-oophorectomy, peritoneal cytology, and pelvic and para-aortic lymphadenectomy are performed.
- Obviously, if intraperitoneal disease is identified at the time of surgery, attempts are made at surgical removal.
- Staging is then determined based on surgical pathologic findings (*see* Staging). Subsequent therapy, if needed, is then determined, depending on the surgical pathological findings of the operative procedure.

Adjuvant Radiotherapy

Radiotherapy may be indicated to reduce the risk of local recurrence (e.g. Brachytherapy to the vaginal vault postoperatively)

Adjuvant Chemotherapy

Platinum based chemotherapy can be considered in stage I G3 with adverse risk factors (patient age, lymph vascular invasion and high tumor volume) and in patients with stages II and III. A variety of chemotherapy regimes exists, a combination of placlitaxel, cisplatin and doxorubicin is now popular because of better toxicity profile.

Treatment of stage IV is variable and patient dependent but typically involves a combination of surgery, radiation therapy, and chemotherapy. Occasionally, hormonal therapy should also be considered.

Hormone Therapy

Hormone therapy with progesterone is recommended only for inoperable or recurrent tumors that are ER/PR receptor positive.

Prognosis

Prognosis is worse with higher-grade tumors, more extensive spread, and older patient age. Average 5-yr survival rates are 70 to 95% with stages I or II and 10 to 60% with stages III or IV. Overall, 63% of patients are cancer-free ≥ 5 yr after treatment.

Keywords

Hereditary nonpolyposis colorectal cancer (HNPCC) syndrome–Lynch syndrome (HNPCC or Hereditary nonpolyposis colorectal cancer) is an autosomal dominant genetic condition which has a high risk of colon cancer as well as other cancers including endometrium, ovary, stomach, small intestine, hepatobiliary tract, upper urinary tract, skin and brain.

Adjuvant therapy: Adjuvant therapy, also called adjuvant care, is treatment that is given in addition to the primary, main or initial treatment. The surgery and complex treatment regimens used in cancer have led the term to be used mainly to describe adjuvant cancer treatments.

EXERCISES

Answer the following questions

1. What is endometrial carcinoma?
2. What is a possible cause of endometrial cancer?
3. What are the examples of hyper estrogenic states associated with development of endometrial carcinoma?

4. Which medical diseases are associated with endometrial carcinoma?

5. Enumerate the risk factors of endometrial carcinoma.

6. What are the histologic subtypes of endometrial carcinoma?

7. How does this cancer spread?

8. Describe the symptoms and signs of endometrial carcinoma.

9. How do you confirm the diagnosis of endometrial carcinoma?

10. What are the other investigations that can be considered in woman suspected for endometrial carcinoma?

11. What are the presurgical evaluation tests?

12. How do you stage the disease?

13. How do you treat endometrial carcinoma?

Fill in the blanks

1. Three main risk factors for endometrial cancer are _____ , _____ , _____ .

2. Risk of endometrial carcinoma is highest with _____ histological pattern of endometrial hyperplasia.

3. Most common histology of carcinoma of endometrium is _____ .

4. Long term tamoxifen may cause _____ carcinoma.

5. Inguinal lymph node involvement in endometrial carcinoma will be staged as _____ disease.

Explain or justify the following statements

1. Unopposed estrogen is a known risk factor for endometrial cancer.

2. Staging of endometrial cancer is surgico-pathological.

Write short notes on

1. Staging of endometrial carcinoma

2. Laboratory diagnosis of endometrial carcinoma.

Questions for practical (read the case summary in the beginning of chapter before answering the questions)

1. Identify the risk factors for endometrial carcinoma that are present in this patient.

2. What is your provisional diagnosis and why?

3. What are the differential diagnoses?

4. How do you investigate her?

5. If her endometrial biopsy suggests endometrial carcinoma, how do you evaluate preoperatively?

6. What are the basic steps in surgical staging?

7. How she should be treated if she is having stage I Grade 1 disease?

Bibliography

1. Mutch DG, Rimel BJ. Endometrial cancer OBG management, Vol. 21 No. 7; July 2009.

2. Elit L. Endometrial cancer Prevention detection management and follow up Can Fam Physician 2000;46:887–892.

3. Colombo N. et al, Endometrial cancer: ESMO Clinical Practice Guidelines for diagnosis, treatment and follow-up Annals of Oncology 22 (Supplement 6): vi35-vi39, 2011.

4. Buchanan E, et al. Endometrial Cancer Am Fam Physician. 2009 Nov 15;80(10):1075–1080.

5. Clinical review: Endometrial cancer BMJ.

6. Mutter G, Ferency A. Endometrial Hyperplasia and Neoplasia: Definition, Diagnosis, and Management Principles Glob. libr. women's med., (ISSN: 1756-2228) 2008.

7. Joseph N. Sanfilippo Primary care for obstetrics and gynecology: a Handbook for physicians.

26

Gestational Trophoblastic Neoplasia

A 20-year-old P 1+1 Muslim woman has presented with irregular vaginal bleeding for last one month. She gives a history of treatment with suction evacuation for molar pregnancy 4 months ago. She did not attend her doctor for follow up as she was well for next few months following evacuation. On examination she has mild pallor and vitals are normal. Gynecological examination reveals a blue-black nodule in suburethral region (Figs 26.2 and 26.3), uterus is normal in size and fornices are free. Ultrasound reveals normal size uterus and cavity is empty. Her serum beta hCG value is 100844 mIU/ml. What is your diagnosis?

In this chapter we will learn:
- What is gestational trophoblastic neoplasia (GTN)
- Its pathophysiology
- Usual clinical presentation
- Investigations
- Work up
- Treatment
- Follow up
- Prognosis

Introduction

Gestational trophoblastic neoplasia (GTN) refers to a pathologic condition that is characterized by aggressive invasion of the endometrium and myometrium by tropho-blastic cells and is divided to four different pathologic entities: invasive mole, gestational choriocarcinoma, placental site trophoblastic tumour and epithelioid trophoblastic tumour. GTN typically develops with or follows some form of pregnancy, but occasionally an antecedent gestation cannot be confirmed with certainty. Most cases follow a hydatidi-form mole. Rarely, GTN develops after a live birth, miscarriage, or termination.

Pathophysiology

A hydatidiform mole is considered malignant when the serum hCG levels plateau or rise during the follow-up period and an intervening pregnancy is excluded. This occurs in 15–20% of hydatidiform moles. Partial moles also have malignant potential, but only 2–3% become malignant.

An invasive mole has the same histo-pathologic characteristics of a hydatidiform mole, but invasion of the myometrium with necrosis and hemorrhage occurs or pulmonary metastases are present.

Choriocarcinoma is a highly anaplastic malignancy derived from trophoblastic elements. Grossly, the tumor has a red, granular appearance on cut section with focal, often extensive central necrosis and hemorrhage (Fig. 26.1).

Histologically, choriocarcinomas have no villi, but they have sheets of trophoblasts and hemorrhage.

In patients with placental site tophoblastic tumor (PSTT), intermediate trophoblasts are found infiltrating the myometrium without causing tissue destruction. The intermediate cytotrophoblasts secrete human placental lactogen (hPL). These patients have persistent low levels of serum hCG (100–1000 mIU/mL).

Epithelioid trophoblastic tumor develops from neoplastic transformation of chorionic type of intermediate trophoblasts. Microscopically these tumors resemble placental site trophoblastic tumor and the cells are smaller and display less nuclear pleomorphisim. Grossly epitheloid trophoblastic tumor grows in a nodular fashion rather than the infiltrative pattern of placental trophoblastic tumor.

Clinical Presentation

History

Most cases of gestational trophoblastic neoplasia are diagnosed when the serum hCG levels plateau or rise in patients being observed after the diagnosis of hydatidiform mole. If metastases are present, signs and symptoms associated with the metastatic disease, such as hemoptysis, abdominal pain, hematuria, and neurologic symptoms, may be present.

Physical Examination

- Metastasis to the lower genital tract present as purple to blue-black papules or nodules (Figs 26.2 and 26.3). These are extremely

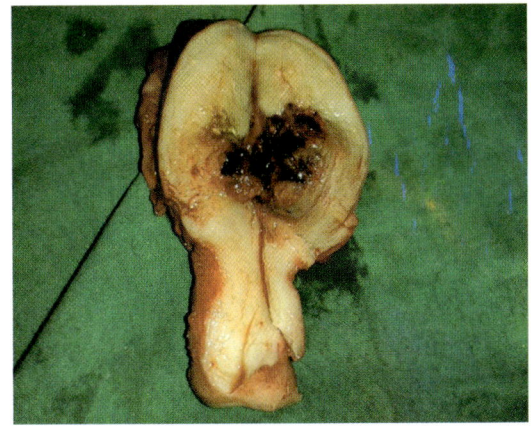

Fig. 26.1: Specimen of uterus showing choriocarcinoma note the areas of myometrial invasion, hemorrhage and necrosis. Patient received prior chemotherapy

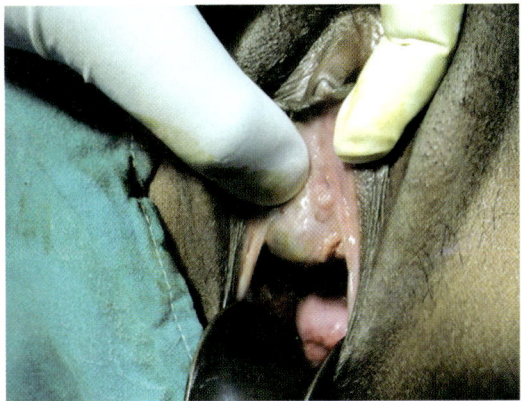

Fig. 26.2: Blue-black nodule in suburethral region

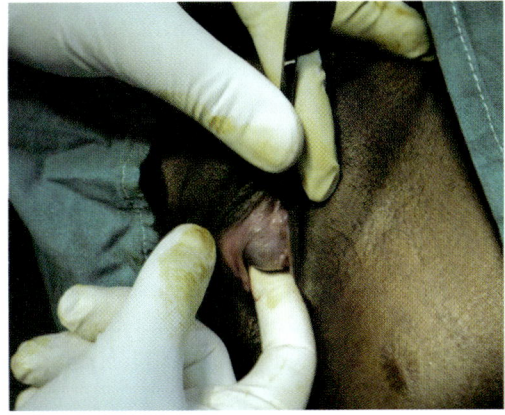

Fig. 26.3: Suburethral blue-black nodule lifted up with index finger

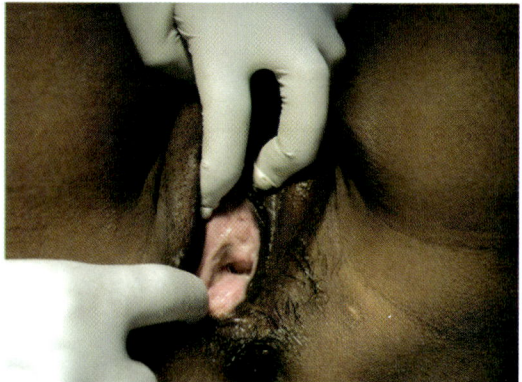

Fig. 26.4: The nodule has disappeared following chemotherapy in same patient of Figs 26.2 and 26.3

vascular and might bleed profusely if biopsied.
- Abdominal tenderness may be present if liver or gastrointestinal metastases have occurred.
- Abdominal guarding and rebound tenderness may be present if a hemoperitoneum has occurred due to bleeding from an abdominal metastasis. Bleeding from a metastasis could also result in signs and symptoms of hemorrhagic shock.
- Neurologic deficits, from lethargy to coma, can be encountered if brain metastasis has occurred.
- Jaundice may be present if liver metastasis causes biliary obstruction.

Clinical pearl
The possibility of metastatic GTN should be considered in any woman of reproductive age group presenting with metastatic disease involving the lungs or distant sites from an unknown primary site of malignancy.

Investigations

- Serum quantitative hCG is used to assess the disease status and response to therapy.
- A CBC may help detect anemia secondary to bleeding.
- Liver enzymes may become elevated in the presence of metastasis to the liver.

- Renal function test
- Thyroid function studies should be performed in all patients with a clinical history or physical examination suggestive of hyperthyroidism. Abnormal thyroid function, manifested as an elevated T4 level, is common in GTN.
- Ultrasonography: A pelvic ultrasound is often useful to detect the extent of uterine involvement and may identify patients who are at risk for uterine perforation or who would benefit from a hysterectomy to reduce tumor burden. An upper abdominal ultrasonography may detect hepatic metatstasis.
- *Chest radiograph:* This test is recommended because the lung is the most frequent site of metastasis.
- *CT scan of the chest (optional):* Micrometastases are present in approximately 40–45% of women with nonmetastatic gestational trophoblastic neoplasia (GTN) who have normal chest radiograph findings. The significance of this is not clear. However, having metastasis elsewhere is extremely rare if pulmonary or lower genital tract metastases has not occurred. If metastases are found on chest CT and not on chest radiograph, they cannot be used for purpose of staging. Additional imaging can be omitted in asymptomatic patients with a negative chest CT given that distant metastases are unlikely in the absence of lung metastases.
- CT scan of the abdomen and pelvis with contrast and MRI of the head (preferable to CT)
  • CT and MRI are recommended if the patient has GTN (hydatidiform mole with metastasis to the lungs, choriocarcinoma, or persistent hydatidiform mole).
  • The lungs, lower genital tract, brain, liver, kidney, and gastrointestinal tract are common sites of metastases.

Work up

Diagnosis: In accordance with the International Federation of Gynecology and Obstetrics (FIGO), GTN is diagnosed after a molar gestation if any of the following is observed:

1. Four values or more of hCG plateau over at least three weeks (days 1, 7, 14, and 21)
2. A rise in hCG of 10% or greater for three or more values over at least two weeks (days 1, 7, and 14)
3. The presence of histologic choriocarcinoma
4. Persistence of hCG six months after molar evacuation.

Staging: The official International Federation of Gynecology and Obstetrics (FIGO) staging of gestational trophoblastic neoplasia is as follows:

- Stage I – Confined to the uterus
- Stage II – Limited to the genital structures
- Stage III – Lung metastases
- Stage IV – Other metastases

Each anatomical stage (roman numeral) is followed by the sum of the prognostic scores (Table 26.1) separated by a colon (e.g., stage III:5).

Prognostic scoring: The currently used prognostic scoring index is a modification of the World Health Organization (WHO) classification. It provides points for the presence of a number of prognostic factors (Table 26.1). The FIGO Oncology Committee at its 2000 meeting recommended that patients could be assigned to a low-risk group if the prognostic score was 0–6 and a high-risk group if the score was 7 or higher.

Treatment: Patients with nonmetastatic GTN or metastatic low-risk GTN are treated with single-agent chemotherapy (Table 26.2). Many clinicians prefer methotrexate. However, actinomycin D can be used in patients with poor liver function. During treatment, the serum hCG levels are monitored every week. One additional course of chemotherapy is administered after a normal serum hCG level. After 3–4 normal serum hCG levels, the levels are observed once per month for 1 year. A switch from methotrexate to actinomycin D is made if the patient receiving methotrexate for nonmetastatic or metastatic low-risk GTN develops rising or plateauing serum hCG levels.

Patients with high risk prognostic score of 7 or higher and who are at high risk of therapy failure are treated with.

- A combination of etoposide, methotrexate, and actinomycin D administered in the first week of a 2-week cycle and cyclophosphamide and vincristine (Oncovin) administered in the second week. This is known as the EMA-CO regimen (Table 26.3).
- Some substitute cisplatin and etoposide for cyclophosphamide and vincristine during the second week. This is known as the EMA-CE regimen. Some reserve the EMA-

Table 26.1: FIGO WHO prognostic scoring system for GTN

Prognostic factor	Score 0	1	2	4
Age (yrs)	< 39	> 39		
Antecedent pregnancy	H mole	Abortion	Term	
Interval (months)[a]	< 4	4–6	7–12	>12
HCG (IU/L)	< 1000	1000–10000	10000–100000	> 100000
Largest tumor (including uterus)	< 3 cm	3–5 cm	> 5 cm	
Site(s) of metastasis	Lung	Spleen, kidneys	GI tract	Liver, brain
No, of metastasis		1–3	4–8	>8
Prior chemotherapy			Single drug	2 or more drugs

[a]Time between end of antecedent pregnancy and start of chemotherapy

Table 26.2: Chemotherapy regimen for nonmetastatic and metastatic low risk GTN

Drug	Administration	Cycle
Methotrexate	1 mg/kg IM /IV days 1, 3, 5, 7	14 days and
Folinic acid	0.1 mg/kg IM/IV days 2,4,6,8	
Actinomycin D	10 µ gm/kg IV daily for 5 days	14 days

Table 26.3: Chemotherapy regimen for high risk GTN

Drug regimen (EMA-CO)		Administration
Course 1	EMA	
Day 1	Etoposide	100 mg/m² IV over 30 mins
	Methotrexate	100 mg/m² IV bolus followed by
		200 mg/m² IV as 12 hr continuous infusion
	Actinomycin D	0.5 mg IV bolus
Day 2	Etoposide	100 mg/m² IV over 30 mins
	Folinic acid	15 mg IV/IM/PO 12 hrly for 4 doses
		Commencing 24 hrs after start of methotrexate
	Actinomycin D	0.5 mg IV bolus
Course 2 (CO)		
Day 8	Cyclophosphamide	600 mg/m² IV over 30 min
	Vincristine (Oncovine)	1 mg/ m² (up to 2 mg) IV bolus

CE regimen for patients in whom EMA-CO fails.

- At least 2 additional courses of EMA-CO or EMA-CE are administered after a normal serum hCG level.
- Patients with metastasis to the brain receive whole brain irradiation (3000 cGy) in combination with chemotherapy. Corticosteroids (dexamethasone) with systemic effect are administered to reduce brain edema.

Surgical care: Scope of surgery in treatment of GTN is limited, however, it is of value in following situations:

- A hysterectomy may be necessary in case of uncontrolled vaginal bleeding. Hysterectomy may reduce the total number of chemotherapy cycles needed to achieve remission.
- Uterine or hypogastric artery ligation or embolization of feeding vessels may be needed to control hemorrhage. Hepatic artery embolization has been used successfully to control hemorrhage from hepatic metastases.

- A repeat D&C in the presence of persistent tissue on pelvic ultrasonography may reduce the number of chemotherapy cycles needed to achieve remission.
- Craniotomy may be needed to control bleeding and provide decompression.
- Resection of solitary metastasis (e.g., thoracotomy) or disease within the myometrium may help achieve a remission.

Treatment of Placental Site Trophoblastic Tumor (PSTT) and Epithelioid Trophoblastic Tumor (ETT)

Hysterectomy is considered as a first-line treatment strategy in women with stage I PSTT and ETT because these are relatively chemoresistant neoplasms. Women with stage I PSTT or ETT are often effectively treated with surgery alone. Patients with

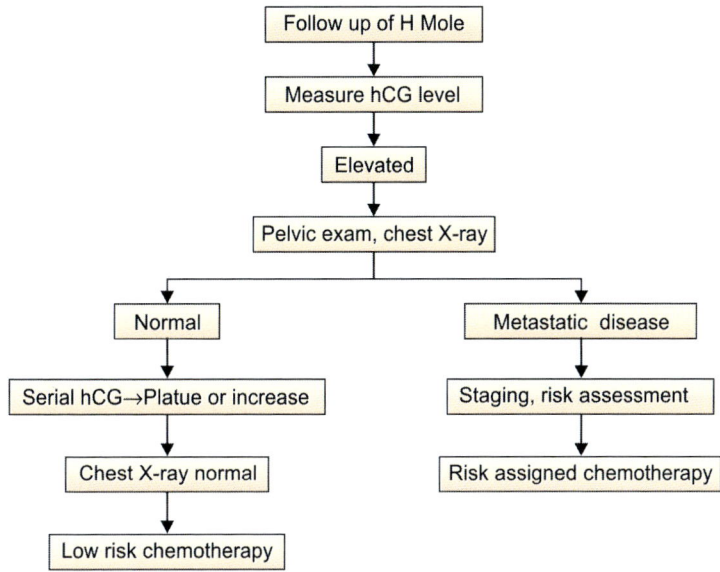

Fig. 26.5: Algorithm for management of GTN

metastatic PSTT may still achieve remission with intensive combination chemotherapy after surgical intervention, particularly when they are diagnosed within 4 years of the antecedent pregnancy. ETT is the rarest variety of GTN, hence there is limited data on the optimal chemotherapy to treat patients with advanced-stage disease.

Follow up: All patients with GTN should be followed with weekly serum quantitative hCG levels until normal for 3 consecutive weeks, then monthly for 12 months. The monthly follow up period is extended to 24 months in patients with stage IV disease given the increased risk of late recurrence in this patient population.

Prognosis

- Nonmetastatic GTN has a cure rate of close to 100% with chemotherapy treatment.
- Metastatic low-risk GTN has a cure rate of close to 100% with chemotherapy treatment (Fig. 26.5).
- Metastatic high-risk GTN has a cure rate of approximately 75% with chemotherapy treatment.

- After 12 months of normal hCG levels, less than 1% of patients with GTN have recurrences.

Keywords

Invasive mole: A condition where molar pregnancy invades the wall of the uterus, potentially spreading and metastasizing to other parts of the body (such as the vagina or lungs).

Choriocarcinoma: A highly malignant trophoblastic tumor tends to be invasive and to metastasize early and widely through both the venous and lymphatic systems. Histologically, choriocarcinomas have no villi, but they have sheets of trophoblasts and hemorrhage.

Placental site trophoblastic tumour: A variety of gestational trophbastic neoplasia which consists of a predominance of intermediate trophoblastic cells with fibrinoid material and vascular invasion.

Methotrexate: Methotrexate is an antimetabolite and antifolate drug, used in treatment of cancer, auto-immune diseases, ectopic pregnancy and for the induction of medical abortion. It acts by inhibiting the metabolism of folic acid.

Folinic acid: Folinic acid or leucovorin, generally administered as calcium or sodium folinate (or leucovorin calcium/sodium), is an adjuvant used in cancer chemotherapy along with methotrexate. Folinic acid is a 5-formyl derivative of tetrahydrofolic acid. It is readily converted to other reduced folic acid derivatives (e.g., tetrahydrofolate), and thus, has vitamin activity that is equivalent to that of folic acid. However, since it does not require the action of dihydrofolate reductase for its conversion, its function as a vitamin is unaffected by inhibition of this enzyme by drugs such as methotrexate. Folinic acid, therefore, allows for some purine/pyrimidine synthesis to occur in the presence of dihydrofolate reductase inhibition, so that some normal DNA replication and RNA transcription processes can proceed.

EXERCISES

1. Answer the following questions

- What is GTN?
- What are the different pathologic entities?
- What are the characteristic features of different histological variety of GTN?
- How GTN is diagnosed?
- Name the investigations you consider in a patient with GTN?
- How do you stage the disease?
- How do you treat GTN?

2. Write short notes on

- Prognostic scoring system in GTN
- FIGO criteria for diagnosis of GTN
- Placental site trophoblastic tumor

3. Fill in the blanks

- GTN refers to pathologic entity namely _____ , _____ , _____ , _____ .
- Most GTN are diagnosed during follow up of _____ .

- Most frequent site of metastasis in GTN is _____ .
- Metastatic low-risk GTN are treated with _____ chemotherapy.

4. Explain or justify the following statements

- Serum quantitative hCG is used to diagnose postmolar GTN
- Chemotherapy is curative treatment for GTN.

5. Questions for practical (read the case summary at beginning of chapter before answering the questions)

- What is your diagnosis?
- What are the points in favour of your diagnosis?
- Which other investigations you consider for this patient?
- How do you stage her disease?
- What is the importance of prognostic scoring for this patient?
- How do you treat her vaginal metastasis?

Bibliography

1. Hammond C, Soper, J. Gestational trophoblastic diseases, Glob. libr. women's med., (ISSN: 1756-2228) 2008; DOI 10.3843/GLOWM 10263
2. ICOG FOGSI recommendations for good clinical practice Management of gestational trophoblastic diseases
3. May T, et al. Current Chemotherapeutic Management of Patients with Gestational Trophoblastic Neoplasia Chemotherapy Research and Practice Volume 2011 (2011), Article ID 806256, 12 pages doi:10.1155/2011/806256.

27

Pelvic Organ Prolapse

A 50-year-old multiparous woman presents with sensation of something coming out of vagina. Symptom worsens with prolonged physical exertions such as lifting, standing. On occasion she can see and feel something bulging from vaginal opening. Increasingly, she is experiencing difficulty in emptying bladder and she need to reduce the bulge with her fingers in order to empty her bladder. She does not have any urinary leakage during physical exercise and coughing. She gives history of chronic cough and constipation. A stage III uterovaginal prolapse with involvement of apex and anterior vaginal wall is diagnosed on pelvic examination. How do you treat this patient?

In this chapter we will learn:
- Definition and types of Pelvic organ prolapse (POP)
- Etiology
- Supports of pelvic organs
- Pathophysiology
- Clinical presentation
- Grading of POP
- Differential diagnosis
- Investigations
- Treatment approach

Definition and Types

Pelvic organ prolapse (POP), also called urogenital prolapse, is the abnormal descent or herniation of the pelvic organs from their normal attachment sites or their normal position in the pelvis. Uterine prolapse is one of the conditions included by the term pelvic organ prolapse (POP), and the names may be used synonymously. The pelvic structures that may be involved include the uterus (uterine prolapse) or vaginal apex (apical vaginal prolapse), anterior vagina (cystocele, urethrocele), or posterior vagina (rectocele, enterocele). In most cases more than one compartment is affected simultaneously. From there the expression: "Prolapse doesn't occur in isolation".

Types (Table 27.1)

1. Anterior Vaginal Wall Prolapse

- *Cystocele:* Urinary bladder descends towards the vagina from its anatomical position and creates a bulge in upper two-third of anterior vaginal wall (Fig. 27.1).

- *Urethrocele:* Urethra descends towards the vagina from its anatomical position and creates a bulge in lower one-third of anterior vaginal wall (Fig. 27.4).
- *Cystourethrocele:* A combination of cystocele and urethrocele.

2. Apical Prolapse (Fig. 27.2)

- *Uterine prolapse:* Descent of the uterus and cervix from its anatomical position (normally external os lies at the level of ischial spine).
  - a. First degree–there is descent of the uterus, but the cervix remains within the upper vagina.
  - b. Second degree–the cervix reaches to the introitus or below on straining, but the uterine body still remains inside vagina (Fig. 27.5).
  - c. Third degree–when the cervix and some or all of the body of uterus is prolapsed outside the vaginal orifice. When whole of the uterus has prolapsed outside the introitus is called procidentia. In practice the fundus of the uterus usually remains within the vagina, but there is an associated inversion of the vagina.
- Vaginal vault prolapse (posthysterectomy)

3. Posterior Vaginal Wall Prolapse

- Enterocoele or pouch of Douglas hernia (Fig. 27.3)—a prolapse of the upper one-third part of the posterior vaginal wall. The hernia contains the peritoneum of the pouch of Douglas often with a loop of bowel or omentum. Enterocoele may occur concurrently with other types of genital prolapse, especially procidentia. It is also seen in prolapse following a hysterectomy (abdominal or vaginal).
- Rectocoele—a prolapse of the middle one-third part of the posterior vaginal wall due to weakness or divarication of the levator ani; the rectum bulges into the vagina (Fig. 27.1).
- Relaxed perineum (perineal body defect)— The perineal body may be deficient and part of the anal canal may bulge into the lower one-third of vagina. It follows inadequately sutured tears after childbirth or by failure of healing in such tears.

Etiology

- Congenital causes
- Acquired causes

Congenital Causes

Symptomatic prolapse occurs in nulliparous women, implying that there may be a

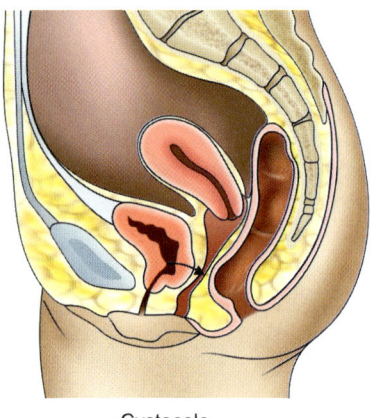

Cystocele
(prolapsed bladder)

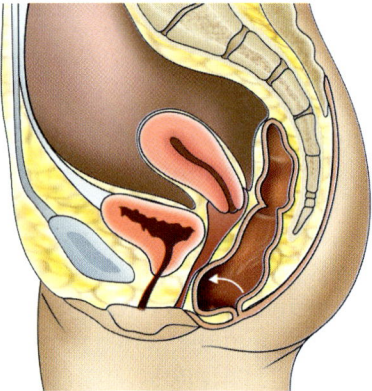

Rectocele
(prolapsed rectum)

Fig. 27.1: Anterior and posterior vaginal prolapse (cystocele and rectocele)

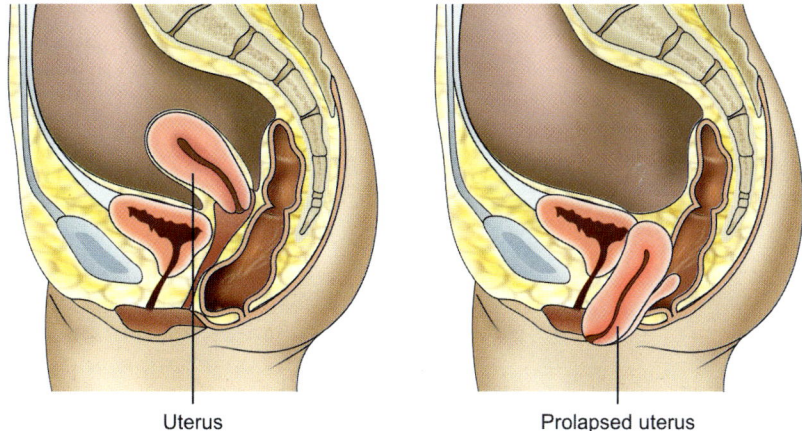

Fig. 27.2: Normal position of uterus and apical (uterine) prolapse

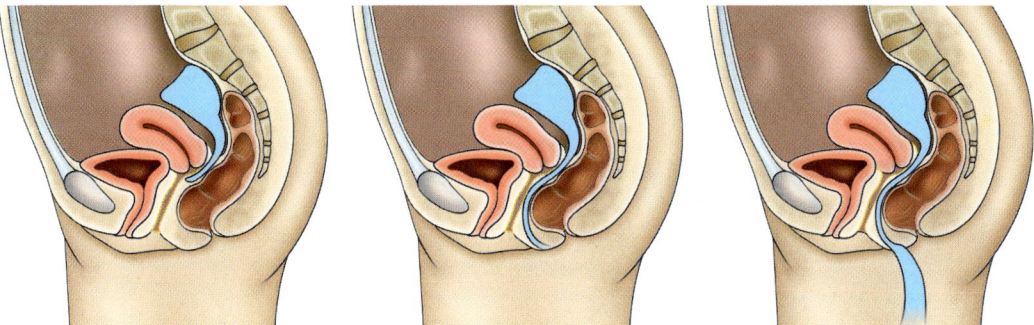

Fig. 27.3: Posterior vaginal wall prolapse (enterocele)

Table 27.1: Pelvic organ prolapse		
Anterior compartment	*Middle compartment*	*Posterior compartment*
Cystocele	Uterine prolapse	Enterocele
Urethrocele	Vault prolapse (posthysterectomy)	Rectocele
Cystourethrocele		Perineal body defect
		(Relaxed perineum)

congenital weakness of connective tissue. In addition, genital prolapse is rare in Afro-Caribbean women, suggesting genetic differences exist. Women with a genetic collagen deficiency (Marfan syndrome, Ehlers Danlos syndrome) have an increased risk of prolapse even if they do not have any of the other risk factors.

Acquired Causes

i. ***Multiparity:*** Vaginal child birth is believed to be the main cause of pelvic organ prolapse. It can occur immediately after pregnancy or 30 years later. Many factors like the weight of the baby, prolonged second stage of labor, episiotomy, forceps delivery, anal

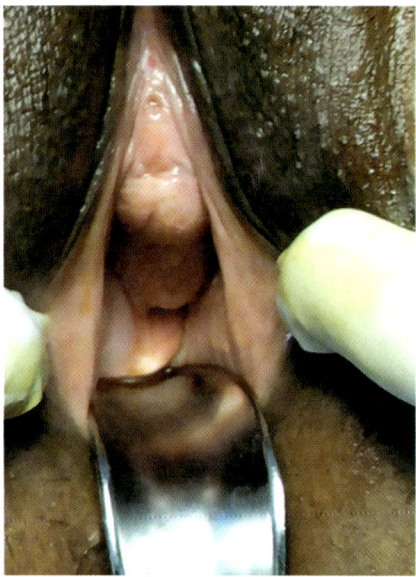

Fig. 27.4: Urethrocele—note the bulge in lower one-third of anterior vaginal wall (12'o clock position)

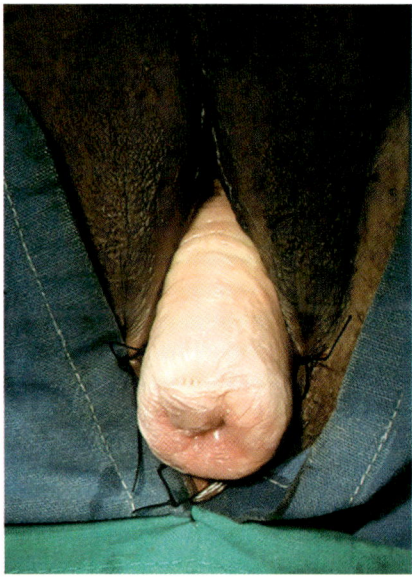

Fig. 27.5: Uterine prolapse with hypertrophy and elongation of cervix

sphincter lacerations and birth stresses can strain the pelvic muscles and ligaments. Investigators suggest that there is damage to the pudendal nerve, connective tissue, and muscle structure during delivery. Some of the damaged muscles and ligaments will never fully regain their strength and elasticity.

  ii. *Ageing and menopause:* The ageing process further weakens the pelvic muscles, and the natural reduction in estrogen at menopause also causes muscles to become less elastic.

  iii. *Increased intra-abdominal pressure:* Chronic coughing, from asthma, or bronchitis, or the straining associated with constipation, increases the risk of prolapse because it may eventually weaken the pelvic support structures.

  iv. *Large fibroids or tumors:* Women who have large fibroids or pelvic tumors are at an increased risk of prolapse.

  v. *Obesity:* Women who are severely overweight are at increased risk of prolapse.

  vi. *Heavy lifting:* Heavy lifting can also strain and damage pelvic muscles, and women in careers that involve regular manual labor or lifting, such as nursing, have an increased risk of prolapse.

  vii. *Previous pelvic surgery:* Poor attention to vaginal vault support at the time of vaginal or abdominal hysterectomy leads to vault prolapse in approximately 1% cases. Pelvic surgery, for example, bladder repair procedures, may damage nerves and tissues in the pelvic area increasing the risk of prolapse.

  viii. *Spinal cord injury and other muscular atrophy conditions:* Spinal cord injury and conditions such as muscular dystrophy and multiple sclerosis increase the risk of prolapse. If the pelvic muscles are paralyzed or movement is restricted, the muscles weaken and cannot support the pelvic organs.

Supports of Pelvic Organs

Pelvic organs are maintained in positions by various factors. The most important of these are:

a. The pelvic diaphragm including the levator ani muscles and the pevic fascia lining these muscles.

Table 27.2: Risk factors associated with prolapse			
Predisposing factors	*Inciting factors*	*Promoting factors*	*Decompensating factors*
Race	Vaginal delivery	Physical exertion	Aging
Anatomy		Chronic cough	Menopause
Morphology		Constipation	Concomitant disease
Histology		Obesity	
Familial genetics		Pelvic surgery	

Fact sheet 1

Uterine prolapse was first recorded on the Kahun papyri (ancient Egyptian text discussing mathematical and medical topics) in about 2000 BC. The first vaginal hysterectomy for the cure of uterine prolapse was self-performed by a peasant woman named Faith Raworth, as described by Willouby in 1670. She was so debilitated by uterine prolapse that she pulled down on the cervix and slashed off the prolapse with a sharp knife. She survived the hemorrhage and continued to live the rest of her life debilitated by urinary incontinence.

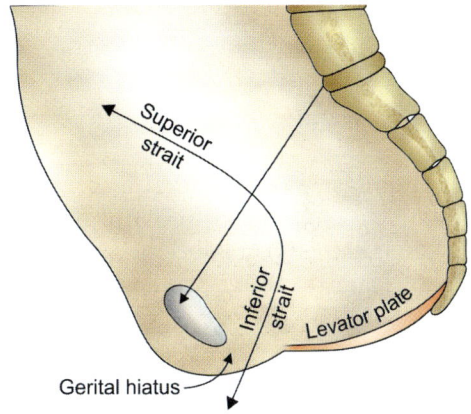

Fig. 27.6: Direction of pelvic axis in erect posture

b. Endopelvic connective tissue and some ligaments.

c. The urogernital diaphragm and the perineal body. These structures normally support the pelvic viscera despite great increments in intra-abdominal pressure that occur with straining, coughing, and heavy lifting when the patient is in the erect position.

Anatomical Consideration

Bony pelvis—In the erect posture, the plane of the pelvic inlet is slanted approximately 50° from the horizontal (Fig. 27.6). As a result, the uterus in normal anteversion is directed toward the sacrum and coccyx by any increase in intra-abdominal pressure.

The Pelvic Diaphragm

The muscles of the pelvic diaphragm primarily provide pelvic support (Fig. 27.7). These muscles form a basin or covering of the pelvic outlet and are often grouped together as the levator ani or levator sling The pelvic diaphragm, or levator ani muscles, consists

of the ischiococcygeal, iliococcygeal, and puborectalis muscles. The urogenital hiatus is the oval opening between the levator crura, through which pass the vagina and urethra, is a site of potential weakness. The urogenital hiatus has the potential to large enough to allow childbirth. This large central opening in the muscular pelvic floor explains why prolapse is such a significant problem. The most medial portion of the pelvic diaphragm is formed by the puborectalis, the muscular boundary of the urogenital hiatus. The levator ani muscle is tonically contracted, providing a firm shelf posteriorly to support the pelvic contents and aiding with urinary and fecal continence. Attenuation of the pubococcygeal and puborectal portions of the levator muscles, whether as the result of a traumatic delivery or of involutional changes, widens the levator gap and converts this potential weakness to an actual defect. If there has been a concomitant injury or attenuation of the

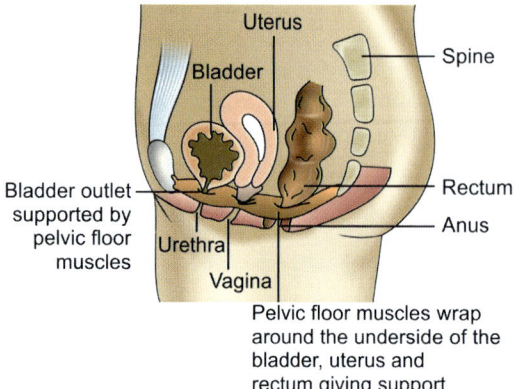

Fig. 27.7: Side view of pelvic organs and their support

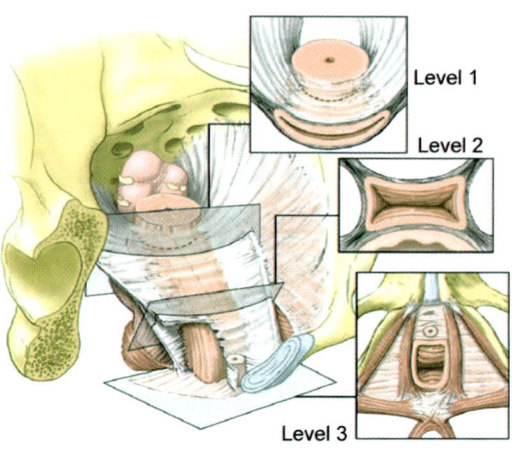

Fig. 27.8: Delancey's three levels of pelvic support—Top most inset Level 1, Middle inset Level 2, Lower most inset Level 3 (for description *see* text)

endopelvic fascia (uterosacral and cardinal ligaments, rectovaginal and pubocervical fascia), heightened intra-abdominal pressure gradually leads to uterine prolapse along with anterior vaginal prolapse, rectocele, and enterocele.

Thus two mechanical principles explain how the pelvic floor prevents prolapse. First, the uterus and vagina are attached to the walls of the pelvis by a series of ligaments and fascial structures that suspend the organs from the pelvic sidewalls. Second, the levator ani muscles constrict the lumina of these organs, forming an occlusive layer on which the pelvic organs may rest. It is a combination of these two factors "suspension of the genital tract by the ligaments and fasciae and closure of the pelvic floor by the levator ani" that holds the vagina over the levator ani muscles and forms a flap-valve closure. This flap-valve mechanism is instrumental in keeping the posterior cul-de-sac closed and preventing the development of an enterocele.

Endopelvic Connective Tissue

Endopelvic fascia is a loose network of connective tissue, small vessels, lymphatics, and nerves, which surrounds and supports the pelvic organs and the vagina. Thickenings of the endopelvic fascia are known as ligaments (e.g., the uterosacral and cardinal ligaments, rectovaginal and vesicovaginal

fascia). The vagina is attached at three levels (Fig. 27.8).

Level 1: The apex of vagina is supported by the cardinal and uterosacral ligaments. Uterine prolapse occurs when the cardinal-uterosacral ligament complex breaks or is attenuated.

Level 2: The arcus tendineous fascia pelvis and the fascia overlying the levator ani muscles provide support to the middle part of the vagina.

Level 3: The urogenital diaphragm and the perineal body provide support to the lower part of the vagina.

Normal vaginal attachments help to keep the pelvic organs (i.e., the uterus, bladder, and rectum) in place.

The Perineal Membrane (Urogenital Diaphragm)

The perineal membrane, a fibromuscular triangular plate lying between the pubic rami, extends posteriorly to the anterior rectal wall. It lies inferior to the levator ani muscles and closes the genital hiatus. With the exception of the deep transverse perineal muscles, the urogenital diaphragm contains few muscle fibers. The diaphragm is most susceptible to injury at the point at which it is traversed by the vaginal canal. Because it is composed mostly of fibrous connective tissue, it cannot accommodate well to the distention and dilation that occur during delivery. The levator muscles that surround the genital hiatus are exposed to the same stress but, if intact, can resume normal position and dimensions within a short time. As a result of childbirth, a transient widening of the genital hiatus occurs, while damage to the perineal membrane is more permanent.

Clinical Presentation

Patients are usually elderly (40 years or more) and multi-parous. There may be presence of other risk factors. Mild cases of uterine prolapse may have no obvious symptoms. If symptoms are present, they are less bothersome in the morning but worsen as the day goes on. Symptoms are often related to the site and type of prolapse.

Symptoms Common to all Types of POP

- A feeling of something coming out of vagina
- Heaviness or pressure in the pelvis

Urinary Symptoms in Anterior Vaginal Wall Prolapse (Cystocele, Urethrocele)

- Difficulty with urination, including involuntary loss of urine(incontinence), or urinary frequency or urgency
- Poor or prolonged urinary stream
- Feeling of incomplete emptying
- Manual reduction to start or complete emptying
- Positional changes to start or complete emptying
- Recurrent urinary tract infections (UTIs)

Bowel Symptoms in Posterior Vaginal Wall Prolapse (rectocele)

- Difficulty in defecation
- Incontinence of flatus, liquid stool, or solid stool

- Urgency of defecation
- Digitation or splinting of vagina, perineum, or anus to complete defecation
- Feeling of incomplete evacuation
- Rectal protrusion during or after defecation (rectal prolapse)

Sexual Symptoms

- Inability to have or infrequent coitus
- Dyspareunia
- Lack of satisfaction or orgasm
- Incontinence during sexual activity

Other Local Symptoms

- Pain in perineum
- Low back pain, which is eased with lying down
- Abdominal pressure or pain
- Blood stained and unusual or excessive discharge from the vagina

Physical Examination

Physical examination should be done with the patient resting and straining in both dorsal and standing positions, to define the extent of the prolapse and establish the segments of the vagina that are affected (anterior, posterior, or apical). Complete gynecological examination, including bimanual examination, is needed for estimating uterus size and cervical length. To determine the type and severity of prolapse, the clinician has two important points to consider:

- Examination must be made with the patient straining (cough or valsalva) forcefully enough that the prolapse is at its maximum.
- The examiner must examine each element of support independently.

Inspection of Perineum

Inspection of the vulva and perineum should focus on evaluation of vulvar architecture, the presence of decubitus ulceration or erosions or of other skin lesions. Inspection of the

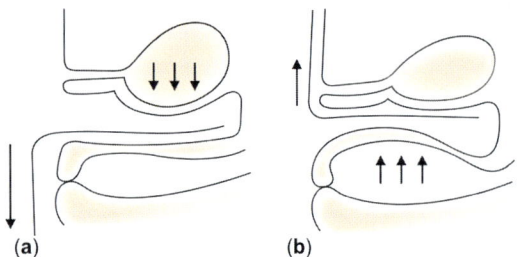

(a)   **(b)**

Figs 27.9a and b: Speculum examinations to demonstrate anterior and posterior vaginal wall prolapse (cystocele and rectocele)

vaginal orifice may reveal a relaxed and open genital hiatus with a thin-walled, rather smooth, bulging mass. Vaginal rugae are normally present. A loss of rugation denotes disruption of the connective tissue attachment below the epithelium. For evaluation for urinary incontinence, a stress test is performed at this initial portion of the examination. The patient should be asked to cough forcefully and any loss of urine noted.

Speculum Examination

A Cusco's speculum is placed in the vaginal vault to visually examine the vagina and cervix. Slowly pull back the speculum and ask the patient to cough or strain, and observe for descent of the cervix or vaginal vault. Vaginal support can then be assessed and the point of maximal protrusion should be noted in centimeters relative to the hymen and recorded. In posthysterectomy patients, the cuff can often be visualized by the presence of "dimples" in the vaginal epithelium at the apex.

The anterior and posterior walls should be examined separately by retracting the opposite wall with the Sim's posterior vaginal speculum (Figs 27.9a and b). For evaluation of the anterior wall compress the posterior wall and have the patient strain. For evaluation of the posterior wall, elevate the anterior wall and have the patient strain. Note the point of maximal descent of the anterior, posterior, and apical walls in relation to the ischial spines and hymen.

Per Vaginal Examination

Place 2 fingers into the vagina such that each finger opposes the ipsilateral vaginal wall, and ask the patient to bear down. After evaluating the lateral vaginal support system, assess the apex (cervix and apical vagina). Next, grade the strength and quality of pelvic floor contraction, asking the patient to tighten the levators around the examining finger. Assess the external genitalia, noting estrogen status, diameter of the introitus, and length of perineal body. Perform a careful bimanual examination and note uterine size, mobility, and adnexa. Decubitus ulcers, if any, are also palpated.

Per Rectal Examination

During rectal examination, assess the external sphincter tone and check for the presence of rectocele or enterocele.

Rectovaginal Examination

During rectovaginal examination, one can evaluate for the presence of concurrent enterocele in addition to a rectocele. The septal defect may involve only the lower third of the posterior vaginal wall, but it often happens that the entire length of the rectovaginal septum is thinned out. The finger in the rectum confirms sacculation into the vagina. A deep pocket into the perineal body may be noted, so that on apposition of the finger in the rectum and the thumb on the outside, the perineal body seems to consist of nothing but skin and rectal wall.

Clinical pearl: Uterine prolapse can occur at the same time as prolapse of the anterior or posterior vaginal compartments

Differentiation Between Rectocele and Enterocele

i. Anatomically, an enterocele extends from the apex of the vagina downward up to upper one-third of posterior vaginal wall, whereas a rectocele typically begins in the middle one-third of the vagina. So, during speculum examination of posterior vaginal wall, slowly pull back the instrument while the patient coughs or strains—bulging of the upper posterior vaginal wall is suggestive of an enterocoele, while bulging lower down is more supportive of a rectocoele.

ii. An enterocele sometimes is evident as a bulge that overrides the more caudal rectocele. Careful inspection of the posterior vaginal wall with a speculum retracting the anterior wall sometimes can suggest that an enterocele is present.

iii. A rectocoele is best diagnosed by a finger in the rectum, demonstrating the defect, as the finger can not reach enterocele. However, the key to detecting an enterocele lies in palpating the small bowel between the vagina and rectum during rectovaginal examination, with the patient straining so that the prolapse is protruding. To do this, a clinician's index finger is placed in the rectum and thumb on the posterior vaginal wall. Small bowel may be palpated between the rectum and vagina, confirming enterocele.

Stages of Pelvic Organ Prolapse

Simultaneous with the demonstration of prolapse at clinical examination, the prolapse is staged, expressing the degree of prolapse. The recommended staging system is the Pelvic Organ Prolapse Quantification (POPQ) system. It is a complicated but an accurate and reproducible system. A summarized version is mentioned here which is easy to apply in clinical practice: Alternately, Baden-Walker system can also be used.

Table 27.3: Critical points of physical examination in women with pelvic organ prolapse

- Vulvovaginal inspection
- Measurement of extent of prolapse in relation to hymen
  - Anterior vagina and urethra
  - Cervix or vaginal apex
  - Posterior vagina and perineum
- Measurement of genital hiatus, perineal body and vaginal length
- Assessment of pelvic muscle and anal sphincter tone

Pelvic Organ Prolapse Quantification (POP Q) Exam System

Stages are based on the maximal extent of prolapse relative to the hymen, in one or more compartment for complete staging.

- *Stage 0:* No prolapse
- *Stage I:* The most distal prolapse is > 1 cm above the level of the hymen
- *Stage II:* The most distal prolapse is between 1 cm above and 1 cm below the hymen (i.e., at the hymen)
- *Stage III:* The most distal prolapse is >1 cm below the hymen but no further than 2 cm less than the total vaginal length.
- *Stage IV:* Represents procidentia/total prolapse.

Baden Walker System

Stages are based only on the most protruding part relative to the hymen.

- *Grade 0:* Normal position for each respective site
- *Grade 1:* Descent halfway to the hymen
- *Grade 2:* Descent to the hymen
- *Grade 3:* Descent halfway past the hymen
- *Grade 4:* Maximum possible descent for each site.

Differential Diagnosis

Differential diagnosis for uterovaginal prolapse is shown in Table 27.4.

Table 27.4: Differential diagnosis of uterovaginal prolapse

Condition	Differentiating symptoms	Differentiating signs/tests
Cervical elongation	• Physical examination is essential for differentiation • Women with pelvic organ prolapse (POP) demonstrate greater descending of the cervix and the vaginal wall when straining	• Vaginal speculum and bimanual examination are the most reliable tests for differentiating between POP and cervical elongation • Vaginal part of cervix is elongated lying below the level of ischial spine • Vaginal fornices are deep and narrow. • Bimanual examination reveals normal size and position of body of uterus
Vaginal cyst (Gartner duct cyst)	• Often asymptomatic • May present with a soft lump in the vaginal wall or protrusion of a lump from the vagina • Superficial dyspareunia may be experienced	• Diagnosis is usually clinical • Well defined, nonreducible cystic lump on anterior or anterolateral vaginal wall • Vaginal mucosa overlying lump is tense with loss of rugosities • Female metal catheter introduced through urethra fails to come underneath the lump. • Vaginal ultrasound is not mandatory but useful to identify the content of the cyst and its topographical relation with adjacent anatomical structure
Uterine polyp	• Often presents with menstrual abnormality such as menorrhagia, metrorrhagia and dysmenorrhoea	• Polypoid mass coming out of introitus without any visible opening on leading part • Bimanual examination reveals pedicle coming out through cervical canal or arising from cervix.

Complications of pelvic organ prolapse: A long standing pelvic organ prolapse may lead to:

 i. Hydonephrosis, hydroureter, renal failure
 ii. Decubitous ulcer that seldom develops carcinoma
 iii. Chronic retention of urine and cystitis

Investigations

If the patient has concomitant incontinence, which is common in advanced POP, assessment of the postvoid residual urine (PVR) volume is a critical evaluation to exclude other causes of urinary retention.

Urinalysis is also useful, as infection is known to exacerbate incontinence symptoms.

Prevention of Pelvic Organ Prolapse

■ The preventive role of obstetric risk factors is unclear-reduced duration of the second stage of labour, decreased use of instrumental deliveries, and episiotomies may help prevent prolapse in the long term.

■ Treatment of conditions that increase intra-abdominal pressure such as constipation, obstructive airway disease, chronic cough, and obesity are primary and secondary prevention strategies

- The role of hormone replacement therapy in preventing prolapse is uncertain
- Pelvic floor exercises after childbirth may help to prevent prolapse in future

Concomitant procedures at the time of hysterectomy, such as closure of the pouch of Douglas with a Moschcowitz's procedure or uterosacral plication, may reduce the incidence of prolapse.

Treatment Approach

The mainstay of treatment is surgery; some women may be managed conservatively.

Clinical pearl: Although prolapse can occur in the anterior, middle, or posterior compartments, the pelvic floor should be considered as a single unit in the treatment of prolapse.

Asymptomatic Patients

Asymptomatic patients or women who have few minor symptoms may have little or no concern as a result of the disorder. Observation or watchful waiting is appropriate. Pelvic floor muscle rehabilitation may be offered despite the lack of data supporting its use to prevent progression.

Conservative Management in Symptomatic Patients

Conservative treatment is indicated for stages I and II prolapse, or more advanced prolapse where surgery is contraindicated for some reason or patient do not want surgery. It consists of the following:

i. Observation

Prolapse is not necessarily a progressive condition. It may progress to a point and then remain stable. Rarely, it may even regress.

Since prolapse is a completely benign condition, it is advisable to wait and follow the patient for 6 months or a year when the indication for surgery is not clear. The patient must be completely convinced of the need for surgery before it is attempted.

ii. Treatment of Symptoms

This approach focuses on the patient's complaints and needs. Examples include vaginal estrogen treatment for improving the quality of the vaginal epithelium (especially in the presence of vaginal ulceration, also known as decubitus ulcer), laxatives and stool softeners together with a healthy diet and exercises for constipation or mild obstructive defecation, and digital reduction of a cystocoele during voiding for complete emptying of the bladder.

iii. Pelvic Floor Exercises

In some patients, improvement of pressure symptoms and of urinary control may be obtained by using pelvic floor muscle exercises, also referred to as Kegel exercises. These exercises are aimed to tighten and strengthen the pubococcygeus muscles. Evidence strongly supports use of Kegel exercises as first-line management in the treatment of urinary and fecal incontinence; however, they may also have some benefit in the relief of POP symptoms. These measures improve the tone and contractility of the pelvic floor muscles, but are unable to improve damaged connective tissue and nerves.

iv. Pessary

A pessary is a rubber or plastic device that fits around or under the cervix, helping to support the uterus and hold it in place (Fig. 27.10). Pessaries are available in a variety of sizes and shapes to suit different patients and are of two main types: support pessaries, and space occupying pessaries. However, a ring pessary is most commonly used (Fig. 27.10). It consists of a ring about 6–7 cm in diameter and is placed obliquely into the vagina where it takes on a horizontal position. Pessaries are held in place by the posterior aspect of the pubic bone and sacrum and prolapse is reduced by lateral stretching with elevation of the vaginal sidewalls. The main indications are:

i. Elderly patients with severe prolapse, unfit for surgery. Typically, it is the woman in a wheelchair.

ii. Women with symptomatic pelvic organ prolapse (POP) who decline surgery

iii. Who need temporary relief of pregnancy-related prolapse or incontinence.

iv. Women who may yet bear children.

Fitting and Managing Pessaries

Patients must be evaluated carefully before pessary placement. All treatment options should be discussed, and the patient should be an active participant in the treatment decision.

Clinicians do a bimanual examination and use the forefinger to measure the distance between the posterior vaginal fornix and external urethral orifice. The measurement of the pessary would be given after deducting 1.5 cm from the former measurement Sometimes trial and error may be the only way to determine which size of pessary should be used, and clinicians should keep a variety of sizes. The largest size that can be comfortably accommodated should be tried (Table 27.5).

After placement of pessary a trial of standing, sitting, walking, and toilet use is done to ensure comfort and correct placement. The patient should also void to be sure that the urethra is not blocked. The most common complications include spontaneous expulsion, irritation of the vaginal wall, ulceration, bleeding, pain, and odor. She should be advised to return in a month's time for a check, but cautioned that if she experiences pain or

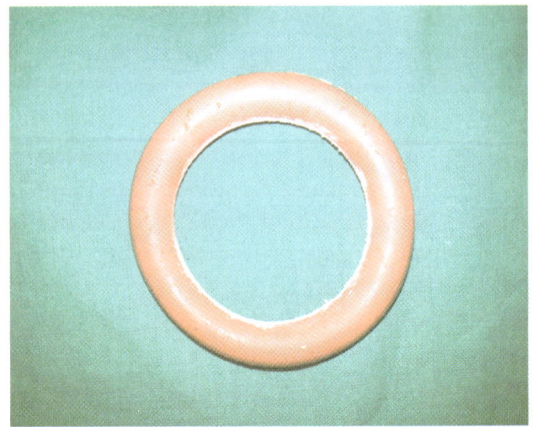

Fig. 27.10: Rubber ring pessary

difficulty in voiding she should return earlier. If there are no adverse symptoms, the pessary can be changed every 9–12 months.

Pessaries work particularly well if the uterus is still intact and no previous surgery for prolapse was performed. Patients are subsequently seen every 3 months, mainly for ruling out vaginal infection or ulceration. When adequate follow up cannot be assured a pessary should not be used, as neglected pessaries can become impacted within the vagina and, rarely, ulcerate into the bladder or bowel.

Fact sheet 2

Although evidence to support the use of pessaries is not strong, they are used by 86% of gynecologists and 98% of urogynecologists in USA.

Surgery

Surgery is indicated under two conditions:

- Stages III and IV prolapse, irrespective of being symptomatic or not

---

Table 27.5: Keypoints for fitting pessaries

- Ensure that the patient's bladder and bowel are empty
- Depress the perineum and posterior vaginal wall with left index finger
- Introduce the pessary being lubricated vertically inside vagina and then rotate to place it properly
- The pessary fits well if a finger can be swept between the pessary and the walls of the vagina
- The goal is to fit the largest pessary that does not cause discomfort

- Stage II prolapse with symptoms where surgery will effectively relieve these symptoms.

General Surgical Principles

- The aims of surgical correction of prolapse are relief of symptoms, restoration of normal vaginal anatomy, and preservation of coitus and urinary and anal continence. Injury after childbirth usually involves all the pelvic floor and pelvic organ supports, although sometimes only one organ may prolapse. When more than one compartment is involved, a combination of procedures is needed. Surgery usually involves a combination of repairs of the anterior vagina, vaginal apex, posterior vagina, and perineum; concomitant surgery may be planned for the bladder neck or anal sphincters.
- Approaches to prolapse surgery include vaginal, abdominal, and laparoscopic routes or a combination of approaches.
- For posterior vaginal prolapse surgery, a transvaginal approach is used. Apical and anterior vaginal prolapse can be approached by either vaginal or abdominal routes.
- Vaginal approach is better than the abdominal approach (i.e., laparotomy), from the perspective of complications and short-term effects on recovery.
- Surgical route is chosen based on the type and severity of prolapse, the surgeon's training and experience, the patient's preference, and the expected or desired surgical outcome.
- The type of surgery is individualized according to type and severity of prolapse, lifestyle, concomitant disease, and age. The first decision is based on whether the patient would like to preserve fertility. Most experts prefer to defer POP surgery until childbearing is complete.
- Procedures for prolapse can be broadly categorized into 3 groups:

1. Restorative, which use the patient's endogenous support structures
2. Compensatory, which attempt to replace deficient support with some type of graft, including synthetic, allogenic, or autologous materials; and
3. Obliterative, which close the vagina.

Surgical Management of Anterior Vaginal Wall Prolapse

i. *Anterior Colporrhaphy*

This operation rectifies a cystourethrocele. In anterior colporrhaphy (anterior repair) the vaginal epithelium is dissected from the underlying fibromuscular connective tissue and bladder, then plicating the vaginal muscularis across the midline. Excess vaginal epithelium is excised and the wound closed.

ii. *Paravaginal Repair*

Paravaginal repair is performed for anterior vaginal prolapse that is confirmed to be a result of detachment of the pubocervical fascia from its lateral attachment at the arcus tendineus fascia pelvis (white line). This defect can be unilateral or bilateral. The surgery can be performed either abdominally or vaginally. Both require identification of the white line and placement of serial sutures from the medial portion of the pubocervical fascia to the lateral sidewall at the level of the white line as it runs from the ischial spine over the obturator internus muscle to the posterior and inferior aspect of the pubic bone on the ipsilateral side.

Surgical Management of Posterior Vaginal Prolapse

Posterior vaginal wall prolapse due to rectocele or relaxed perineum are repaired by colpoperineorrhaphy or perineorrhaphy.

- Colpoperineorrhaphy involves posterior midline incision. The vaginal epithelium is separated off the underlying fibromuscular layer and endopelvic fascia. Repair often includes plication of the levator ani muscles and bulk lateral plication of tissue oversewing the rectovaginal fascia.

Perineum: The perineum provides distal support to the posterior vaginal wall and anterior rectal wall and anchors these structures to the pelvic floor. A disrupted perineal body will allow descent of the distal vagina and rectum and will contribute to a widened levator hiatus.

- Perineorrhaphy is often done in conjunction with posterior repair to recreate normal anatomy. During surgery, the perineum is rebuilt through midline plication of the perineal muscles and connective tissue. Overly aggressive plication can narrow the introitus, create a posterior vaginal wall ridge, and lead to entry dyspareunia. However, in a woman who is not sexually active, high perineorrhaphy with intentional introital narrowing is believed to decrease the risk of posterior wall prolapse recurrence.

Surgical Management of Apical Vaginal Prolapse

Apical vaginal prolapse includes uterine prolapse with or without enterocele and vaginal vault prolapse, typically with enterocele.

- Any degree of uterine prolapse in elderly women—The standard treatment for symptomatic uterine prolapse is vaginal hysterectomy with procedure(s) to suspend the vaginal apex, anterior colporrhaphy and colpoperineorrhaphy, repair of enterocele when indicated (Ward-Mayo's operation), and perform antiincontinence procedures as needed.
- Uterine prolapse in young women— Fothergill's operation is performed for preservation of uterus in symptomatic uterovaginal prolapse.

Principles of this operation include:
- Cervical dilatation and curettage

- Amputation of cervix with reconstruction of new cervical os with vaginal flaps.
- To shorten and fix (plication) Mackenrodt ligaments to the front of the cervix, so that uterus is elevated and anteverted.
- Anterior colporrhaphy to restore the bladder supports
- Colpoperineorrhaphy to rebuilt the perineum
- To repair the enterocele, if there is any.

Repair of Apical Defects

Repair of apical defects may be performed transvaginally or transabdominally, with laparotomy or laparoscopy.

There is a growing appreciation that support of the vaginal apex provides the cornerstone for a successful prolapse repair.

Transvaginal Repairs

- *Sacrospinous ligament fixation:* In this procedure vaginal apex is attached with the sacrospinous ligament, the tendinous component of the coccygeus muscle. Initially described as a unilateral procedure, later series reported bilateral fixation.
- Iliococcygeal vaginal suspension. Iliococcygeal vaginal suspension involves attachment of the vaginal apex to the iliococcygeus muscle and fascia, usually bilaterally.
- Uterosacral ligament suspension. Originally described by McCall in 1938, surgical variations of the uterosacral ligament suspension can be used prophylactically at hysterectomy or therapeutically for vaginal apical suspension.

Abdominal Repairs

Abdominal Sacral Colpopexy (Laparoscopy / Lapaotomy). Abdominal sacral colpopexy uses graft material attached to the anterior and posterior vaginal apex and suspended to the anterior longitudinal ligament of the sacrum for repair of apical prolapse.

Enterocele repair: Enterocele repair can be performed by vaginal, abdominal, or laparoscopic route. The enterocele is repaired by sharply dissecting the peritoneal sac from the rectum and bladder. A purse-string suture can be used to close the peritoneum as high (cephalad) as possible. The redundant peritoneum is excised. In addition to closing the enterocele sac, approximation of the anterior to the posterior fibromuscular connective tissue of the vagina is also done. Suspension of the vaginal apex is almost always necessary, except in rare cases when the enterocele occurs in the presence of adequate apical support.

Clinical peal: Surgical treatment for pelvic organ prolapse should incorporate procedures to prevent recurrence.

Other Procedures

Vaginal Obliterative Procedures

  i. Partial (Le Fort) colpocleisis
  ii. Total colpocleisis, these operations are indicated for patients who are not able to tolerate general anesthesia or long surgical procedures, and who are not contemplating sexual activity.

With the Le Fort colpocleisis, a rectangular portion of anterior and posterior vaginal mucosa is removed. The anterior pubocervical septum is sutured to the posterior rectovaginal septum using Lembert inverting sutures and, as the approximation is continued progressively on each side, the most dependent portion of the prolapse is gradually inverted. A perineorrhaphy is also usually performed to support the inverted vagina and help prevent pelvic organ prolapse recurrence.

Operations for Nulliparous Uterovaginal Prolapse

Cervicopexy or sling operation (Purandare's operation) is performed in congenital or nulliparous prolapse. The operation is performed through abdominal route. Two fascial strips of rectus sheath are passed extra-peritoneally and are stitched in front of cervix so that cervix is pulled up.

Mesh

Mesh has revolutionized prolapse surgery. Newer techniques for pelvic organ prolapse repair include complete vaginal mesh kits that consist of synthetic mesh placed using small incisions with minimal dissection. More refined meshes have resulted in improved results and this process of development is continuing. The classification of mesh is as follows:

a. Biological mesh (natural tissue)
b. Synthetic mesh:
   Type 1: Macroporous (containing pores > 75 μ in diameter)
   Type 2: Microporous (< 10 μ)
   Type 3: Macro-microporous (multifilament)
   Type 4: Submicronic pores (no visible pores)

Currently, type 1 monofilament synthetic mesh is commonly in use. It remains in situ permanently as it is insoluble. Generally, it delivers excellent results, but may cause the following problems:

Mesh erosion: The mesh erodes through the vaginal epithelium, appearing visibly on the surface. It may be accompanied by a discharge, bleeding or pain. The incidence is 5–15%, but in > 90% of cases the exposed mesh can easily be excised in the consulting room.

Infection, rejection and expulsion: when mesh becomes infected, the body sequestrates it by forming a fibrotic tunnel in which the mesh lies. A sinus forms into the vagina through which pus drains.

Excessive fibrosis and pain: Rarely, excessive fibrosis may cause stenosis of the vagina with pain, including dyspareunia. This is a difficult problem to treat.

The latest development in mesh technology is the production of more affordable biological

Table 27.6: Operations for pelvic organ prolapse

Compartment	Vaginal route	Abdominal route (laparotomy/laparoscopy)
Anterior	Anterior colporrhaphy (with or withot mesh) Paravaginal repair	Paravaginal repair
Middle	Vaginal hysterectomy Vault (enterocele) repair Uterosacral ligament suspension Sacrospinous fixation Ileococcygeous fixation	Sacrocolpopexy, sacrohysteropexy, sling operation
Posterior	Colpoperineorrhaphy with or withou mesh	Mesh interposition, sacrocolpopexy with mesh interposition

mesh. These meshes are much better tolerated with equally good results for the correction of prolapse. In the future, this type of mesh might completely replace synthetic mesh.

Suspensory

i. Anterior sacrospinous fixation with variations such as Anterior Prolift®

ii. Posterior sacrospinous fixation with variations such as Posterior Prolift®

iii. Sacrocolpopexy (with mesh)

In (i), (ii) and (iii) mesh is placed either between the bladder and vagina, and/or between the rectum and vagina. The mesh is then suspended and fixed somewhere inside the pelvis (pulling up the prolapsed vagina).

Keywords

Arcus tendineus fascia pelvis or white line: A thickening of the parietal fascia of the pelvic sidewall along a line between the ischial spine and pubic tubercle. Along this line, the pubocervical septum attaches to the pelvic sidewall.

POPQ system: Pelvic Organ Prolapse Quantification (POP-Q) system refers to an objective, site-specific system for describing, quantifying, and staging pelvic support in women. The hymen acts as the fixed point of reference throughout the POPQ system.

There are six defined points for measurement in the POPQ system (Fig. 27.11)—Aa, Ba, C, D, Ap, Bp and three others landmarks: gh, tvl, pb. Each is measured in centimeters above or proximal to the hymen (negative number) or below or distal to the hymen (positive number) with the plane of the hymen being defined as zero (0). The hymen was selected as the

reference point rather the introitus because it is more precisely identified.

The terminology avoids assigning a specific label, such as cystocele or rectocele, to the prolapsing part of the vagina, acknowledging that the actual organ(s) above the prolapse frequently cannot be determined by physical examination. There are three reference points anteriorly (Aa, Ba, and C) and three posteriorly (Ap, Bp, and D). Points Aa and Ap are 3 cm proximal to or above the hymenal ring anteriorly and posteriorly, respectively. Points Ba and Bp are defined as the lowest points of the prolapse between Aa anteriorly or Ap posteriorly and the vaginal apex. Anteriorly, the apex is point C (cervix), and posteriorly is point D (pouch of Douglas). In women after hysterectomy, point C is the vaginal cuff and point D is omitted. Three other measurements are taken: the vaginal length at rest, the

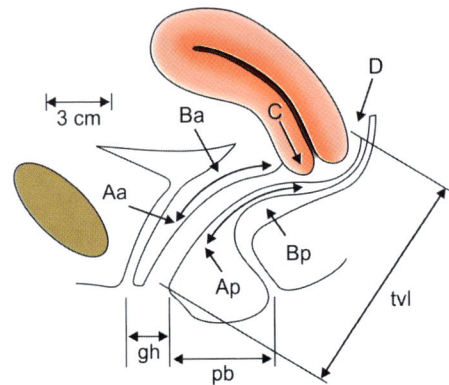

Fig. 27.11: Points and landmarks for POP-Q system examination. Aa, point A anterior, Ap, point A posterior, Ba, point B anterior; Bp, point B posterior; C, cervix or vaginal cuff; D, posterior fornix (if cervix is present); gh, genital hiatus; pb, perineal body; tvl, total vaginal length

genital hiatus (gh) from the middle of the urethral meatus to the posterior hymenal ring, and the perineal body (pb) from the posterior aspect of the genital hiatus to the midanal opening.

Gartner's duct cyst: A Gartner's duct cyst (sometimes incorrectly referred to as vaginal inclusion cyst) is a benign vaginal cystic lesion that arises from the vestigial remnant of a mesonephric duct or Gartner's duct.

EXERCISES

Answer the following questions

1. What is pelvic organ prolapse?
2. What are the common POP abnormalities? Describe each defect—Cystocele, urethrocele, rectocele, enterocele, relaxed perineum, vault prolapse.
3. What are the different degrees of uterine prolapse? What is procidentia?
4. What are the risk factors of POP?
5. How child birth is responsible for development of POP?
6. Defects in which pelvic floor muscles/ the supporting structures allow POP?
7. How does pelvic organ prolapse occur?
8. What is most common symptom of POP?
9. How does one evaluate pelvic organ prolapse?
10. How do you differentiate rectocele and enterocele?
11. Whar are the grading systems for pelvic organ prolapse?
12. How do you differentiate Gartner duct cyst and anterior vaginal prolapse/ cystocele?
13. How do you differentiate elongated cervix and uterine prolapse?
14. How do you differentiate fibroid polyp and uterine prolapse?
15. Name some measures that may be helpful to prevent POP.
16. What is the management of asymptomatic POP?
17. What is the traditional procedure for anterior vaginal wall prolapse (cystocele)? What dose it involve?
18. What are the different surgical options for treatment of apical prolapse?
19. What is the traditional procedure for posterior vaginal wall prolapse (rectocele)? What does it involve?
20. When is a hysterectomy warranted?

Write short notes on

1. Supports of pelvic organs
2. Pelvic organ prolapse quantification (POPQ) system
3. Conservative management of symptomatic POP

Explain or justify the following statement/s

1. Vaginal child birth is the main cause of pelvic organ prolapse.
2. Surgery for POP may be performed through vaginal, abdominal and laparoscopic routes

Fill in the blanks with appropriate word/s

1. Normally external os is at the level of _____ .
2. Following vaginal or abdominal hysterectomy _____ prolapse may occur.
3. Levator ani muscles, consists of the _____ , _____ , and _____ muscles.
4. _____ operation is performed for preservation of uterus in symptomatic uterovaginal prolapse in young parous women.
5. _____ operation is performed in congenital or nulliparous prolapse.

Questions for practical examination (Look at figure 27.10 before answering the following questions)

1. Identify the instrument.
2. What are the two main types of pessaries.
3. In which group iris pessary belongs?
4. How does it act?
5. What are their main indications of use?
6. How do you determine size of pessary for a particular woman?
7. How pessary should be fitted?

8. What are its complications?

9. How frequently pessary should be changed?

Questions for practical examination (read the case summary mentioned at the beginning of chapter before answering the following questions)

1. Identify the risk factors of POP that are present in this patient

2. Apart from the symptoms mentioned here, which other symptoms she might have?

3. What do you mean by stage III uterovaginal prolapse?

4. How do you demonstrate the findings of anterior vaginal wall prolapse?

5. How do you demonstrate findings of uterine prolapse?

6. Name the operation that should be performed in this patient.

7. How the support of vaginal apex is to be restored?

Bibliography

1. Blueprints of Obstetrics and Gynecology by Tamera L.

2. Cronje HS. Pelvic Organ Prolapse.

3. Cundiff GW, Weidner AC, Visco AG, Bump RC. Addison WA. A survey of pessary use by members of the American Urogynaecologic Society. Obstet Gynecol 2000;95:931–5.

4. Kuncharapu I, Majorini B, Johnson DW. Pelvic organ prolapse Am Fam Physician. 2010;81(9): 1111–1117, 1119–1120.

5. Office urogynecology—practical pathways in Obstetric and Gynecology 1st ed. New York (NY): McGraw-Hill; 2004.

6. Oshani A, Teo REC, Mayne C, et al. Uterine prolapse BMJ 2007;335:819–23.

7. Pelvic organ prolapse Current Obstetrics and gynecology, Mc Grew Hill.

8. Pelvic organ prolapse Williams Gynecology Mc Grew Hill 2008.

9. Porges R. Abnormalities of pelvic support Glob. libr. women's med.(ISSN: 1756-2228) 2008; DOI 10.3843/GLOWM.10056.

10. Porges RF, Porges JC, Blinick G. Mechanisms of uterine support and the pathogenesis of uterine prolapse. Obstet Gynecol 15:711, 1960

11. Srohbehn K, Richter HE. Operative management of pelvic organ prolapse Danforth Obstetrics and Gynecology Lippinkott Williams and Wilkins 19th edition 2008.

12. Thaker R, Stanton S. Management of genital prolapse BMJ 324 : 1258 doi: 10.1136/bmj.324. 7348.1258.

13. Uterovaginal prolapse Ash Monga Ed Gynecology by Ten Teachers 18 th edition.

14. Weber Am, Richter AH. Pelvic organ prolapse Obstet Gynecol Vol. 106, no. 3, September 2005.

28

Urinary Incontinence

A 45-year-old P 3+0 female presents at gynecology outdoor with 10 years history of urinary leakage with coughing or sneezing. Urine leakage began shortly after her third vaginal delivery and has gradually become more frequent. It also occurs during physical exertion and sexual intercourse. She is greatly embarrassed with her problem and limited her social activities as a result. A medical history and medication review are noncontributory. How do you approach this patient?

In this chapter we will learn:
- What is incontinence
- Different types of incontinence
- Causes of urinary incontinence in women
- Diagnosis of incontinence
- Investigations
- Treatment

Introduction

Urinary incontinence is defined as a condition of involuntary loss of urine that is objectively demonstrable and is a social or hygienic problem. The incidence of urinary incontinence in women is about 5–7% in 15–44 yrs age group and range between 8 and 12% after 45 yrs of age. It affects quality of life and leads to complications like urinary retention, lower urinary tract infection and vesicoureteral reflux leading to greater morbidity. It may be of two types:

1. *True incontinence:* This type of urinary incontinence occurs when there is continuos involuntary loss of urine as in urinary fistulae. These fistula may be congenital or acquired and depending upon the organ involved may be vesico-vaginal or ureterovaginal (*see* Chapter 29).

2. In false incontinence there is involuntary loss of urine only under certain conditions.

   a. *Stress incontinence*—When there is involuntary loss of urine (whether a few drops or in spurts) during coughing, sneezing or under condition of stress of increased intra-abdominal pressure. This is due to defective support of bladder neck or urethra (Fig. 28.1).

   b. *Urge incontinence*—In urge incontinence there is marked urgency to pass urine and before the woman can reach the toilet there is involuntary escape of urine.

This is more common than stress incontinence. The vesical sphincter is normal but there is trigonitis or cystitis.

c. *Detrusor instability (over active bladder, unstable bladder)*—This is a psycho-somatic or functional disorder often mistaken for stress incontinence. The bladder objectively contracts (spontaneously or on provocation) during the filling phase while the patient attempts to inhibit micturition. It may be due to hyperexcitability of detrusor muscle cells or a neuropathy involving the para-sympathetic innervation. The symptoms include urgency, urge incontinence, frequency, and stress incontinence. Detrusor instability can only be diagnosed by subtracted filling cystometry, although cystometry is not always necessary before treatment.

d. *Overflow incontinence:* In overflow incontinence the blader overfills with urine and is not able to release it. The patient typically has a large overdistended bladder but dribbles urine either continuously or with stress maneuvers like coughing or bearing down (Fig. 28.1). In this condition the detrusor muscle no longer contracts (usually due to local nerve injury) or there is a blockage preventing the urine from emptying (postoperative urinary retention).

e. Functional incontinence is urine loss due to cognitive or physical impairments (e.g. due to dementia or stroke) or environmental barriers that interfere with control of voiding. For example, the patient may not recognize the need to void, may not know where the toilet is, or may not be able to walk to a remotely located toilet. Neural pathways and urinary tract mechanisms that maintain continence may be normal.

f. Mixed incontinence is any combination of the above types. The most common combinations are urge with stress incontinence and urge or stress with functional incontinence.

Etiology

Urinary continence depends upon coordinated urethral sphincter relaxation and bladder contraction. Initiation of these processes is under the control of the parasympathetic nervous system, and is triggered by signals that originate from S2–S4 of the spinal cord and travel through the hypogastric nerves. Once stimulated, these nerve endings release the neurotransmitter acetylcholine, which in turn binds to muscarinic receptors located in

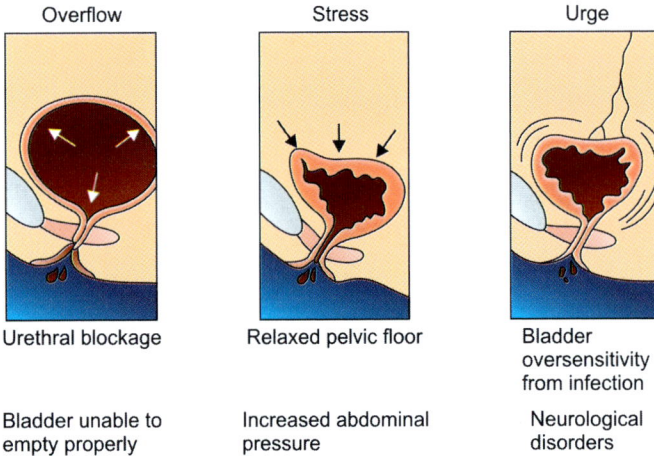

Overflow	Stress	Urge
Urethral blockage	Relaxed pelvic floor	Bladder oversensitivity from infection
Bladder unable to empty properly	Increased abdominal pressure	Neurological disorders

Fig. 28.1: Common types of urinary incontinence

the bladder. Contraction of smooth muscle of bladder, the detrusor muscle, occurs and results in urinary flow through relaxed urethra (Figs 28.2 and 28.3).

Inhibition of voiding is controlled by the pontine storage center, which receives afferent signals from the distended bladder. These signals are then mediated through a branch of the sympathetic nervous system that originates in T11-L2 of the spinal cord. These nerves release norepinephrine, which binds to beta receptors on the bladder wall and alpha receptors at the bladder neck and urethra. Binding of norepinephrine triggers smooth muscle relaxation at the level of the bladder, inhibiting detrusor contraction. Meanwhile, sympathetic stimulation at the alpha receptors causes muscle contraction. This coordinated event inhibits micturition (Fig. 28.3).

Thus voiding begins with relaxation of the urethra, followed by activation of the spinal reflex pathways. This reflex pathway is coordinated by the pons and parasympathetic transmissions to the bladder that initiate detrusor contraction. Whereas these same pathways act to inhibit sympathetic and pudendal outflow to the urethra, maintaining urethral relaxation. Detrusor contraction raises the intravesical pressure sufficiently to allow the bladder from emptying.

Urge incontinence is believed to be caused by any disruption to the well-coordinated process of micturition. Current theories propose either a neurogenic or a myogenic origin. A commonly used treatment regimen targets the muscarinic receptors of the bladder. By contrast, stress urinary incontinence tends to be caused by an

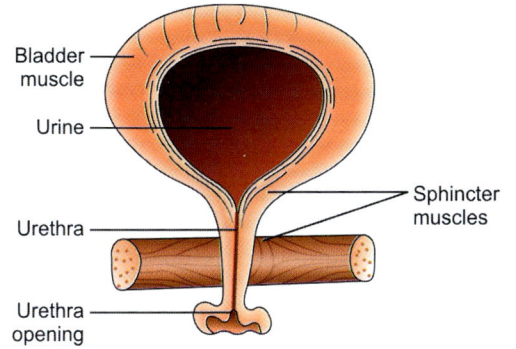

Fig. 28.2: Neurological innervations of urinary bladder

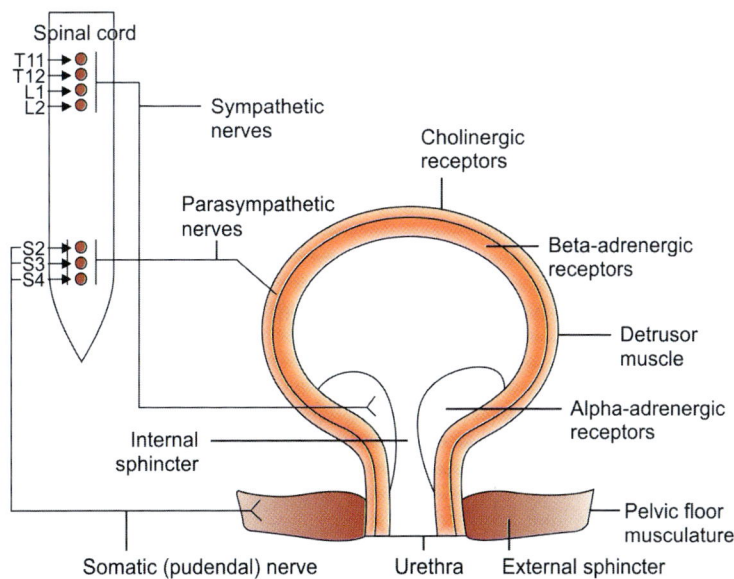

Fig. 28.3: Urinary bladder and sphincter muscles

anatomic abnormality, such as cystocele or urethral hypermobility. The support structures of the bladder and/or urethra may alter the system in such a way that urethral closure pressure is no longer maintained, or no longer exceeds intra-abdominal pressure during strenuous activity, which creates a pressure gradient favoring loss of urine, albeit involuntarily.

The disorder tends to differ among age groups. With aging, bladder capacity decreases, ability to inhibit urination declines, involuntary bladder contractions (detrusor overactivity) occur more often, and bladder contractility is impaired. Thus, voiding becomes more difficult to postpone and tends to be incomplete. Postvoid residual volume increases, probably to ≤ 100 mL (normal < 50 mL). Endopelvic fascia weakens. In post-menopausal women, decreased estrogen levels lead to atrophic urethritis and atrophic vaginitis and to decreasing urethral resistance, length, and maximum closure pressure. In younger patients, incontinence often begins suddenly, may cause little leakage, and usually resolves quickly with little or no treatment. Often, incontinence has one cause in younger patients but has several in the elderly.

Conceptually, categorization into reversible (transient incontinence) or established causes may be useful. However, causes and mechanisms often overlap and occur in combination.

Transient incontinence: There are several causes of transient incontinence. A useful mnemonic for many transient causes is DIAPPERS (with an extra P): Delirium, infection (commonly, symptomatic UTIs), atrophic urethritis and vaginitis, pharma-ceuticals (e.g. those with α-adrenergic, cholinergic, or anticholinergic properties; diuretics; sedatives), psychiatric disorders (especially depression), excess urine output (polyuria), restricted mobility, and stool impaction.

Diagnostic Approach

The aim of diagnosis is to identify the type of incontinence (i.e. stress, urge and mixed) and to rule out the presence of a complex or potentially life threatening underlying condition (e.g. spinal cord compression, multiple sclerosis). In most instances, urinary incontinence are diagnosed on the basis of history alone. The main complaint of the disorder is almost always confirmed by physical signs or clinical testing. However, most patients are embarrassed to mention incontinence and do not volunteer information about it. So women should therefore be screened with a question such as "Do you ever leak urine?"

Evaluation

- History
- *Examination:* Neurologic, pelvic, rectal
- *Testing:* Urinalysis, postvoid residual urine volume; sometimes urodynamic testing

History: History focuses on duration and patterns of voiding, bowel function, drug use, and obstetric and pelvic surgical history. Particular attention to the obstetric and gynecologic history is important to determine any predisposing risk factors. The obstetric risk factors include number of pregnancies, mode of delivery, history of assisted delivery and obstetric trauma.

Other factors and urinary symptoms that should be included are:

- Involuntary urine leakage on effort, exertion, sneezing, or coughing (suggestive of stress incontinence)
- Involuntary urine leakage accompanied by urgency (suggestive of urge incontinence)
- Fluid and caffeine intake
- History of chronic constipation
- Dysuria, hematuria or known history of recurrent urinary tract infection
- Frequency of urination
- Postvoid dribbling

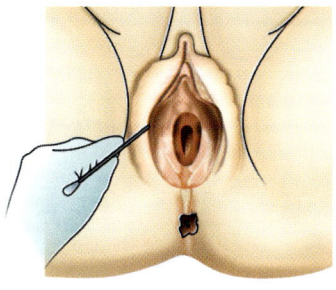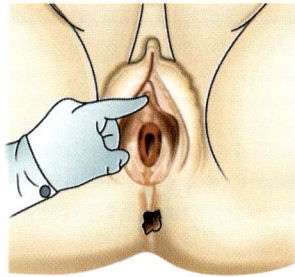

Fig. 28.4: (Left) Bulbocavernosus and (Right) clitoral sacral reflexes. Lightly tapping the clitoris or brushing the labia majora should produce a reflex contraction of the external anal sphincter muscle

- History of child hood enuresis
- Nocturia
- Fecal incontinence
- Family history of incontinence
- Mental state is also evaluated particularly in elderly women dementia, depression and other cognitive impairment may be linked with incontinence.
- History of smoking, alcoholism.
- History of back injury and fall
- Use of drugs such as antihistamines, antidepressants, and antipsychotics, calcium channel blockers and alfa adrenergic agonists
- Chronic medical conditions, such as chronic cough, multiple sclerosis, chronic heart failure, and diabetes mellitus.

Physical examination: Neurologic, pelvic, and rectal examinations are the focus.

Neurologic examination involves assessing mental status, gait, and lower extremity function and checking for signs of peripheral or autonomic neuropathy, including orthostatic hypotension. Neck and upper extremities should be checked for signs of cervical spondylosis or stenosis. The spinal column should be checked for evidence of prior surgeries and for deformities, dimples, or hair tufts suggesting neural tube defects.

Innervation of the external urethral sphincter, which shares the same sacral roots as the anal sphincter, can be tested by assessing (Fig. 28.4):

- Perineal sensation
- Voluntary anal sphincter contraction (S2 to S4)
- The anal wink reflex (S4 to S5), which is anal sphincter contraction triggered by lightly stroking perianal skin
- The bulbocavernosus reflex (S2 to S4), which is anal sphincter and labia majora contraction triggered by brushing the labia majora.

However, the absence of these reflexes is not necessarily pathologic.

Pelvic examination: Pale, thin vaginal mucosae with loss of rugae indicate atrophic vaginitis. Urethral hypermobility can be seen during coughing when the posterior vaginal wall is stabilized with a speculum. Presence of cystocele, an enterocele, a rectocele, or uterine prolapse suggests pelvic floor weakness. Pooling of urine in the vagina during examination may be due to the presence of any fistulous tract, particularly in patients who have undergone pelvic surgery or pelvic radiation. A bimanual examination also provides valuable information about the size and position of the pelvic organs. Mechanical compression of the bladder by an enlarged, bulky uterus may cause urinary urgency and frequency by constricting the bladder's ability to distend in already occupied pelvis.

Rectal examination can identify fecal impaction, rectal masses and sphincter tone.

If stress incontinence is suspected, urinary stress testing can be done on the examination table; it has a sensitivity and specificity of > 90%. The bladder must be full; a patient sits upright or close to upright with the legs spread, relaxes the perineal area, and coughs vigorously once. Immediate leakage that starts and stops with the cough confirms stress incontinence. Delayed or persistent leakage suggests detrusor over activity triggered by the cough. If cough triggers incontinence, the maneuver can be repeated while the examiner places 1 or 2 fingers inside the vagina to elevate the urethra (Marshall-Bonney test); incontinence that is corrected by this maneuver may respond to surgery. Results can be false-positive if patients have an abrupt urge to void during the test or false-negative if patients do not relax, the bladder is not full, the cough is not strong, or a large cystocele is present. In presence of large cystocele, the test should be repeated with the patient supine and the cystocele reduced, if possible.

Investigations: Urinalysis and postvoid residual urine estimation are initial tests to order. Urinalysis can help to identify underlying medical conditions that may contribute to urinary incontinence. For example, UTIs and glycosuria-induced polyuria, as seen in diabetes mellitus, can produce overactive bladder symptoms. Urine culture, blood urea nitrogen and serum creatinine estimation may be required in some women. Postvoid residual measurement assesses the volume of urine in the bladder after a void. It is measured by sterile catheterization or ultrasound with good accuracy, and can differentiate between adequate bladder emptying and urinary retention. Postvoid residual volume plus voided volume estimates total bladder capacity and helps to assess bladder proprioception. A post void residual urine volume < 50 mL is normal; < 100 mL is usually acceptable in patients > 65 but abnormal in younger patients; and > 100 mL may suggest detrusor underactivity or outlet obstruction.

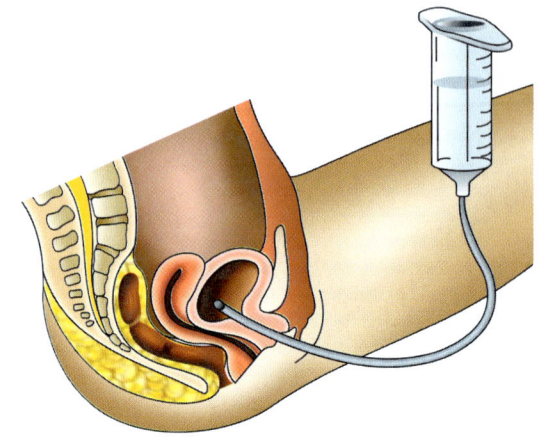

Fig. 28.5: Simple cystometry

After a history review, examination, and simple tests, most women with uncomplicated urinary incontinence can be given a preliminary diagnosis and have treatment initiated.

Urodynamic testing is indicated when clinical evaluation combined with the appropriate tests is not diagnostic or when abnormalities must be precisely characterized before surgery.

Cystometry measures bladder pressure during filling and can be undertaken by any clinician. Cystometry (Fig. 28.5) may help to diagnose urge incontinence, but sensitivity and specificity are unknown. Sterile water is introduced into the bladder in 50 mL increments using a 50 mL syringe and a 12- to 14-F urethral catheter until the patient experiences urgency or bladder contractions, detected by changes in fluid level in the syringe. If < 300 mL causes urgency or contractions, detrusor overactivity and urge incontinence are likely.

Additional testing: In cystometrography, pressure-volume curves (Fig. 28.6) and bladder sensation are recorded while the bladder is filled with sterile water; provocative testing (with bethanechol or ice water) is used to stimulate bladder contractions. Electromyography of perineal muscle is used to assess

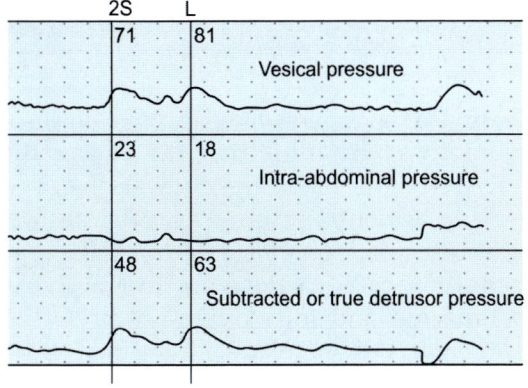

Fig. 28.6: Detrusor instability is demonstrated in multichannel cystometrogram

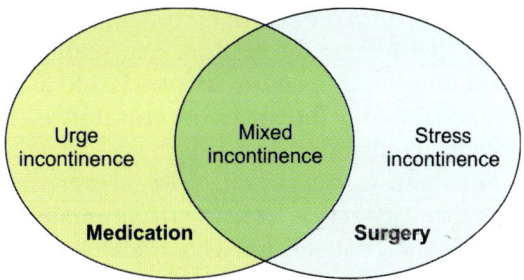

Fig. 28.7: Principle of treatment of incontinence

sphincter innervation and function. Urethral, abdominal, and rectal pressures may be measured. Pressure-flow video studies, usually done with voiding cystourethrography, can correlate bladder contraction, bladder neck competency, and detrusor-sphincter synergy, but equipment is not widely available. Urethral function could be assessed by electrophysiological studies, real-time ultrasonography, or MRI, and although we do not discuss these approaches in detail, they are often used in research settings.

Clinical pearl: In most cases, a preliminary diagnosis of urinary incontinence can be made and treatment initiated based on findings of the medical history, physical examination and simple laboratory testing.

Treatment

- Bladder training
- Kegel exercises
- Drugs
- Surgery

After obtaining a complete history and performing a physical examination, it is appropriate to initiate treatment without referral for specialized testing in most cases. Behavioral approaches and lifestyle changes are the preferred initial treatment for this condition. Reducing weight, and caffeine and fluid intake, can improve symptoms.

Improvement of pelvic muscle function and bladder retraining, where appropriate, can also help

For stress incontinence, pharmacotherapy and surgery can be considered in severe cases. For urge incontinence, additional treatment may include pharmacotherapy, neuromodulation, or onabotulinumtoxin A. For mixed incontinence, treatment should be determined by the predominant symptoms or according to urodynamic test results. That is, if symptoms primarily suggest stress incontinence (e.g., involuntary urine leakage on effort, exertion, sneezing, or coughing), or urodynamic testing reveals a diagnosis of stress incontinence, patients should be treated as for stress incontinence; if symptoms primarily suggest urge incontinence (e.g., involuntary urine leakage accompanied by or immediately preceded by urgency), or urodynamic testing reveals a diagnosis of detrusor overactivity, patients should be treated as for urge incontinence (Fig. 28.7).

General measures: Patients may benefit from bladder training (to change voiding habits) and changes in fluid intake. Bladder training usually involves timed voiding (every 2 to 3 h) while awake. Prompted voiding is used for cognitively impaired patients; they are asked about every 2 h whether they need to void or whether they are wet or dry. A voiding diary helps establish how often and when voiding is indicated and whether patients can sense a full bladder. Patients are instructed to limit fluid intake at certain times (e.g., before going out, 3 to 4 h before bedtime), to avoid fluids that irritate the bladder (e.g., caffeine-containing fluids), and to drink 1500 to 2000 mL of fluid a day (because concentrated urine irritates the bladder).

Pelvic muscle exercises (e.g., Kegel exercises) are often effective, especially for stress incontinence. Patients must contract the pelvic muscles (pubococcygeus and paravaginal) rather than the thigh, abdominal, or buttock muscles. The muscles are contracted for 10 sec, then relaxed for 10 sec 10 to 15 times tid. Re-instruction is often necessary. In women <75 yr, cure rate is 10 to 25%, and improvement occurs in an additional 40 to 50%, especially if patients are motivated; do the exercises as instructed; and receive written instructions, follow-up visits for encouragement, or both. Pelvic floor electrical stimulation is an automated version of Kegel exercises; it uses electrical current to inhibit detrusor overactivity and contract pelvic muscles. Advantages are improved compliance and contraction of the correct pelvic muscles, but benefits over behavioral changes alone are unclear.

Clinical pearl: All incontinent patients should be offered pelvic floor exercises because they supplement all forms of treatment and have no adverse side effects. Some patients benefit from a biofeedback session in order to correctly identify and contract appropriate muscle group.

Drugs

Pharmacologic Agents for Urge Incontinence

Pharmacologic agents may improve detrusor overactivity by inhibiting the contractile activity of the bladder. Medications used include anticholinergics, tricyclic antidepressants, and musculotropic drugs. For urge incontinence with detrusor overactivity, oxybutynin and tolterodine are preferred treatments. If these treatments are ineffective, solifenacin, trospium, darifenacin, fesoterodine, and propantheline may be used.

Pharmacologic Agents for Stress Incontinence

In stress incontinence caused by urethral sphincter insufficiency, the first-line pharmacologic therapy is pseudoephedrine, if there are no contraindications. This is also useful in patients who are considered a high surgical risk. Estrogen can be used as an adjunct in postmenopausal women with stress incontinence.

Imipramine is recommended if first line drugs have not been effective. Imipramine, tricyclic antidepressant, has both anticholinergic and alfa-adrenergic properties and is useful in treating both urge and stress urinary incontinence by suppressing bladder contraction and increasing urethral contracti-

Table 28.1: Common medications used to treat urinary incontinence	
Drug	Dosage
Stress Incontinence	
Pseudoephedrine	15 to 30 mg, three times daily
Vaginal estrogen cream	0.5 to 1 g, apply in vagina every night
Urge incontinence	
Oxybutynin ER	5 to 15 mg, every morning
Generic oxybutynin	2.5 to 10 mg, two to four times daily
Tolterodine	1 to 2 mg, two times daily
Imipramine	10 to 75 mg, every night
Dicyclomine	10 to 20 mg, four times daily
Hyoscyamine	0.375 mg, two times daily
Darifenacin	5–10 mg daily

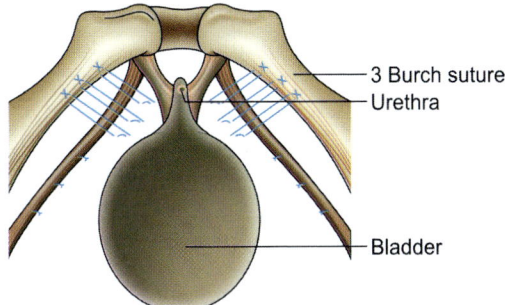

Fig. 28.8: Burch colpo suspension

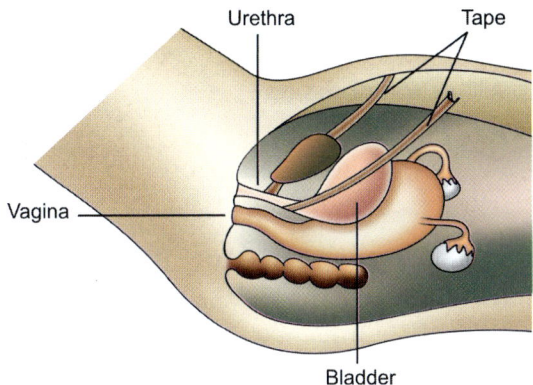

Fig. 28.9: A TVT in place supporting the urethra

lity. Duloxetine, has been widely studied and found to be effective. Local estrogen can be added if the patient is postmenopausal. Estrogen causes engorgement of the periurethral blood supply and subsequent thickening of the urethral mucosa.

Surgery

Surgical Treatment for Stress Incontinence

Recommended for stress incontinence. Surgery is indicated if conservative treatment fails or patient requests more definitive therapy. Retropubic urethropexies (i.e., Burch colposuspension and Marshall-Marchetti-Krantz [MMK] procedures) and suburethral slings have long-term success rates consistently reported in the 80 to 96 percent range and are clearly superior to other procedures (Fig. 28.8).

A new minimally invasive suburethral sling ["tension-free vaginal tape (TVT)"] has been shown to cause less postoperative morbidity than traditional surgeries while achieving long-term (five-year) cure rates greater than 86 percent (Fig. 28.9). The sling is placed during surgery under local anesthesia on an outpatient basis. While the tension-free vaginal tape sling is a nonabsorbable polypropylene mesh, and concern may exist regarding erosion and/or infection of this material; to date, few cases have been reported.

Periurethral bulking is used when stress incontinence exists in the absence of urethral hypermobility, as second-line therapy after failed anti-incontinence surgery, or in patients who are poor surgical candidates. Many consider glutaldehyde cross-linked bovine collagen the gold standard bulking agent. A collagen skin test is required prior to therapy. Autologous fat, usually harvested from the lower abdomen, has been shown to be comparable to placebo. It can be rapidly autolyzed, making it a less than durable option. Case reports of fatal fat emboli have been reported. Macroplastique is a silicone polymer that has shown very promising results, although long-term results are pending. Coaptite is calcium hydroxyapatite in a gel medium that can also be used.

Clinical pearl: Stress incontinence may be treated surgically but behavioral treatment (including pelvic floor exercise) is first line treatment.

Other Considerations

Neuromodulation is a newer treatment option that has been used in the management of overactive bladder (detrusor overactivity) refractory to pharmacotherapy. It can be delivered percutaneously to target the afferent input of the tibial nerve (Urgent PC), or via the sacral nerve directly.

Injection of onabotulinumtoxin A (formerly known as botulinum toxin type A) into the bladder wall has also been shown to be effective for detrusor overactivity. This may be considered as an alternative to neuromodulation if pharmacotherapy is unsuccessful.

Transurethral radiofrequency therapy is a nonsurgical in-office treatment for patients with stress urinary incontinence without intrinsic sphincter deficiency. It may be offered to the patient who cannot undergo surgery due to either physical or time constraints. Radiofrequency is used to denature and remodel collagen at the bladder neck, resulting in decreased elasticity and compliance, reducing exertion-related urine loss.

Keywords

Urinary incontinence: Any involuntary loss of urine.

Stress incontinence: Stress incontinence is losing urine during physical activity, such as coughing, sneezing, laughing, or exercise.

Urge incontinence: Urge incontinence is the strong, sudden need to urinate due to bladder spasms or contractions.

Cystometry: Cystometry is a test of bladder function in which pressure and volume of fluid in the bladder is measured during filling, storage, and voiding.

Urodynamic study: Urodynamics is the investigation of the function of the lower urinary tract with regard to bladder filling/storage and emptying. It measures bladder pressures, volumes, and flows.

Kegel exercise: An exercise devoloped by Dr. Arnold Kegel designed to strengthen the muscles of the pelvic floor—especially the pubococcygeal (PC) muscles—to increase vaginal muscle tone, improve sexual response, and limit involuntary urine loss due to stress urinary incontinence.

EXERCISES

1. Answer the following questions

- Define urinary incontinence.
- What are its different types?
- How do you differentiate between overflow, urge and stress incontinence?
- What are the causes of transient incontinence?

- What is the mechanism of development of urge and stress incontinence?
- How do you clinically evaluate a case of urge or stress incontinence?
- How do you investigate such patients?
- How do you treat stress and urge incontinence?
- Give some examples of urge incontinence medications?
- What are the main side effects of all these medications?
- What is mixed urinary incontinence?
- How should it be treated?
- What is overflow incontinence?

2. Write short notes on

- Kegel exercise
- Pharmacologic treatment of urge incontinence

3. Explain or justify the following statements

- Incontinent patients should be offered pelvic floor exercises
- Stress incontinence may be treated surgically

4. Fill in the blanks

- Detrusor muscle contraction is triggered by _____ segment of spinal cord.
- Inhibition of voiding is mediated through _____ segment of spinal cord.
- Postvoid urine volume is normal if it is _____ .
- Drugs that are used to treat urege incontinence are _____ , _____ , _____ .

5. Questions for practical (read the case summary in the beginning of chapter before answering the following questions)

- What are the causes of urinary incontinence in women?
- What kind of incontinence this patient might have?
- What elements of the physical examination are important to obtain?

- What other evaluation can be performed to confirm the diagnosis?
- How she should be treated?

Bibliography

1. Carol Havens, Nancy D. Sullivan Manual of out patient Gynecology.
2. Culligan P. Urinary Incontinence in Women: Evaluation and Management Am Fam Physician 2000;62:2433-44,2447,2452.
3. Frank C, et al. Office management of urinary incontinence among older patients Can Fam Physician 2010;56:1115–20.
4. Homma Y, et al. Urodynamics Japan.
5. Ming ping Yu Urodynamic study in urogynecology.
6. Norton P. Urinary incontinence in women Lancet 2006; 367: 57–67.
7. O'Neil B. Approach to urinary incontinence in women Diagnosis and management by family physicians Can Fam Physician vol 49: may 2003.
8. Paul D. Urinary incontinence in women Marke Manual 2008.
9. Thaker R, Stanton S. Management of urinary incontinence in women Volume 321, Number 7272BMJ 321: 1326 doi: 10.1136/bmj.321.7272.1326 (Published 25 November 2000).

29

Vesicovaginal Fistula

A 17-year-old P 1+0 woman has presented to the gynecology OPD with continuous passage of urine per vagina for last 3 months. She belongs to low socioeconomic status and educated up to class IV. She had a home delivery 3 months back and delivered a dead baby. From her fifth day following child birth she has noticed continuous passage of urine and she has no urge to pass urine. On general examination she is short stature with height 140 cm. On gynecological examination, her perineum is wet with urine smell and a large fistula of 3 cm diameter was noted in anterior vaginal wall. How she should be managed?

In this chapter we will learn:
- Definition of VVF and its causes
- Types of urogenital fistula
- Classification and clinical presentation of VVF
- Investigations
- Prevention
- Treatment

Introduction

A vesicovaginal fistula (VVF) is an abnormal communication between the urinary bladder and the vagina that results in the continuous involuntary discharge of urine into the vaginal canal. Vesicovaginal fistula (VVF) is a subtype of female urogenital fistula (UGF) (Table 29.1). Regardless of the etiopathology, physically, psychologically and socially, it is major source of distress for the patient due to continuous urine leakage through vagina. The earliest evidence of a VVF was found in 1923, when a large VVF was detected in a mummified body of queen Henhenit(11th dynasty who reigned around 2050 BC). In 1845, James Marion Sims developed the surgical techniques of VVF repair and established sound surgical principles of fistula repair.

Etiology

The causative factors leading to VVF formation can be broadly categorized into congenital and acquired (Table 29.2) causes. Majority of VVF fall into the obstetric trauma and iatrogenic subcategories.
- Obstetric trauma—most cases (up to 80%) of VVF occur during a prolonged obstructed labor. In obstructed labour the soft tissues

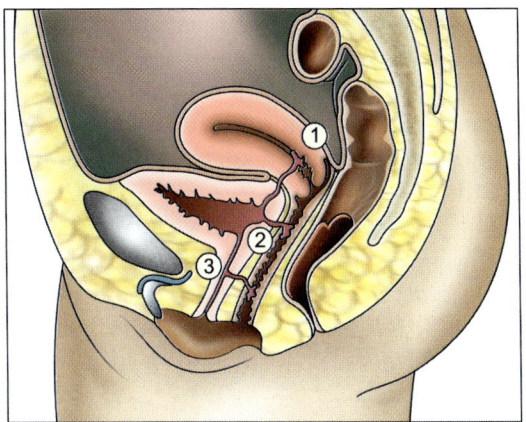

1: Vesicouterine fistula   3: Urethrovaginal fistula
2: Vesicovaginal fistula

Fig. 29.1: Different types of fistula

of the pregnant woman's vagina, bladder, and rectum are compressed between the fetal head and the maternal pelvic bones by the contractions of the uterus. As the fetal head is forced tighter and tighter into the pelvis, the blood supply to the mother's soft tissues is progressively constricted, and, ultimately is shut off completely. This results in tissue necrosis of vesicovaginal wall due to ischemia which ultimately sloughs out resulting in development of fistula formation. This type of VVF is also called obstetric fistula, and is often seen during unattended and/or prolonged labor, in very young women whose pelvis is still too small for harboring a baby, or in malpresentation of the baby, or due to poor uterine contractions during labor. It can also be the result of a cesarean section or a difficult forceps delivery.

Following is the obstetric fistula pathway-its origin and consequences:

Low socioeconomic status of the women → Lack of education, early marriage → child-bearing before pelvic growth is completed → Relatively large fetus or mal presentation → Cephalopelvic disproportion → Lack of emergency obstetric services → Obstructed labor → Obstructed labor injury complex → VVF → Isolation and loss of social support

- *Hysterectomy or other* gynecological surgery to the pelvic area (Table 29.2 and Fig. 29.1). Occasionally, a VVF can occur accidentally during surgery in the pelvic area, especially, during extensive tumor surgery in case of a cancer of cervix or hysterectomy following previous myomectomy.

Numerous authors highlight the risk of various types of bladder trauma during pelvic surgery. Such injuries include unrecognized intraoperative laceration of the bladder, bladder wall injury from electrocautery or mechanical crushing, suture placement through bladder wall and the dissection of the bladder into an incorrect plane, causing avascular necrosis. Other types of pelvic surgery (e.g. urologic, gastrointestinal surgery) also contribute to the incidence of VVFs; such surgeries include suburethral sling procedures, surgical repair of urethral diverticulum, electrocautery of bladder papilloma, and surgery for pelvic carcinomas. Minimizing the risk of injury at the time of surgery is the goal of surgeon. Measures that can minimize fistula formation following pelvic surgery are mentioned in Table 29.3.

- Other less common causes of VVFs include pelvic infections (e.g. tuberculosis, syphilis,

Table 29.1: Types of urogenital fistula based on anatomical communication

Genital tract	Urinary tract		
	Ureter	Bladder	Urethra
Vagina	Ureterovaginal	Vesicovaginal	Urethrovaginal
	Vesicoureterovaginal		
Cervix	Ureterocervical	Vesicocervical	Urethrocervical
Uterus	Ureterouterine	Vesicouterine	----

Table 29.2: Causes of vesicovaginal fistula

1. Congenital
   - Cloacal abnormality
2. Acquired
   a. Noniatrogenic
      1. Obstructed labor (obstetric trauma)
      2. Infection
      3. Locally advanced pelvic malignancy
      4. Foreign body
      5. Pelvic trauma/fracture
   b. Iatrogenic
      A. Postsurgical
         i. Hysterectomy
         ii. Pelvic laparoscopy
         iii. Incontinence procedure
         iv. Anterior colporrhaphy
         v. Cesarean section
         vi. Intravesical formalin instillation
      B. Radiation therapy

Table 29.3: Surgical techniques for minimizing lower urinary tract injuries during gynecological surgery

- Proper positioning of the patient to allow abdominal and vaginal access
- Adequate exposure and lighting of operative field
- Surgeon familiarity of the anatomy of the space entered
- Continuous bladder drainage for abdominal operation.
- Performance of sharp and blunt dissection where appropriate. Blunt dissection is appropriate along certain spaces in pelvis (i.e. vesicovaginal space) but sharp dissection is required to enter into the space. When unsure always use sharp dissection.
- Be aware about the course of ureter and position of bladder and protect them from injury.
- Control bleeding with pressure, suction, identification of source and correction.
- Minimize use of electrocautery in the area of the bladder in proximity to the vaginal cuff.

lymphogranulomavenereum), vaginal trauma, and vaginal erosion with foreign objects (e.g., neglected pessary) and radiation therapy. Lastly, a congenital urogenital abnormality may exist that includes a VVF.

- Risk factors that predispose to VVFs include prior pelvic (commonly prior caesarean delivery) or vaginal surgery, previous PID, ischemia, diabetes, arteriosclerosis, carcinoma, endometriosis, anatomic distortion by uterine myomas, and infection, particularly postoperative cuff abscess.

The development of a VVF has severe psychological consequences for the patient, as she is embarrassed about her incontinence, and often rejected by the community due to her impairment.

Classification

Proper classification of a vesicovaginal fistula can help in planning the appropriate surgical treatment. Obstetric vesicovaginal fistulas may be classified depending on their location, cause, complexity, or site of obstruction. Gynecologic fistula is classified as simple or complicated and may have important implications for surgical approach as well as prognosis for cure. Although the simple vesicovaginal fistulas are usually uncomplicated surgical cases with good prognosis, complicated vesicovaginal fistulas are challenging even for the most experienced and skilled surgeon (Table 29.4).

Table 29.4: Classification of vesicovaginal fistulae due to gynecologic cause

Classification	Description
Simple	• Fistula is less than 2 to 3 cm in size and near the cuff (supra-trigonal)
	• Patient has no history of radiation or malignancy
	• Vaginal length is normal
Complicated	• Patient has had previous radiation therapy
	• Pelvic malignancy is present
	• Vaginal length is shortened
	• Fistula is greater than 3 cm in size
	• Fistula is distant from cuff or has trigonal involvement

Clinical Presentation

Patient profile: Patients will typically present at variable time intervals after the antecedent event (childbirth, pelvic surgery, radiation therapy, etc.). If related to obstructed labor, most patients experience urine leakage within the 4–10 days following delivery. Patients are young and primipara. Following pelvic surgery, symptoms will usually present within 7–30 days after surgery. In contrast, radiation induced fistulas have a slow development process secondary to slowly progressive devascularization necrosis and may present between 30 days and 30 years following the antecedent event.

Symptoms

- *Continuous leakage of urine from the vagina:* This is the most common presenting feature of VVFs. The size and location of the fistula determine the degree of leakage. Patients with small fistulas may void normal amounts of urine and notice only slight position-dependent drainage. Alternatively, they may have leakage only at maximal bladder capacity. Those with larger fistulas may not void trans urethrally and may have total incontinence. Urinary leakage may make the patient socially isolated, disrupt sexual relations, and lead to depression, low self-esteem, and insomnia.

- *Symptoms of urinary tract infections:* The patient may experience recurrent cystitis or pyelonephritis; unexplained fever; hematuria; flank, vaginal, or suprapubic pain; and abnormal urinary stream.

- The leakage of urine may cause irritation of the vagina and vulvar mucosa, and perineum and usually produces a foul ammonia odor. Phosphate encrustations may be noted in more neglected cases. These crystals serve to further irritate what can be already compromised tissue.

Physical Examination

Inspection of perineum: Pooling of fluid in the vagina with urine smell may be noted, clothing may be wet, and fluid should be sent for analysis if the diagnosis is unclear. The perineum may show wetness, redness and marks of scratches.

Vaginal speculum examination: A careful speculum examination allowing visualization of the entire anterior vaginal wall should be performed to identify the fistula tract. In many cases, the fistula is grossly visible. The location of the fistula in relation to the vaginal apex and bladder trigone should be inspected and the quality of the surrounding tissue (inflammation, edema, or infection) noted. In some cases of small fistula, no obvious tract may be noted.

Bimanual examination: Bimanual examination with careful palpation of the anterior wall may help isolate the location with palpation of a surrounding zone of induration.

Clinical pearls: A patient who complains urine leaking from her vagina following pelvic surgery should be presumed to have a fistula unless proved otherwise

Investigations

1. *Exmination of vaginal fluid:* If the presence of a vesicovaginal or ureterovaginal fistula is in doubt, vaginal secretions and fluid pooling in the vaginal vault should be sent for creatinine level evaluation. Serum creatinine should be drawn simultaneously, and that level should be compared with the fluid creatinine. If the fluid creatinine level is significantly higher than the serum creatinine, this confirms that the fluid is urine. If fluid creatinine test result is equivocal but a fistula is still suspected, proceed with a complete fistula workup, as discussed below.

2. Double dye test
   - Frequently, the double dye test is useful for diagnosing vesicovaginal fistula.

- In this test, the patient ingests oral phenazopyridine (Pyridium), and indigo carmine or methylene blue is instilled into the bladder via a urethral catheter. Pyridium turns urine orange, and methylene blue (or indigo carmine) turns urine blue.

  A tampon is placed into the vagina. If the tampon turns blue, suspect vesicovaginal fistula. If the tampon turns orange, suspect ureterovaginal fistula. If the tampon turns blue and orange, suspect a combination of vesicovaginal and ureterovaginal fistulas.

3. *Three swab test (Moir 1973):* As an alternative to double dye test a three swab test can also be performed

   In this test three cotton wool swabs are placed sequentially inside vaginal canal, one at the vault, one in the middle and one just above the level of introitus. A diluted solution of Methylene blue dye is instilled inside the bladder through a urethral catheter. The woman is asked to walk for five minutes. Then the swabs are removed serially from the vagina and inspected for presence of dye. If the upper most swab is wet but not stained with dye, indicates ureterovaginal fistula. If the upper most swab is stained with methylene blue dye, a vesicovaginal or a vesicocervicovaginal fistula is present. If middle swab is stained with dye the interpretation is vesicovaginal fistula and if the lower most swab is stained with dye then urethrovaginal fistula is present.

4. *Cystoscopy:* A VVF can be diagnosed by performing a so-called cystoscopy, a flexible or rigid optical tube which is inserted through the urethra into the urinary bladder, in order to examine the interior walls of the bladder.

5. *IVP:* Intravenous pyelography (IVP) or CT urography is done to rule out coexisting ureterovaginal fistula or ureteral obstruction. When a ureter is involved in the margin of the vesicovaginal fistula, IVP may demonstrate a standing column of contrast within the ureter, extravasation of contrast around the distal ureter, or hydronephrosis.

6. Urinalysis and urine culture are used to rule out coexisting urinary tract infection.

7. Complete blood cell (CBC) count is used to rule out systemic infection.

Differential Diagnosis

The differential diagnosis of a VVF includes:

- Urge or stress incontinence
- Urethrovaginal fistula
- Ureterovaginal fistula
- Vaginal discharge secondary to infection

Prevention of Vesicovaginal Fistula

The best strategy in dealing with obstetric fistula is to prevent them entirely. This has been shown by the developed countries by improved obstetric care where obstetric fistula is rare. Elimination of obstetric fistula from developing world will require the following measures:

- Adequate childhood nutrition and delay in child bearing until full pelvic growth is achieved before childbearing begins.
- Universal basic education for women.
- Supervision and monitoring of every labor by trained personnel with use of partogram to detect cephalopelvic disproportion early and to prevent the development of obstructed labor.
- Prompt and universal access to emergency obstetric care at the first referral site.

  Gynecological fistulas are also preventable. Surgical techniques that can minimize the development of urogenital fistula formation are mentioned in Table 29.3.

Treatment

Symptomatic vesicovaginal fistula requires appropriate treatment as spontaneous closure is uncommon. Appropriate treatment will depend on various factors including size and location of the fistula, timing from the antecedent event, and severity of symptoms, quality of surrounding tissue, and clinician experience and surgical skills.

Conservative Management

A small number of fistulas may heal following prolonged bladder drainage through a transurethral or suprapubic catheter if diagnosed within the first few days of gynecological surgery. There is increased chance of success if the fistula is diagnosed within seven days of index surgery, is less than 1 cm in size, is simple without associated carcinoma or radiation, and is subject to at least four weeks of constant bladder drainage. Persistent, large, or complex fistulas are best treated with surgical intervention.

Surgical Management

The treatment of vesicovaginal fistula is surgical repair.

- General principles of surgical repair of vesicovaginal fistula include adequate exposure, good hemostasis, wide mobilization of the bladder and vagina, resection of devascularized tissue and removal of foreign body, multilayered tension free closure, and confirmation of a water tight seal on bladder closure, and postoperative bladder drainage for 10–14 days.
- Traditionally, an interval of 3–6 months has been recommended between the fistula repair and index event or surgery so that local infection and inflammation is controlled and up to 1 year in cases of radiation induced fistula. However, early repair of simple, iatrogenic fistulae has been found to be highly successful and minimizes the physical and psychological disruption to the patient's life. The basic rule for fistula repair is that the first operation has the best chance of success, and surgeons should use the approach with which they feel most comfortable.

Vaginal Approach

Most vesicovaginal fistulas can be surgically corrected using a vaginal approach. Traditionally, fistulectomy with flap splitting closure, or a Latzko partial colpocliesis have been advocated.

Flap splitting closure: This procedure begins with excision of the fistulous tract to expose healthy tissue at the wound margins. The fistulous opening is then closed in a multilayer fashion beginning with the bladder mucosa, bladder serosa, pubo-cervical fascia, and vaginal mucosa. Care should be taken to avoid tension on suture lines. A fascial flap is created to prevent opposition of the incision planes and reduce risk of recurrence.

Latzko partial colpocleisis: This operation is used to repair a VVF that develops following hysterectomy operation. After identification of the fistulous tract, a circumferential incision is made in the vagina approximately 2 cm from the fistulous tract. The vagina is mobilized and then closed over the fistulous tract with delayed absorbable suture in double layer without disturbing the bladder mucosa. The vaginal mucosa is then closed, completing the repair.

Abdominal/Laparoscopic Approach

Although most vesicovaginal fistulas can be surgically corrected via the vaginal approach, the abdominal route may be preferred for high and inaccessible fistulas, large complex fistulas, multiple fistulas, concurrent uterine or bowel involvement, or need for ureteral reimplantation. Laparoscopic VVF repair technique has not gained widespread acceptance due to the technical challenges it poses even to skilled laparoscopic surgeons.

Postoperative Management

- Continuous bladder drainage for 10–14 days via a self retaining Foley catheter is vital. This ensures that the repair is kept tension-free during healing and allows tissue integrity to re-establish. The placement of an additional suprapubic catheter is desirable in all transabdominal repairs, where the bladder has been opened as part of the procedure. In the post-operative period catheters must be checked regularly to ensure that they remain patent. The advantage of both suprapubic and urethral catheter placement is that bladder drainage is maintained even if one catheter blocks. Inadequate bladder drainage is a common cause of failure of the repair.

- Bladder spasms can be treated effectively with anticholinergic drugs. There is a concern that these spasms may compromise healing as well as being a source of patient discomfort.
- Urinary antibiotics are given to prevent infection.

Complications

The success of VVF repair at the first attempt is approximately 85% for both transabdominal and transvaginal techniques. Complications include recurrent fistula formation, ureteric injury or obstruction, vaginal stenosis, reduced bladder capacity and irritative lower urinary tract symptoms.

EXERCISES

1. Answer the following questions

- What do you mean by vesicovaginal fistula?
- What are the different types of urogenital fistula?
- What are the different causes of vesico-vaginal fistula?
- What is the commonest cause of VVF in our country?
- What is the mechanism of development of obstetric fistula?
- Name some iatrogenic causes of VVF.
- Name some risk factors that predispose VVF formation during pelvic surgery .

- How risk of VVF can be minimized during pelvic surgery?
- How do you classify gynecologic VVF?
- Describe the clinical presentation of a case of VVF.
- Name the investigations that can be considered in a case of VVF.
- How do you collect urine for routine examination and culture of urine?
- What is the role of conservative manage-ment for treatment of VVF?
- What are the general principles of fistula repair?
- Following development of obstetric fistula when should it be repaired and why?
- Outline the different surgical options for treatment of VVF.
- Name the complications of VVF repair.

2. Write short notes on

- Three swab test
- Obstetric VVF

3. Explain or justify the following statement

- Vesicovaginal fistulas are mostly preventable.

4. Fill in the blanks with appropriate word/s

- _____ developed the surgical techniques of VVF repair and established sound surgical principles of fistula repair.
- In most cases, VVF occur during _____ .
- If VVF is related to obstructed labour, most patients experience urine leakage within _____ days.
- Two vaginal approaches of surgical repair of VVF are _____ and _____ .
- Continuous bladder drainage following VVF repair should be continued for _____ days.

5. Questions for practical examination (read the case summary mentioned at the beginning of chapter before answering the following questions)

1. Identify the risk factors present for develop-ment of uro genital fistula in this case.

2. What is the cause of fistula in this case?

3. What are the differential diagnosis?

4. Name the tests you consider for her?

5. How she should be treated?

6. What is the success rate of the operation?

7. What are the postoperative measures you take following fistula repair?

Bibliography

1. Arrowsmith SD, Briggs ND, Browning N, Lassy A. The Obstetrcvesicovaginal fistula in the developing world.

2. Chesson RR, Ibeanu OA. Ostergard's urogynecology and pelvic floor dysfunction, Fistula and urethral diverticulum

3. Kohli N, Miklos J. Managing vesico vaginal fistula Women's Health & Education Center

4. Rackley RR, Apple RA. Vesicovaginal fistula repair current approach. AUA Update series 1998;21:161–168

5. Vesico vaginal fistula OBG Management. August 2003.

6. Wall LL. Obstetric vesicovaginal fistula as an international public health problem Global sisterhood network.

7. Wall L Lewis. Obstetric vesicovaginal fistula as an international public-health problem.

30

Anal Incontinence—Old Complete Perineal Tear (CPT)

A 22-years-old P 1+0 woman from low socioeconomic status has presented with inability to hold stool and flatus since after her difficult child birth at home 1 month back. Her general examination findings reveal no abnormality. On inspection of her perineum, the appearance resembles as shown in Figures 30.1 and 30.2. How she should be managed?

In this chapter we will learn:
- What is anal and fecal incontinence?
- Different degrees of perineal tear and risk factors associated with complete perineal tear (CPT)
- Clinical presentation of old complete perineal tear
- Differential diagnosis, pre operative investigations and treatment of old CPT.
- Postoperative management ,complications and follow up following surgical repair of old CPT

Introduction

Anal incontinence (AI) is defined as an involuntary loss of flatus, liquid, or solid stool that causes a social or hygienic problem. The definition of anal incontinence includes incontinence of flatus, whereas that of fecal incontinence (FI) does not. This condition may lead to poor self-image and social isolation, thus significantly impairing quality of life. There are two factors most commonly involved in anal incontinence. One is colonic contraction or motility, and the other is the sphincter injury or sphincter defect. Sphincter injury or sphincter defect usually results from inadequate repair or poor healing of obstetric perineal injuries. It is the most common cause of anal incontinence in young women. The overall risk of obstetric anal sphincter injury is 1% of all vaginal deliveries.

Other causes include perineal trauma from surgical procedures such as perineorrhaphy, hemorrhoidectomy, fissurectomy, or radical oncologic procedures. Rectal prolapse is a very common cause in older women. Anal incontinence may even occur as the result of a primary neoplastic process. Less frequently, anal incontinence may result from congenital anomalies, neurologic disorders affecting the perineum and anal sphincter, or demyelinating diseases that alter multiorgan systems. Anal incontinence is not common as either an acute or chronic side effect of radiotherapy.

This chapter addresses obstetric sphincter injury that results in anal incontinence due to inadequate repair or poor healing of obstetric perineal injuries. Anal incontinence due to systemic, malignant, or neurologic disease processes lie outside the scope of this chapter.

Perineal Tear and Old Complete Perineal Tear

Many women, 8–9 out of 10 (85%), have a perineal tear during childbirth. The tear, which is usually due to overstretching of the soft tissue of the birth canal, may vary in severity and may be identified as follows:

1st degree tears: Injury to perineal skin only; these are small, and may heal naturally. Some women do not require stitches.

2nd degree tears: Injury to perineum that affects the perineal muscles but not the anal sphincter; these are slightly deeper, affecting the perineal muscles as well as the skin. All second degree tears require stitches.

Third degree: Injury to perineum that affects partial or complete disruption of the anal sphincter muscles; it can affect the external anal sphincter (circular fibres) or the internal anal sphincter (longitudinal fibres), or both:

3a: Less than 50% of external anal sphincter torn

3b: More than 50% of external anal sphincter torn

3c: Both external and internal anal sphincter torn

Fourth degree: Injury to perineum involving the anal sphincter complex and anal epithelium.

Thus both third and fourth degree perineal tears result in injury to the anal sphincter(with or without anal mocosa) and called complete perineal tear . There are several identified risk factors associated with obstetric anal sphincter injury which are shown in Table 30.1.

However, most of the risk factors identified cannot readily be used to prevent or predict the occurrence of a complete perineal tear.

Third- and fourth-degree perineal tear— Complete perineal tear seen within 24 hours of delivery should be repaired at once. This is not a minor operation. The patient's future continence depends on the skill of the repair. If the repair cannot be performed or not detected immediately, or the repair breaks down, it is best to wait for several weeks, arbitrarily 3 months. After three months following childbirth complete perineal tear is termed as old complete perineal tear and surgical repair is recommended. This delay in surgical repair provides sufficient time for resolution of the inflammatory response, return of an adequate blood supply to the margins of the defect, and return of optimum viability of the perineal tissues.

Clinical pearl: Clinicians need to be aware of the risk factors for obstetric anal sphincter injury but also recognise that known risk factors do not readily allow its prediction or prevention.

Clinical Presentation

History

Patient profile: The patient is a young primipara with history of home delivery or delivery at institution with risk factors of anal sphincter injury. On occasions, anal sphincter injuries may not be recognised or may be incorrectly classified by a doctor or midwife at the time of vaginal delivery possibly because of poor understanding of perineal

Table 30.1: Risk factors for obstetric anal sphincter injury (complete perineal tear)	
Antenatal risk factors	*Intrapartum risk factors*
Birth weight > 4000 g	Instrumental delivery (forceps delivery)
Nulliparity	Midline episiotomy
Induction of labour	Second stage of labour longer than one hour
Persistent occipitoposterior position	Face to pubis delivery
	Shoulder dystocia
	Epidural analgesia

anatomy or the perineal injury classification system.

Complaints

- Inability to have voluntary control of flatus and feces (incontinence of flatus and feces)- while incontinence of flatus is always present, presence of fecal incontinence depends on the extent of anal sphincter damage. If the damage is less there is incontinence of loose stool (external sphincter damage only) and if the damage is more there is incontinence of both hard and loose stool (damage of both internal and external sphincter). A thorough history should include incontinence duration and frequency, stool consistency, timing of incontinent episodes, use of sanitary protection, and social impact of incontinence.
- Other symptoms that may be present after persistent sphincter defect following third and fourth degree tear include perineal pain, dyspareunia and fecal urgency. Urgency of stool resulting in a rush to the toilet and urge faecal incontinence are thought to indicate damage to the external sphincter, whereas the passive leakage of faeces or flatus is associated with internal sphincter damage.

Obstetric history: Obstetric history should include mode of delivery, length of second stage, use of forceps/vacuum, episiotomies or lacerations, any wound complications, and birth weight of the baby.

Physical examination: Examination begins with careful inspection of the posterior vaginal wall, perineum and anal region.

Inspection of Perineum

- It is important to note the presence or absence of fecal material and whether or not there is discoloration and irritation of perianal skin, which is commonly seen in patients with significant incontinence.

- There may be the loss of the perineal body; the vaginal introitus and the anus almost open together (Figs 30.1 and 30.2—vaginal mucosa is pink and anal mucosa is red). There is loss of the corrugated appearance surrounding the anus. There are cutaneous dimples—one on either side of the anus due to retracted torn ends of the sphincter ani externus.
- Normally the perianal skin creases or folds should completely encircle the anus. In cases of complete anal sphincter disruption, a dovetail sign is usually present in which

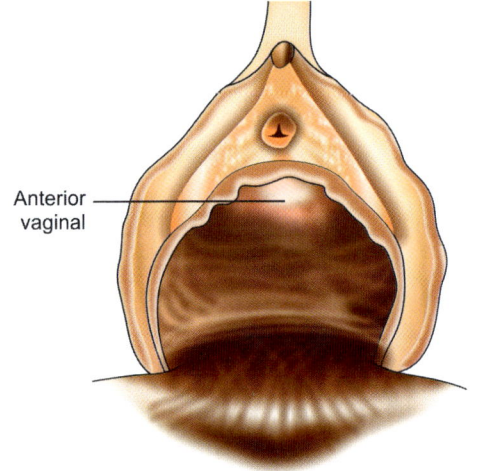

Anterior vaginal

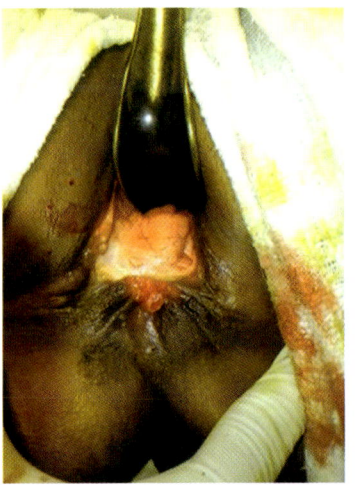

Figs 30.1 and 30.2: Complete perineal tear—Note the disruption of the perineal body and anterior anal sphincter complex secondary to obstetric injury in the past

the normal radial distribution of the anal creases is absent anteriorly but is present laterally and inferiorly.

- Any prior episiotomies, lacerations, or surgical scars should be noted.

Vaginal examination: The levator ani should be palpated for strength and symmetry. Any scarring or retraction of the posterior vaginal wall should be noted.

Rectal examination

A rectal examination is performed to assess anal sphincter tone at rest and during sphincter contraction. An anterior sphincter defect may be easily detectable as the loss of the palpable muscular ring and the anal canal is separated from the vagina by the recto-vaginal septum only. In normal condition, when the patient is asked to tighten the sphincter around the finger, a circumferential contraction and tightening should be felt in addition to some upward movement of the rectum and posterior compartment.

Differential Diagnosis

Recto vaginal fistula may produce similar symptoms and must be differentiated from complete perineal tear. A rectovaginal fistula is usually easily diagnosed by careful inspection of the posterior vaginal wall. By spreading the labia, a low fistula can be seen, usually involving the area of a previous episiotomy or obstetric laceration. The vaginal opening of a fistula may be localized by the presence of feces in the vagina or by the dark red rectal mucosa seen protruding at the fistulous opening contrasting with the lighter vaginal mucosa. A per rectal examination makes the fistulous opening more obvious. A small probe can be pushed gently from the vaginal side of the fistula and the tip felt on a rectally placed finger (Fig. 30.3).

Investigations

Most of the patients will have an obvious diagnosis and be ready to proceed to

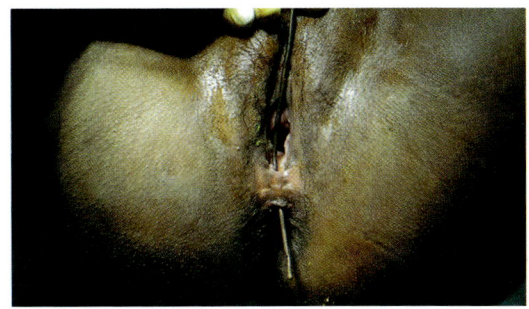

Fig. 30.3: A case of rectovaginal fistula

treatment after their history and physical examination. For them the pre operative evaluation includes a complete blood count and urinalysis, with chest radiography, electrocardiography, renal function test, and blood sugar estimation, and routine examination of stool. In few women endoanal ultrasonography may be required to identify sphincter injury.

Endoanal Ultrasonography

This technique is now the primary diagnostic imaging technique to evaluate the integrity, thickness, and length of the internal and external anal sphincters. This tool allows diagnosis of sphincter defects in women with occult defects from obstetric trauma who in the past were labeled as having "idiopathic" fecal incontinence. High-resolution images of the separate sphincter muscles are obtained using a rotating endoprobe, and anatomic defects can be identified as a loss of continuity of the muscle rings (Fig. 30.4).

Preoperative Preparation

- *Preoperative bowel preparation:* An oral bowel preparation to empty all solid fecal material should be given the evening before surgery is scheduled. An isotonic bowel preparation such as polyethylene glycol (Peglec) is administered by dissolving in 2 litre of water.

- *Vaginal douche:* On the evening before surgery a vaginal cleansing douche with antiseptic solution is applied to clean the operative field.

- *Intestinal antiseptics:* Three doses of oral erythromycin 500 mg and neomycin 1 g are given orally on the day before surgery.

Surgical Procedure

The treatment of complete perineal tear is surgical repair. There are different techniques of repair of complete perineal tear such as layered method of repair, Warren flap method or the Noble operation. Regardless of which approach is taken to repair a complete perineal laceration, it is the sphincteroplasty itself that is the keystone to the repair. Layer repair is commonly employed nowadays and described below (Fig. 30.5):

- A transverse incision is made at the junction of the vaginal and rectal mucosa and extended up the midline of the posterior vaginal wall.

- The vaginal mucosa is separated from the rectal mucosa in the midline, and this plane is extended laterally. The external sphincter muscle fibers are identified and dissected free and grasped with Allis tissue forceps. The internal anal sphincter can be seen between the external anal sphincter and the anorectal mucosa as an area of white fibrous tissue.

- All scar tissue is excised from the margins of the anorectal mucosa, and the defect in the anal mucosa is closed using a continuous or interrupted suture of 3-0 delayed-absorbable material. The internal anal sphincter then is reapproximated over a length of 3 to 5 cm.

- The external sphincter then is brought together over the repaired internal sphincter with two rows of two horizontal mattress sutures of delayed-absorbable suture material. Plication of the superior puborectalis muscle loop with an interrupted 0 delayed-absorbable suture adds additional support to the repair.

- The bulbocavernosus and superficial transverse perinei muscles are reattached to the perineal body, and the vaginal mucosa is closed with a continuous locking stitch of 3-0 delayed-absorbable suture that was continued subcuticularly to approximate the perineal skin.

Postoperative Care

- *Antibiotics:* Intravenous antibiotics (Cefuroxime 1.5 g and Metronidazole 500 mg) should be given stat intra-operatively. Change to oral antibiotics on the ward. Antibiotics are continued for 10 day because of high risk of wound dehiscence and infection.

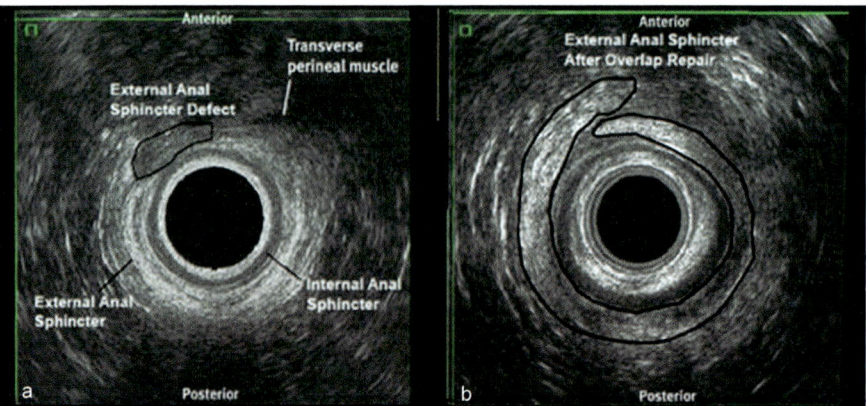

Fig. 30.4: (a) A preoperative endoanal ultrasound scan showing an external anal sphincter defect at 12 o'clock; **(b)** a postoperative endoanal ultrasound scan showing an "overlapping" repair of the external anal sphincter

- *Urinary catheter:* Urinary catheterization should continue overnight or until the patient becomes fully ambulatory. Severe perineal discomfort is a known cause of urinary retention and following regional anaesthesia it can take up to 12 hours before bladder sensation returns. Moreover, urine will not wet the perineal stiches.

- *Diet:* Specific dietary restrictions are commonly used postoperatively. Normal feeding is delayed and the patient is kept on clear liquid diets or soft low residue foods for first four days. Preferably, no solid fecal evacuation should challenge the repair until late in the postoperative period.

- *Bowel care:* Daily stool softeners (Lactulose 15 mls bd) and a bulking agent (Metamucil 2 × 5 ml spoonfuls bd) are started when solid diet is begun and cotinued for at least 6 weeks.

Complications

- *Wound break down:* The most common complication is superficial separation of skin and subcutaneous tissues, and the frequency rate is as high as 25% in some series.

- *Wound haematoma:* Bleeding and hematoma formation are also possible complications. Bleeding can usually be controlled with pressure achieved with packing. Hematoma formation into the perirectal space can go unnoticed and result in the sequestration of large amounts of blood. Treatment requires evacuation of the hematoma and surgical hemostasis.

- *Infection and abscess formation:* Risk of infection is 3–5%. Opening the wound to allow for drainage and treatment with antibiotics may allow the physician to save the surgical repair.

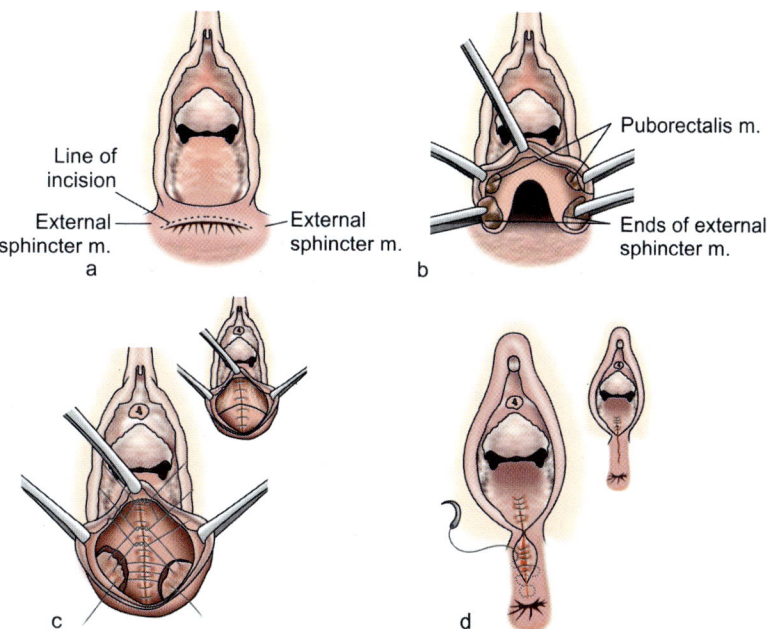

Fig. 30.5: Layered repair. **(a)** A transverse mucosal incision exposes the severed ends of the external sphincter muscle. **(b)** The vaginal mucosa is sharply dissected from the underlying rectal mucosa, and the external sphincter muscles are identified. **(c)** The rectal mucosa is reapproximated. All three loops of the external anal sphincter are plicated. **(d)** The perineal muscles, skin, and vaginal mucosa are closed

- *Stenosis of vaginal introitus* may lead to dyspareunia or introital and perineal body pain.
- *Anal incontinence:* Anal incontinence may recur following failure of repair.
- *Rectovaginal fistula:* Fistula formation occurs in fewer than 1% of the patients, but it is more common in those cases in which infection develops.

Keywords

Anal incontinence: Involuntary loss of flatus, liquid, or solid stool through the anus that is perceived as a social or hygienic problem.

Fecal incontinence: Involuntary loss through the anus of liquid or solid stool only; excludes flatal incontinence.

External anal sphincter: Striated muscle sphincter, that is responsible for much of the squeeze pressure in the anal canal and under voluntary control.

Internal anal sphincter: Thickened continuation of the circular smooth muscle layer of the bowel, under autonomic control, that is responsible for much of the resting pressure in the anal canal.

Puborectalis muscle: Medial portion of the levator ani muscle that is responsible for maintaining and increasing the anorectal angle and contributes to the squeeze pressure in the anal canal.

Rectovaginal fistula: Epithelial lined tract between the vagina and rectum or anal canal.

EXERCISES

Answer the following questions

1. Define anal incontinence. How definition of fecal incontinence differs from that of anal incontinence?
2. Enumerate the causes of anal sphincter injury resulting in anal incontinence?
3. What are the different degrees of perineal tear?
4. What is complete perineal tear?
5. When it is called old?
6. Describe the clinical presentation of a patient with old complete perineal tear.
7. What is the significance of control of solid stool but incontinence of liquid stool in history?

8. What are the special pre operative preparation of old complete perineal tear repair?
9. Describe the steps of operation in layered method of repair of old complete perineal tear.
10. What are the special postoperative care following repair of old complete perineal tear?
11. Name the complications of surgical treatment of old CPT?

Write short notes on

1. Risk factors of obstetric sphincter injury

Explain or justify the following statement

1. A low rectovaginal fistula can be easily differentiated from old CPT by clinical examination.

Fill in the blanks with appropriate word/s

1. If both external and internal anal sphincter are torn without involvement of anal mucosa the degree of perineal injury is _____ .
2. The most common complication of repair of old complete perineal tear is _____ .

Questions for practical (read the case summary at the beginning of the chapter before answering the questions below)

1. What is your diagnosis?
2. Which perineal inspection findings are helpful to reach this diagnosis?
3. What is the degree of perineal injury in this case?
4. How do you identify the position of torn sphincter?
5. What is dovetail sign? Why it appears?
6. What is the per rectal findings in this case?
7. Which preoperative investigations you consider for her?
8. What should be the optimum time for surgical intervention following obstetric sphinctor injury repair failure?

9. What is its rationality?
10. Name the different operations that can be considered for her?

Bibliography

1. Abott D, Atere - Roberts N, Williams A, et al. Obstetric anal sphincter injury BMJ 2010;341;3414.

2. Fecal incontinence E Medicine

3. Leeman L, Spearnah N, Rogers R. Repair of obstetric perineal laceration Am Fam Physician 2003; 68:1585–90

4. Mayer, A, Nelson, B, et al. Anal incontinence Glob. libr. women's med., (ISSN: 1756-2228) 2009; DOI 10.3843/GLOWM.10072

5. Perineal tears Northern Lincolnshire and Goole Hospital

6. Perineal tear—third and fourth degree Auckland District health board 2011

7. RCOG Green Top Guidelines No. 29, March 2007. Third and Fourth-degree Perineal Tears, Management

8. Repair of anal sphincter injury Practical obstetric fistula surgery

31

Menopause and Hormone Therapy

A 51-year-old schoolteacher has presented with complain of hot flushes, night sweating, palpitation and difficulty in sleeping. She has also noticed a decrease in libido and discomfort during sexual activity. Her husband complains that she is more irritable now a day. Her menstrual periods had been getting heavier and her cycles have shortened to three weeks. Now she has not had her periods for three months. On pelvic examination, vaginal mucosa is slightly pale and she finds insertion of speculum uncomfortable. However, rest of her physical examination is entirely unremarkable. How should her case be managed?

In this chapter we will learn:
- What is menopause
- Its pathophysiology
- Clinical effects of menopause
- Diagnosis
- Management of menopause
- Hormone therapy

Introduction

Menopause is defined as permanent cessation of menstruation resulting from the loss of ovarian follicular activity. Because 12 months amenorrhea ensures a cessation of ovarian function in older women, diagnosis of menopause is usually made retrospectively after 12 months of final menstrual period. A standardized system for chronology and terminology of menopause has been developed by experts. Menopausal transition is defined as the period of time from first variation in menstrual cycle length and elevated follicle stimulating hormone (FSH)

to the final menses. Menopause is the year after the final period. Perimenopause includes the transition phase and menopause itself. Postmenopause includes the remaining lifetime after menopause (Table 31.1). In healthy women, menopause is the natural event that usually occurs between 40 and 60 years of age. The average age of menopause in India is 49 years. Menopause before the age of 40 years is known as premature menopause and may occur spontaneously or because of surgery, radiation in the pelvis, chemotherapy, autoimmune disease, fragile X syndrome or idiopathic causes.

Table 31.1: STRAW staging system (modified) (*Adapted from* Soules MR, Sherman S Parrot, E Rebar. Executive summary: Stages of reproductive aging workshop (STRAW), fertility sterility 2001;874–878)

Terminology	Reproductive period	Menopause transition	Menopausal 1 year	Postmenopause
		Perimenopause		
Menstrual cycles	Regular	Variable cycle length	Amenorrhea 12 months	None
Endocrine	Normal FSH	Increased FSH	Increased FSH	Increased FSH

Pathophysiology

Women are born with a set number of oocytes. The oocytes in the ovaries undergo atresia throughout a woman's life cycle, resulting in a decline in both the quantity and quality of follicles. As these supply of oocytes becomes depleted in women in their early 40s, ovarian production of estrogen and progesterone begins to decline. As the ovarian productions of steroid hormone falls , there is loss of negative feedback at the hypothalamus and pituitary. The earliest evidence of these endocrine changes is a mild increase in FSH levels toward the upper limit of normal. During the course of perimenopausal transition, the menstral cycle interval often shortens (because of shorter follicular phase) and gradually these cycles are mixed together with abnormally long menstrual cycle (secondary to anovulatory cycle).

When menstrual cycle caease, the secretion of steroid hormones and gonadotrophins changes dramatically. The FSH level rises sharply and estradiol level falls. The ovaries no longer produce estrogen and progesterone but continue to produce androstenedione until women reach approximately age 65. In postmenopausal period some androstenedione is converted to estrone by peripheral adipose tissue.

Vaginal tissue is an estrogen sensitive tissue and therefore declining estrogen level is associated with symptomatic urogenital atrophy of postmenopausal women. There may be vaginal epithelial thinning, decreased secretions, reduction in vaginal size, and increase in PH of vaginal fluid (> 6). This may be the cause of more painful intercourse, more frequent vaginal infections and UTIs. During menopausal transition, bone resorption accelerates resulting in rapid decline in bone density in 3–5 years after the final menstrual period.

Fact sheet: It is estimated that more than 40 million people will experience menopause during the next 20 years. For most women, one-third of their life will occur in postmenopausal period.

Clinical Effects of Menopause

The hypoestrogenic state seen at menopause is manifested in many women by signs and symptoms of hormonal deficiency in tissues containing estrogen receptors. Estrogen sensitive tissues that are affected are the ovary, endometrium, vaginal epithelium, urethra, hypothalamus, and skin. The most common complaints are vasomotor disturbances characterized by hot flushes, genital atrophy, and neuropsychiatric symptoms. The decline in estrogen also causes an increased risk of osteoporosis.

Perimenopausal changes in menstruation usually begin during a woman's 40s. Menstrual flow and cycle length can vary. Menses become irregular, then are skipped. Large daily fluctuations in estrogen levels usually begin at least 1 yr before menopause and are thought to cause perimenopausal symptoms. Symptoms can last from 6 months to over 10 years and range from nonexistent to severe.

Symptoms and Signs

Vasomotor

Hot flushes (flashes) and sweating due to vasomotor instability affect 75 to 85% of women and usually begin before menses stop. Hot flushes continue for > 1 yr in most women and for > 5 yr in 50%. The hot flush is characterized by a sensation of warmth and heat that starts in the chest and spreads upward over the neck and head. This sensation is accompanied by regional vasodilation, which causes flushing of the neck and face and produces body heat loss. The core temperature falls an average of 0.2°C, resulting in perspiration and the episodic flush, which may last from 30 sec to 5 min. Flushes may manifest during the night as night sweats. The withdrawal of estrogen seems to alter the hypothalamic thermo-regulatory system such that the "set point" lowers, the patient vasodilates to meet this temperature setting, and changes in neural activity alter hormonal secretions (Fig. 31.1).

Genital

Decreased estrogen leads to vaginal and vulvar dryness and thinning, which may result in inflammation of the vaginal mucosa (atrophic vaginitis). Atrophy may cause irritation, dyspareunia, and dysuria and may increase vaginal pH. The labia minora, clitoris, uterus, and ovaries decrease in size.

Neuropsychiatric

Neuropsychiatric changes (e.g., poor concentra-tion, memory loss, depression, anxiety) may accompany menopause but are not directly related to decreased estrogen. Recurrent night sweats, which can disrupt sleep, can contribute to insomnia, fatigue, irritability, and poor concentration.

Other

Although menopause is normal, health problems can occur, and for some, quality of life may decrease. Risk of osteoporosis increases because estrogen is decreased,

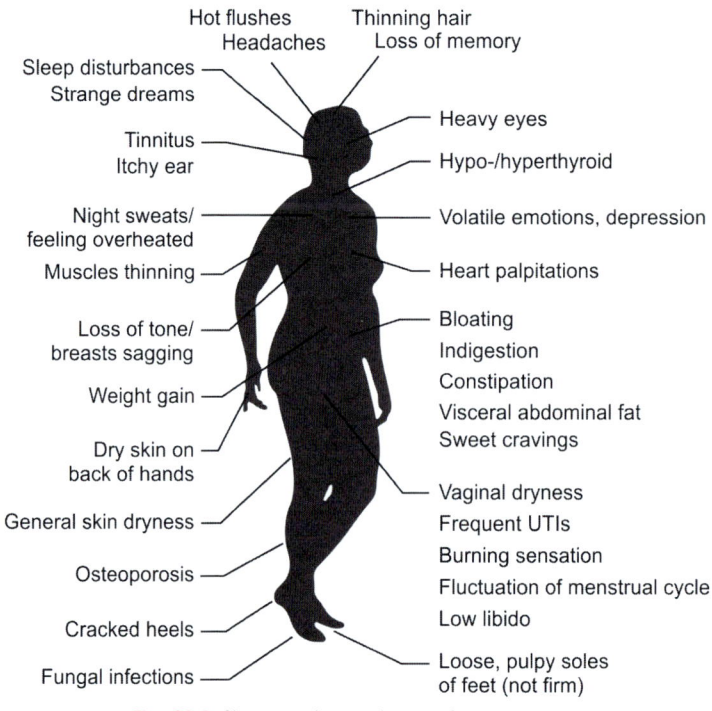

Fig. 31.1: Signs and symptoms of menopause

increasing bone resorption by osteoclasts. The most rapid loss occurs during the first 2 yr after estrogen begins to decrease. The hypoestrogenic state may be a significant factor in the development of ischemic heart disease. Premenopausal females are relatively protected against atherosclerosis and coronary heart disease compared with males the same age. Women rarely suffer heart attacks until after the menopause, when the risk of cardiovascular disease approximates that of men by age 65.

Diagnosis

- *Clinical evaluation*—Diagnosis is clinical. Menopause is likely if menses have gradually decreased in frequency and have been absent for 6 months to one year. Complaints of vasomotor instability, genitourinary symptoms and other non-specific symptoms help to reach to diagnosis.
- *FSH levels rarely needed*—FSH levels may be measured, but this test is rarely necessary. Consistently elevated levels (30 IU/L) predict menopause, sometimes many months to a year in advance.
- Women with amenorrhea are examined to exclude pregnancy if they are < 50.

Management of Menopause

Many women manage the menopause by themselves and only 10% seek help from health care providers. Treatment is indicated if menopausal symptoms interfere with woman's daily activities or quality of life. The prevailing symptoms should be clarified and different options from lifestyle changes to drug therapy with its benefit and risk to be explained.

The menopause and postmenopause can be managed with or without hormones.

Non-hormonal Management

- *Lifestyle changes:* Women may be encouraged to lose weight (where appro-

priate) and to increase exercise, both of which are beneficial for overall wellbeing but may not have a direct impact on hot flushes. For hot flushes, avoiding triggers (e.g. hot drinks, spicy food, staying in cold rooms), wearing clothing in layers that can be removed as needed, use of hand held fans and drinking cold waters may be helpful. Regular exercise, stress avoidance, and relaxation techniques may improve sleep and reduce irritability; relaxation techniques can also reduce vasomotor symptoms including hot flushes. Paced respiration, a type of slow, deep breathing, may decrease the incidence of hot flushes by 50%.

- *Nonhormonal drug treatment:* For women who are unable to take estrogen because of risk factors or inability to tolerate hormone therapy, or who have received short duration estrogen therapy but still having hot flushes, may be considered for non hormonal drug therapy. Nonhormonal drugs that can be used for treatmet of hot flushes include selective serotonin reuptake inhibitors (SSRIs, e.g. fluoxetine, paroxetine, sertaline) and serotonin-norepinephrine-reuptake inhibitors (SNRIs, e.g. velnafexine). Dose requirements for SSRIs and SNRIs vary; starting doses can be lower than those used to treat depression. Clonidine, an alfa adrenergic agonist, when taken orally or transdermally results in reduction in hot flushes ranging from 20–80%. It is not clear whether Gabapentin is effective or not.

For treatment of hot flushes, soy protein has been used, but its efficacy has not been confirmed. Black cohosh, other medicinal herbs, vitamin E, and acupuncture do not appear helpful. Vaginal lubricants and moisturizers may help to relieve vaginal dryness.

Red clover which contains 4 phyto-estrogens has also to be found ineffective in treatment of hat flushes in well designed randomized controlled trial.

Clinical pearl: Although it is reasonable to discuss lifestyle changes (e.g., dressing in layers and lowering room temperature), such strategies are unlikely to be adequate in women with severe hot flushes.

Hormone Therapy

Hormone therapy (HT) is the treatment with prescription of hormonal medications-namely, estrogen alone or estrogen in combination with progestogen to restore a woman's declining hormone levels. Hormone therapy can be used if the patient has no contraindication and when lifestyle changes alone have failed to relieve moderate to severe menopausal symptoms. Forms may be oral, transdermal (a patch, lotions, or gels), or a tablet inserted vaginally. Women who have a uterus, if given estrogen in any form or type, are also given a progestin (as combination therapy) because unopposed estrogen increases risk of endometrial cancer (and possibly ovarian cancer if unopposed estrogen is taken > 10 yr). Estrogen is used alone in women who have undergone hysterectomy. A progestogen is not indicated when estrogen is used locally.

There is no absolute contraindication of hormone therapy. However, hormone therapy is relatively **contraindicated** in patients with:

- History of breast carcinoma
- History of endometrial carcinoma
- Severe active liver disease
- Porphyria
- Thromboembolic disorders
- Undiagnosed vaginal bleeding
- Endometriosis
- Fibroid uterus

Indications: Estrogen, either oral or transdermal, is the most effective treatment of vasomotor symptoms, reducing hot flushes 80–90%. Estrogen is also the most effective treatment of moderate to severe vaginal and vulvar atrophy.

Duration of use: HT is associated with a reduced risk for fractures but it is associated with potentially increased risk of breast cancer, stroke, thromboembolic and cardiovascular events. The general approach is to take lowest effective dose for the shortest time. Recommendations for duration of use of HT differ for estrogen and estrogen progestogen therapy. For estrogen progestogen therapy, duration of use is limited by breast cancer risk with use for 3 to 5 years. For estrogen therapy, there is more flexibility in duration of use because the risk for breast cancer is not increased after 7 years of follow-up.

Dosage schedule: There are 3 common combination regimens, progestins for a minimum of 10–14 days each month is recommended for endometrial protection.

1. A continuous combination regimen of both estrogen and progestins daily
2. A cyclic sequential regimen in which estrogen and progestin given daily on day 1 day 25 of month followed by an withdrawal bleeding on day 26– day 31.
3. A cyclic sequential regimen in which estrogen is given on days 1 to 21 of the month then no estrogen for 7 days, progestin is added on day 7– day 21 and then stopped on the same day as the estrogen. Withdrawal bleeding occurs on day 22– day 30.

The dosage varies but the most commonly prescribed HT is combined estrogen and progestin in the form of 0.625 mg/d CEE with 2.5 mg/d MPA in women with an intact uterus. Lower dose preparations that contain 1.5 mg/d of MPA with either 0.45 mg or 0.3 mg/d of CEE are becoming increasingly popular.

The estrogens most commonly prescribed are conjugated equine estrogens (CEE, natural estrogen) or synthetic, micronized 17β estradiol, and ethinyl estradiol. The progestins that are used commonly are medroxyprogesterone acetate (MPA) and norethindrone acetate.

Clinical pearls

- Hormone therapy remains an appropriate treatment for moderate to severe menopausal symtoms
- Hormone therapy should not be used for prevention of chronic diseases
- HT is associated with a reduced risk for fractures and increased risks for ischemic stroke, thromboembolism, and breast cancer.

Keywords

Menopause: Menopause is diagnosed retrospectively after 12 months of amenorrhea due to loss of ovarian follicular activity .

Hot flush: A hot flush is a sudden feeling of warmth that is generally most intense over the face, neck, and chest. The duration is variable but averages about 4 minutes. It is often accompanied by sweating that can be profuse and followed by a chill

Hormone therapy: Hormone therapy refers to treatment with estrogen or estrogen plus progesterone with progesterone taken at least 10–14 days per month.

EXERCISES

Answer the following questions

1. Define—Menopause, menopausal transition, perimenopause, postmenopause
2. What is premature menopause? what are its causes?
3. What hormonal changes occur in perimenopause?
4. Describe sex sreroid production in postmenopausal period.
5. What are the symptoms of menopause?
6. What are vasomotor symptoms?
7. What causes hot flushes?
8. How long vasomotor symptoms continued?
9. What are the genital and neuropsychiatric changes in menopause?
10. How you diagnose menopause?
11. How do you manage menopausal symptoms?

Write short notes on

1. Pathophysiology of menopause
2. Hormone therapy
3. Menopausal symptoms

Explain or justify the following statements

1. Menopause can be managed with lifestyle changes
2. Hormone therapy should be used carefully in post menopausal women.

Fill in the blanks

1. Menopause before _____ years is known as premature menopause.
2. After menopause ovaries continue to secrete _____ hormone.
3. After menopause the vaginal PH is _____ .
4. Long term complications of hypoestrogenic state following menopause are _____ , _____ .
5. Consistently elevated level of FSH above _____ ml/L predicts menopause
6. Indication of using hormone therapy is _____ .
7. Three contraindications of hormone therapy are _____ , _____ , _____ .
8. Major side effects of hormone therapy include _____ , _____ , _____ .

Questions for practical (read the case summary at the beginning of chapter before answering the questions)

1. How do you explain the symptoms of this patient?
2. Why vaginal mucosa is pale and speculum insertion is uncomfortable?
3. Which laboratory investigation may be considered for her?
4. How do you treat her ?
5. When do you consider her for hormone therapy?

Bibliography

1. Beckmann C R B Obstetrics and Gynecology 6th edition Lippincott Williams Wilkins 2010.
2. Gass MLS, Rebar RW. The Menopause Glob. libr. women's med., (ISSN: 1756-2228) 2008; DOI 10.3843/GLOWM.10079
3. Guidelines for Counseling Women on the Management of Menopause Produced in

Collaboration with The National Committee for Quality Assurance. The American College of Obstetricians and Gynecologists, and The North American Menopause Society February 2000.

4. Hendrix LS Menopause Merk Manual 2007

5. Mbilu J N K Essentials of Obstetrics and Gynecology for clinical officers and midwives Volume II universe 2002.

6. Practical gynecology a guide for primary care physician

7. Roberts H. Managing the menopause BMJ 2007;334;736–741.

8. Ryden J , Blumenthal PD Practical gynecology A guide for primary care physician ACP press 2009.

9. Ward C, Bowen- Simpkins P Transcript of learning module Menopause: a guide to symptoms and diagnosis Available online at: http://learning.bmj.com/learning/moduleintro/. html?moduleId=10023568

32

Postmenopausal Vaginal Bleeding

A 65-year-old woman has presented with complaint of vaginal bleeding for the first time since her natural menopause 13 years ago. The bleeding began 2 weeks ago, mild in flow and stopped spontaneously after five days. She had no pain and any other symptom. She had never received hormone therapy. On examination she was obese, hypertensive and without pallor. Her pelvic examination revealed no abnormality. How should her case be investigated?

In this chapter we will learn:
- What is postmenopausal vaginal bleeding (PMB)
- Its causes
- Clinical approach to a patient with PMB
- Differential diagnosis
- Investigations in postmenopausal bleeding per vagina
- Treatment

Introduction

Postmenopausal bleeding per vagina is a common clinical problem. Menopause is marked by 12 months of amenorrhea after the last menstrual period (*see* Chapter 31). Postmenopausal bleeding, then, is any vaginal bleeding that occurs more than 12 months after the onset of menopause. Any postmenopausal bleeding is abnormal and should be investigated because of increased risk of reproductive tract cancers in women in this age group. The most common cause of postmenopausal bleeding, however, is endometrial or vaginal atrophy and not cancer. However, endometrial cancer is responsible for 10–15% of all postmenopausal bleeding.

Abnormal bleeding in postmenopausal women who are using hormone therapy can be difficult to assess. Women on continuous estrogen and progestogen hormone therapy can expected to have irregular vaginal bleeding especially for first six months. This bleeding should cease after one year. Women on cyclical estrogen and progestogen hormone therapy should have a regular withdrawal bleeding after stopping of progestogen. Thus women will require evaluation if:

- Any postmenopausal bleeding, spotting or vaginal discharge if not on hormone therapy
- On continuous combined hormone therapy who have bleeding six months after starting treatment

- On cyclical hormone therapy who have bleeding outside the expected time of withdrawal bleed.

Clinical pearl: Postmenopausal bleeding should always be investigated as 10% patient will have endometrial carcinoma. PMB may also be the presenting symptom of cervical cancer, particularly in our country.

Causes

In order to approach the management of a patient with postmenopausal bleeding the differential diagnosis should be considered. The causes of postmenopausal bleeding are summarized in Table 32.1. Endometrial or vaginal atrophy are most common causes of PMB but more threatening causes of the bleeding such as carcinoma must first be ruled out. Common causes of PMB are discussed below.

1. *Endometrial atrophy:* The endometrium, can become very thin after menopause because of diminished estrogen levels, and may cause unexpected bleeding

2. *Endometritis* is inflammation of the endometrial lining of the uterus. In addition to the endometrium, inflammation may involve the myometrium and occasionally, the parametrium.

3. *Atrophic vaginitis:* Atrophic vaginitis is inflammation of lining of vagina due to the lower level of circulating hormone, estrogen, at this time. It is considered as the most common cause for the postmenopausal bleeding. Severe loss of estrogen results in

secondary infection caused by yeast (Candida) overgrowth or bacterial infection secondary to a host of opportunistic bacteria that are normally in or around the vagina but start to overgrow because of injury or inability of the vagina to defend itself.

4. Endometrial hyperplasia. In this condition, the endometrium may undergo hyperplasia as a result of too much estrogen and too little progesterone, and bleeding may occur as a result. Atypical endometrial hyperplasia (complex variety) will progress to adeno carcinoma in 29% cases

5. *Urethral caruncle.* Urethral caruncles, which often originate from the posterior lip of the urethra, may be described as fleshy outgrowths of distal urethral mucosa. They are usually small but can reach 1–2 cm in diameter. Most urethral caruncles are asymptomatic; however, some may be painful, and others may be associated with dysuria. Larger necrotic lesions may bleed. Some caruncular lesions may look like urethral carcinoma.

6. *Cervical cancer.* Cervical cancer appears to have a bimodal age distribution. Many women with cervical cancer, in our country, present with postmenopausal bleeding as the women are not screened for pre malignant lesions with pap smear in their reproductive age.

7. *Endometrial cancer:* Bleeding after menopause can be a sign of endometrial cancer. Endometrial cancer is the most common type of uterine cancer. Although

Table 32.1: Causes of postmenopausal bleeding per vagina	
Vaginal	Atrophy, inflammation, tumor, ulceration (e.g. decubitous ulcer in genital prolapse)
Cervical	Carcinoma, cervicitis, polyp
Uterine	Endometrial atrophy, hyperplasia, carcinoma, polyp, submucosal leiomyoma, uterine sarcoma
Ovarian	Hormone producing ovarian tumors
Vulvar	Carcinoma, ulceration or laceration, urethral caruncle
Endocrinologic	Exogenous estrogen, peripheral conversion of androgens perimenopausal ovarian functions
Others	Coagulation disorders, rectal lesions, urinary tract infections

the exact cause of endometrial cancer is unknown, increased levels of estrogen appear to play a role. Patients at risk of endometrial cancer are those who are obese, hypertensive, diabetic, nulliparous, on exogenous estrogen (including tamoxifen) or those who experience late menopause.

Approach to a Patient with Post-menopausal Bleeding per Vagina

Primary objective of diagnosing postmeno-pausal bleeding is to find out cause of bleeding and to exclude malignancy. Sometimes bleeding per rectum and hematuria may be confused with bleeding per vagina. This must be cleared from history as our concern is primarily for vaginal bleeding.

History

Important areas that should be enquired in history include amount of bleeding, number of episodes, any associated symptoms such as pain in lower abdomen or something coming out per vagina, age of menopause and menarche, menstrual bleeding pattern prior menopause, history of hormone intake, use of tamoxifen or anticoagulants. It is also important to enquire about nonprescription medication such as phyto-estrogens. In addition the presence of other co morbid conditions such as diabetes, hypertension should also be recorded.

Examination

General physical examination should include presence of pallor, obesity and hypertension. **Abdominal examination** should look for presence of any abdominal masses. Presence of lower abdominal lump may be indicative of Pyometra, uterine sarcoma or ovarian malignancy. **Inspection of perineum** is done to detect prolapsed uterus with decubitous ulcer or any vulval ulcer or growth. During palpation, urethral meatus is examined separating the labia for any curuncle.

A **speculum examination** should be performed to detect atrophic vaginitis and to rule out malignant lesions of vagina, cervix and cervical polyps, ulcer. **Bimanual examination** should be performed to assess uterine size, mobility and position. Cervical or vaginal masses that were not seen in speculum examination may be palpated, as well as detection of adnexal masses. **Recto-vaginal examination** allows detection of nodularity in pouch of doughlus.

Clinical pearl: Abnormal bleeding should NEVER be an excuse, on the part of either the patient or the doctor, not to perform a pelvic examination, as it is usually indicative of a problem.

Differential Diagnosis

Atrophic vaginitis/endometritis: Atrophic vaginitis can be diagnosed by direct inspection of vagina. The patient may complain of soreness or pain in vagina on intercourse with or without bleeding. Speculum examination reveals a thin friable vaginal wall that may bleed upon opening the speculum. Vagina looks atrophic, thin and red and may show evidence of bleeding. If the vagina is atrophic, endometrium is also atrophic. Endometrial atrophy with dysfunctional shedding of endometrium is the commonest cause of post-menopausal bleeding, accounting for up to 80% of cases. This diagnosis can only be made after evaluation of endometrium to exclude uterine cancer. Women with atrophic endometritis usually have been post-menopausal for over 10 years. There is often minimal tissue or mucous or blood in endometrial biopsy.

Cervical polyps: Cervical polyps can originate from endocervix and ectocervix as a result of focal hyperplasia. They are composed of a central vascular and connective tissue stroma covered by squamous, columner or squamo-columner epithelium. The surface epithelium may show squamous metaplasia. And tissue at the tip of polyp is often necrotic. They most often are found in women in their reproductive years but can occur at menopause. Asymptomatic polyps are found on routine vaginal examination or may present with postcoital, inter menstrual or postmenopausal bleeding.

Endocervical polyps are more common than ectocervical polyps. They appear as red protrusions from the cervical os. They can vary in length and diameter from few millimeter up to 3 cm.

Ectocervical polyps are less vascular and more fibrous than endocervical polyps. They are paler and smoother in appearance and less likely to bleed than endocervical polyps.

They can easily be removed by grasping with sponge forceps and twisting on their pedicle. The polyp should be sent for histopathological examination.

Endometrial polyps: The incidence of endometrial polyp varies with age reaching a peak in the fifth decade of life. Because they are estrogen sensitive, their incidence decline after menopause. They are also associated with tamoxifen use and are most common endometrial abnormality seen with Tamoxifen use. Rarely endometrial polyp may undergo malignant change into carcinoma or sarcoma.

Most polyps occur in fundal region and project down into the endometrial cavity. Larger polyp can extend up to the vaginal introitus. They are composed of a central fibrous stroma containing large vascular channels covered by endometrial epithelium.

In postmenopausal women endometrial polyp can cause postmenopausal bleeding that is usually light. Sometimes a polyp may infarct and there is more sudden onset bleeding accompanied by crampy abdominal pain. Hysteroscopy can indentify endometrial polyp by direct visualization. Saline infusion sonograms have been used to indentify the polyps that show up as filling defects. Pelvic ultrasound does not reveal endometrial polyps unless they are particularly large.

Endometrial hyperplasia: Endometrial hyperplasia cover a wide range of pathological changes in the uterine glands and stroma. Hyperplasia can be simple or complex with or without atypia. The presence of atypia is the most worrisome feature as approximately 20% of those with atypical hyperplasia will have a concomitant endometrial carcinoma and another 25% will develop endometrial carcinoma within two years if the condition remain untreated.

Endometrial carcinoma: Over 90% of women with endometrial carcinoma presents with vaginal bleeding. The diagnostic accuracy of endometrial biopsy by endometrial sampling (see below) for endometrial cancer is over 90% when compared to dilatation and curettage (D&C).

Clinical pearl: Assessment of endometrium is essential even in the presence of obvious atrophic vaginitis or cervical polyp.

Investigations

The cause of majority of the cases with PMB can be identified with history, clinical exanimation, cytology and biopsy procedures. It may be necessary to look for blood in stool or urine if the source of bleeding is not clear. Hemoglobin estimation with full blood count is needed if the bleeding is prolonged or heavy. If the physical examination does not reveal the cause for PMB, it is necessary to evaluate the endometrium.

Papanicolaou smear: A papanicolaou smear should be done in any women presenting with postmenopausal bleeding. The presence of dysplastic cells, atypical glandular cells or endometrial cells necessitates evaluation of cervix and endometrium with colposcopy and biopsy.

Ultrasonography: Transvaginal ultrasound gives better visualization of the endometrium than does transabdominal ultrasound and allows measurement of endometrial thickness.

It also provides an opportunity to evaluate the pelvis for any related or incidental pathology especially in ovaries. It is in general true that thicker the endometrium of a postmenopausal woman the higher the likely hood of endometrial cancer be present. According to the most recent evidences, an endometrial thickness of more than 3 mm is considered abnormal and further investigation will be required (except for women on sequential combined hormone therapy cut off point of 5 mm or less is normal).

The transabdominal ultrasound may be used as a complimentary examination if the uterus is significantly enlarged or a wider view of pelvis and abdomen is required. In some women where transvaginal ultrasound may be technically difficult and trans-abdominal ultrasound may be considered.

Biopsy: The gold standard for diagnosis of any malignancy is biopsy. Histopathological examination of any abnormality of the genital tract is mandatory in this age group. Any growth, present in vulva, vagina or cervix should be biopsied for histopathological examination. The techniques used for endometrial biopsy include:

- Endometrial sampling
- Endometrial curettage
- Hysteroscopy and biopsy

Endometrial sampling: Endometrial biopsy can be obtained using endometrial samplers (e.g. Pipelle endometrial sampling). A plastic tube like device is inserted into the uterine cavity and the plunger is withdrawn and the negative pressure permits aspiration of tissue into the device. When there is small focus of malignancy, endometrial sampling is more likely to miss it, because it samples a small percentage of the endometrial area.

Dilatation and curettage (endometrial curettage): This involves curetting of the endometrial cavity in a systematic fashion. The technique is blind and operator cannot assess whether lesion have been missed or not.

Hysteroscopy and biopsy: Hysteroscopy allows the operator to directly visualize the endometrial cavity. A biopsy of the endometrium is generally taken following hysteroscopy either with a sampler or by curettage. Hysteroscopy and biopsy should be reserved for cases in which endometrial sampling cannot be performed due to cervical stenosis or patient discomfort or where bleeding persists following a negative biopsy or where an inadequate specimen was obtained.

Saline infusion sonography (SIS): In saline infusion sonography, saline is infused through a catheter in to the endometrial cavity during ultrasound to improve the image. The saline separates the two walls of endometrium, allowing their thickness to be measured. It also allows the clinician to evaluate the uterus for intracavitory lesion such as fibroid or polyp.

Treatment

Treatment of postmenopausal bleeding is directed towards the organic cause which is diagnosed. If no cause is detected and there is minimal bleeding, patient can be observed carefully. In case of repeated episode of post-menopausal bleeding, it is better to perform hysterectomy with bilateral salpingo-oopho-rectomy, even when diagnosis can not be established by endometrial biopsy.

A brief out line of treatment of common causes of postmenopausal bleeding is mentioned below.

Treatment of cervical polyp: Most cervical polyps can be treated by grasping the pedicle with sponge forceps and twisting it until the polyp is avulsed (polypectomy). Polyp in which the pedicle is not visible are removed best by a dilatation and curettage (D and C) which allows the pedicle to be visualized and the whole polyp is removed.

Treatment of endometrial polyp: Treatment is removal during hysteroscopy. The specimen should always be sent for histopathological examination.

Treatment of atrophic vaginitis: Treatment is topical or systemic estrogens. The addition of progestogen is needed if we use systemic estrogen with intact uterus. It is not necessary to use progestogen in conjunction with topical estrogen, although the estrogen cream should be used on cyclical basis. The patient should be instructed to apply estrogen cream every night for 3 weeks, followed by a treatment free week. The cyclical regimen can be continued or the patient can reduce use to a maintenance level at which she remains asymptomatic. There is evidence that topical estrogen does not increase the risk for endometrial cancer but it is prudent to use the lowest dose of estrogen so that the vaginal tissue is maintained and cancer risk is not increased.

Treatment of endometrial hyperplasia: Endometrial hyperplasia in patients without cytologic atypia responds well to progestin therapy (response rate 80%). It is reasonable to start with 20 mg of medroxyprogesterone acetate twice a day for 3–6 months and then an endometrial biopsy is repeated. If hyperplasia is still present, a hysteroscopy and biopsy should be performed. If hysteroscopy confirms presence of hyperplasia, an additional 3 months of progesterone therapy can be given followed by another endometrial biopsy or a hysterectomy may be performed. Hyperplasia with atypia responds less well to progesterone treatment and definitive treatment in postmenopausal women should be hysterectomy. Those patients medically unfit for surgery can be treated with high dose progesterone but need to be reassessed frequently with endometrial sampling for reversal of changes.

Treatment of cervical cancer: Surgery, radiotherapy and chemoradiation are different treatment options depending upon the stage of the disease.

Treatment of endometrial cancer: Surgery with a total abdominal hystetrectomy with bilateral salpingo-oophorectomy is the mainstay of treatment. Subsequent treatment with radiation or chemotherapy depends on staging of the tumor.

Keywords

Postmenopausal bleeding: Vaginal bleeding occurring at least one year after onset of menopause.

Atrophic vaginitis: Thinning and inflammation of vaginal wall due to a decline in estrogen level.

Polyp: Any growth or mass protruding from mucous membrane. Polyp may be attached with a membrane by a thin stalk (pedunculated polyp) or they may have broad base (sessile polyp).

Endometrial sampling: Endometrial sampling, is a technique of removing a piece of tissue from the endometrium for histopathological examination. This less invasive diagnostic procedure was introduced by Novak in 1935 as an alternative to dilatation and curettage. Pipelle sampling has been shown to be as effective as D and C in diagnosing malignancy.

Hyperplasia without atypia: Glands are crowded without cytologic atypia; these have a < 1% progress to carcinoma.

Simple hyperplasia: Glands are not back-to-back

Complex hyperplasia: Glands are back-to-back Hyperplasia with atypia Glands are crowded with cytologic atypia; Risk of endometrial carcinoma in simple hyperplasia with atypia and complex hyperplasia with atypia is 8% and 29% respectively.

EXERCISE

Answer the following questions

1. What is postmenopausal bleeding?
2. What are its causes?
3. Which are common causes?
4. How do you clinically approach to a patient with PMB?
5. When do you investigate a women with PMB if she is on hormone therapy?
6. What are the investigations available for evaluation of endometrium?
7. What are their advantages and disadvantages?

8. How do you treat a case of post-menopausal bleeding?

Write short notes on

1. Atrophic endometritis
2. Endometrial hyperplasia
3. Cervical polyp
4. Endometrial polyp

Fill in the blanks with appropriate word/s

1. Commonest cause of PMB is _____ .
2. Endometrial cancer is responsible for _____ % of PMB.
3. Carcinoma cervix may present with PMB as it has _____ age distribution and not screened in our country.
4. Endometrial hyperplasia may be _____ or _____ with or without atypia.
5. A transvaginal endometrial thickness more than _____ mm is considered abnormal in presence of PMB.
6. The techniques of endometrial biopsy include _____ , _____ , and _____.
7. Endometrial hyperplasia with atypia should be treated with _____ .

Explain or justify the following statements

1. PMB should always be investigated
2. Endometrium in case of PMB can be evaluated by noninvasive methods.

Questions for practical (read the case summary at the beginning of chapter before answering questions)

1. What are the possible causes of bleeding in this case?
2. Which one is likely cause and why?
3. Which investigations you will consider for her and why?
4. How do you treat her?

Bibliography

1. Bindra V, Paul B Practical manual of Obstetrics and Gynecolgy for residents and fellows Jaypee 2011.
2. Brand AH. The woman with post menopausal bleeding Australian Family Physician Vol. 36, No. 3, March 2007.
3. Breijer MC, et al. Diagnostic strategies in post menopausal bleeding Obstetrics and Gynecology International 2010.
4. Callahan T L , Caughey A B Blueprints Obstetrics and Gynecology Lippincott Williams and Willkins 2013.
6. Evaluation of postmenopausal bleeding Indian Menopause Society Guideline number 4 2010.
7. Goldstein RB. Evaluation of the Woman With Postmenopausal Bleeding Society of Radiologists in Ultrasound-Sponsored Consensus Conference Statement American Institute of Ultrasound in Medicine o J Ultrasound Med 20:1025–1036, 2001.
8. Mbilu JNK. Essentials of Obstetrics and Gynecology for clinical officers and midwives Volume II universe 2002.
9. Munsey AL. Post menopausal bleeding Evaluation and management Clinics in Family Practice; Volume 4; Number 1; March 2002.
10. Obstetrics and Gynecology clinical cases uncoverd.
13. Obstetrics and gynecology Phelan and Chiang.
14. Phelan St, Phelan ST, Chiang S. Obstetrics Gynecology Hayes Barton Press 2003.
15. Practical manual of obstetrics and gynecology for residents and fellows.
16. Ramsay P. Investigation of post menopausal bleeding.
17. Ultrasonography in obstetrics and Gynecology - a practical approach Kruger M , Botha H Clinical Gynecology Juta Pulishers 2011.

Contraception

Introduction

Contraception means avoidance of pregnancy in sexually active couple. Contraception is practiced for many reasons, such as pregnancy planning, limiting the number of children, avoiding medical risks of pregnancy (especially with heart disease, diabetes mellitus) and controlling the world population. A wide variety of effective contraceptive methods is currently available. None is completely without side effects or categorically without danger—for example, an intrauterine device (IUD) can cause perforation of uterus and may enter in peritoneal cavity. However, contraception poses less risk than does pregnancy.

Counselling

Counselling enable clients to make contraceptive choices that best fit their values and needs; it should lead to greater satisfaction and more correct and longer use of contraception, particularly when partners are involved. The World Health Organization identifies four types of clients according to their counselling needs:

■ New clients with no method in mind
■ New clients with a method in mind
■ Returning clients with no problems
■ Returning clients with problems.

Family planning providers must therefore be both knowledgeable and skilled in communicating information. Decision-making concerning contraception is, for many people, a deeply personal and sensitive issue, often involving religious or philosophical convictions. Thus, it is important for the clinician to approach the client with particular sensitivity, empathy, maturity, and non-judgmental behaviour. The GATHER technique is one such method used to organize the elements of the counselling process. This acronym is designed to remember important points in an effective counselling session. GATHER is one approach to counselling; in practice, counselling should be tailored to the woman's individual needs and circumstances and thus may follow a different sequence or require other techniques. GATHER means:

G Greet Greet the woman
A Ask Ask her about herself
T Tell Tell her about family planning
H Help Help her select a method
E Explain Explain how to use the method
R Return visit/Refer

Contraceptive Methods

Methods of variable effectiveness that are in use include:

- *Behavioural*
  i. Withdrawal method
  ii. Periodic abstinence
  iii. Lactational amenorrhoea method
- *Barrier methods*
  i. Male condom
  ii. Female condom
  iii. Diaphragm
  iv. Cervical cap
  v. Spermicidal (nonoxynol-9).

- *Hormonal contraception*
  i. Combined oestrogen/progestogen contraception (pills, patch, or vaginal ring)
  ii. Progestogen-only contraception (pill, injection, implant, or progestogen intrauterine device [IUD]).
- *Intrauterine devices*
  i. Copper IUD
  ii. Progestogen (progestin) IUD
- *Sterilization*
  i. Tubectomy
  ii. Vasectomy
- *Emergency contraceptives*
  i. Progestogen-only emergency contraception: levonorgestrel
  ii. Oestrogen/progestogen emergency contraception
  iii. Copper IUD
  iv. Selective progesterone-receptor modulator (ulipristal).

Table 33.1: Contraceptive failure rates during first year of use		
Method	% of women with pregnancy Typical use	% of women with pregnancy Perfect use
No method	85	85
Withdrawal	27	4
Periodic abstinence	-	3–5
Lactational amenorrhoea method	5	2
Condom		
Male	15	2
Female	1	2
Diaphragm	16	6
Sponge		
Parous women	32	20
Nulliparous	16	9
Combined pill and progestogen only pill	8	0.3
Contraceptive patch, contraceptive ring		
Depo-Provera	3	0.3
Implanon	0.05	0.05
IUD		
Copper T 380A	0.8	0.6
LNG IUS (Mirena)	0.2	0.2
Female sterilization	0.5	0.5
Male sterilization	0.15	0.1

Source: Trussell J. Contraceptive efficacy. In: Hatcher RA, Trussell J, Nelson AL, Cates W, Stewart FH, Kowal D. Contraceptive technology: nineteenth revised edition. New York NY: Ardent Media, 2007.

Contraceptive Effectiveness

Effectiveness is related to the acceptability of the contraceptive method and to compliance. "Typical use" is considerably less effective than "perfect use" (correct and consistent use). Failure rates and effectiveness of different methods are shown in Tables 33.1 and 33.2.

Fact sheet: Even though a wide variety of contraceptive choices are available in India, contraceptive prevalence in the country is only 56% as per the WHO Global Health Statistics 2012.

Behavioural Methods

Withdrawal Method or Coitus Interruptus

One of the oldest contraceptive methods is withdrawal of the penis before ejaculation. This process results in deposition of the semen outside the female genital tract. It has the disadvantage of demanding sufficient self-control by the man so that withdrawal precedes ejaculation. Although the failure rate probably is higher than that of most methods, reliable statistics are not available. Even when performed perfectly, the withdrawal method may fail if there are live sperm in the man's pre-ejaculate. Risk of failure may be reduced if the man urinates before intercourse.

Periodic Abstinence

It has long been known that women are fertile for only a few days of the menstrual cycle. The periodic abstinence (rhythm or natural family planning) method of contraception requires that coitus be avoided during the time of the cycle when a fertilizable ovum and motile sperm could meet in the fallopian tube. Following are the methods based on this principle:

a. *Calendar methods:* Calendar-based methods require abstaining from unprotected intercourse during the woman's fertile period, which is estimated from the typical length of her menstrual cycle and from assumptions about the timing of ovulation, the length of time the ovum is capable of being fertilized, and the length of time sperm can survive in the female genital tract. One method estimates the fertile period to be from the length of the shortest cycle –18 to the length of the longest cycle –11. For example, if the woman's shortest cycle was 25 days and her longest cycle was 29 days, her fertile period (i.e., when abstinence is required) would be from day 7 through day 18.

b. *Cervical mucus method:* The cervical mucus method requires checking the quality and quantity of cervical mucus each day; the fertile period is indicated by clear, wet, and slippery mucus. Abstinence from unprotected intercourse is necessary during the preovulatory period (as intercourse interferes with interpreting the cervical mucus signs), and from the time fertile mucus appears through 3 days after the last day of fertile mucus.

c. *Basal body temperature method:* The basal body temperature method is based on temperature changes throughout the menstrual cycle. A rise of 0.4° F to 0.8° F above the mean temperature of the pre-

Table 33.2: Comparing family planning methods		
Most effective and easiest to use	Very effective but must be carefully used	Effective but must be carefully used
Female sterilization	Breastfeeding method (LAM)	Male condom
Vasectomy	Pills	Female condom
IUD	Injectables	Withdrawal method
Implants		Calendar method
		Symptothermal method

ovulatory phase for 3 days indicates ovulation has occurred. Therefore, abstinence is required from the time of menses until 3 days after the rise in temperature.

d. *Symptothermal method:* The symptothermal method is the use of at least two of the previously described methods simultaneously and also may rely on other physiologic changes during the menstrual cycle, including midcycle pain and bleeding as well as position and texture of the cervix.

Lactational Amenorrhea Method (LAM)

The conditions under which breastfeeding can be used safely and effectively for birth-spacing purposes are developed for the use of lactational amenorrhoea in family planning. These conditions include the following three criteria, all of which must be met to ensure adequate protection from an unplanned pregnancy:

1. Amenorrhoea
2. Fully or nearly fully breastfeeding
3. Less than six months postpartum.

Another contraceptive method must be used as soon as these criteria are no longer fulfilled. Lactational amenorrhea is 95 to 98% effective for pregnancy prevention (typical to perfect use). The beneficial effects of exclusive breastfeeding on the infant are important additional advantages.

Barrier Methods

Male Condom (Fig. 33.1)

The condom, or contraceptive sheath, serves as a cover for the penis during coitus and prevents the deposition of semen in the vagina. The most common material used for male condom manufacture is latex, although condoms are also made from polyurethane material. The **advantages** of the condom are that it provides highly effective and inexpensive contraception as well as protection against sexually transmitted

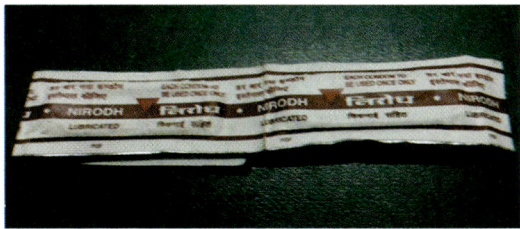

Fig. 33.1: Male condoms

infections (STIs). Male condoms can also help to prevent early ejaculation. Some condoms now contain a spermicide, which may offer further protection against failure, particularly if the condom breaks. The male condom is 85 to 98% effective for pregnancy prevention (typical to perfect use). A new condom must be used each time a couple has intercourse. Method of using condom is shown in Figs 33.2a to e. Adverse effects and disadvantages include:

- Latex allergy
- Loss of sensation
- Inconvenience/interruption of sexual intercourse
- Slippage/breakage.

Female Condom (Fig. 33.3)

The female condom is made of thin polyurethane material with 2 flexible rings at each end. The open ring remains outside the vagina, and the closed internal ring is fitted under the symphysis like a diaphragm. Female condoms have the advantage of being under the control of the female partner and of offering some protection against STIs. In vitro tests have shown the condom to be impermeable to human immunodeficiency virus, cytomegalovirus, and hepatitis B virus. It has a 0.6 percent breakage rate. Significant disadvantages may be their cost and overall bulkiness. Adverse effects and other disadvantages include:

- Friction/noise during intercourse
- Loss of sensation
- Inconvenience/interruption of sex

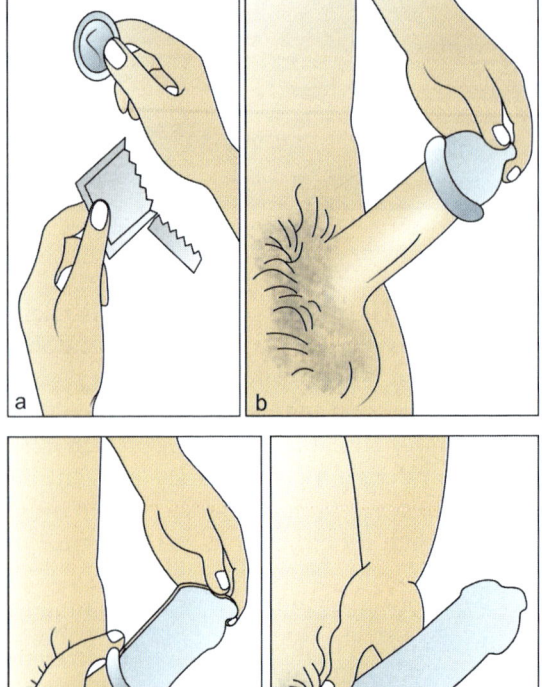

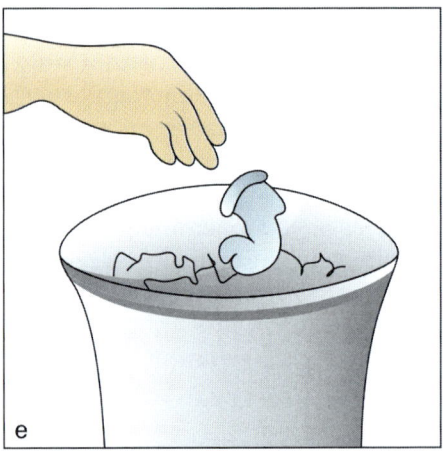

Fig. 33.2: **(a)** Use a new condom for each sex act; **(b)** Before any contact, place condom on tip of erect penis with rolled side out; **(c)** Unroll condom all the way to base of penis; **(d)** After ejaculation, hold rim of condom in place, and withdraw penis while it is still hard; **(e)** Use only once and throw away used condom safely

- Slippage/breakage (has a higher risk of slippage than the male condom).

Comparisons of the female condom with other female barrier methods such as the diaphragm and cervical cap indicate that typical use failure rates are comparable. The female condom is 75 to 95% effective for pregnancy prevention (typical to perfect use).

Vaginal Diaphragm

The diaphragm is a latex, dome-shaped cup with a flexible spring rim that acts a mechanical barrier between the vagina and the cervical canal. Diaphragms range in size from 5 to 10 cm and require fitting by a physician or a trained paramedical personnel. A contraceptive jelly or cream should be placed on the cervical side of the diaphragm before insertion because the device is ineffective without it. An appropriately placed diaphragm should completely cover the cervix; the posterior rim should lie in the posterior fornix, and the anterior rim should be just behind the symphysis pubis, with about 1 cm between the rim and the symphysis pubis. In general, the largest diaphragm that is comfortable for the woman should be prescribed. The diaphragm can be inserted up to 6 hours prior to intercourse and

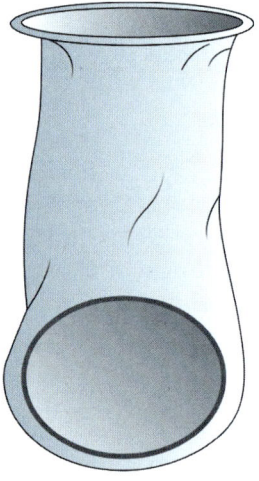

Fig. 33.3: Female condom

should be left in place for at least 6–24 hours after intercourse. When the diaphragm is of proper size (as determined by pelvic examination and trial with fitting rings) and is used according to directions, its failure rate is as low as 6 pregnancies per 100 women per year of exposure. With typical use, however, the pregnancy rate is 15–20 pregnancies per 100 woman-years. As with condoms, diaphragms offer some protection against STDs. The only side effects are vaginal wall irritation, usually with initial use or if the device fits too tightly, and an increased risk of urinary tract infections due to pressure of the rim against the urethra and alterations in the composition of the vaginal flora.

Cervical Cap

The cervical cap is a latex cup with a firm rim that covers the cervix and fits snugly around its base. To provide a successful barrier against sperm, they must fit tightly over the cervix. Because of variability in cervical size, individualization is essential. The device is used with spermicide placed in the cap before insertion and is effective for 48 hours after insertion. It should be removed no longer than 48 hours after insertion to reduce the risk of toxic shock syndrome. With proper use, the efficacy of the cervical cap is similar to that of the diaphragm, with dislodgment being the most frequently cited cause of failure in most reports.

Spermicide (nonoxynol-9)

Spermicidal vaginal jellies, creams, gels, suppositories, vaginal sponge, and foams, in addition to their toxic effect on sperm, act as a mechanical barrier to entry of sperm into the cervical canal. The spermicide contains nonoxynol 9, which is a long-chain surfactant that is toxic to spermatozoa. Spermicide must be inserted each time a couple has intercourse. Spermicides can be used alone or in conjunction with a diaphragm or condom. In general, when used alone, spermicides have a failure rate of approximately 15% per year with perfect use but double that rate with typical use. These chemical agents may irritate the vaginal mucosa and external genitalia. Recent evidence indicates that spermicides containing nonoxynol 9 are not effective in preventing cervical gonorrhea, chlamydia, or HIV infection.

Hormonal Contraception

Hormonal contraception includes:
- Combined oestrogen/progestogen contraception (pills, patch, or vaginal ring, injections)
- Progestogen-only contraception [pill, injection, implant, or progestogen intrauterine device (IUD)].

Combined Estrogen/ Progestogen Contraception

Oestrogen/progestogen contraceptives work primarily by suppressing ovulation. They are available in 4 forms:
- Combined oral contraceptive (COC) pill
- Patch
- Vaginal ring
- Injectables

Combined Oral Contraceptives

Pharmacology: The oral contraceptive pill consists of either:
- A fixed-dose combination progestogen (monophasic) usually with 30 micro gm of ethinyl oestradiol
- A combination of oestrogen and progestogen in a phasic form given daily for 3 weeks.

The estrogen that is used is ethinyl estradiol (less commonly its 3-methyl ether, mestranol). Almost all currently available progestins are 19-nortestosterone derivatives, but one is an aldosterone derivative. The progestin component of COCs varies and may include a first-generation progestogen (estranes) such as norethindrone, norethindrone acetate, ethynodiol diacetate, and norethynodrel; a second-generation progestogen (gonanes), including levonorgestrel and norgestrel; or a third-generation progestogen such as desogestrel, norgestimate, and gestodene. A newer contraceptive uses drospirenone, a spironolactone derivative, as its progestin. Drospirenone has some antimineralocorticoid activity and has been shown to decrease the water retention, and appetite changes that commonly are associated with menstrual cycle changes. Monophasic pills have constant doses of estrogen and progestin, whereas multiphasic pills vary the doses of estrogen, progestin, or both throughout the cycle. Hormonal content of commonly used monophasic combined oral contraceptive pills are shown in Table 33.3.

Mechanism of Action

Combined oral contraceptives act both centrally and peripherally:

- The primary mechanism of COCs is inhibition of ovulation by suppressing follicle-stimulating hormone(FSH) and luteinizing hormone (LH). Suppression of FSH and LH results in absence of follicular development within the ovary and therefore ovulation.

- Peripheral effects include:
  - Making the endometrium atrophic and hostile to an implanting embryo
  - Progestin thickens the cervical mucus, inhibiting the ascent of sperm into the upper genital tract
  - Progestin also alters tubal motility.

Formulations

There are many different formulations and brands of COC. Most modern preparations contain the estrogen, ethinyl estradiol, in a daily dose of between 20 and 35 microgram. Since most adverse effects are dose related, side effects have decreased with modern pill dosages. However, those containing lower dosages are associated with slightly poorer cycle control. Those containing a higher daily dosages, e.g. 50 microgram of ethinyl estradiol, are generally now only prescribed in special situations, discussed below. Higher dosages of estrogen are strongly linked to increased risks of both arterial and venous thrombosis (*see* below). Most COC contains progestogens that are classed as second or third generation. Commonly prescribed formulations are listed in Table 33.3. Monophasic pills contain standard daily dosages of oestrogen and progestogen.

Table 33.3: Hormonal content of commonly used monophasic combined oral contraceptive (COC) pills

Estrogens	Progestogens
Ethinyl estradiol 20,30,35,50 microgram	**First generation** Norethindrone Norethindrone acetate
	Second generation: Norgestrel levonorgestrel 0.15, 0.25 mg
	Third generation: Gestodene 0.075 mg Desogestrel 0.15 mg Norgestimate 0.25 mg
	Anti-mineralocorticoid and anti-androgenic: Drospirenone 3 mg

Biphasic or triphasic preparations have two or three incremental variations in hormone dose. Current thinking is that biphasic and triphasic preparations are more complicated for women to use and have few real advantages. Most brands contain 21 pills; one pill to be taken daily, followed by a 7-day pill-free interval. There are also some every-day (28 pills) preparations that includes even placebo pills that are taken instead of having a pill-free interval. Some newer products contain fewer placebo pills (e.g., 24 active pills and 4 placebo pills), with the goal of reducing the number of unintended pregnancies that occur when women miss one of the first few pills in a pack. Finally, in USA, an extended COC regimen consisting of 84 days of active pills and seven days of nonhormonal pills have been marketed containing levonorgestrel and ethinyl estradiol (Seasonale). For maximum effectiveness, COC should always be taken regularly at roughly the same time each day.

Side Effects

The vast majority of women tolerate COC well, with few problems. However, a large number of potential side effects exist, the most important relating to cardiovascular disease. Many minor side effects will settle within a few months of starting COC.

There are two major adverse effects of oral contraceptives. The first is an increased incidence of thromboembolic disease, especially in smokers (4–5 times nonusers). The death rate from thromboembolic disease in users is 3/100,000. The second is the increased incidence of coronary artery disease (Myocardial infarction) (2.7 times nonusers age 30–39 and 5.7 times nonusers age 40–44) in women who smoke. This association is so strong that oral contraceptives are contraindicated in women aged 35 who smoke.

All side effects are reduced with lower-dose products. Even so, the estrogenic components occasionally cause depression, mood changes, sleepiness, nausea, breast tenderness, fluid retention (usually 3–4 lbs), hypercoagulability (ethinyl estradiol), and hypertension (transient). Indeed, the occurrence of hypertension warrants checking (4–6 weeks, then annually) the blood pressure after initiation of therapy. Progestogens may cause weight gain, acne, nervousness, or failure of withdrawal bleeding. Both act to cause chloasma.

Use of combined oral contraceptives is associated with an increased risk of stroke, gallbladder disease, glycometabolic imbalance in women with diabetes, carcinoma of the cervix, hepatocellular carcinoma, and to a lesser degree-breast cancer in current users. Oral contraceptive use does not interfere with future pregnancies.

Drug Interaction

Certain drugs may interfere with the absorption, metabolism or efficacy of oral contraceptives. Drugs like phenytoin, rifampicin, barbiturates decrease the contraceptive effectiveness of COCs because of their liver enzyme inducing effects. Higher dose oestrogen pills containing 50 microgram ethinyl estradiol may need to be prescribed. Some broad-spectrum antibiotics can alter intestinal absorption of COC and reduce its efficacy. Additional contraceptive measures should therefore be recommended during antibiotic therapy and for 1 week thereafter. Another agent, vitamin C, competes for active sulfate in the intestinal wall and increases the bioavailability of ethinyl estradiol. Thus, erratic use of vitamin C can result in breakthrough bleeding.

Contraindications of COC

The absolute contraindications (Medical eligibility criteria—MEC category 4 conditions and relative (MEC category 3 conditions) to the combined pill and patch are listed in Tables 33.4 and 33.5 respectively.

Table 33.4: WHO Medical Eligibility Criteria category 4 conditions (absolute contraindications) for use of the combined oral contraceptive pill

Pregnancy
Undiagnosed genital bleeding
Breast cancer
Past or present circulatory disease (for example, arterial or venous thrombosis, ischemic heart disease, and cerebral haemorrhage)
Thrombophilia
Pill induced hypertension
Migraine with aura
Active liver disease, cholestatic jaundice, Dubin-Johnson syndrome, acute porphyria
Systemic lupus erythematosus
Haemolytic-uremic syndrome
Thrombotic thrombocytopenic purpura

Table 33.5: WHO Medical Eligibility Criteria category 2 or 3 conditions (relative contraindications) for use of the combined oral contraceptive pill

Smoker aged over 35 years
Hypertension (blood pressure above 140/90 mm Hg)
Diabetes
Hyperprolactinemia
Gallbladder disease
Migraine without aura
Otosclerosis
Sickle cell disease

Noncontraceptive Benefits of Combined Oral Contraceptive Use

Benefits that are reasonably established include reduction in risk of ovarian and endometrial cancer, ectopic pregnancy, pelvic inflammatory disease (PID), menstrual disorders (menorrhagia, dysmenorrhea, premenstrual syndrome), benign breast disease, iron deficiency anemia and acne. Emerging benefits include protection against bone mineral density loss, development of colorectal cancer, and progression of rheumatoid arthritis. However, COCs do not offer protection against lowergenital tract infections such as gonorrhea or chlamydia and HIV infection. While low-dose contraceptives have not been shown to affect the size of pre-

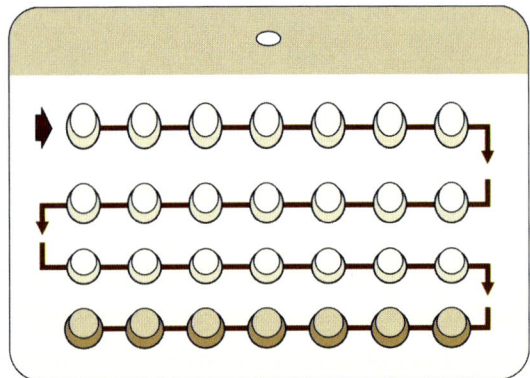

Fig. 33.4: Combined oral contraceptive pills - 21 hormonal pills (white) with 7 placebo pills

existing leiomyoma or lead to new ones, they can be effective in controlling menstrual bleeding due to leiomyoma.

Clinical Aspect

- For a woman to take COC successfully there must be careful explanation of the method, supplemented by information leaflets. Before COC is prescribed, a detailed past medical and family history should be taken. Examination should include a record of blood pressure and body weight. The breasts, heart and abdomen should be examined. A pelvic examination should be made to exclude pelvic pathology. However, routine weighing, breast and pelvic examinations are not mandatory and should not be forced on young women requesting COC. According to WHO international guidelines, the minimum requirements before starting contraception with a combined oestrogen-progestogen product consists of asking for a personal and family history of deep vein thrombosis and measuring blood pressure at baseline and follow-up.
- The pill is taken for 21 days followed by a 7-day break when withdrawal bleeding usually occurs. Everyday (ED) preparations contain 28 tablets, in which seven placebo tablets are taken during the pill free interval (PFI), may improve compliance (Fig. 33.4)

- The choice of oral contraceptive pill often depends on the doctor's preference; the list of available pills is extensive. In general:
  i. 20 microgram pills are best kept for the very thin women
  ii. 50 microgram pills are only used as emergency contraception or for women with epilepsy
  iii. The choice lies between and 30 or 35 microgram pill to be taken either continuously or as one of the triphasic pills.
- Watch for interacting drugs that are also being taken.
- Most women are given a 3-month supply of COC in the first instance, and 6-monthly reviews thereafter. Woman need clear advice about how to initiate pill taking and what to do if they miss taking their pills (*see* below).
- There may be some side-effects such as early morning nausea, breast tenderness and slight bleeding during the first cycle.

When can a woman start combined oral contraceptives (COCs)? (according to WHO Guideline)

Having Menstrual Cycles

- She can start COCs within 5 days after the start of her menstrual bleeding. No additional contraceptive protection is needed.
- She also can start COCs at any other time, if it is reasonably certain that she is not pregnant. If it has been more than 5 days since menstrual bleeding started, she will need to abstain from sex or use additional contraceptive protection for the next 7 days.

Amenorrheic

- She can start COCs at any time, if it is reasonably certain that she is not pregnant.

She will need to abstain from sex or use additional contraceptive protection for the next 7 days.

Postpartum (breastfeeding)[1]

- If she is more than 6 months postpartum and amenorrhoeic, she can start COCs as advised for other amenorrhoeic women.
- If she is more than 6 months postpartum and her menstrual cycles have returned, she can start COCs as advised for other women having menstrual cycles.

Postpartum (Non-breastfeeding)

- If her menstrual cycles have not returned and she is 21 or more days postpartum, she can start COCs immediately, if it is reasonably certain that she is not pregnant. She will need to abstain from sex or use additional contraceptive protection for the next 7 days.
- If her menstrual cycles have returned, she can start COCs as advised for other women having menstrual cycles.

Postabortion

She can start COCs immediately postabortion. No additional contraceptive protection is needed.

What can a woman do if she misses combined oral contraceptives (COCs) (according to WHO guideline)?

Missed 1 or 2 active (hormonal) pills or if she starts a pack 1 or 2 days late

- She should take an active (hormonal) pill as soon as possible[2] and then continue taking pills daily, 1 each day.
- She does not need any additional contraceptive protection.

---

[1]Women less than 6 weeks postpartum who are primarily breastfeeding should not use COCs. For women who are more than 6 weeks but less than 6 months postpartum and are primarily breastfeeding, use of COCs is not usually recommended unless other more appropriate methods are not available or not acceptable.

[2]If a woman misses more than 1 active (hormonal) pill, she can take the first missed pill and then either continue taking the rest of the missed pills or discard them to stay on schedule. Depending on when she remembers that she missed a pill(s), she may take 2 pills on the same day (one at the moment of remembering, and the other at the regular time) or even at the same time.

Missed 3 or more active (hormonal) pills or if she starts a pack 3 or more days late

- She should take an active (hormonal) pill as soon as possible[2] and then continue taking pills daily, 1 each day.
- She should also use condoms or abstain from sex until she has taken active (hormonal) pills for 7 days in a row.
- If she missed the pills in the third week, she should finish the active (hormonal) pills in her current pack and start a new pack the next day. She should not take the 7 inactive pills.
- If she missed the pills in the first week and had unprotected sex, she may wish to consider the use of emergency contraception.

Missed any inactive (nonhormonal) pills

She should discard the missed inactive (nonhormonal) pill(s) and then continue taking pills daily, 1 each day.

Contraceptive Patch

The oestrogen/progestogen patch contains hormones that are absorbed transdermally. It releases 20 mcg of ethinyl estradiol and 150 mcg of norelgestromin per day. Its mechanism action is same as OCPs. Each package contains 3 patches. The patch is applied weekly for three weeks, followed by a patch-free week during which withdrawal bleeding occurs. Because each patch releases adequate hormone levels to last 9 days, women who change their patch 1 to 2 days late do not increase their risk of unintended pregnancy. Recommended application sites include the upper arm, buttocks, lower abdomen, and upper torso (excluding the breasts). The most common adverse effects of the patch include:

  i. Spotting
  ii. Skin irritation
 iii. Nausea.

Most adverse effects improve after the first 2 or 3 cycles; persistent adverse effects often resolve when a patient changes to a different oestrogen/progestogen formulation. The patch is 92 to 99% effective for pregnancy prevention (typical to perfect use).

Contraceptive Vaginal Ring

A combined contraceptive vaginal ring (Nuvaring, Organon) is now licensed in India. It is a flexible polymer ring with an outer diameter of 54 mm and an inner diameter of 50 mm. Its core contains ethinyl estradiol and the progestin, etonogestrel. The ring releases ethinyl estradiol at a rate of 15 mcg per day and etonogestrel at a rate of 120 mcg per day, and is placed in the vagina for three weeks. The ring works in a similar manner as OCPs, but daily action by the patient is not required. The ring is initially placed within 5 days of the onset of menses. It is removed after 3 weeks of use for 1 week to allow withdrawal bleeding. After this, a new ring is inserted. Breakthrough bleeding is uncommon. Almost 20 percent of women and 35 percent of men reported being able to feel the ring during intercourse. If this is bothersome, the ring may be removed for coitus, but should be replaced within 3 hours. In all other respects, including efficacy, the ring is no different from the pill.

Combined Injectable Contraceptive

Combined injectable contraceptives (CICs) provide for the release of a natural estrogen plus a progestogen and act through the inhibition of ovulation. Two CIC formulations, both given at four-week intervals, are considered here: (1) Cyclofem = medroxyprogesterone acetate 25 mg plus estradiol cypionate 5 mg (2) Mesigyna = norethisterone enantate 50 mg plus estradiol valerate 5 mg. CICs contain the naturally occurring estrogen, estradiol. Estradiol is less potent, has a shorter duration of effect and is more rapidly metabolized than the synthetic estrogens. Serum estradiol values reach a peak level by 3 to 4 days postinjection and then decline, leading to withdrawal bleeding 20 to 25 days after injection. Clinical trials have shown this contraceptive method to be highly effective, with life-table failure rates of 0 to 0.2 pregnancies per 100 women-years. However, CICs are a relatively new contraceptive method, and there are few epidemiological data on their long-term effects.

Clinical pearls: Combined oestrogen and progestogen contraceptives inhibit ovulation. Their biological effects and safety profiles are similar regardless of route of administration

Progestogen-only Contraception

Progestogen-only contraceptions are available in the form of pill, injection, implant, or progestogen intrauterine device (IUD). Progestogen-only preparations may be given to women in whom oestrogens are contra-indicated.

Progestogen-only Pill (POP)

Progestogen-only pills are also known as mini-pills and are taken daily without any pill free interval. A number of types of progestogen-only pills (POP) are available. The older formulations of POP contain a very low dose of second generation progestogen which inconsistently inhibits ovulation. Instead, their effectiveness depends more on cervical mucus alterations and effects on the endometrium. The newest POP (Cerazette) contains the third generation progestogen, 75 microgram desogestrel at a dose sufficient to inhibit ovulation in almost every cycle .

Benefits-progestogen only pills have minimal if any effect on carbohydrate metabolism or coagulation, and they do not cause or exacerbate hypertension. They may be ideal for some women who are at increased risk of cardiovascular complications. Ideal candidates include older women who smoke; women with sickle cell anemia, women with a history of thrombosis, migraine headache, hypertension, or systemic lupus erythematosus; or women with mental retardation. In addition, the mini-pill is an excellent choice for lactating women as it does not impair milk production.

When can a woman start progestogen-only pills (POPs)? (according to WHO guideline)

Having menstrual cycles

- She can start POPs within 5 days after the start of her menstrual bleeding. No additional contraceptive protection is needed (Fig. 33.5).
- She also can start POPs at any other time, if it is reasonably certain that she is not pregnant. If it has been more than 5 days since menstrual bleeding started, she will need to abstain from sex or use additional contraceptive protection for the next 2 days.

Amenorrheic

- She can start POPs at any time, if it is reasonably certain that she is not pregnant. She will need to abstain from sex or use additional contraceptive protection for the next 2 days.

*Postpartum (breastfeeding)**

- If she is between 6 weeks and 6 months postpartum and amenorrheic, she can start POPs at any time. If she is fully or nearly fully breastfeeding, no additional contraceptive protection is needed.
- If she is more than 6 weeks postpartum and her menstrual cycles have returned, she can start POPs as advised for other women having menstrual cycles.

Postpartum (non-breastfeeding)

- If she is less than 21 days postpartum, she can start POPs at any time. No additional contraceptive protection is needed.**

*For women who are less than 6 weeks postpartum and primarily breastfeeding, use of POPs is not usually recommended unless other more appropriate methods are not available or not acceptable.

**It is highly unlikely that a woman will ovulate and be at risk of pregnancy during the first 21 days postpartum. However, for programmatic reasons, some contraceptive methods may be provided during this period.

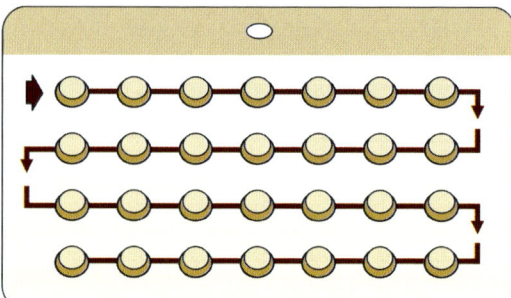

Fig. 33.5: Progestogen-only pill

- If she is 21 or more days postpartum and her menstrual cycles have not returned, she can start POPs at any time, if it is reasonably certain that she is not pregnant. She will need to abstain from sex or use additional contraceptive protection for the next 2 days.
- If her menstrual cycles have returned, she can start POPs as advised for other women having menstrual cycles.

Postabortion

She can start POPs immediately postabortion. No additional contraceptive protection is needed.

The progestogen-only pill comes in monophasic monthly packs (28 pills) without placebo pills (Fig. 33.4). To maximise efficacy, women must take each pill at the same time daily.

What can a woman do if she misses progestogen-only pills (POPs)?

Having menstrual cycles (including those who are breastfeeding) and missed 1 or more pills by more than 3 hours (12 hrs for desogestrel containing pill)

- She should:
  - Take 1 pill as soon as possible.
  - Continue taking the pills daily, 1 each day.
  - Abstain from sex or use additional contraceptive protection for the next 2 days.

- She may wish to consider the use of emergency contraception if appropriate.

Breastfeeding and amenorrhoeic and missed 1 or more pills by more than 3 hours (12 hrs for desogestrel containing pill)

- She should:
- Take 1 pill as soon as possible.
- Continue taking the pills daily, 1 each day.
- If she is less than 6 months postpartum, no additional contraceptive protection is needed.

Disadvantages: Women may or may not have a monthly menstrual period while taking the progestogen-only pill. Common adverse effects include:

- Spotting (may persist beyond the first few cycles)
- Hair or skin changes
- Headaches
- Depression
- Decreased libido.

Fertility returns quickly when women stop taking the pill.

Progestogen Injections

Depot medroxyprogesterone acetate (Depo-Provera) and norethindrone ethanthate (Norgest) are two progestogen injections that are in use. Long-acting injections of nor ethisterone-enanthate (NETEn) and depot medroxyprogesterone acetate (DMPA, Depo-Provera) are both highly effective. Depo-Provera is given by deep intramuscular injection, 150 mg every 12 weeks. Depo-povera should be begun within 5 days of the onset of menses. NET-En is administered every 8 weeks (at least initially). Their mechanisms of action are similar to those for oral agents: ovulation inhibition, increased cervical mucus viscosity, and stimulation of an endometrium unfavourable for ovum implantation.

Depot medroxyprogesterone is injected deeply into the upper outer quadrant of the buttock or into the deltoid muscles without massage to ensure that the drug is released slowly. The usual dose is 150 mg every 90 days. An additional contraceptive method should be used for at least 2 weeks after the initial injection.

Progestogen injection lowers the risk of ovarian and endometrial cancer. After 2 or more cycles, many women become amenorrhoeic. Common adverse effects include:

- Vaginal spotting (most common)
- Weight gain
- Hair or skin changes
- Headaches
- Depression
- Decreased libido. Progestogen injections cause a temporary decrease in bone density. Bone density stabilises after 2 years of use and returns to baseline levels after the method is discontinued.

Implant

The first contraceptive implant that becomes available was Norplant. Implanon, is a single rod, containing 68 mg 3-keto-desogestrel (a metabolite of desogestrel) providing contraception for 3 years. The initial release rate of 60–70 μg/day falls gradually to around 25–30 μg/day at the end of 3 years. Implanon is preloaded into a sterile disposable inserter and is inserted subdermally on the inner aspect of the non-dominant arm above the elbow. It is inserted and removed using local

anaesthetic by a clinician trained in its use. The implant is 99% effective for pregnancy prevention. Many women become amenorrhoeic after a few months. Common adverse effects include: Vaginal spotting (most common; may persist for years), weight gain, hair or skin changes, headaches, depression, decreased libido. Fertility returns quickly when the implant is removed.

> *Clinical pearl:* Progestogen-only methods act by various mechanisms and can be used by women in whom oestrogens are contraindicated.

INTRAUTERINE DEVICES

Two types of IUD are available now a days:

- *Copper IUD:* Multiload Cu250, multiload Cu375, CuT 380A,
- *Progestogen (progestin) IUD:* Levonorgestrel releasing intrauterine system (LNG-IUS)

Description of Devices

Copper IUD (Fig. 33.6): At present the most commonly used IUD is the copper T 380A. The CuT380A IUD (WHO specification 2010) consists of a T-shaped frame made from low-density polyethylene with barium sulphate added for X-ray opacity. The device is 32 mm wide and 36 mm long, with a plastic ball at the bottom of the vertical stem to guard against cervical penetration. A small hole may be located on the vertical stem near to its junction with the horizontal arms to act as an

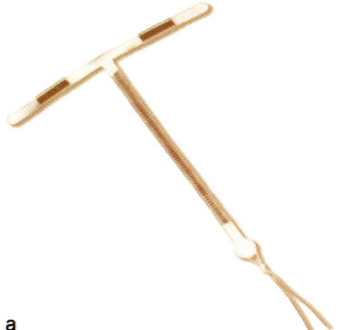

a

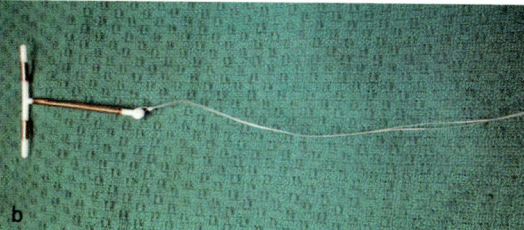

b

Figs 33.6a and b: CuT 380 A

anchor forthe copper wire. The IUD has solid copper collars on each of its two horizontal arms. Each of these collars has a surface area of 35 mm². Copper wire with a surface area of 310 mm² is wound tightly around the vertical stem, giving a total surface area of 380 mm² of copper, as indicated in the name of the device. A pigmented polyethylene filament is tied in a knot through a small hole in the ball to provide two equal-length threads as ameans to locate and remove the device.

Progestogen IUD (Figs 33.6 and 33.7): The progestin-releasing releases 20 mcg of levonorgestrel per day for 5 years and known as LNG IUS (Levonorgestrel releasing intra uterine system) or Mirena. It is a T-shaped polyethylene structure that has its stem wrapped with a cylinder made of poly dimethyl siloxane and levonorgestrel. A permeable membrane surrounds the mixture to regulate the rate of hormone release. A monofilament brown polyethylene thread is attached to a small loop at the distal end of the device's vertical body.

Mechanism of Action

- The primary mechanism of action of IUDs is to prevent fertilization. The intense local inflammatory response induced in the uterus, especially by copper-containing devices, leads to lysosomal activation and other inflammatory reactions. This leads to decreased sperm transport, inability of sperm to fertilize the ovum, and may be spermicidal.
- IUDs may also act to prevent implantation if fertilization occurs.

In the progestin-releasing IUD, the hormone also acts on the cervical mucus, endometrium and ovarian function. The progestin interferes with sperm penetration by making cervical mucus thickened. The endometrium becomes atrophic and the ovulation may be inhibited, but not consistently.

Candidates for Use

Modern IUDs are appropriate for women seeking reversible contraception, as well as by those who have completed their families. Previously (before 2005), ideal candidate for IUDs were multiparous women with a monogamous relationship without any history of PID. However, recent evidences suggest IUD use in nulliparous women is not associated with tubal infertility, and there is no delay in return to fertility after IUD removal. Moreover, the risk of pelvic infections is markedly reduced with the currently used monofilament string along with techniques to ensure safer insertion. Thus, the modern IUDs can safely be used in women who are nulliparous, nonmono-gamous, or have a past history of PID. These women are not at increased risk of infertility. However, if a potential IUD user is at risk of sexually transmitted infections, then she, like all at-risk contraceptive users, should be encouraged to use condoms.

Contraindications

Conditions for which women should not use an IUD include the following (World Health Organization Medical Eligibility Criteria—Category 4 conditions, absolute contra-indications):

- Pregnancy
- Puerperal sepsis
- Immediate postseptic abortion
- Unexplained vaginal bleeding
- Malignant gestational trophoblastic disease
- Cervical cancer (awaiting treatment)
- Breast cancer (≤ 5 years)
- Endometrial cancer
- Uterine fibroids with distortion of the uterine cavity
- Distorted uterine cavity
- PID ≤ 3 months
- Current purulent cervicitis, chlamydial infection or gonorrhea
- Known pelvic tuberculosis

Timing of Insertion

Timing of insertion is influenced by the ease of placement as well as the pregnancy and expulsion rates. Ideally, IUDs insertion should occur within the first 7 days of menstrual cycle to decrease the risk of concurrent pregnancy. However, IUDs can be inserted at any time during the menstrual cycle if the woman is not pregnant.

Postpartum IUD Insertion

(WHO recommendation) IUDs (both copper bearing and LNG IUS) (Figs 33.7 and 33.8) can be inserted within 48 hrs of delivery, including immediately after delivery of placenta (within 10 minutes). If the delivery is by caesarean section, IUDs can be placed after delivery of the placenta, before closing the uterus. The IUD also can be inserted after 4 weeks postpartum without an increased risk of perforation or expulsion.

Insertion after elective or spontaneous abortion (WHO recommendation): Following an uncomplicated first-trimester abortion, an IUD can be inserted immediately without increased risk of infection or perforation. However, the expulsion risk is higher with second-trimester abortions compared to first-trimester abortions.

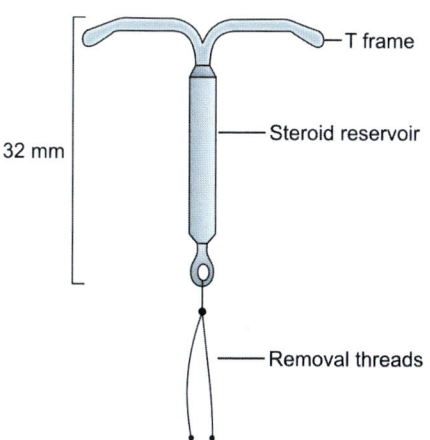

Fig. 33.7: LNG IUS—Total length of system is 32 mm

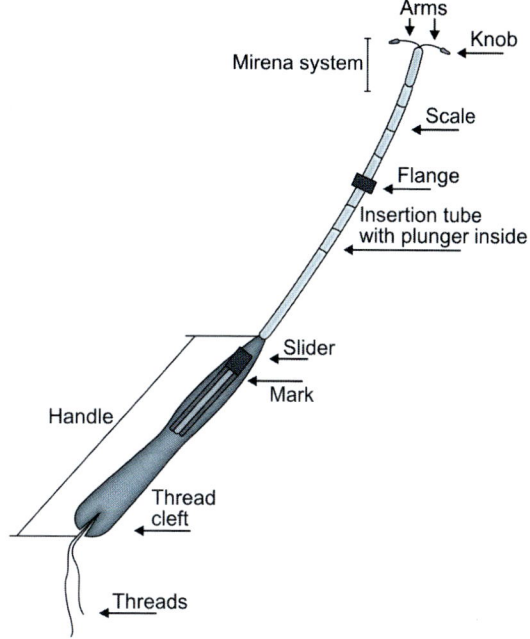

Fig. 33.8: LNG IUS with inserter

IUD for emergency contraception: The copper IUD is safe and effective for use as an emergency contraceptive if inserted within 5 days of unprotected intercourse.

Technique of Insertion

Equipment

- The equipment necessary for insertion include the IUD and package contents. The TCu380A IUD is supplied sterile in a sealed primary pack together with an insertion device. The insertion device consists of insertion tube, insertion rod, and a moveable flange (Fig. 33.9). The moveable plastic flange is positioned on the insertion tube to control the depth of insertion and to locate the IUD correctly within the uterus during insertion. The insertion rod keeps the TCu380A IUD correctly positioned within the uterus while the insertion tube is withdrawn.
- Other equipment include a speculum, an Allis tissue forceps or volsellum, an uterine sound, antiseptic solution, cotton balls,

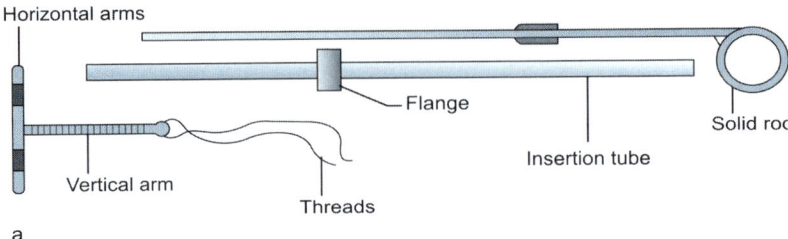

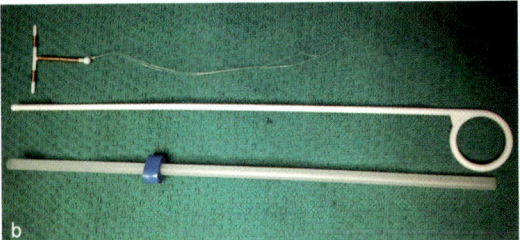

Figs 33.9a and b: Copper releasing intrauterine device Cu T 380 A

sponge holding forceps, sterile gloves, and scissors. If insertion occurs in the immediate postpartum period, ring forceps are needed.

Anesthesia

No anesthesia or analgesia is indicated for insertion of the copper T380A.

The technique for insertion of the CuT 380A is as follows:

1. Determine whether there are contraindications, counsel the woman regarding various problems associated with device use, and obtain written consent.
2. After emptying the bladder the patient is placed in comfortable lithotomy position.
3. Aseptic technique is critical. Thoroughly clean the vulva, vagina with a suitable antiseptic solution
4. Do a bimanual exam to establish the size and position of the uterus, to detect other genital contraindications, and to exclude pregnancy.
5. Gently insert a vaginal speculum to visualize the cervix.
6. Clean the cervix with antiseptic solution. Grasp the anterior lip of the cervix with a Allis tissue forceps and apply gentle traction to align the cervical canal with the uterine cavity.
7. Gently insert a uterine sound to measure the length of the uterine cavity, confirm its position.
8. The copper T380A packaging is opened by an assistant, taking care to maintain the sterility of the package contents.
9. Load the IUD into the insertion tube. This is accomplished by slightly withdrawing the insertion tube and folding the horizontal arms of the IUD down along

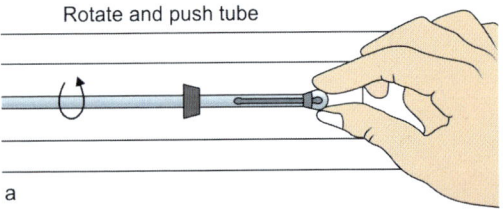

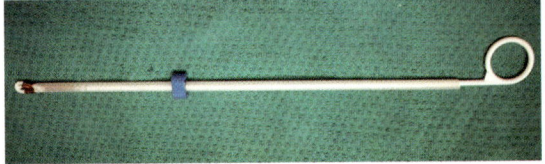

Figs 33.10a and b: Loading of Cu T

the vertical arm using the thumb and index finger. The insertion tube is then advanced so that the horizontal arms sit securely within the insertion tube..

10. Place white insertion rod into the insertion tube at the end opposite to arms and advanced to the point that it touches the bottom of the IUD.

11. Ensure blue flange is set at the distance of measured length of uterine cavity by the uterine sounds. The insertion tube is then rotated so that the horizontal arms of the IUD are parallel to the long axis of the blue flange (Figs 33.10a and b).

12. The loaded insertion tube is passed through the cervical canal until resistance is met at the uterine fundus and the blue flange should be at the external cervical os (Fig. 33.11).

13. With the solid insertion rod steady, the insertion tube is withdrawn approximately 1 cm, releasing the IUD (Fig. 33.12).

14. Advance the insertion tube slowly back into uterus until flange touches cervix to ensure correct positioning (Fig. 33.13).

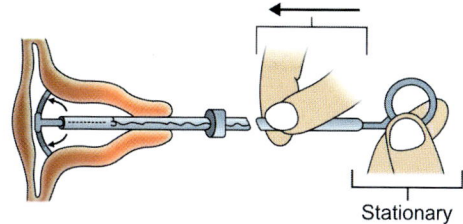

Fig. 33.13: The insertion tube is advanced for placement of the copper-releasing intrauterine device

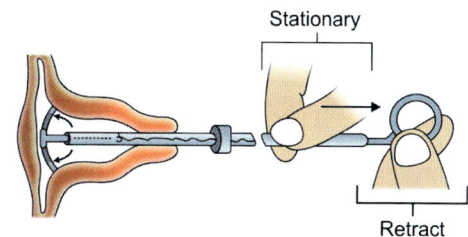

Fig. 33.14: The insertion rod of the copper-releasing intrauterine device is withdrawn

15. Remove the insertion rod entirely by holding the insertion tube in place (Fig. 33.14).

16. Then remove the insertion tube and Allis tissue forceps.

17. Cut the threads to 3 cm from the cervix

After care

- Teach patient how to locate IUD threads after the insertion
- Strings should be checked after each menses
- Follow up should be arranged after the next menses (1 month) to check threads with the patient, address any concerns or adverse effects.

Replacement

The Cu T 380A device is approved for 10 years of continuous use and the LNG IUS (Mirena) device for 5 years.

Effectiveness

The IUD is a highly effective form of long-term, reversible contraception (as effective as

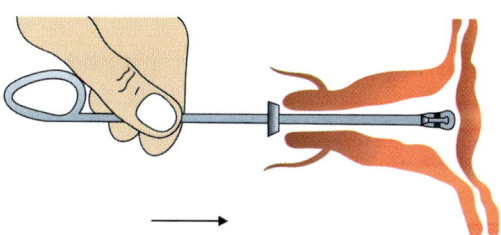

Fig. 33.11: Insertion tube reaches the fundus

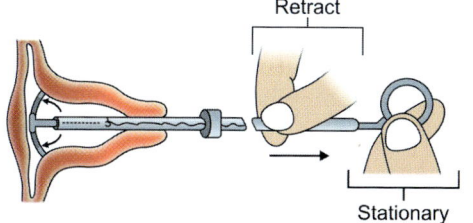

Fig. 33.12: The arms of the copper-releasing intrauterine device are released by withdrawal technique

tubectomy), with an associated failure (pregnancy) rate of less than 1% (0.8%) in the first year of use (Trussell 2004a). In a long term, international study sponsored by the WHO, the average annual failure rate was 0.4% or less.

Side Effects and Health Risks

Side effects of IUD may be unpleasant but are not harmful and in most women these subside or resolve within a few months after insertion. Some women may experience the following:

- *Menstrual changes:* There may be increase in the duration/amount of menstrual bleeding or spotting or light bleeding during the first few days or months after insertion. These usually subside with symptomatic treatment.
- Discomfort or cramps during IUD insertion and for the next few days which subsides indue course.

Potential health risks associated with the IUD, which are uncommon or rare, are discussed below:

- Uterine perforation during IUD insertion is a rare complication which occurs in 0.5 to 1.5 per 1000 insertions and is associated with level of provider's skill and experience.
- Expulsion is influenced by the skills and experience of the provider and the timing of insertion. Spontaneous expulsion is about 2–8% (Trieman et al 1995) and is most likely to occur during the first three months after insertion, and during menstrual periods. Nulliparity, heavy menstrual flow and insertion immediately postpartum or after second trimester abortion increases the chances of expulsion.
- Infection following IUD insertion is less than 1%. This minimal risk is highest during the first 20 days after IUD insertion, especially if aseptic precautions have not been taken, rather than due to the IUD itself.
- If pregnancy occurs with Copper T in situ, there is a risk of spontaneous abortion,

sepsis and ectopic pregnancy; however, IUD is not found to be having any adverse effects on the fetus.

Indications of IUD Removal

- Personal reasons (offers no reason at all)- The woman has a right to discontinue the method at any time, regardless of the reason.
- Wants another child
- At the end of effective life of intrauterine device-after of 10 years following CuT 380A insertion and after 5 years of LNG IUS insertion.
- Medical reasons (e.g., pregnancy, heavy menstrual bleeding)
- Menopause
- Evidence of IUD displacement

However, it should be ensured that she understands the following key points about having her IUD removed:

- She can get pregnant again immediately after IUD removal.
- If she does not want to become pregnant, she should immediately have another IUD inserted or
- Start another contraceptive method.

IUD Removal

Routine removal of IUDs is straightforward. The tail strings are grasped close to the external os with straight artery forceps. Gentle traction on the strings generally delivers the IUD with ease.

Management of Missing Thread/String

When the thread cannot be visualized, the possible causes are:

- The device may have been expelled
- The device may have perforated the uterus
- The thread simply may be coiled up in the uterine cavity along with a normally positioned device. In first two possibilities, pregnancy is possible.

Rule Out Pregnancy

Once pregnancy has been ruled out from history, examination and/or urine pregnancy test: Probe the cervical canal using a sterile long artery forceps to locate the threads, and gently draw them out so that they are protruding into the vaginal canal.

If the threads are not retrievable, ultrasound can localize the IUD to rule out expulsion or perforation. If the findings are negative or inconclusive for device visualization, then a plain radiograph of the abdomen and pelvis may be obtained with a uterine sound inserted into the endometrial cavity for orientation. Instillation of radiocontrast for hysteron-salpingography may also be done. Hysteroscopy is yet another alternative. Obviously none of these invasive maneuvers should be performed if a woman is pregnant and does not desire termination.

Uterine Perforation

An extrauterine copper-bearing device induces an intense local inflammatory reaction and adhesions. Copper-bearing devices are more firmly adhered and laparotomy is necessary for removal.

Pregnancy with Retained IUD

Early identification of pregnancy is important in these women. Pregnancy is identified from:
- Delayed or missed menstrual period
- Other signs/symptoms of pregnancy.

The first step in management is to confirm pregnancy and to exclude ectopic pregnancy. Up to about 14 weeks, the tail of the device may be visible through the cervix. If seen, it should be removed. If the woman does not wish to continue her pregnancy and she is in permissible period of termination (i.e. up to 20 weeks), her pregnancy should be terminated. If she wishes to continue the pregnancy and IUD can not be removed, she should be informed regarding possible complications in pregnancy like second-trimester miscarriage, infection, and preterm delivery. She should be closely monitored throughout the pregnancy and look for expelled IUD at the time of abortion/delivery.

FEMALE STERILIZATION

Female sterilization is the surgical procedure that involves blocking (commonly referred to as occluding) the fallopian tubes so that the ovum and sperm cannot meet and as a result a woman's ability to become pregnant comes to an end.

Candidate for Sterilization

Female sterilization is suitable for most women who are certain that they want no more children and need a reliable contraceptive method. From a medical perspective, the procedure is most appropriate for women who have no contraindications to surgery or anaesthesia. According to national guideline clients should fulfil following criteria:
- Clients should be married (including ever-married).
- Clients should be below the age of 49 years and above the age of 22 years.
- The couple should have at least one child whose age is above one year unless the sterilization is medically indicated.
- Clients or their spouses/partners must not have undergone sterilization in the past (not applicable in cases of failure of previous sterilization).
- Clients must be in a sound state of mind so as to understand the full implications of sterilization.
- Mentally ill clients must be certified by a psychiatrist, and a statement should be given by the legal guardian/spouse regarding the soundness of the client's state of mind.

Timing of Sterilization

- Interval sterilization should be performed within 7 days of the menstrual period (in the follicular phase of the menstrual cycle).

- Postpartum sterilization should be done after 24 hours up to 7 days of delivery (preferably within 48 hours after delivery), or during a caesarean section delivery.
- Sterilization with medical termination of pregnancy (MTP) or following spontaneous abortion can be performed concurrently.

Laparoscopic tubal ligation should not be done concurrently with second-trimester abortion and in the postpartum period.

Surgical Approaches or Procedures

Two common approaches, both through the abdomen, are used to reach the fallopian tubes:

- *Mini laparotomy* involves a small abdominal incision (Fig. 33.15) through which a surgeon usually lifts the fallopian tubes out of the abdomen to block them. The incision is 2–5 cm above the pubic hairline when a woman has not recently been pregnant or 1.5–3 cm just below the navel or umbilicus for postpartum procedures. This procedure is appropriate for women during interval, postabortion and immediate postpartum periods. During interval minilaparotomy, the provider may use a uterine elevator, a metal instrument which is inserted into the vagina to raise the uterus. This makes it easier to move the pelvic structures so that the tubes are near the incision site.
- *Laparoscopy* a laparoscope, is inserted through a small puncture near the navel,

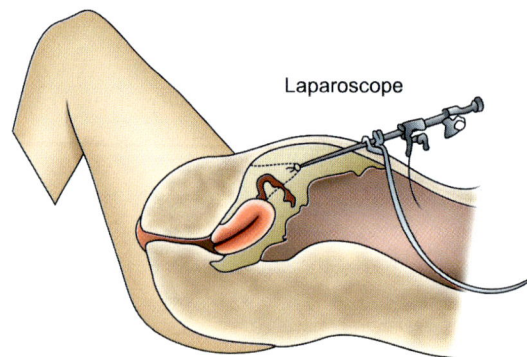

Fig. 33.16: Laparoscope illuminating the abdominal cavity

or umbilicus (Fig. 33.16). The same opening, or sometimes a second puncture, is used to manipulate the organs and block the tubes. It is recommended only for women in the interval period or following first-trimester abortion (when gestation is less than 12 weeks). Laparoscopy should not be performed on women during the postpartum period because of the orientation and the vascular nature of the postpartum uterus.

Eligibility of Providers for Performing Sterilization Operation

- Minilap services can be provided by trained MBBS doctor.
- Laparoscopic sterilization can be performed by doctors trained in laparoscopic sterilization with DGO, MD (obstetric and gynecology), or MS (Surgery) degree.

Common Techniques of Sterilization Operation

The choice of the blocking method depends upon several factors, including type of surgical approach (mini laparotomy or laparoscopy), the timing of the sterilization (postpartum or interval), provider's training, and availability of supplies. Once the provider reaches the uterine tubes, the tubes can be blocked (Fig. 33.17) by two commonly used methods:

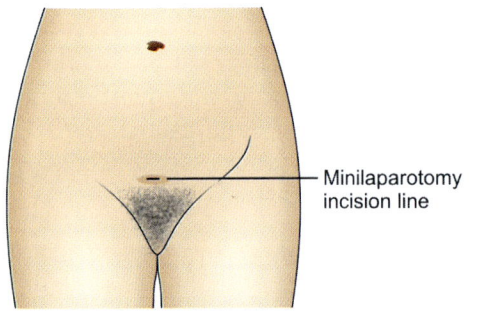

Minilaparotomy incision line

Fig. 33.15: Incision site for mini laparotomy female sterilization, interval procedure

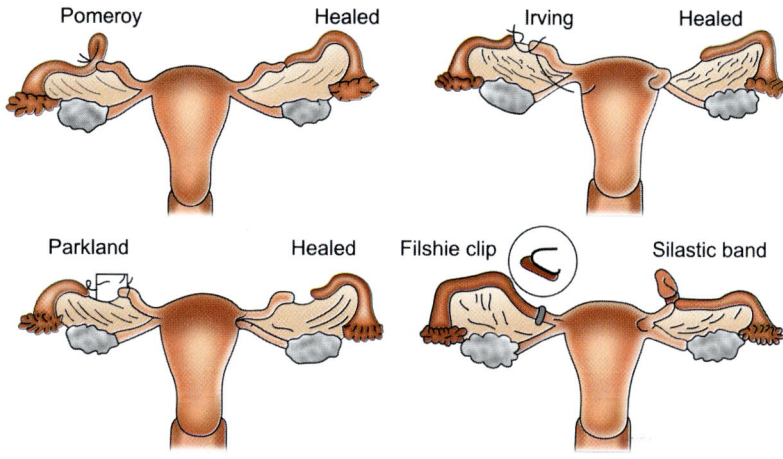

Fig. 33.17: Selected blocking techniques of sterilization

Ligation and Division

Ligation is used only with mini laparotomy (both postpartum and interval cases), this method involves tying each fallopian tube with suture material and then cutting and removing a section. The operating surgeon should identify each fallopian tube clearly, following it right up to the fimbria. The site of the occlusion of the fallopian tube must always be within 2–3 cm from the uterine cornu in the isthmal portion (this will improve the possibility of reversal if required in the future). Care must be taken to avoid damage to the blood vessels, ovaries, and surrounding tissues. Excision of 1 cm of the tube should be done. Use of cautery and crushing of the tube should be avoided.

The most common method is the Pomeroy technique, in which a segment of the fallopian tube is tied in a loop and then the top portion of the loop is cut and removed. Another method: the Parkland technique—involves tying the tube at two points and removing the intervening segment.

Two other ligation and division techniques used previously are the Uchida and Irving techniques. Both are very effective but require large incisions (the Irving has been done during caesarean section) and because of their more complicated nature, take a relatively long time to perform.

Mechanical Devices

The preferred choice for use with laparoscopy, this involves placing a device (hinged or spring clips or a small ring or band made of silicone rubber), to close and seal each tube. The various mechanical methods, which are suitable for interval cases using laparoscopy, require a specialist surgeon trained in laparoscopy. The rates of failure and complications may increase if training is inadequate or skills not maintained by routine practice of the procedure.

Electrical Methods

Electrocoagulation is used with a laparoscope to burn and block the tubes. This method is no longer recommended because research shows a greater risk for internal burns during the procedure and for ectopic pregnancy after the operation.

Complications

- **Short term:** Complications are rare and the types of complications vary by the type of surgical procedure. Complications of mini laparotomy include wound infection, bladder or intestinal injury and uterine perforation with uterine elevator. Complications of laparoscopy may involve anesthesia problems, tears and transections of the tubes, and injuries to organs from instruments such as the uterine elevator, insufflation needle or trocar.

- *Long-term:* Failure of sterilization is rare. However, when pregnancy occurs in a woman who has undergone sterilization, it is likely to be an ectopic (tubal) pregnancy. Subsequent regret about the sterilization decision is another possible consequence.

MALE STERILIZATION

Vasectomy provides permanent, non-reversible protection against pregnancy. In this operation, through a small incision in the scrotum, the lumen of the vas deferens is disrupted to block the passage of sperm from the testes. It is 99% effective for pregnancy prevention.

Eligibility of Providers for Performing Male Sterilization

Both conventional vasectomy and nonscalpel vasectomy can be performed by trained MBBS doctor.

Candidate for Male Sterilization

According to national guideline the following criteria should be fulfilled before male sterilization operation:

- Clients should be ever-married.
- Clients should ideally be below the age of 60 years.
- The couple should have at least one child whose age is above one year unless the sterilization is medically indicated.
- Clients or their spouses/partners must not have undergone sterilization in the past (not applicable in the cases of failure of previous sterilization).

- Clients must be in a sound state of mind so as to understand the full implications of sterilization.
- Mentally ill clients must be certified by a psychiatrist, and a statement should be given by the legal guardian/spouse regarding the soundness of the client's state of mind.

Timing of Surgical Procedure

Male sterilization can be done at any convenient time on healthy clients.

Surgical Techniques

Anaesthesia: Local anaesthesia is recommended for vasectomy procedures. The local anaesthetic to be used is 1% lignocaine without adrenaline. The maximum dosage is 200 mg or 20 ml of 1% lignocaine or 10 ml of 2% lignocaine (10 ml solution of 2%, to be diluted with an equal amount of distilled water).

Conventional Vasectomy

Incision: The vasectomy operation is to be performed either with two incisions located at the root of the scrotum on either side, or with one incision on the midline. The length of each incision should not be more than 2 cm. Smaller incisions will minimize the chances of complication.

Site of vasectomy: The mid-scrotal part of the vas should be removed. It must not be cut close to the epididymis, over the convoluted part of the vas deferens. Excision of vas: The vas must be separated from the tissues and excised in all cases. The portion excised should not be more than 1 cm in length. Removal of the excess length of the vas may make a re-canalization operation difficult, if it is required in the future.

Tying of cut ends of vas: The cut ends of the vas must be tied with 2′0′ silk, and the sheath of the vas (Spermatic fascia) should be interposed between the two cut ends.

Closing skin incision: The skin incision should be closed with non-absorbable sutures and covered with a piece of sterile gauze. Before closing the wound, all bleeding points must be tied so as to ensure compete hemostasis and to prevent bleeding or hematoma formation. Use of tincture of benzoin causes excoriation of the scrotal skin and should therefore be avoided for dressing.

Scrotal support: The patient should wear a suspensory bandage for one week, until the stitches are removed.

No-scalpel Vasectomy (NSV)

The basic difference between the NSV procedure and the conventional technique is in the surgical approach to the vas, which is through a small puncture in the scrotum rather than by a cut with a scalpel.

Fixation, puncture, and delivery of vas: The site of fixation and puncture of the vas will be at the junction of the upper and the middle third of the scrotum on the midline. The vas is fixed in the midline at the junction of its upper one-third and lower two-third by a vas fixation forceps. This is done by the three-finger technique. The skin is then punctured with a vas dissection forceps, the vas is dissected out, the bare vas is delivered out of the puncture hole, and is ligated and excised

Excision of vas: About 1 cm length of the bare vas should be ligated and excised. The removal of the excessive length of vas may make the re-canalization operation difficult, if it is required by the client in the future.

Ligature of vas: The cut ends of the vas should be tied with non-absorbablesuture material (2'0' black silk), and the sheath of the vas should preferably be interposed between the two cut ends.

Delivery of the opposite vas: The opposite vas must be fixed exactly in the same manner using the three-finger technique at the lower end of the previously made puncture hole. It should be punctured and delivered in the same way through the earlier hole without increasing its size.

Skin wounds: After the excision and ligature of both the vas, inspect the puncture site for any bleeding. If there is none, the puncture site should be dressed with a small piece of gauze. This should be retained for 48 hours. No stitch is applied since the puncture contracts and is nearly invisible after the removal of the instruments.

Scrotal support: The client should wear his normal snugly fitting underwear, or use scrotal support with suspensory bandage.

Disadvantage

A disadvantage of vasectomy is that sterility is not immediate. Complete expulsion of sperm stored in the reproductive tract beyond the interrupted vas deferens takes about 3 months or 20 ejaculations. So azoospermia should be documented after 3 months by semen analysis and another form of contraception must be used during this period.

Complications

Intraoperative Complications

- Convulsion or reaction to local anaesthetic agent
- Vasovagal attack
- Injury to the testicular artery

Immediate Postoperative Complications

- Swelling of scrotal tissue, bruising and pain
- Hematoma formation
- Infection—stitch abscess, wound sepsis, orchitis

Delayed Complications

- Wound granuloma
- Psychological problem
- Failure of vasectomy

There is no association of prostatic or testicular cancer and cardiovascular disorder with vasectomy.

EMERGENCY CONTRACEPTION (POSTCOITAL CONTRACEPTION)

Definition

Emergency contraception refers to contraception taken to prevent pregnancy after unprotected sexual intercourse or a potential contraceptive failure.

Situations at which emergency contraception to be used: Emergency contraception can be used in a number of situations following sexual intercourse:

- When no contraceptive has been used.
- When there is a contraceptive failure or incorrect use, for example:
  - Condom breakage, slippage, or incorrect use
  - Three or more consecutively missed combined oral contraceptive pills
  - The progestogen-only pill (mini pill) taken more than three hours late (or more than 12 hours late if taking a 0.75 mg desogestrel-containing pill)
  - Failed withdrawal (e.g. ejaculation in the vagina or on external genitalia)
  - Failure of a spermicide tablet or film to melt before intercourse
- In cases of sexual assault when the woman was not protected by an effective contraceptive method.

Methods of Emergency Contraception

There are broadly two methods of emergency contraception:

Emergency Contraception Pills (ECPs)

- *Progestogen-only emergency contraception:* Levonorgestrel
- Oestrogen/progestogen emergency contraception
- Selective progesterone-receptor modulator (ulipristal).

Copper-bearing Intrauterine Devices (IUDs)

Progestogen-only emergency contraception: WHO recommends levonorgestrel for emergency contraceptive pill use.

Dosage schedule: Women may take a single oral dose of levonorgestrel 1.5 mg within 72 hours of unprotected intercourse, or as a dose of levonorgestrel 0.75 mg followed by 0.75 mg 12 hours later. This medication is more effective the sooner it is taken, but it retains some efficacy up to 5 days after unprotected intercourse.

Mode of action: Levonorgestrel emergency contraceptive pills prevent pregnancy by preventing or delaying ovulation. They may also work to prevent fertilization of an ovum by affecting the cervical mucus or the ability of sperm to bind to the ovum. Levonorgestrel emergency contraceptive pills are not effective once the process of implantation has begun, and they will not cause abortion.

Effectiveness: Taken within 72 hours of unprotected intercourse, this method reduces the risk of pregnancy by 89%. The regimen is more effective the sooner after intercourse it is taken.

Safety: Levonorgestrel-alone emergency contraception pills are very safe and do not cause abortion or harm future fertility. Side-effects are uncommon and generally mild. Adverse effects include nausea, spotting and change in timing of menstruation. There are no medical contraindications to the use of levonorgestrel emergency contraception pills.

Oestrogen/progestogen emergency contraception: This method is also known as Yuzpe regimen.

Dosage schedule: In this regimen two 50 µg ethinyl-estradiol/250 µg levonorgestrel (LNG) pills, taken twice at 12 h intervals, as soon as possible within 72 h following unprotected intercourse.

Mode of action: Oestrogen/progestogen emergency contraception works primarily by preventing or delaying ovulation.

Effectiveness: Taken within 72 hours of unprotected intercourse, this method reduces the risk of pregnancy by 75%. This method does not disrupt an implanted pregnancy.

Safety: This method is equally safe but causes more nausea than progestogen-only emergency contraception. Adverse effects include: nausea, vomiting, spotting and change in timing of menstruation.

Ulipristal acetate: Ulipristal is a selective progesterone-receptor modulator. It has agonist and antagonist effects on progesterone receptors.

Dosage schedule: It is used as a single dose of 30 mg, to be taken within five days (120 h) of the first unprotected sexual intercourse regardless of the number of coital acts occurred over that period. This method is yet to be available in India.

Mode of action: The primary mechanism of action is inhibition of ovulation. In addition it may delay ovulation by suppressing lead follicles when given just before ovulation, including during the luteinising hormone surge. It may alter the endometrium resulting in impaired implantation.

Effectiveness: Ulipristal appears to be more potent than levonorgestrel in inhibiting ovulation. Taken within 5 days of unprotected intercourse, it reduces the risk of pregnancy by about 90%.

Safety: WHO has not yet made a statement on ulipristal. Because its safety has not been widely evaluated, the manufacturer advises avoidance if there is any risk of an implanted

pregnancy or hepatic dysfunction; it also advises caution in women with asthma that is inadequately controlled with oral glucocorticoids and in those who have hereditary problems with lactose metabolism. It is not yet known whether ulipristal is excreted in breast milk so breastfeeding is not recommended for up to 36 hours. Moreover, Ulipristal significantly increases their vulnerability to pregnancy for the rest of the cycle. So Ulipristal acetate may not be the first-line emergency contraceptive for all users of hormonal contraceptives. However, if users are willing to use back-up barrier contraception until the next menses and free of medical illness, UPA should be recommended. Side effects include headache, dizziness, and abdominal pain.

Copper IUD

WHO recommends that a copper-bearing IUD, as an emergency contraceptive, be inserted within five days of unprotected intercourse. This may be an ideal emergency contraceptive for a woman who is hoping for an ongoing, highly effective contraceptive method.

Mode of action: As emergency contraception, the copper-bearing IUD primarily prevents fertilization by causing a chemical change that damages sperm and ovum before they can meet.

Effectiveness: When inserted within five days of unprotected intercourse, a copper-bearing IUD is over 99% effective in preventing pregnancy. This is the most effective form of emergency contraception available. Once inserted, the woman can continue to use the IUD as an ongoing method of contraception, and she may choose to change to another contraceptive method in the future.

Safety: A copper-bearing IUD is a very safe form of emergency contraception. The risks of infection, expulsion or perforation are low.

EXERCISES

Answer the following questions

1. What is contraception?
2. How many Indian eligible couple use contraceptives?
3. What are the two measures for effectiveness of a contraceptive method?
4. What are the main five classes of contraceptive methods?
5. Rank the following contraceptives from the highest to the lowest with respect to actual effectiveness—Condom, Combined oral contraceptive pills, Cu T 380A, Tubectomy. What is the failure rate associated with each?
6. What are the different behavioural methods of contraception?
7. What three methods can be used to predict fertility and which days are women presumed to be fertile?
8. What is lactational amenorrhea method? Name three criteria to be fulfilled for use of LAM? How effective it is?
9. What are the types of barrier methods available?
10. What are the advantages of condom over other methods? What are its disadvantages?
11. What is the female condom and how is it used? What are its advantages and disadvantages?
12. How are the diaphragm and cervical cap used?
13. Name the spermicide that is used in vaginal sponge?
14. What are their disadvantages?
15. What are the different types of hormonal contraception?
16. What is the general mechanism of action of hormonal methods of contraception?
17. Do hormonal contraceptives protect against STIs?
18. What are the types of oral contraceptive pills?
19. What are the different types of estrogen progestogen contraception?
20. How are combined oral contraceptive pills dosed?
21. What are the mechanism of actions of COC?
22. What are the different preparation of COC available?
23. What are the side effects of COC pills? Which are estrogenic side effects and which are progestogenic side effects?
24. Name some drugs that may interfere with absorbtion/metabolism/efficacy of COC pills?
25. What are the absolute and relative contraindications of COC pills?
26. What instruction to be given to the patient regarding intake of COC?
27. When should COC pills be started?
28. What instruction to be given to the patient if she misses one or two consecutive pills?
29. What is the contraceptive patch?
30. How contraceptive patch is administered?
31. What is contraceptive vaginal ring?
32. How is it used?
33. What are the combined injectable contraceptives?
34. How they are used?
35. What is POP?
36. Who are suitable candidates for POP use?
37. When it should be started and how it is administered?
38. What instruction to be given to the woman if she misses one plll?
39. What are its disadvantages?
40. What injectable contraceptive is available in India?
41. How is DMPA administered?
42. What are IUDs?
43. What are the two types of IUD available and how do they work?
44. Who are the ideal candidates of IUD insertion?
45. What are its contraindications?
46. When IUD can be inserted in nonpregnant state, postpartum, postabortion?
47. How frequently Cu T 380 A should be replaced?

48. What are the risks of IUD insertion ?
49. What are the indications of IUD removal?
50. How an IUD can be removed?
51. What are the causes of missing thread?
52. How do you manage when a woman presents with complaint of missing thread?
53. How you manage a case of pregnancy with retained IUD?
54. What methods are available for sterilization?
55. Who are the suitable candidates for female sterilization?
56. What are the different procedures for female sterilization?
57. When should sterilization operation be performed following vaginal delivery/abortion/nonpregnant state?
58. Who can perform sterilization?
59. What are the short and long term complications of sterilization?
60. Who are the candidates for male sterilization?
61. What is the disadvantage of vasectomy ?
62. What are its complications?
63. What do you mean by emergency contraception?
64. Name the situations where emergency contraception is used?
65. What are the different methods of emergency contraception?

Write short notes on

1. Contraception counselling
2. LNG IUS
3. Nonscalpel vasectomy
4. Pomeroys technique
5. Progestogen only emergency contraception

Fill in the blanks with appropriate word/s

1. The chemical agent which acts as spermicide is _____ .
2. Third generation progestogens used in COC are _____ , _____ , and _____ .

3. Progestogen with antiminerelocorticoid and antiandrogenic activity used in COC is _____ .
4. Drugs that may reduce contraceptive effectiveness are _____ , _____ , and _____ .
5. Newest progestogen only pill contains _____ .
6. In CU T 380 A device, 380 stands for _____ .
7. LNG IUS releases _____ microgram of _____ for _____ years.

Explain or justify the following statements

1. There are many non contraceptive benefits of COC pills.
2. There are many methods of tubectomy during minilaparotomy operation

Questions for Orals

Look at the Fig. 33.1 before answering questions

1. Idetify the contraceptive.
2. What type of contraceptive is it?
3. With which material it is made off?
4. What are its advantages and dis-advantages?
5. What are the noncontraceptive benefits of this method?
6. What is its failure rate?
7. How it should be used?

Look at Fig. 33.4 before answering the following questions

1. Identify the contraceptive.
2. What are its contents?
3. How many pills are there?
4. Why the pills are of different colour?
5. How does it act?
6. Who are the ideal candidates?
7. When the woman should start pill?
8. What instruction you give to the woman regarding intake of pills?
9. What she will do if she misses one or two white pills?

10. What are its side effects?

11. How effective the method is?

Look at the Fig. 33.5 before answering questions

1. Identify the contraceptive.

2. What is its content?

3. Who are the ideal candidates for this contraceptive?

4. When this pills can be started?

5. How it should be taken?

6. What can a woman do if she misses pill?

Look at Fig. 33.9 before answering questions

1. Identify the contraceptive device?

2. What are the components of the pack?

3. How does it act?

4. Tell the technique of insertion.

5. What are its complications?

Bibliography

1. A guide to family planning for community health workers and their clients. World Health Organization 2012.

2. Ami JJ, Tripathi V Contraceeption for women: an evidence based overview BMJ 2009;339:b2895 doi: 10.1136/bmj.b2895

3. Baird D T, Glasier A F. Contraception BMJ Vol 3 19;1999: 969-972

4. BATUR P Emergency contraception Separating fact from fiction clevel and clinic journal of medicine volume 79 number 11 november 2012.

5. Emergency contraception World Health Organization 2012.

6. Herndon E, Zieman M. New contraceptive options Am Fam Physician 2004;69:853–60.

7. IUCD reference manual for medical officers Ministry of Health and Family Welfare Government of India, July 2007.

8. Liao PM, Dollin J. Half a century of oral contraceptive pill Historical review and view to the future Can Fam Physician 2012;58:e757–60

9. LNG IUS training manual for family planning ICA Foundation International contraceptive access.

10. Medical eligibility criteria for contraceptive use - 4th ed. World Health Organization 2010.

11. Milton HS, Chelmow D. Intrauterine device insertion E Medicine.

12. Mittal S, Agarwal P Interventions for emergency contraception The WHO reproductive Health Library 2012.

13. Nelson, A. Intrauterine contraceptives Glob. libr. women'smed.May 2008.

14. Prabaker I. Emergency contraception BMJ 2012;344:e1492doi: 10.1136/bmj.e1492 (Published 19 March 2012)

15. Selected Practice Recommendations for Contraceptive Use 2008 update; World Health Organization 2008.

16. Selected practice recommendations for contraceptive use Department of Reproductive Health and Research Family and Community Health World Health Organization, Geneva, 2004

17. Stika, C, Emergency Postcoital Contraception Glob. libr. women's med 2008.

18. The TCu380A Intrauterine Contraceptive Device (IUD): Specification, requalification and Guide-lines for Procurement, 2010 World Health Organization, UNFPA, UNAIDS and FHI, 2011.

34

Common Minor Gynecological Operations

In this chapter we will learn:
• Name of common minor gynaecological operations, their indications, contraindications, steps of operations and complications

DILATATION AND CURETTAGE

Definition

Dilatation and curettage (D & C) is an operative procedure in which the cervix is dilated and the endometrium is scraped away. "Curettage" refers to the scraping or removal of endometrium with a surgical instrument called a curette. The procedure is usually performed in a blind fashion. However, the procedure can be performed under ultrasound guidance or in conjunction with visualization of the uterine cavity by a hysteroscope.

Indications

Indications of dilatation and curettage can be divided as diagnostic indications and therapeutic indications.

Diagnostic Indications

- Abnormal uterine bleeding: Menorrhagia, metrorrhagia, menometrorrhagia, DUB - D and C will help.
  - To identify the histologic type of endometrium (proliferative or secretory)
  - To exclude pathology like endometrial-carcinoma, polyps, or hyperplasia.
  - As a therapeutic measure of menorrhagia
- Postmenopausal bleeding—D and C will exclude endometrial carcinoma and identify the histologic type of endometrium
- Evaluation of infertility—Secretory change of the endometrium in second half of mens identifies ovulation and dating of endometrium helps to diagnose luteal phase defect.
- Follow up of previously diagnosed endometrial hyperplasia
- Abnormal PAP smear with atypical cells favouring endometrial origin
- Evaluation of patient with amenorrhea

Therapeutic Indications

- Menorrhagia unresponsive to hormone therapy.
- In conjunction with endometrial ablation for histologic evaluation of the endometrium
- During polypectomy

Contraindications

- Pregnancy
- Acute pelvic inflammatory disease
- Clotting disorders (coagulopathy)
- Acute cervical or vaginal infections
- Cervical stenosis and obstructive cervical lesion (cervical carcinoma)

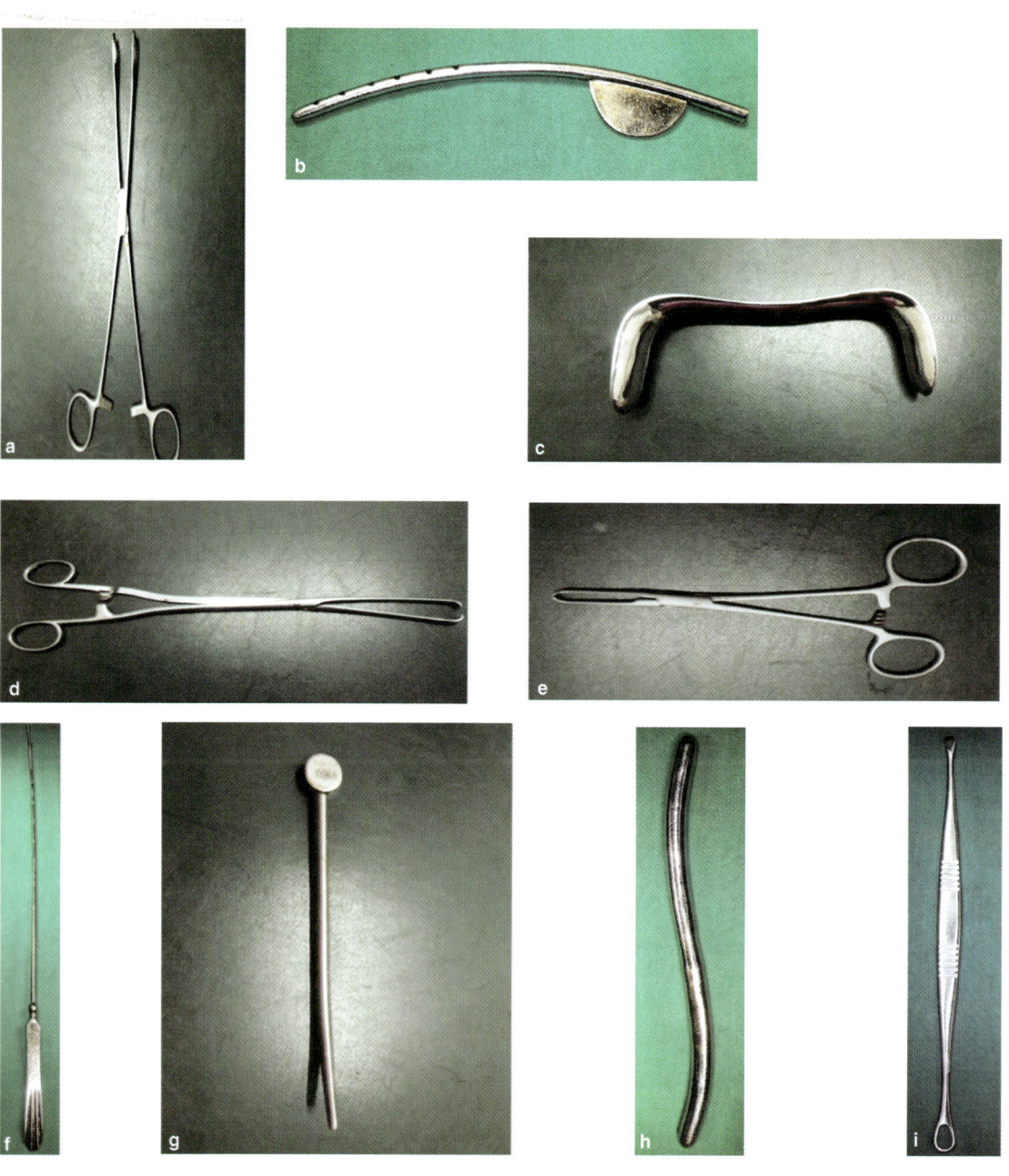

Fig. 34.1: Some of the instruments used in dilatation and curettage. **(a)** Sponge holding Forceps; **(b)** Female metal catheter; **(c)** Sim's Speculum; **(d)** multiple teeth vulsellum; **(e)** Allis tissue forceps; **(f)** Uterine sound; **(g)** Hawkin-Ambler's cervical dilators; **(h)** Hegar's Cervical dilator; **(i)** sharp and blunt uterine curette

Procedure

Equipment: The following materials are required to perform dilatation and curettage:

- Formalin container (for specimen)
- Drape
- Cotton balls soaked in povidone iodine
- Gloves
- Gauge
- Sponge holding forceps
- Female catheter
- Vaginal speculum
- Uterine sound
- Cervical dilators
- Endometrial curette
- Vulsellum/Allis tissue forceps to grasp cervix (Fig. 34.1)

A Sim's vaginal speculum is used to visualize the cervix. The Hawkin-Ambler cervical dilator has the most gradual taper and ranges in size from 3/6 to 18/21 sizes.. The tips of the Hegar and Das dilators are more blunt and may therefore require greater force to dilate the cervix. This could increase the risk of cervical laceration or uterine perforation, particularly in an inelastic cervix.

Position: The procedure is typically performed in the dorsal lithotomy position.

Anesthesia: The procedure can be done using general, regional, or local block anesthesia. The type of anesthesia chosen depends upon the indication of the procedure.

Steps of Operation (Fig. 34.2)

1. An aseptic solution is applied to the vulva and vagina and appropriate sterile drapes are placed. The bladder is drained with a catheter. Bimanual examination is performed to determine the uterine size and position. This step allows instruments to be inserted along the long axis of the uterus to avoid perforation.

2. A Sim's speculum is introduced to visualize the cervix. The anterior lip of the cervix is cleaned with iodine solution and grasped with a volsellum or tenaculum and gentle outward traction is given to stabilize the uterus. A uterine sound is held as a pencil with the thumb and first two fingers. The sound is passed slowly through the cervical os, into the uterine cavity, and up to the fundus. Importantly, instruments should not be forced because this increases the risk of perforation. Once gentle resistance is met at the fundus, the distance from the fundus to the external os is measured by score marks along the length of the sound. Passing the uterine sound provides confirmatory information about the position of the uterus, the length of the uterine cavity, and the angulation between the cervical canal and the uterine cavity. It acts as a first dilator as well.

3. Cervical dilatation—Each dilator is grasped with the first finger and thumb, similar to the grasp used with the uterine sound. It is held at its mid portion and inserted into the cervical os just past the internal cervical os. It should not be inserted up to the fundus since this may traumatize the endometrium and may increase the chance of uterine perforation. Dilation should continue until the appropriate diameter of the curette to be inserted has been achieved.

4. Uterine curettage—A 4" × 4" gauze is placed between the vaginal speculum and the external os to receive the endometrial curettings. Then the uterine curette is inserted and advanced to the fundus, following the long axis of the uterus. On reaching the fundus, the sharp surface of the curette is positioned to contact the adjacent endometrium. Pressure is exerted against the endometrium as the curette is pulled toward the internal cervical os. After reaching the os, the curette is redirected to the fundus and positioned immediately adjacent to the path of the first curettage pass. In this manner, the surgeon attempts to sample the entire uterine surface. After several serial passes, tissues collected in the

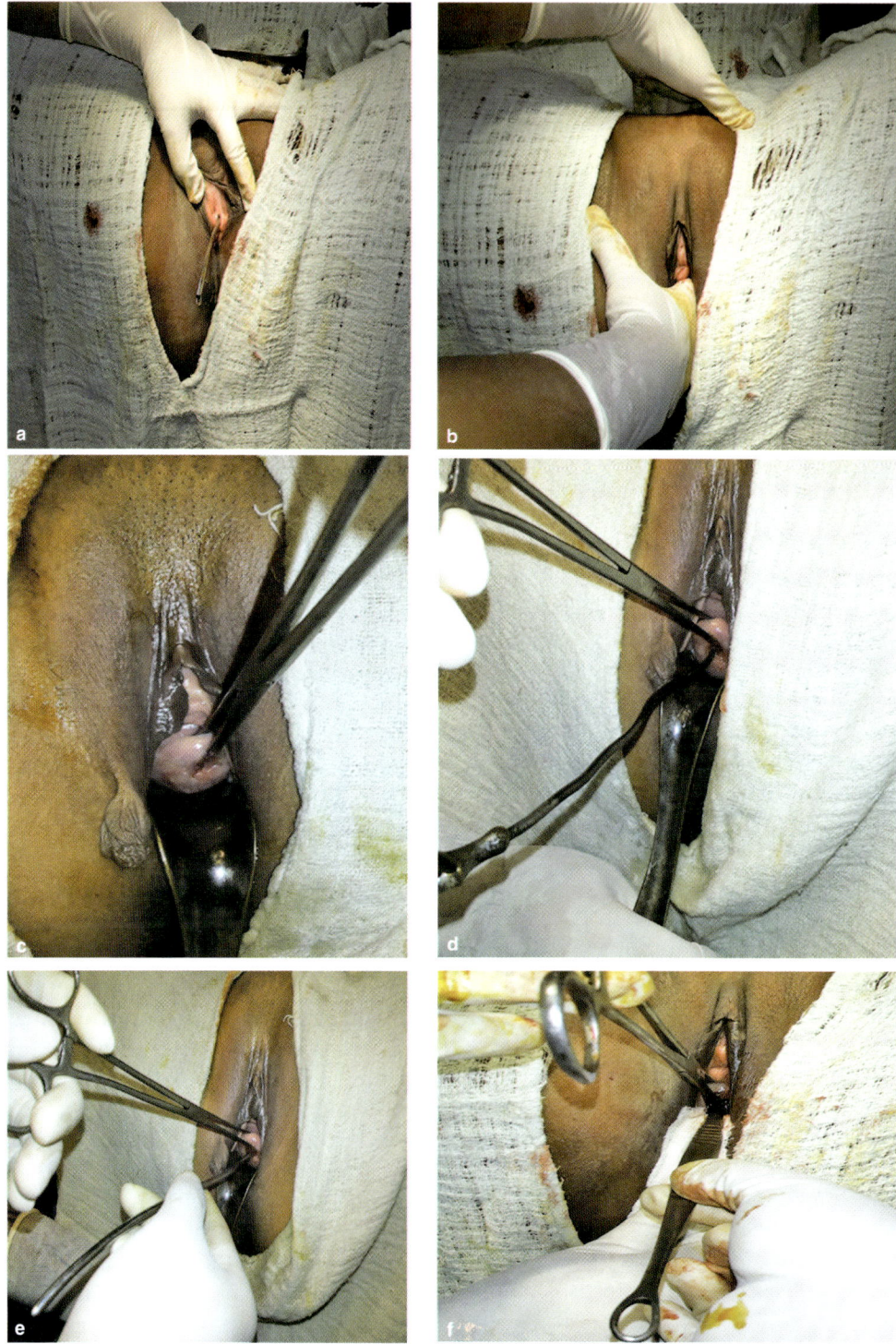

Fig. 34.2: (a) Catheterisation of urinary bladder; **(b)** bimanual examination; **(c)** Sim's speculum is introduced and anterior lip of cervix is grasped with Allis tissue forceps; **(d)** Uterine sound is passed through the cervix; **(e)** cervix is dilated using Hegar's cervical dilator; **(f)** uterine curette is introduced for curettage

isthmus region are scraped out onto the gauze piece.

5. The volsellum or tenaculum is gently removed. Excess blood and povidoneiodine solution are wiped from the vagina, and the vaginal speculum is removed.

Complications

Complications can occur at the time of dilatation and curettage. Possible complications include the following:

- Bleeding or hemorrhage
- Cervical laceration
- Uterine perforation
- Postprocedural infection
- Postprocedural intrauterine synechiae (Asherman's syndrome)
- Anesthetic complications

Management of Complications

Cervical Laceration

Cervical laceration occurs when the resistance of cervical dilation exceeds the strength of the external os where the volsellum is placed. If the cervix is bleeding at the end of the procedure, a suture may be required for hemostasis.

Uterine Perforation

Uterine perforation may occur and is suspected when:

- Sudden loss of resistance
- The instrument travels deeper than previously measured
- Instrument is freely mobile.

The instruments most commonly associated with uterine perforation are the uterine sound or dilators and occasionally curette. If perforation is known to have occurred with a blunt instrument (uterine sound or dilator), operation should be stopped and observation of vital and peritoneal signs for several hours is all that is needed. If suspicion that a sharp instrument, such as a curette, has perforated the uterus or if the fat has been retrieved by curettage, then intra-abdominal injury must be excluded by laparoscopy. Active bleeding may necessitate a laparotomy.

Late complication: Asherman's Syndrome

During vigorous curettage the basal layer of the endometrium may be destroyed. Healing will result in synechiae (adhesions) between the walls of the uterus. The patient presents with amenorrhea. Diagnosis is made by hysterosalpingography, and therapy is hysteroscopic lysis of adhesions and estrogen therapy to stimulate endometrial growth.

HYSTEROSALPINGOGRAPHY

Hysterosalpingography (HSG) is a radiographic imaging of the cervical canal, uterine cavity, fallopian tubes, and peritoneal cavity following the injection of a contrast agent. This examination reveals the size, shape of the uterine cavity and inside of the fallopian tubes.

Information obtained by HSG includes:

- The width of the cervical canal
- The contour of the uterine cavity
- An outline of the lumen of the fallopian tubes and cornu
- The presence or absence of spillage of contrast from the fimbriated ends of the tubes.

Indications

The most common indication for HSG is:

- Infertility to know the patency of fallopian tubes; other indications include
- Congenital abnormalities and/or anatomic variants of uterus (e.g. bicornuate uterus)
- Patients' prior to or after tubal surgery such as tubal recanalization or other intervention.
- Uterine leiomyoma (fibroid)
- Postoperative uterine cavity, for example, myomectomy.

Contraindications and Cautions

- HSG should not be performed on a woman who is pregnant or who could be pregnant. This is usually avoided by scheduling the examination in the follicular phase of the menstrual cycle, after menstrual flow has ceased but before the patient has ovulated, HS6 is done usually on day 7 to 10 of the menstrual cycle.

- HSG should not be performed when ongoing pelvic infection or active vaginal bleeding is present. If pelvic infection is of concern, premedication with antibiotics should be considered.

- History of allergy or idiosyncratic reaction to iodinated contrast media is a relative contraindication, and may require premedication with steroids and/or other medications.

Procedure

Equipment: Instruments required for hysterosalpingogram (HSG, Fig. 34.3) are:
- Sponge holding forceps
- Antiseptic solution
- Contrast medium in disposable syringe
- Sim's speculum
- Allis tissue forceps/vulsellum
- HSG cannula

Analgesia: No analgesic is recommended as analgesics can not relieve pain or discomfort during the procedure.

Contrast medium: Both oil-based and water-based iodinated contrasts are used for HSG.

Water-soluble dyes have been found to provide better detail of the uterine cavity and fallopian tubes and are more quickly eliminated. Oil-based dyes have been associated with less post-procedure vaginal bleeding, but in animal models oil-based dyes are reported to cause temporary granulomatous formation of the pelvic peritoneum.

Steps of the Procedure

- After emptying bladder patient is placed on the X-ray table in the lithotomy position.
- A Sim's speculum is introduced to visualise the cervix .
- The cervix is cleansed with an antiseptic solution and the anterior lip of the cervix grasped with an Allis tissue forceps or vulsellum.
- The HSG cannula is completely filled with the warm contrast medium before injection to avoid introducing air into the endometrial cavity. The cannula is then applied into the cervical canal and the tip of the cannula should not protrude further than 2 cm into the cervical canal. The tip should be fitted so as to prevent reflux of the contrast medium.
- Speculum is removed and patient is placed beneath a X-ray machine.
- Five to 10 ml of contrast media is then injected through cannula. To decrease uterine spasm, the media should be warmed to body temperature and injected slowly.
- About 1 mL of the contrast is introduced into the endometrial cavity, and then an X-ray is obtained. The film is then developed and used to decide whether further injection is necessary or hazardous. This process is repeated until the tubes are filled and intraperitoneal spill is obtained. Thus a series of at least 4 more images are captured as the contrast spreads through the genital tract.
- After the images are made, cannula is removed.

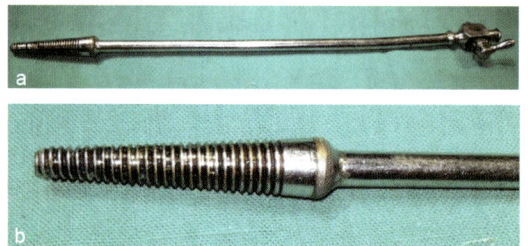

Fig. 34.3: (a) HSG cannula; **(b)** Tip of HSG cannula

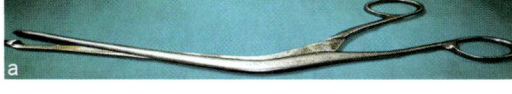
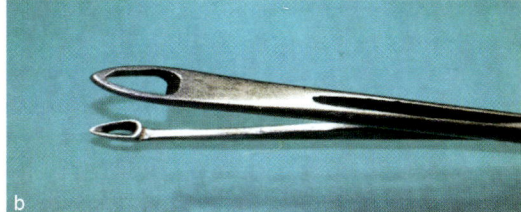

Fig. 34.4: **(a)** Punch biopsy forceps; **(b)** Tip of punch biopsy forceps

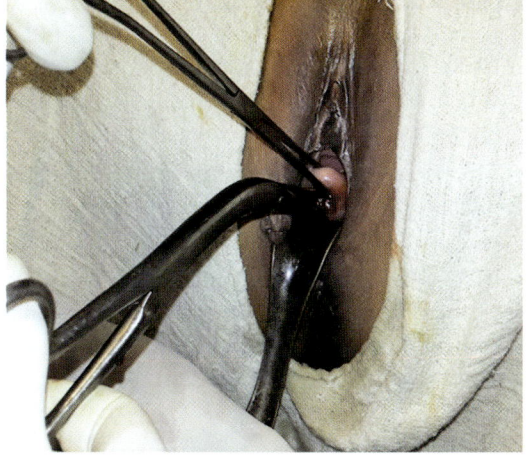

Fig. 34.5: Cervical biopsy using punch biopsy forceps

Complications

Complications from HSG are rare.

The common adverse effects include syncopal attack, lower abdominal pain and slight vaginal bleeding. More serious complications from HSG include injury to cervix, pelvic infection and allergic reactions from contrast media.

CERVICAL BIOPSY

Definition

A cervical biopsy is an operative procedure performed to remove tissue from the cervix for histopathological examinations.

Types

Types of cervical biopsies (Figs 34.4 and 34.5) include:

- Punch biopsy. A small piece of tissue is removed from the cervix. One or more punch biopsies may be performed on different areas of the cervix.
- Cone biopsy or conisation. A large cone-shaped piece of tissue is removed from the cervix by using a scalpel or laser.
- Endocervical curettage (ECC). A curette is used to scrape the lining of the endocervical canal, an area that cannot be seen from the outside of the cervix.

Indications

A cervical biopsy is usually performed to detect cancer of the cervix or precancerous lesions of the cervix. Situations are:

- Abnormal Pap test result
- A lesion over cervix during pelvic examination
- During a colposcopic procedure.

A cervical biopsy may also be used to diagnose and assist in the treatment of the following conditions:

- Genital warts, which may indicate infection with human papilloma virus (HPV), a risk factor for developing cervical cancer.
- Diethylstilbestrol (DES) exposure in women whose mothers took DES during pregnancy, as DES exposure increases the risk for cancer of the reproductive system.

Methods to identify abnormal area of the cervix: A cervical biopsy is usually done after a procedure called as colposcopy. A colposcopy allows the gynecologist to do a detailed examination of the tissues in the cervix so as to identify abnormal or diseased tissues. Colposcopic examination is neither needed nor particularly effective for a gross cervical lesion, but can be helpful when there is a small surface lesion to identify the most abnormal area for directed biopsies. There are two well-known methods that can identify an abnormal area of the cervix. The first method involves removing the mucous from the cervix with an acetic acid solution, which helps to highlight the areas that are diseased or abnormal. Applying 3- to 5-percent acetic acid to mucosal epithelium results in the acetowhite change characteristic of neoplastic lesions as well as some non-neoplastic conditions. The second method, also called the Schiller's Method, involves staining the cervix with iodine. Lugol iodine solution stains mature squamous epithelial cells mahogany in estrogenized women due to high cellular glycogen content. Due to attenuated cellular differentiation, dysplastic cells have lower glycogen content and fail to fully stain, appearing various shades of yellow.

Position: The procedure is typically performed in the dorsal lithotomy position.

Anesthesia: Generally, no anesthesia is required for a simple cervical biopsy. The procedure, however, can be done using general, regional, or local block anesthesia.

Steps of Operation

- After emptying bladder patient is placed on the operation table in the lithotomy position.
- An aseptic solution is applied to the vulva and vagina and appropriate sterile drapes are placed.
- A Sim's speculum is introduced to visualise the cervix.
- The cervix is cleaned and soaked with an acetic acid solution. This solution helps make the abnormal tissues turn white and become more visible. A colposcope, may be used to identify the area of cervix for taking biopsy. Alternately an iodine solution may be used to coat the cervix, called the Schiller test.
- The type of biopsy performed will be determined by the size, shape, location, and other characteristics of the abnormalities.
- A vulsellum or Allis tissue forceps may be used to hold the cervix so to steady for the biopsy.

- For a punch biopsy, one or more small samples of tissue will be removed using a punch biopsy forceps. It is important to obtain a specimen where frank stromal invasion can be demonstrated, not from the exophytic portion where no benign stroma is present. Cells from the inside of the cervical canal may be sampled with an endocervical curette or an endocervical brush.
- For a cone biopsy, a larger cone-shaped piece of tissue is removed from the cervix. The loop electrosurgical excision procedure (LEEP) or the cold knife cone biopsy procedure may be used. With the cold knife cone biopsy, a laser or a surgical scalpel is used to remove tissue. This procedure requires the use of regional or general anesthesia.
- The tissue samples are then sent to a pathologist for detailed examination.
- Bleeding from the biopsy site may be treated with electrocauterization (use of a probe with high frequency electrical signals to stop bleeding) or sutures, or packing the vagina with pressure dressing.

Complications

As with any surgical procedure, complications may occur but rare. Possible complications may include:

- Infection
- Bleeding

In addition, cone biopsies may increase the risk for infertility and miscarriage because of the changes and scarring in the cervix that may occur as a result of the procedure.

EXERCISES

Answer the following questions

1. Enumerate the indications of dilatation and curettage.
2. Why D&C is done in women with DUB/ menorrhagia?

3. Why D&C is done in postmenopausal women?
4. Why D&C is done in infertile women?
5. Name the instruments required to perform D&C.
6. Name the different types of cervical dilators that are used in D & C.
7. What is the position of the patient during D & C operation?
8. What are the steps of operation?
9. Why do you perform bimanual examination before starting the procedure?
10. Why uterine sound is used?
11. How much cervical dilatation is required at the time of D&C?
12. Name some complications of D& C.
13. When do you suspect uterine perforation at the time of doing D & C operation?
14. How do you manage uterine perforation during D & C operation?
15. Why Asherman's syndrome develops following D & C?
16. What is hysterosalpingography?
17. What are its indications? What is the commonest indication of HSG?
18. When HSG should be performed in relation to menstrual cycle and why?
19. Which contrast medium is used in HSG?
20. Describe the steps of operation?
21. What are its adverse effects?
22. What are the different types of cervical biopsy?
23. Why it is done?
24. Describe the steps of operation.
25. How do you identify the sites from where cervical biopsy to be taken?

Identify the instruments and mention their use

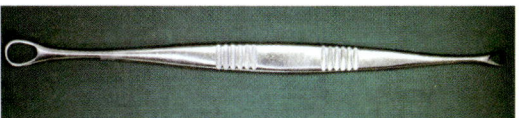

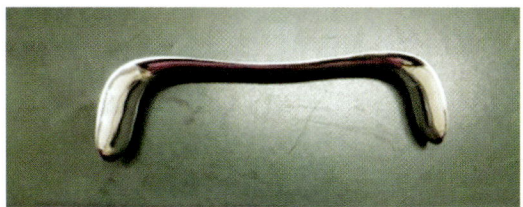

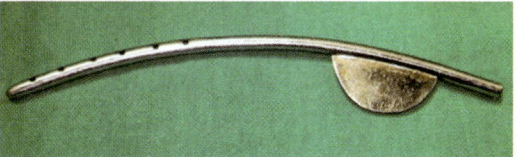

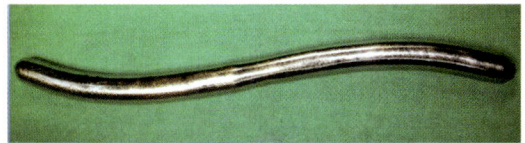

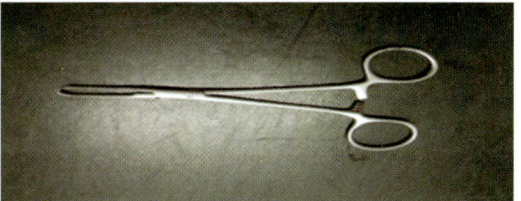

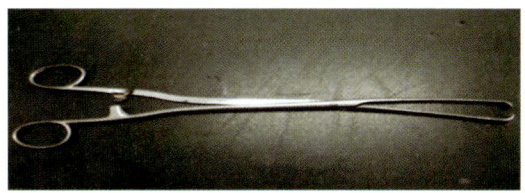

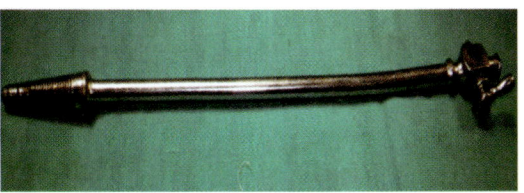

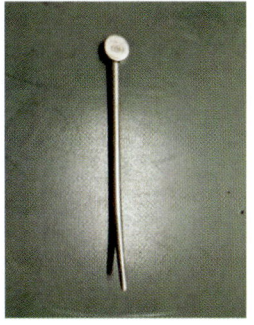

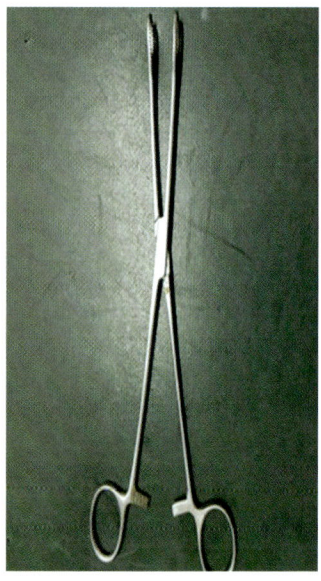

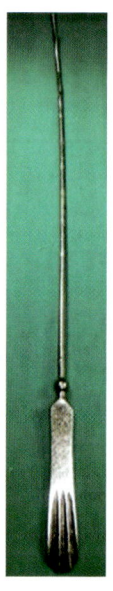

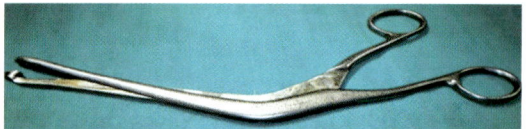

Bibliography

1. Barad DH. Tests for gynaecologic disorders 2013.
2. Kuntz C. Endometrial biopsy Can Fam Physician. 2007 January; 53(1): 43–44.
3. Hulka JF. Dilatation and curettage Glob lib of Medicine.
4. Dilatation and curettage overview up-to-date 2013.
5. Zuber T. Endometrial biopsy Am Fam Physician 2001; 63:1131-5,1137-8,1139–41.
6. Bacon JL, et al. Diagnostic dilatation and curettage Medscape 2013.
7. Vorvick JL. Colposcopic directed biopsy 2012.

35

Major Operations in Gynecology

In this chapter we will learn:
- Preoperative evaluation before common major gynecological operations
- Name of common major operations, their indications, steps of operative procedure, and complications

Consent for Surgery

Informed consent means that the gynecologist has explained the need for the surgery, the risks, and possible alternatives, and that the patient has understood these facts and agreed to the surgery. All discussions about indications, risks, and alternatives as well as the patient's response must be documented in the chart.

Preoperative care: Most gynecologic surgery is elective and low risk. Surgery in oncology carries more risks as geriatric patients, who may have multiple medical problems. There are two groups of indications for gynecological surgery: absolute—when surgery must be undertaken, when its cancellation is life-threatening, and relative—when surgery can be postponed till the most appropriate occasion for its performing. Before making a decision on surgery, one of the three requirements must be fulfilled: relief of pain and suffering, preservation of life, correction of an existing deformity. If none of the three goals can be achieved by surgery, the surgery

should be given up. The main objective of the preoperative assessment is to make sure that the patient is fit for the appropriate surgery and that the patient understands the indications, benefits, risks, and alternatives for the planned procedure.

1. *Preoperative evaluation:* A detailed history and physical examination are essential to evaluate the patients' fitness for surgery. Further consultation and investigations will be planned accordingly. Preoperative consultation with an anesthesiologist is important for the medically compromised patient.

2. *Preoperative testing:* Preoperative testing requires some routine preoperative laboratory tests and additional specialist examinations guided mostly by positive findings on the history and physical examination. For patients older than 40 years, laboratory analyses of the blood involves blood group determination, complete blood count, bleeding and coagulation time. Renal function is checked (urea, creatinin) and liver function as well

(bilirubin, serum alanine-aminotransferase, serum aspartate aminotransferase). Glucose in the blood is determined as well. Routine analysis of the urine and urine culture is performed, if required. An ECG and chest radiograph are also done. A pregnancy test is usually done for women of reproductive age to exclude pregnancy. For patients younger than 40 years, a CBC is usually required.

3. *Preoperative management*
a. *Antibiotics before gynecologic surgery:* Prophylactic use of antibiotics have been found to be more successful for vaginal compared to abdominal operations. A recommended regimen for patients undergoing vaginal hysterectomy, abdominal or radical hysterectomy consists of a dose of i.v. ceftriaxone (1 g) at the induction of anesthesia, or aminoglycosides with metronidazole.

b. *Bowel preparation.* Reduction of GI contents provides additional room in the pelvis and abdomen and facilitates surgery. Reduction in the number of pathogenic flora in the colon reduces the risk of infection if bowel surgery is performed. Mechanical bowel preparation with oral gut lavage using an agent such as polyethylene glycol electrolyte solution (Peglec) and a clear liquid diet for 24 hours the day before surgery is commonly used.

c. *Medications.* Antihypertensive and thyroid medications should be taken with a sip of water on the morning of surgery. Diabetic patients are co-managed with consultation of physicians.

d. *Deep venous thrombosis (DVT) prophylaxis.* The best DVT prophylaxis is early ambulation after surgery. Below-the-knee elastic stockings and pneumatic compression devices may be used for patients undergoing gynecologic surgery. In high-risk patients (oncologic patients, obese patients, patients with a history of previous DVT or pulmonary embolism, or patients for whom prolonged pelvic surgery is anticipated), 5000 U of unfractionated heparin is given subcutaneously (SC) 30 minutes before surgery and every 8 hours postoperatively until the patient is mobile. Alternative regimens include the use of low-molecular-weight heparin formulations such as enoxaparin sodium 40 mg/day SC starting 2 hours preoperatively or postoperatively.

e. *Autologous blood donation.* Information regarding the possibility and risk of a blood transfusion must be part of the informed consent procedure. In healthy adult patients, blood loss up to 500–700 mL can usually be tolerated.

f. *Prophylaxis for subacute bacterial endocarditis:* Women undergoing surgery with cardiac disease are candidates for prophylaxis for subacute bacterial endocarditis. Prophylaxis is recommended only for those in the high- and moderate-risk categories.

HYSTERECTOMY

Definition

Hysterectomy is the surgical removal of the uterus. Different portions of the uterus, as well as other organs, may be removed at the same time.

Types of Hysterectomy

- *Total hysterectomy:* It includes the removal of the entire uterus, including the body and the cervix, but not the tubes or ovaries. This is the most common type of hysterectomy.

- *Subtotal hysterectomy* (supracervical hysterectomy): Removal of the body of the uterus while leaving the cervix intact.

- *Hysterectomy with salpingo-oophorectomy:* Includes the removal of one or both ovaries, and the fallopian tubes, along with the uterus. **Pan hysterectomy** means hysterectomy with bilateral salpingo-oophorectomy.

- *Radical hysterectomy* includes the removal of the uterus, cervix, the top portion of the vagina and parametrium (most of the tissue that surrounds the cervix in the pelvic cavity), and may include the removal of the pelvic lymph nodes. This is done in some cases of malignancies.

Indications of Hysterectomy

A. *Benign diseases*

- Dysfunctional uterine bleeding in perimenopausal women.
- Uterine leiomyomas
- Symptomatic adenomyosis
- Symptomatic endometriosis
- Pelvic inflammatory disease
- Chronic pelvic pain
- Pelvic organ prolapse
- Pregnancy related conditions, e.g. severe postpartum hemorrhage, rupture uterus.

B. *Malignant diseases*

- Cervical intraepithelial neoplasia
- Invasive cervical cancer
- Atypical endometrial hyperplasia
- Endometrial cancer
- Ovarian cancer
- Fallopian tube cancer
- Gestational trophoblastic neoplasia.

Routes of Hysterectomy

There are different surgical techniques used to perform a hysterectomy. The uterus can be removed via the abdominal route, transvaginally, or laparoscopically. Surgical hysterectomy techniques include:

1. *Abdominal hysterectomy.* The uterus is removed through the abdomen via a surgical incision about six to eight inches long. The incision can be made either vertically, from the umbilicus to the pubic bone, or transversely, along the top of the pubic hairline.

2. *Vaginal hysterectomy.* The uterus is removed through the vaginal opening. This procedure is most often used in cases of uterine prolapse, or when vaginal repairs are necessary for related conditions. No external incision is made, which means there is no visible scarring.

3. *Laparoscope-assisted vaginal hysterectomy/robot-assisted laparoscopic hysterectomy.* Vaginal hysterectomy is performed with the aid of a laparoscope. The uterus is removed in sections through the laparoscope or through the vagina. In a robot-assisted laparoscopic hysterectomy, the surgeon inserts the laparoscope and other instruments, then uses a computer station to control the instruments.

4. *Total laparoscopic hysterctomy.*

Steps of Abdominal Hysterectomy

- The patient is placed in the supine position on the operating table.
- The patient is anesthetized.
- The vagina and perineum are cleaned with antiseptic solutions and a Foley catheter is inserted.
- The abdomen then is dressed with antiseptic solution from the anterior thighs to the xiphoid, and sterile drapes are applied.
- In most instances, abdomen is opened through a low transverse incision; most gynecologists prefer a Pfannenstiel's incision, which is cosmetically appealing and strong.
- After confirming the pathology, the patient is put in a slight Trendelenburg position, a self-retaining retractor is placed, and the bowel packed superiorly to afford good exposure of the pelvis.
- Straight clamps are placed alongside the uterus near cornu (include the round ligament, fallopian tube and utero-ovarian ligaments.) to elevate the uterus out of the pelvis by giving adequate traction.
- *Round ligament transection:* The right round ligament is visualised and clamped and divided and tied.

- The broad ligament is opened.
- *Ovarian conservation:* The fallopian tube and utero-ovarian ligament are doubly clamped and divided and doubly ligated.
- The same procedure is performed on the left.
- *Oophorectomy:* If the adnexa are to be removed, the tube and ovary are grasped with a Babcock clamp and elevated away from the infundibulopelvic (IP) ligament. The infundibulopelvic ligament is doubly clamped, and the ovarian vessels are cut between the clamps. The proximal pedicle is ligated with a free tie followed by a transfixion suture ligature.
- *Bladder flap:* The peritoneal incisions from one round ligament to other are connected from the broad ligament over the bladder at the point of the vesicouterine reflection. The loose connective tissue is pushed down from the bladder to expose the endopelvic fascia over the anterior portion of the cervix. 1–2 cm of the entire anterior vaginal wall below the level of the vaginal transection must be exposed.
- *Uterine arteries:* Next, the uterine arteries are identified along the lateral aspects of the uterus at the level of the isthmus. A Kocher (or equivalent) clamp is placed on the side of the cervix at approximately at 45° angle at the position of the uterine artery. The tissue is divided close to the cervix. The pedicle is doubly ligated.
- *Cardinal ligament transection:* These ligaments lie lateral to the uterus and are inferior to the uterine vessels. A straight clamp is used to clamp the cardinal ligament A scalpel is used to transect the portion of the cardinal ligament held between the clamp. The clamp is replaced by a transfixing suture.
- *Uterosacral ligament transection:* At this point, attention is directed to the posterior aspect of the uterus and to the uterosacral ligaments. Each ligament is grasped with a straight clamp close to its uterine attachment.

The ligament is divided medial to the clamp, a transfixing suture is placed, and the clamp is removed.

- *Vaginal entry:* The vagina is incised and curved clamps are used to grasp the anterior and posterior vaginal walls at the point just below the cervix. The vaginal tissue above these clamps then is incised. The uterus is removed.
- *Vaginal vault closure:* The vaginal vault is sutured, either using figure of eight sutures or as a continuous running suture with careful attention to each angle.
- The pelvic peritoneum should be included in the suturing of the vagina to aid hemostasis.
- *The pelvis is inspected for hemostasis:* Reperitonealisation is not necessary, but may aid hemostasis.
- The packs are removed and the abdomen is closed.

Steps of Vaginal Hysterectomy

- The patient is put under general or regional anesthesia.
- The patient is placed in lithotomy position.
- Antiseptic dressing and draping is done. Bladder is catheterised. Bimanual examination is done to reconfirm preoperative findings.
- *Vaginal wall incision:* The cervix and vaginal mucosa may be injected with 10–15 mL of a dilute saline solution containing vasopressin (20 units diluted in 20 mL of saline) or 0.5 percent lignocaine and epinephrine (1:200,000 dilution). Injection of vasocontrictors decreases bleeding during dissection and aids in defining tissue planes. The vaginal wall above the cervix then is circumcised. To avoid dissection into the cervix, this incision is kept at a depth superficial to the pubo-cervical fascia.
- *Anterior peritoneal entry:* The bladder is dissected off the anterior aspect of the uterus and displaced anteriorly. The

vesicouterine fold is grasped and elevated to place this peritoneal layer on tension. The peritoneum then is incised.

- *Posterior entry:* The posterior lip of cervix is lifted anteriorly to expose the posterior vaginal vault, and an Allis forceps is placed on the incised edge of the posterior vaginal wall. The Allis tissue forceps is pulled downward to create tension across the exposed posterior peritoneum. The posterior vaginal vault is cut with curved Mayo scissors, and the Douglas cul-de-sac is entered.
- Curved Kocher clamps are inserted into the pouch of Douglas to take the uterosacral pedicles first vertically angled and then horizontally. The uterosacral ligament is then transected, and ligated with 0-gauge delayed-absorbable suture using a transfixing stitch. After ligation of the uterosacral ligaments, the cardinal ligaments similarly are clamped, cut, and sutured.
- The uterine pedicles are then clamped, cut and ligated.
- The uterus is delivered through the vagina.
- Clamps are, then, placed across the utero-ovarian and round ligaments and fallopian tubes. Each pedicle is doubly ligated with a simple suture.
- The uterus is removed.
- The peritoneum is then closed in a purse string to include the uterine vessels and uterosacral pedicles and pouch of Douglas peritoneum.
- The vaginal vault is closed, either as an inverted 'Y' or horizontally as a continuous locking suture, securing the uterosacrals into the vaginal mucosa.

Postoperative management of hysterectomy patient: The details of postoperative care are dictated by the indications for hysterectomy, route of hysterectomy, i.e. vaginal or abdominal and the individual patient's overall medical condition. Following vaginal hysterectomy, there is faster return of normal bowel function, easier ambulation, and decreased analgesia requirements in comparison to abdominal hysterectomy. General guidelines include the following:

- Intravenous fluid—Physiologic fluids such as 5% dextrose and lactated Ringer's solution are administered and maintained at approximately 125 mL/hour (2–3 L/day). When to stop the IV maintenance fluids will depend on the patient's dietary tolerances.
- A Foley catheter is left indwelling for 24 hours.
- Prophylactic antibiotics are given within the first 24 hours postoperatively.
- Adequate analgesia is given parenterally. Pain is typically managed initially with parenteral narcotics. The choice will vary from surgeon to surgeon but usually includes pethidine hydrochloride or meperidine sulfate. Once the patient can tolerate a regular diet, she can be switched to oral analgesics.
- Sips of water may be given the first night, followed by clear liquids or regular diet on the next postoperative day depending on the patient's appetite. The diet is advanced based on return of bowel sounds and appetite, toleration of the diet, and the passage of flatus.
- Ambulation is begun on the first postoperative day.

Complications of Hysterectomy

Hysterectomy is one of the safe surgical procedures. But as with any surgery complication may occur:

- *Peroperative complications:* Injury to the bowel, bladder, ureter or major vessels. Excessive bleeding, complications due to anesthesia
- *Early postoperative complications:* Postoperative hemorrhage usually from the angle of vault of vagina, wound infection and febrile morbidity, pelvic hematoma and abscess formation, deep vein thrombosis, wound complications.

MYOMECTOMY

Definition

Myomectomy means surgical removal of leiomyomas from their surrounding myometrium in an attempt to relieve symptoms of leiomyoma such as abnormal uterine bleeding, pelvic pain, and infertility.

Indications

Myomectomy is indicated for women with symptomatic leiomyoma who are willing for fertility or willing to retain uterus. Following are the situations where myomectomy is indicated:

- Infertility with distortion of endometrial cavity or tubal occlusion
- Recurrent pregnancy loss with distortion of endometrial cavity
- Abnormal uterine bleeding not responding to medical treatment
- Pain and pressure symptoms that interfere with quality of life
- Urinary symptoms (frequency and/or symptoms of obstruction)
- Iron deficiency anemia secondary to menstrual blood loss.

Contraindications

Myomectomy is not indicated if:
- The patient has no desire for fertility or uterine preservation
- The patient is pregnant
- Asymptomatic women with possible exception of unexplained infertility.

Routes of Myomectomy

a. Myomectomy by laparotomy or abdominal laparotomy (*see* below)
b. Myomectomy by laparoscopy. Laparoscopic myomectomy is a safe and effective option for women with a small number (< 4) of moderately sized (5–7 cm) uterine leiomyomas who do not desire future fertility (ACOG). When compared with abdominal approach, laparoscopic myomectomy is associated with less blood loss, shorter hospital stay and lower overall complication rate. However laparoscopic myomectomy is more time consuming, larger myoma are more difficult to remove, and may be associated with uterine rupture during pregnancy if inadequately repaired.
c. *Myomectomy by hysteroscopy:* This is the first line procedure when intracavitory leiomyoma is present and fertility is desired.

Steps of Abdominal Myomectomy

Preliminary steps of operations are same as in abdominal hysterectomy.

- Abdomen is opened through a Pfannenstiel incision or through a vertical midline incision depending upon the size of uterus.
- *Delivery and inspection of uterus:* The uterus is delivered as far as possible out of the abdominal cavity and the size and position of myoma/s are noted to select the best site of incision/s over uterus .
- *Measures to reduce blood loss:* Myomectomy is associated with profuse hemorrhage. So to minimise blood loss during operation, tourniquets are used to temporarily occlude blood flow through the uterine and ovarian arteries. Alternately dilute solutions of vasopressin are injected directly into the myoma, raising a circumferential wheal and causing vasoconstriction.
- *The primary incision in the uterus:* Attempt should be made to place incisions on the anterior uterine wall and number of incisions should be minimized to avoid postoperative risks of adhesion formation. For most patients, a midline vertical uterine incision allows removal of the greatest number of leiomyomas through the fewest incisions
- *Removal of a solitary leiomyoma:* Incision over the uterine leiomyoma is carried down to the point at which leiomyoma clearly bulges into the incision. Sharp and

blunt dissection of the pseudocapsule surrounding the leiomyoma frees the tumor from the adjacent myometrium. Small bleeding points in the base of the cavity are individually tied.

- *Obliteration of the cavity:* The cavity should be obliterated with series of circler mattress suture until the whole space is obliterated. Serosal incision should be closed using a running baseball suture with 4-0 or 5-0 monofilament delayed-absorbable suture to limit adhesion formation.

Complications

Myomectomy is a technically difficult operation and may be associated with hazards. The major potential complication is peroperative hemorrhage. Although it is not common, uncontrolled intraoperative hemorrhage may require a hysterectomy. Because it is difficult to predict preoperatively which patients will require this procedure, all patients should be warned of the risk. Additional potential complications include those of any pelvic surgery: bowel obstruction; adhesion formation; damage to bowel, bladder, fallopian tube, and ureter; general anesthesia; wound infection; and wound separation. Roughly 20 to 25% of patients undergoing myomectomy require another pelvic operation, usually hysterectomy. Recurrent myomas are common, especially in patients with multiple myomas. Significant febrile morbidity results, and it is often difficult to distinguish infection from fever caused by the release prostaglandins during myomectomy. Nonsteroidal anti-inflammatory agents are often useful in preventing this type of fever.

LAPAROSCOPY

Definition

Laparoscopy (Gr: *Laparo*-abdomen, *scopein*-to examine) is a transperitoneal endoscopic technique that provides excellent visualization of the abdominal contents with an illuminated telescope and often permits the diagnosis and management of gynecologic disorders without laparotomy.

Equipment

A number of instruments are used to facilitate operative laparoscopic procedures.

a. *Viewing system:* The video equipment includes a three-chip camera, a processor, a 300-watt xenon light source with fiber-optic cable (Fig. 35.1), a high-resolution monitor, and a video recorder. The three-chip camera provides a sharper, brighter image with higher resolution than the older single-chip cameras.

b. *Insufflator:* Pneumatic insufflator is used to monitor the rate, pressure, and volume of the gas used for inflation. For most procedures, the pneumoperitoneum may be maintained with an insufflator that flows at a rate of 2 to 7 L per minute. Insufflator controls intra-abdominal pressure rather than flow, and this should be set at 12–15 mmHg; a higher pressure of up to 25 mm Hg is acceptable during the intial phase of trocar entry (Fig. 35.2).

c. *Laparoscopes:* Laparoscopes are telescopes that vary in size from 4–12 mm in diameter. Viewing angles are available in 0-, 30-, 45-, and 70-degree increments. The choice is operator dependent. The instrument has an effective length of over 25 cm and can be utilized with a fiberoptic light box. In order to facilitate visualization, CO_2 must be instilled into the peritoneal cavity to distend the abdominal wall (Fig. 35.3).

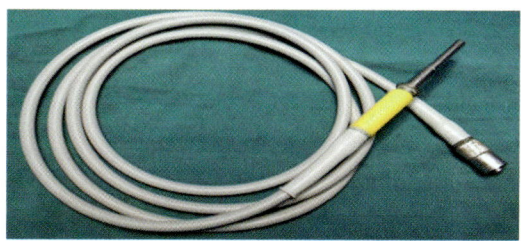

Fig. 35.1: Fiberoptic cable of xenon light source

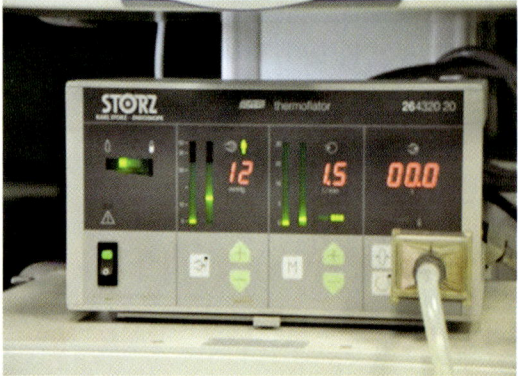

Fig. 35.2: Carbon dioxide insufflators showing normal working pressure

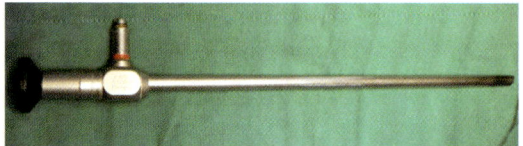

Fig. 35.3: Thirty degree laparoscopes

d. *Operating table:* An operating room table that allows 30 degrees of flexion (Trendelenburg position) is ideal for visualization of the deep pelvis (Fig. 35.4).

e. *Veress needle:* Veress needle is used to insufflate the abdomen with gas at the start of laparoscopy (Fig. 35.5).

f. *Trocars and cannulae:* Trocars and cannulae act as a conduit for the laparoscope and other instruments. They come in a variety of sizes depending on the diameter of the instrumentation to be accommodated, with 5 mm and 10–12 mm

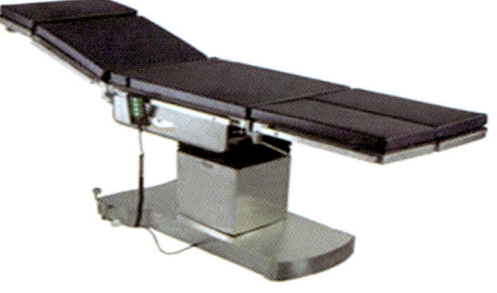

Fig. 35.4: Operation table for laparoscopy

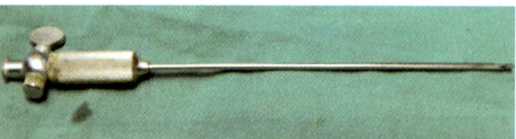

Fig. 35.5: Veress needle

ports being the most commonly required (Fig. 35.6).

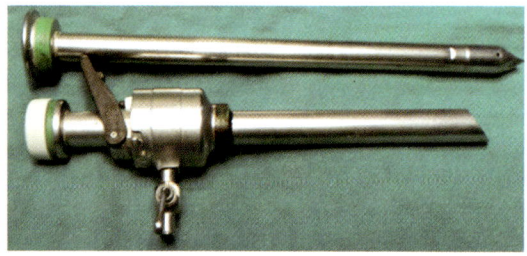

Fig. 35.6: Sharp trocar 10 mm with cannula

g. *Suction and irrigation system:* During laparoscopic surgery, irrigation and suctioning of electrosurgical smoke, blood, or irrigation fluids is often required. It can also be used to aspirate ovarian cysts, sucking out ectopic pregnancy and for hydrodissection in difficult cases (Fig. 35.7).

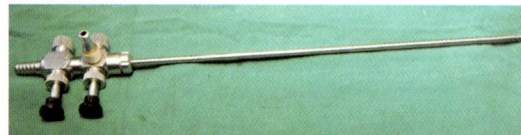

Fig. 35.7: Suction and irrigation system

h. *Ancillary instruments:* There is an enormous range of disposable and non-disposable instruments available for laparoscopy of various designs and sizes. A standard laparoscopy set should include (Fig. 35.8):

- Atraumatic grasping forceps—for holding the tissues
- Bipolar forceps
- Pointed Metzenbaum scissors and blunt saw toothed scissors

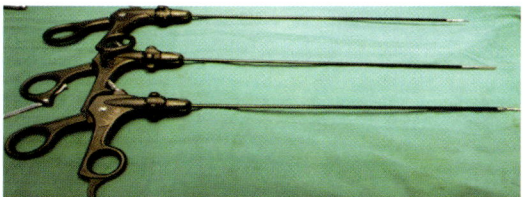

Fig. 35.8: Laparoscopy hand instrument

- Cyst aspiration needle
- Uterine manipulator.

An advanced laparoscopy set may include:
- Needle holders
- Knot pusher
- Vaginal delineator
- Babcock atrumatic grasper
- Endoscopic specimen retrieval bag
- Corkscrew
- Morcellator
- Microbipolar forceps.

Indications of Laparoscopy

Diagnostic

- Acute and chronic pelvic pain
- Infertility
- Endometriosis
- Pelvic inflammatory disease
- Evaluation of uterine perforation
- Genital anomalies, e.g. ovarian dysgenesis, uterime maldevelopment

Therapeutic

- Tubal sterilization
- Ectopic pregnancy
- Lysis of adhesions
- Fulguration of endometriosis
- Ovarian cystectomy and aspiration of small ovarian cysts
- Myomectomy
- Laparoscopy assisted vaginal hysterectomy, laparoscopic subtotal hysterectomy, laparoscopic hysterectomy
- Removal of extruded intrauterine device
- Uterosacral ligament division (denervation)

Contraindications of Laparoscopy

Absolute contraindications:
- Generalised peritonitis
- Intestinal obstruction
- Massive hemorrhage i.e. shock

Relative contraindications
- Severe cardiac or pulmonary disease
- Previous periumbilical surgery
- Intrauterine pregnancy after the first or early second trimester
- Presence of a large mass
- Inflammatory bowel disease
- Presence of known severe intraperitoneal adhesions

Clinical pearl: Laparoscopic procedure has replaced open surgery for many commonly performed gynecologic procedure such as tubal sterilization, treatment of ectopic pregnancy, ovarian cystectomy, treatment of endometriosis.

Steps of Laparoscopy

- *Anaesthesia and patient positioning:* The patient is put under general anesthesia and is placed in a low dorsal lithotomy position. The abdomen and the vagina is surgically prepped, and bladder is catheterised .
- *Uterine manipulator placement:* Sim's speculum is introduced in vagina to display the cervix, and a volsellum is placed on the anterior cervical lip. An uterine manipulator then is inserted into the external cervical os.
- *Veress needle placement:* A vertical incision is made through the skin corresponding to the size of the trocar, either within the umbilicus or at the base. The Veress needle is inspected for sharpness and a spring mechanism. The anterior abdominal wall inferior to the umbilicus is grasped with the non-dominant hand, and the umbilicus is lifted up. The tip of the Veress needle is held in the dominant hand between the thumb and forefinger while the ulnar palm rests on the patient's abdomen. The needle is

inserted carefully at a 45–90 degree angle, through the base of the umbilicus, millimeter by millimeter, until a click is heard and resistance is no longer felt, identifying intra-abdominal placement. Saline-filled 10-cc syringe is attached to the Veress needle and aspirated, inspecting for blood or bowel contents. If only bubbles are visible, saline is injected and observed to fall from the trough on the needle into the peritoneal cavity.

- *Carbon dioxide insufflation:* The syringe is removed, the insufflation tubing (with CO_2 turned on low flow) is attached, and the initial intra abdominal pressure is observed. If the pressure is <10 mm Hg, the needle is intra-peritoneal. Once intra-peritoneal placement is confirmed, a CO_2 pneumoperitoneum is obtained to reach an initial intra-abdominal pressure of 20 to 25 mm Hg. This temporary increase in intra-abdominal pressure increases the distance between abdominal viscera and the anterior abdominal wall (in the absence of adhesions) during primary sharp trocar placement through the umbilicus.

- *Primary Trocar insertion:* The end of the sharp trocar is held in the palm of the dominant hand, with the forefinger extended along the shaft as close to the sharp tip as possible. The tip is inserted through the umbilical incision until the fascia at the base of the umbilicus is felt. After placement of the primary trocar, the intra-abdominal placement is confirmed visually with the fiberoptic laparoscope. The intra-abdominal pressure is reduced to 12 to 15 mm Hg.

- *Insertion of ancillary ports:* Once the laparoscope has been inserted, the patient can be placed head down to facilitate the bowel out of the pelvis and lower abdomen. A quick check is made of the abdominal cavity, and one or two ancillary ports are inserted in the lower abdomen. Additional operative cannulas are needed to insert

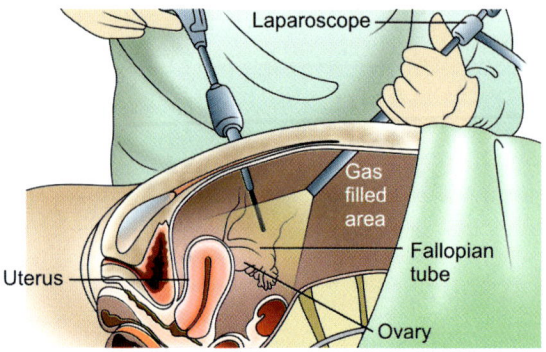

Fig. 35.9: Laparoscopy procedure

instruments into the abdomen. The number, location, and size of these cannulas will vary depending on the surgical instruments required for the laparoscopic procedure.

- *Inspection of pelvis and abdomen and laparoscopic procedure:* After checking the upper abdomen, pelvis is inspected. The indicated procedure then may be performed (Fig. 35.9).

- *Ending the procedure:* The ancillary ports should be removed under direct vision followed by deflation of the abdomen via the port used for the laparoscope.

Complications

Diagnostic laparoscopy is a safe procedure with published complication rates of 2–4 per 1000. However, following laparoscopic gynecologic operations, the complication rate is variable with a range from 0.2–10.3%. Complications of laparoscopic surgery include:

- *Intraoperative complications:* Bowel injury, vascular injury, bladder injury, ureter injury, surgical emphysema, and anesthetic complications.

- *Postoperative complications:* Unrecognized visceral or vascular injury, venous thromboembolism, infection and port site hernia.

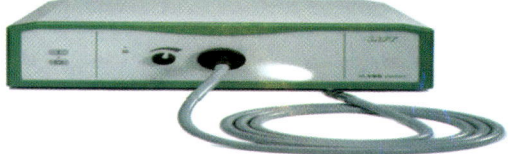

HYSTEROSCOPY

Definition

Hysteroscopy is a surgical intervention of viewing and operating in the endometrial cavity from a transcervical approach.

Equipment for Hysteroscopy

1. *Hysteroscope:* The telescope consists of 3 parts: the eyepiece, the barrel, and the objective lens. Hysteroscopes are available in different styles, including rigid and flexible hysteroscopes, contact hysteroscopes, and microcolpohysteroscopes. Majority of gynecologists prefer rigid hysteroscope because the image tends to be superior, the equipment is more robust, it can be used with a resectoscope, and not least, the purchase cost is much less. Rigid hysteroscopes come in different sizes in terms of their outer diameter, 4 and 2.9 mm being popular sizes. They are available at 0°, 12°, 15° or 30° angles of view (Fig. 35.10).

2. *Light source:* Each hysteroscope is attached to an internal or external light source for illumination at the distal tip. Energy sources include tungsten, metal halide, and xenon. A xenon light source with a liquid cable is considered the superior option (Fig. 35.11).

3. *Uterine distension media:* The uterine cavity must be distended for panoramic inspection of the uterine cavity. The medium opens the potential space of the otherwise narrow uterine cavity. To achieve this, gas (CO_2), low-viscosity fluids (e.g. N/

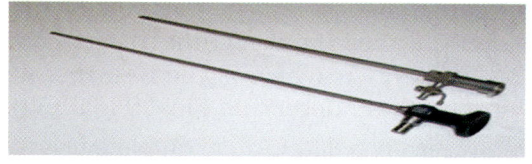

Fig. 35.10: Hysteroscope 4 mm

saline, 5% dextrose, 1.5% glycine, 3% sorbitol, 5% mannitol) or high-viscosity fluid (e.g. Hyskon, which is 32% dextran 70 in dextrose) can be used.

4. *Surgical instruments:* Surgical instruments are available in both rigid and flexible forms to be inserted through the operating channels of the scopes. Examples of surgical instruments (Fig. 35.12) and their uses are:
   - *Scissors:* To incise a septum, excise a polyp, or lyse synechiae
   - *Biopsy forceps:* To perform directed biopsy for pathologic review
   - *Grasping instruments:* To remove foreign bodies
   - *Roller ball, barrel, or ellipsoid:* To perform endometrial ablation and/or desiccation (this instrument is used with a resectoscope)
   - *Loop electrode:* To resect a fibroid or polyp or endometrium (this instrument is used with a resectoscope)
   - *Scalpel:* To cut or coagulate tissue, with high power density at its tip (this instrument is used with a resectoscope)
   - *Vaporizing electrodes:* To destroy endometrial polyps, fibroids, intrauterine adhesions, and septa; also used for endometrial ablation (this instrument is used with a resectoscope)
   - *Morcellator:* To cut and remove endometrial polyps or fibroids

5. *Resectoscope:* If resection of intrauterine tissues is required, then a resectoscope may be used. This instrument consists of inner and outer sheaths. The inner sheath houses 3 to 4 mm telescope and a channel for fluid medium inflow, whereas the 8 to

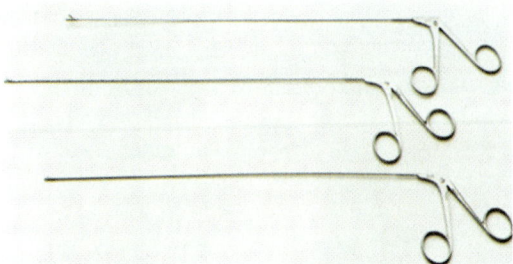

Fig. 35.12: Surgical instruments (top to bottom): Scissors, biopsy forceps, grasping forceps

10 mm outer sheath allows fluid pass out from the uterus through a series of small holes near the sheath's distal end. By means of a spring mechanism, the resection loop can be extended and then retracted to shave off contacted tissues.

Indications of Hysteroscopy

- Postmenopausal bleeding
- Abnormal uterine bleeding, e.g. menorrhagia, menometrorrhagia
- Abnormal pelvic ultrasound finding, e.g. endometrial polyp, submucous fibroid
- Recurrent pregnancy loss
- Congenital uterine anomaly
- Asherman's syndrome
- Lost intrauterine device

Contraindications

- Pregnancy
- Pelvic infection
- Cervical cancer

Fact sheet: Diagnostic hysteroscopy has become a basic investigation in modern gynecology and has essentially replaced the time honoured D & C (dilation and curettage).

Steps of Hysteroscopy

1. *Anesthesia and patient positioning:* Diagnostic hysteroscopy can be performed under local analgesia with or without intravenous sedation. For extensive procedures or for patients with a low pain tolerance, general or regional anesthesia is indicated. The patient is placed in a dorsal lithotomy position. The abdomen and the vagina is surgically prepped, and bladder is catheterised.

2. *Examination under anesthesia:* Bimanual examination is performed to assess the size and position of uterus and thus preventing perforation.

3. *Cervical dilation:* A vaginal speculum is introduced, and the anterior lip of cervix is grasped with a single-tooth tenaculum. The cervical canal is then gradually dilated to number 7 or 8 Hegar, depending on the outer diameter of the instrument.

4. *Hysteroscope introduction:* After the cervix is dilated, the hysteroscope attached to its light source, is inserted into the endocervical canal and advanced into the uterine cavity (with the distention medium flowing) under direct visualization to limit the risk of perforation. Pressure exerted by the distention medium opens the endocervical canal and allows hysteroscope entry.

5. *Hysteroscopic evaluation:* The tenaculum on the cervix is left in place to help in manipulating the uterus, and the vaginal speculum is removed to increase maneuverability of the hysteroscope. Once in the uterine cavity, it is simply a matter of systematically inspecting the fundus, tubal areas and the four walls of the uterus by a combination of rotating (if using an oblique-view hysteroscope) and moving the hysteroscope up/down and left/right. If the view is poor, it is usually because the intrauterine pressure is too low, either because the distending medium is at a relatively low pressure or pressure is lost through cervical leakage. Once the uterine cavity has been inspected, the hysteroscope is withdrawn which is the best time to inspect the endocervical canal (Fig. 35.13).

6. *Specific procedure:* After complete inspection, if specific lesions are identified, they

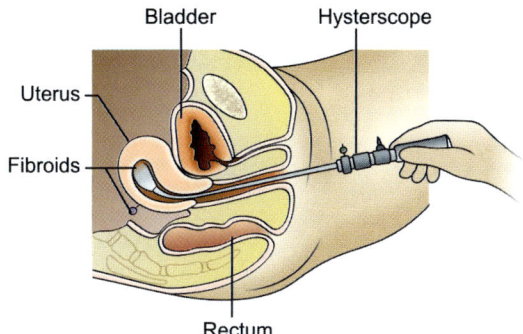

Bladder   Hysterscope

Uterus

Fibroids

Rectum

Fig. 35.13: Hysteroscopy procedure

typically are biopsied with hysteroscopic forceps.

7. *Procedure completion:* At the end of the procedure, the flow of distending medium is stopped, and hysteroscope and tenaculum are removed.

Complications

Diagnostic hysteroscopy is a safe procedure, and complications are uncommon. Uterine perforation, fluid overload from distending media, infection, and associated injuries related to laser or electrosurgical energies are the most common complications related to operative hysteroscopy.

Keywords

Pfannenstiel incision: The skin incision for a Pfannenstiel's incision is elliptical (concavity upwards) just above the symphysis pubis. The skin, subcutaneous fat, and rectus sheath of the abdominal wall are incised transversely. The rectus sheath is separated from the rectus muscle superiorly, inferiorly, and laterally. Small perforating vessels require ligation or coagulation. The rectus muscles are separated in midline. The peritoneum is usually entered vertically.

Trendelenburg position: With the patient on the operating table in the supine position, the head is lowered below the level of the pelvis.

Lithotomy position. A supine position with buttocks at the end of the operating table, the hips and knees being fully flexed with feet strapped in position.

Veress needle: A spring-loaded needle designed to allow entry into body cavities without trauma to underlying organs during laparoscopy.

EXERCISES

Answer the following questions

1. What do you mean by informed consent?
2. Name the routine investigations that are performed before major gynecological operations?
3. What preoperative measures you take before major gynecological operations?
4. What do you mean by hysterectomy?
5. What are its different types?
6. Namer the indications of hysterectomy. Which are common indications?
7. What are the different routes of hysterectomy?
8. During abdominal hysterectomy which structures are clamed and divided?
9. Where you plaxce clamps if you wish to remove the ovaries?
10. Which structures are clamped during vaginal hysterectomy?
11. How do you manage hysterectomy patients during postoperative period?
12. What are the complications of hysterectomy?
13. What is myomectomy? What are its indications?
14. What are the drawbacks of myomectomy?
15. What is laparoscopy?
16. Name the instruments used in laparoscopy?
17. What are the diagnostic and therapeutic indications of laparoscopy?
18. How do you perform diagnostic laparoscopy?
19. What are the complications of laparoscopy?
20. What is hysteroscopy? What are its indications and contraindications?
21. How do you perform diagnostic hysteroscopy?
22. What are its complications?

36

Medical Termination of Pregnancy (MTP)

A 28-year-old P 2+0 woman has come to OPD with amenorrhea for 35 days. Her urine for pregnancy test is positive. Her menstrual history reveals she had a cycle length of 28 days. Her blood pressure is 120/70 mm Hg and she is not anemic . She wants MTP by medicines. How she should be managed?

In this chapter we will learn
- Medical termination of pregnancy (MTP) Act
- Methods of MTP in first trimester
- Methods of MTP in second trimester
- Complications of MTP

Introduction

Abortion refers to the termination of pregnancy before the fetus is viable. Induced abortion means purposely causing an abortion. Termination of pregnancy refers to a procedure, whether medical or surgical, that results in expulsion of the products of conception. As per the Indian abortion law, only qualified doctors under certain stipulated conditions can perform an abortion on a woman in an approved hospital or clinic. The Indian abortion law is called MTP Act: Medical Termination of Pregnancy Act.

Medical Termination of Pregnancy Act

The Medical Termination of Pregnancy Act was enacted by the Indian Parliament in 1971 and came into force from 01 April, 1972. The MTP act was again revised in 1975. Further, MTP act was amended in 2002 and the Central Government made the Medical Termination of Pregnancy Rules 2003.

The MTP Act lays down the condition under which a pregnancy can be terminated, the persons and the place to perform it.

i. When pregnancy may be terminated by registered medical practitioners?

a. Where the length of the pregnancy does not exceed twelve weeks if at least one medical practitioner agrees, or
b. Where the length of the pregnancy exceeds twelve weeks but does not exceed twenty weeks, if at least two registered medical practitioners agree to do MTP.

ii. When pregnancy can be terminated?

a. The continuation of the pregnancy would involve a risk to the life of the pregnant woman, or risk of grave injury to her physical or mental health.

b. There is a substantial risk that if the child were born, it would suffer from such physical or mental abnormalities as to be seriously handicapped.

c. Where, any pregnancy alleged by the pregnant woman to have been caused by 'Rape'.

d. Where any pregnancy occurs as a result of failure of any device or method used by any married woman or his husband for the purpose of limiting the number of children.

iii. Consent of the woman

In case of a 'major' woman, i.e. who has attained the age of 18 years, consent in writing in consent form, 'Form C' (Rule 9) is required before MTP. In case of a 'minor', i.e. less than 18 years of age, {Sec. 4 (a)} or in case of 'mentally ill person' even she has attained the age of 18 years—consent of the guardian is required.

Clinical pearls

- For termination of pregnancy that exceeds 12 weeks and not 20 weeks, opinion of two registered medical practitioners are required.
- MTP should not be denied irrespective of the woman's decision to concurrent contraception.

iv. Who can do MTP?

a. Must be MBBS (or equivalent) in accordance with MCI Act 1956 (registered medical practitioner, RMP).

b. *Experience (MTP Rules 2003, Rule 4):* The medical practitioner must have any of the following experience:
   i. DGO or MS Gynecology
   ii. 6 months' House Job in Obstetrics and Gynecology.
   iii. 1 year's practice in Obstetrics and Gynecology at any Hospital.
   iv. Has assisted in performance of 25 cases of which at least 5 are done by him/herself in a hospital maintained/approved by Government for such training. (Qualified to do only 1st Trimester abortions.)

v. Where pregnancy may be terminated?

a. A hospital established or maintained by government, or

b. A place approved by 'District Level Committee' (DLC). *Provided:* That the DLC shall consist of 3 to 5 members including the Chairperson.

vi. Approval of place

a. Up to seven weeks, MTP may be done with medicines such as with Mifepriston and Misoprostol. Any 'RMP', may prescribe it at his/her clinic, provided: such RMP has access to a place, approved and display such certificate of access at some conspicuous place obtained from the owner of the 'approved place'.

b. *Up to 12 weeks MTP:* Place may be approved with following facilities: {Rule 5 1(ii)} gynecology examination table/labour table, resuscitation and sterilization equipment, drugs and parental fluids, backup facilities for treatment of shock, and facilities for transportation.

c. *Up to 20 weeks MTP:* Place may be approved with following facilities: {Rule 5 1(ii) a, b, c}

   - An operation table and
   - Instruments for performing abdominal or gynaecological surgery;
   - Anaesthetic equipment, resuscitation and sterilization equipment; and
   - Drugs and parental fluids for emergency use, as notified by government of India from time to time.

Fact sheet 1: In India, statistics state that there are 11 million MTPs are carried out annually and 20 thousand women die due to induced abortion. Morbidity and mortality from unsafe abortions remain a serious problem for Indian women even 40 years after the introduction for a legal abortion was liberalised in India. The reason this act came into legal acceptance and governance was to decrease septic abortions. But, it gradually gave rise to the biggest menace our country is facing Sex Selective termination, which is grossly affecting our sex ratio. However, to check the above mentioned problem, the PNDT Act came into force, which states that prenatal tests-like USG, conducted to determine the sex of the fetus is criminalised by Indian law since 1994.

METHODS OF MTP

The duration of pregnancy (gestation duration) in respect to medical termination of pregnancy is conventionally divided into two trimesters: First trimester MTP, up to 12 weeks of gestation since the first day of the last menstrual period; second trimester MTP, 12–20 weeks. First trimester surgical abortion (up to 12 weeks) and medical abortion (up to seven weeks) should be performed as outpatient procedures.

A. METHODS OF MTP IN FIRST TRIMESTER

Medical termination of pregnancy can be accomplished by surgical or medical techniques in first trimester. The phrase "medical abortion" refers to early abortion (usually before 7 weeks' gestation), not for medically induced second-trimester terminations, which are referred to as induction of abortion. Currently the medical abortion in India is approved up to 7 weeks of amenorrhea. Surgical techniques in the first trimester consist virtually exclusively of vacuum or suction techniques. The term "suction evacuation" is used interchangeably with "uterine aspiration" or "vacuum aspiration"; all refer to evacuation of the uterus by suction, regardless of the source of the suction. Manual vacuum aspiration is the term commonly applied to uterine evacuation using a hand-held syringe as the source of the vacuum. The methods that are available for MTP in first trimester are:

a. *Medical method:* Medical abortion with mifepristone and misoprostol
b. *Surgical methods:*
   a. Manual vacuum aspiration

b. Electrical vacuum aspiration or suction evacuation
c. Dilataion and evacuation.

A comparison of medical method and surgical method is shown in Table 36.1.

Medical Abortion

Background

- Mifepristone is a progesterone antagonist which binds to progesterone receptors and prevents the effects of progesterone on the uterus. It interferes with implantation and placental development resulting in fetal demise. It also increases uterine sensitivity to prostaglandins.

- Misoprostol is a prostaglandin E-1 analogue which induces uterine contractions, cervical dilatation and ripening. Its use in conjunction with misoprostol is very effective (> 96%) in bringing about termination in early pregnancy.

- Misoprostol in the first trimester of pregnancy has been shown to double the risk of congenital malformations. For this reason women should be informed of the importance of follow-up and in the rare event of ongoing pregnancy are recommended to undertake further abortion procedure when medical abortion has failed.

- Mifepristone is approved for use with misoprostol to terminate pregnancy up to 49 days (7 weeks) gestation. Its use up to 63 days (9 weeks) gestation remains off-label but is widely established as a safe alternative to surgical termination of pregnancy.

Indication

Medical abortion should be offered to all women seeking termination of pregnancy up to 7 weeks period of gestation (49 days from the first day of the last menstrual period in women with regular cycle of 28 days).

Safety and Efficacy

Medical abortion is successful in 95–98% of cases. It is a safe method of termination of pregnancy so long the contraindications are not disregarded. A few cases of failure are due to:

a. 1% women may require surgical evacuation for heavy bleeding.
b. 1% may fail to abort
c. 2–3% may be incomplete abortion resulting in surgical evacuation

Contraindications

a. Suspected/confirmed ectopic pregnancy/undiagnosed adnexal mass
b. Anemia—hemoglobin < 8 gm%
c. Coagulopathy or women on anticoagulant therapy
d. Chronic adrenal failure or current use of systemic corticosteroids (as mifepristone suppresses adrenal function for 3–4 days due to its competitive antagonism at glucocorticoid receptors)
e. Uncontrolled hypertension with BP > 160/100 mmHg
f. Lack of access to 24 hours emergency services.
g. Allergy to mifepristone and/or misoprostol
h. Intrauterine device in situ
i. Pelvic infection.

The following information should be given to all those women who are suitable and who wish to have medical abortion:

- She will require visit to hospital/clinic on three occasions.
- Following use of this method of abortion, vaginal bleeding usually occurs for 10–14 days; it is more like a heavy, prolonged menses. Sometimes, a small embryo may be visible in the blood clot.
- In case of failure (2–5%) of this method, she will require to undergo surgical abortion by suction evacuation (vacuum aspiration) as it will not be advisable to continue pregnancy.
- In case of heavy bleeding any time, she will have to report to her doctor/clinic immediately to decide whether a suction evacuation is needed to control bleeding.
- Her next menses may be delayed by one to two weeks, but subsequent menses will come on time.
- She has full option of choosing suction evacuation for terminating her pregnancy if she does not want to use medical abortion.
- During treatment and, preferably, till the next menses, she will have to avoid intercourse.
- She will have to sign a consent form after being satisfied with all the information provided, and after getting satisfactory answers to any doubts that she may have in mind.

Pre-abortion Workup and Investigations

- Careful history
- General examination
  - Pallor, blood pressure, cardiovascular and respiratory system
  - Bimanual examination to confirm the duration of pregnancy
- Rule out fibroid (if clinically significant) and ectopic pregnancy
- Pregnancy test (optional)
- *Optional investigations:* Hb%, urine examination, ABO and Rh blood group (necessary in primigravidae and if facilities available).
- Ultrasound is not required except in few conditions.
  - Ultrasound dating of pregnancy may be done in women who are:
  - Unsure of dates
  - Have conceived during lactational amenorrhoea have irregular cycles
  - Have a discrepancy between history and clinical findings.
- Women having any medical or psycho-social contraindication are not offered

termination of pregnancy with mifepristone (RU-486) and misoprostol.

Standard dose for mifepristone is 200 mg given orally followed by 400 µg misoprostol oral/vaginal according to the discretion of the clinician.

a. *Clinical protocol*
First visit (day 1)

- After a careful history, the woman is examined to confirm the uterine size, is counseled and an informed written consent is obtained.
- Mifepristone 200 mg is administered orally.
- Anti-D (50 µgm) given to Rh negative women with pregnancy > 6 weeks.

Second visit (day 3)

- History of any bleeding or side-effects should be noted.
- Oral/vaginal misoprostol 400 µg (2 × 200 microgram tablets) is given.
- For vaginal use, misoprostol tablet should be moistened with a few drops of water and the women must lie in bed for half an hour. Misoprostol usually acts quickly and the women can expect to pass products of conception within the next few hours, but bleeding usually continues for several weeks
- She should be observed for 4 hours in the clinic/hospital.
- Pulse and blood pressure are to be monitored and any side-effects noted.
- The time of start of bleeding and expulsion of products is noted.
- A pelvic examination is done before the woman leaves the clinic and if cervix is open and products are partially expelled, these are digitally removed.
- Drugs for pain relief or nausea vomiting are prescribed if required.
- Patient should be advised to abstain from intercourse, or to use condoms, till the next visit.

- She is instructed to take adequate rest and avoid going out of station.
- She should report in case of excessive pain or bleeding.

Third visit (day 15)

- A clinical history and pelvic examination should be done to ensure that there are no complications.
- Ultrasonography is required if history and examination do not confirm expulsion of products of conception.
- If she is still having irregular bleeding, curettage may be required.
- She should come for a check-up if she does not get period in 6 weeks.
- Contraceptive advice is given and appropriate contraception provided.

Fact sheet 2: Mifepristone + Misoprostol (1 tablet of 200 mg Mifepristone and 4 tablets of 200 microgram Misoprostol) combipack has been approved by the Central Drugs Standard Control Organization, Directorate General of Health Services for medical abortion of pregnancy (MTP) for up to 63 days gestation in December 2008. The Ministry of Health and Family welfare, Government of India is taking action on modifying the MTP rules in accordance with this approval.

Surgical Termination of Pregnancy

Indications

Women seeking termination of pregnancy at a gestational age of 12 weeks or less. The alternative is medical termination with mifepristone/misoprostol if < 7 weeks Surgical abortion can be performed by aspiration (using an electric pump or a manual syringe) or by dilatation and evacuation (D&E) which is not a preferred method.

a. *Manual vacuum aspiration:* Manual vacuum aspiration requires a single or double valve syringe: the vacuum (at least 55 mm Hg) is generated by a 60 mL hand-held syringe which accommodates flexible plastic cannula ranging from 4 mm to at least 12 mm in diameter.

b. *Electric vacuum aspiration (Suction evacuation):* This uses an electric pump. The technique is fundamentally the same as with manual vacuum aspiration.

Safety and efficacy of vacuum aspiration— Vacuum aspiration is very safe and effective method for first trimester MTP and successful in over 98% cases. Specific safety benefits of vacuum aspiration include a significantly reduced necessity of cervical dilatation, reduced risk of cervical injury, or uterine perforation, a reduced risk of infection and a reduced risk of blood loss, all resulting in a reduced need of anesthesia and a shortened hospital stay. The rates of major complications of conventional dilatation and evacuation/ curettage are two to three times higher than those of vacuum aspiration.

Preoperative Preparation

a. Fast from food for six hours before the procedure
b. Administer preoperative misoprostol for cervical preparation (400 microgram orally 3 hr before surgery). Cervical preparation reduces the need for mechanical cervical dilatation as well as reducing the risk of an incomplete evacuation
c. Administer a single dose of oral antibiotic such as ampicillin 1 gm or a suitable alternative.

Procedure

a. The woman is placed in the lithotomy position after emptying of bladder.
b. Povidone Iodine or chlorhexadine solution to the pubic area, vulva, perineum and vagina.
c. Drape with sterile sheet.
d. Insert sims speculum to expose cervix and clean cervix with povidone iodine solution.
e. Vulsellum forceps or Allis tissue forceps are applied to the anterior lip of the cervix to control the position of the cervix.

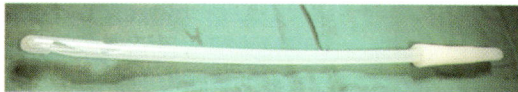

Fig. 36.1: Suction cannula (Karman's, disposable single use)

f. *Inject cervical local anaesthetic:* (2% lignocaine with adrenaline at 3 o'clock and 9 o'clock positions).
g. Dilate cervix with Hegar or Hawkin/ Ambler dilators starting with smallest dilator to a size appropriate for gestation. As a general rule, the dilator size will be equivalent to the number of weeks of gestation).
h. Choose appropriate suction cannulae (Fig. 36.1) and attach to the tubing. Either flexible or rigid suction cannulae are used. Insert into the uterus up to the fundus with the suction hole open. Then, apply suction and move the cannulae with a circular motion while slowly withdrawing it until the uterus is empty. Uterine evacuation is done with 60–80 mm Hg of negative pressure for an electric pump, or full vacuum for a 60 cc manual syringe (Fig. 36.2). When the uterus is empty, a strong uterine contraction can be felt as the uterus grips the cannula, making the aspiration more difficult. Bubbles and red foam appear in the cannula. The surgeon can detect a rough sensation in the uterus. These signs indicate that the uterus is empty and that the procedure is complete.

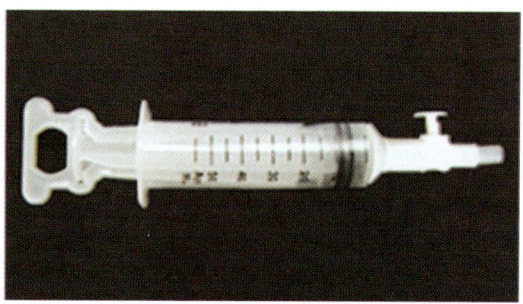

Fig. 36.2: IPAS single valve aspirator

Clinical pearl: Vacuum aspiration is the recommended technique of surgical abortion for pregnancies of up to 12 to 14 weeks of gestation. The procedure should not be routinely completed by sharp curettage. Dilatation and sharp curettage (D&C), if still practised, should be replaced by vacuum aspiration—WHO recommendation

B. METHODS OF MTP IN SECOND TRIMESTER

1. *Medical methods*

a. *Intra-amniotic instillation*—(i) hypertonic saline. (ii) Urea, (iii) Intra-amniotic prostaglandins, (iv) Intra-amniotic medication combination, e.g. prostaglandins plus urea

b. *Extra-amniotic instillation*—(i) Prostaglandins, (ii) Ethacridine lactate

c. Intravenous oxytocin

d. Vaginal and oral prostaglandins

e. Mifepristone in combination with prostaglandin analogue

2. *Surgical methods:* Hysterotomy, dilatation and evacuation by trained personnel.

Medical Methods

1. *Intra-amniotic Instillation*

a. ***Hypertonic saline:*** Taking aseptic precautions, a spinal needle is passed through the abdominal wall into the amniotic cavity. A variable amount of the amniotic fluid surrounding the fetus is removed and

Table 36.1: Advantages and disadvantages of medical and surgical abortion

Medical abortion

Advantages
- Avoids surgery and anesthesia
- More 'natural', like menses
- Emotionally easier for some women
- Client controlled; more privacy and autonomy; can be home-based
- Better than surgical abortion in very early gestation, or with severe obesity (body mass index >30) without other cardiovascular risk factors, or in the case of fibroids, uterine malformations or previous cervical surgery
- No risk of cervical/uterine injury

Disadvantages
- Bleeding, cramping, nausea, diarrhea and other side-effects of medicines
- Waiting, uncertainty
- More clinic visits
- Drugs are costly
- Can only be used up to 7 weeks

Surgical abortion

Advantages
- *Quicker*
- More likely to have a complete abortion
- Emotionally easier for some women
- Takes place in a health care centre, clinic or hospital
- Can be used up to 14 weeks (12–14 weeks by experts only)
- Sterilization can be concurrent

Disadvantages
- *Invasive*
- Small risk of cervical or uterine injury
- Risk of infection
- Less privacy and autonomy
- Can be costly

replaced by 150 to 250 ml of 20% sodium chloride solution that will induce abortion. *Effectiveness:* 81% will abort by 48 hours, with a mean time to abortion of 30 hours. *Complications:* Significant complications includes hemorrhage, clinical coagulopathy including disseminated intravascular coagulopathy, hypernatremia, renal failure and cervical laceration.

b. *Urea:* Safer agent than hypertonic saline for intra-amniotic instillation. When an inadvertent intravascular injection occurs, urea rapidly traverses cell membranes and acts as an osmotic diuretic. *Dose:* Intra-amniotic instillation of 40% urea solution (80 gm of urea in 200 ml of distilled water) is used with intravenous oxytocin drip. *Effectiveness:* 85–97% will abort within 48 hours with use of oxytocin.

c. *Intra-amniotic prostaglandins:* Instillation of prostaglandin inside the amniotic fluid acts as a reservoir, slowly allowing the prostaglandin to cross the sac to stimulate the myometrium. Natural prostaglandins such as PGE2 and PGF2α are commonly used. *Dose:* 5–10 mg of PGE2 and 2.5 mg–50 mg of PGF2α. *Effectiveness:* Abortion rate for PGE2 is 88–90% within 24 hrs. Abortion rate for PGF2α is 72–76% at 24 hours and 93–96% at 48 hours. *Side effects:* Vomiting, hemorrhage, genital injury including cervical laceration, infection and retained placenta.

2. Intra-amniotic Medication Combinations

In order to further improve efficacy of second trimester inductions and to decrease the induction to abortion interval, combinations of intrauterine agents have been investigated such as hypertonic saline plus prostaglandin F2α and urea plus prostaglandin F2α.

3. Extra-amniotic Instillation

a. *Prostaglandins:* Extra-amniotic PGE2 is instilled via a catheter through the internal os into the extra-amniotic space. *Dose:* 0.75 mg–2.5 mg of PGE2 gel. Intravenous oxytocin may be added after 6 hrs to improve effectiveness. *Effectiveness:* 78–90% abortion occurs within 24 hrs depending upon the dose used. *Side effects:* Vomiting, diarrhea, retained placenta.

b. *Ethacridine lactate:* Ethacridine lactate is a yellow dye with antiseptic properties. It is thought to stimulate endogenous prostaglandin production and subsequent uterine contractions. 0.1% solution of ethacridine lactate is instilled via a Foley catheter into the extra-amniotic space at a dose of 10 mL per gestational week to a maximum of 200 mL. A no 16 Foley catheter is passed through external os for about 10 cm from internal os between the membranes and deciduas and the balloon is inflated with 30 ml water. Intravenous oxytocin is often administered concomitantly to expedite fetal expulsion. *Effectiveness:* The abortion rate is 45% at 24 hours, 72% at 48 hours, and 93% at 72 hours. The mean induction abortion interval is 30 hours. *Side effects:* Hemorrhage, retained placenta.

4. Intravenous Oxytocin

A concentrated high-dose oxytocin regimen begins with a dose of 100 units per 500 mL of 5% dextrose in normal saline (D5NS), the 500 mL is infused over 3 hours, and then 1 hour is allowed for diuresis to preclude water intoxication. The dose of oxytocin is increased 50 units per 500 mL of D5NS until delivery is achieved, to a maximum of 300 units. *Effectiveness:* Abortion rate is 91% with a mean time to abortion of 8.2 hours.

5. Vaginal and Oral Prostaglandins

Misoprostol, a PGE1 analogue, has been has been shown to be effective in inducing second trimester abortion. This preparation has the advantage of being stable at room temperature and inexpensive. It is absorbed orally, vaginally, sublingually, buccally and rectally.

An ideal dosing regimens for misoprostol in second trimester induction of labor remains unclear vaginal misoprostol is more effective than oral misoprostol as vaginal misoprostol results in more sustained serum levels. However, sublingual and buccal misoprostol have also been widely used, as they are more convenient to administer and may be preferred by patients. *Dosage:* Studies suggest that the ideal dose of vaginal misoprostol for second trimester induction is between 200 and 600 µg and the ideal dosing interval is between 3 and 12 hours. A regimen comprising 400 µg misoprostol applied vaginally every 3–6 hrs with a maximum of 5 doses resulted in 95% success in induction of abortion with mean induction to abortion interval of 13 hrs (Government of India recommendation, Chaudhuri et al, 2009). *Side effects:* Vomiting, diarrhea, fever, retained placenta. Uterine rupture is rare but may occur in scarred uterus.

6. Mifepristone in Combination with Prostaglandin Analogue

The most dramatic improvement in second trimester induction abortion technology has come with the introduction of mifepristone. It sensitizes the myometrium of the uterus to prostaglandin. The induction to abortion interval has been dramatically reduced when mifepristone is used before prostaglandin analogues. *Dosage:* Mifepristone 200 mg followed 36–48 h later by: Misoprostol 800 µg vaginally followed by misoprostol 400 µg orally every 3 h up a maximum of 4 doses (WHO). It is highly safe and effective (97% success rate) method and adverse effects are similar to that of misoprostol only regimens.

> **Clinical pearl:** The World Health Organization (WHO) recommends medical method for pregnancies of gestational age more than 12 weeks is 200 mg mifepristone administered orally followed 36 to 48 hours later by repeated doses of misoprostol.

Surgical Methods

1. *Dilatation and evacuation:* Dilatation and evacuation (D&E) is the standard method at gestations above 13 weeks in many parts of the world but infrequently practised in India. It is the safest and most effective surgical technique, where skilled, experienced providers are available. D&E requires preparation of the cervix using osmotic dilators or pharmacological agents and evacuating the uterus using 12–16 mm diameter cannulae and long forceps. Depending on the duration of pregnancy, preparation to achieve adequate cervical dilatation can require from 2 hours to 2 days.

2. *Hysterotomy:* Hysterotomy is an operative procedure in which the products of conception is removed before viability by making an incision on anterior uterine wall Hysterotomy has limited role in present abortion practice since its morbidity is markedly higher than medical methods. However, at times hysterotomy may be considered such as: (i) Failed second trimester medical induction, (ii) Presence of uterine anomaly (iii) Scarred uterus and woman is willing for tubectomy. *Complications:* Peroperative bleeding, anesthetic hazards, abdominal wound infection, scar endometriosis, scar rupture in future pregnancy.

Complications of MTP

- *Ongoing pregnancy:* Failed abortion with ongoing pregnancy can occur following either surgical or medical methods of MTP, although it is more common after medical abortions. Women with clinical signs of failed abortion should be offered a uterine evacuation procedure as early as possible.

- *Incomplete abortion:* Incomplete abortion is also more common following medical abortion than following vacuum aspiration when the abortion is performed by a skilled provider. Common symptoms include vaginal bleeding and abdominal pain, and signs of infection may be present. Vacuum aspiration is recommended over D&C for uterine evacuation, as it is associated with less blood loss, less pain and shorter procedure times. Incomplete abortion may also be treated using misoprostol. The recommended misoprostol dose and route of administration for this indication is either 600 μg oral or 400 μg sublingual.

- **Hemorrhage:** Hemorrhage can result from retained products of conception, trauma or damage to the cervix, coagulopathy or, rarely, uterine perforation. Depending on the cause of the hemorrhage, appropriate treatment may include re-evacuation of the uterus and administration of uterotonic drugs to stop the bleeding, intravenous fluid replacement, and, in severe cases, blood transfusion, replacement of clotting factors, laparoscopy or exploratory laparotomy.

- **Infection:** Infection rarely occurs following properly performed abortions. Common signs and symptoms of infection include fever or chills, foul smelling vaginal or cervical discharge, abdominal or pelvic pain, prolonged vaginal bleeding or spotting, uterine tenderness, and/or an elevated white blood cell count. When infection is diagnosed, administer antibiotics and, if retained products of conception are a likely cause of the infection, re-evacuate the uterus. Women with severe infections may require hospitalization.

- **Uterine perforation:** Uterine perforation during the performance of suction evacuation or dilatation evacuation is a potentially serious complication that can result in hemorrhage or visceral injury. However, perforations are frequently unrecognized and frequently benign. Perforation commonly occur during introduction of uterine sound or dilator and common site of perforations is the junction of the cervix and the lower uterine segment. Perforation can be suspected when there is sudden loss of resistance with free mobility of the instrument, no tissue is obtained, when instruments are inserted deeper than expected, or when obviously maternal tissues such as omentum are obtained. Treatment of perforation depends on the expected location, the woman's vital signs and condition, and whether the abortion is complete. When the uterus is already empty before a perforation is first suspected and the perforation is thought to be midline, then intraperitoneal bleeding is unlikely. If the pain and bleeding continue to be minimal, repeated pelvic examinations are negative, and vital signs and repeat hematocrit are stable, antibiotic treatment and observation for several hours are all that is necessary. Under any other circumstance, she should be admitted to a hospital for observation and possible laparoscopy or laparotomy. If the laparoscopy examination and/or the status of the patient give rise to any suspicion of damage to the bowel, blood vessels or other structures, a laparotomy to repair the damaged structures may be needed. If the abortion is not complete at the time perforation is suspected, abortion should be completed with the aid of laparoscopy.

- **Uterine rupture:** Uterine rupture is a rare but catastrophic complication that can result in hysterectomy. It is associated with later gestational ages and uterine scar, but has also been reported in women without these risk factors. The risk of rupture for women with a prior cesarean delivery is 0.28%. Uterine rupture has been reported with almost all agents used to cause abortion by medicines , including high-dose oxytocin, hypertonic saline, PGF2α, ethacridine lactate, and with misoprostol.

- **Anesthesia related complications:** Local anesthesia is safer than general anesthesia, both for vacuum aspiration in the first trimester and for D&E in the second trimester.

EXERCISES

1. Answer the following questions

- What do you mean by abortion, induced abortion, termination of pregnancy?
- Till how many weeks of gestation medical termination of pregnancy is permissible in India?
- What are the conditions when pregnancy can be terminated according to MTP act?
- When consent from the guardian is required for MTP?
- What are the different methods available for first trimester MTP?
- What are the different methods available for second trimester MTP?
- Till how many weeks medical abortion is indicated in first trimester?
- What are its contraindications?
- What are the mechanism of action of mifepristone and misoprostol for medical abortion?
- What is the dosage schedule of medical abortion?
- Who are candidates for surgical termination of pregnancy in first trimester?
- Describe the steps of vacuum aspiration (suction evacuation) operation.
- How do you manage uterine perforation occurred during vacuum aspiration?

2. Write short notes on

- MTP Act
- Medical abortion in first trimester
- Complications of MTP

3. Fill in the blanks with appropriate word/s

- MTP act was passed in the parliament in the year _____ and came into force in the year _____ .
- For medical abortion in first trimester woman will require to visist hospital/clinic at least _____ occasions.

- _____ mm Hg pressure is generated in manual vacuum aspiration by a _____ ml hand held syringe.
- Drugs that are used for intra-amniotic instillation in second trimester MTP are _____ , _____ , _____ .
- Drugs that are used for extra-amniotic instillation for second trimester MTP are _____ , _____ .

4. Explain or justify the following statements

- Medical abortion should be offered to all who seek MTP within 49 days.
- Medical methods are more commonly used than surgical methods in second trimester MTP.

Bibliography

1. Borgatta, L, Kattan, D, et al. Surgical techniques for first trimester abortion Glob. libr. women's med., (ISSN: 1756-2228) 2012; DOI 10.3843/GLOWM.10440.
2. Borgatta, L. Labor induction termination of pregnancy Glob. libr. women's med., (ISSN: 1756-2228) 2011; DOI 10.3843/GLOWM.10444 December 2011.
3. Chaudhuri S, et al. Comparison of two regimens of misoprostol for mid trimester MTP Tropical Doctor 2009.
4. Clinical guideline South Australian perinatal practice guideline First trimester medical and surgical termination of pregnancy Nov 2013.
5. Comprehensive abortion care Training and service delivery guidelines Ministry of Health and Family Welfare Government of India.
6. Guideline for medical abortion in India Material circulated by CASSA during the state-level Workshop on Review of MTP act 1971 in the context of Woman's Right to abortion and halting sex selective abortion, held in Chennai 2007.
7. Induced abortion guideline SOGC Clinical Practice Guidelines 2006.
8. International Planned Parenthood Federation First trimester abortion guidelines and protocols Surgical and medical procedures.
9. Johnston HB. Abortion practice in India—a review of literature Mumbai 2002.

10. Lalitkumar S, et al. Mid trimester induced abortion—a review Human Reproduction Update, Vol.13, No.1 pp. 37–52, 2007.

11. MTP Act Ministry of Health and Family Welfare (Department of Family Welfare) Notification New Delhi, the 13th June, 2003.

12. Safe abortion. Technical and policy guidance for health system World Health Organization 2012.

13. The Medical Termination of Pregnancy Act, 1971 (Act No. 34 of 1971).

14. Wildschut H, Both MI, Medema S, Thomee E, Wildhagen MF, Kapp N. Medical methods for mid-trimester termination of pregnancy. Cochrane Database of Systematic Reviews 2011, Issue 1. Art. No.: CD005216. DOI: 10.1002/14651858.CD005216.pub2.

15. Yadav M, Kumar A. Medical termination of pregnancy (amendment) act, 2002 an answer to mother's health & 'female foeticide' JIAFM, 2005: 27 (1). ISSN 0971-0973.

37

Instruments, Specimens and X-rays

In this chapter we will learn:
- To identify an instrument and to describe its uses
- To describe a specimen and to diagnose a disease and to identify the type of operation that was done
- To describe a HSG/ X-ray plate and to diagnose a disease

INSTRUMENTS

1. Female Metal Catheter (Fig. 37.1)

Use

a. To empty the urinary bladder before vaginal gynecological operations, e.g. D&C, vaginal hysterectomy, PFR
b. To differentiate between a cystocele and Gartner duct cyst—in cystocele catheter tip can be felt below the bulge.
c. During PFR operation—to know the lower limit of bladder before making an incision over anterior vaginal wall and before dividing vesicocervical ligament.

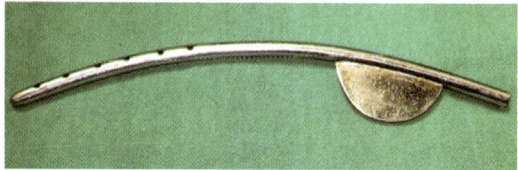

Fig. 37.1: Female metal catheter

2. Uterine Curette (Figs 37.2a to c)

Uterine curette may be of different types:
- Sharp at one end and blunt on other end

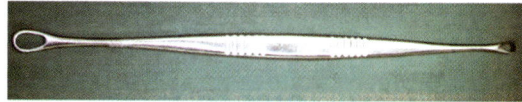

Fig. 37.2a: Sharp and blunt uterine curette. Double ended: Sharp and blunt uterine curette is available in three sizes small (4 mm), medium (6 mm) and large sizes (8 mm)

- Sharp at one end with handle
- Sharp or blunt on both ends
- Sharman's curette
- Flushing curette.
  Uterine curette is used for scraping of the endometrial cavity to obtain sample for histopathology or therapeutic purpose during dilatation and curettage operation (D&C) or dilatation and evacuation operation (D & E). Endometrium is curetted from the fundus to internal os starting from 12 o' clock position and then anticlockwise fashion until one round of whole endometrial cavity is curetted. In general, sharp end of curette is used in non-pregnant uterus and blunt end is used in

382

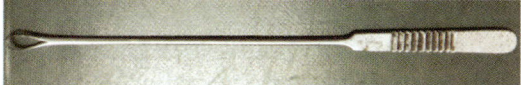

Fig. 37.2b: Uterine curette—sharp at one end with handle

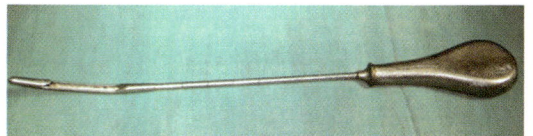

Fig. 37.2c: Sharman's curette—used for curettage in Infertility where only strip of endometrium is enough to study hormonal change of endometrium (secretory change in ovulatory cycle)

pregnant uterus or when the uterus is soft, e.g. choriocarcinoma, pyometra.

3. Cervical Dilators (Figs 37.3a to e)

Cervical dilators are of different varieties:
- Hegar's cervical dilator—single or double ended
- Das's cervical dilator (named after Sir Kedar Nath Das)
- Hawkin Ambler cervical dilator.

Uses:

Cervical dilators are used for cervical dilatation in procedures like D&C, D&E, Fothergill's operation, hysteroscopy, cervical stenosis, treatment of primary dysmenorrhea, Copper T insertion, drainage of pyometra, hematometra, lochiometra.

4. Punch Biopsy Forceps (Figs 37.4a and b)

Use: To take biopsy from cervix.

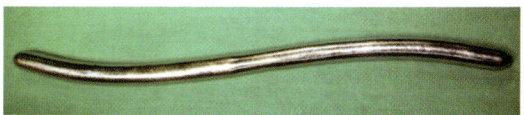

Fig. 37.3a: Hegar's cervical dilator–long rod like instrument with tapering end and gentle curve. Hegar's dilators are double ended. There are 12 sets, smallest one, 1–2 mm

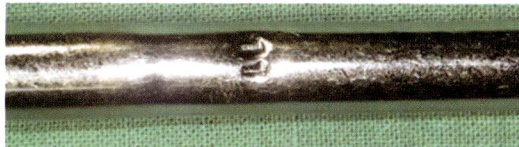

Fig. 37.3b: Number 11 Hagar's cervical dilator—the dilators are numbered as per outer diameter - no 11 means diameter of 11 mm on that end. For D&C operation, dilatation up to 8 mm and for MTP dilatation up to 12 mm may be done

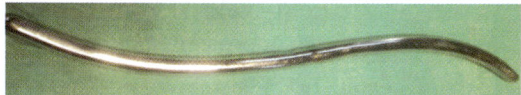

Fig. 37.3c: Das's cervical dilator

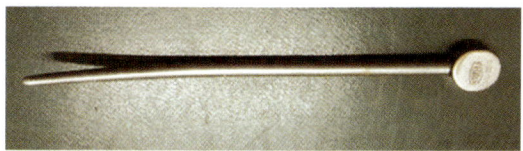

Fig. 37.3d: Hawkin Ambler's cervical dilator. There are 16 sets starting from 3/6 mm to 18/21 mm size. 3/6 means outer diameter at the tip of dilator is 3 mm and 6 mm at the base.

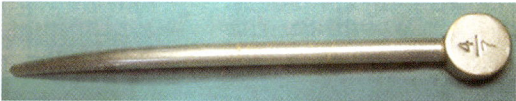

Fig. 37.3e: Number (4/7) on Hawkin Ambler cervical dilator

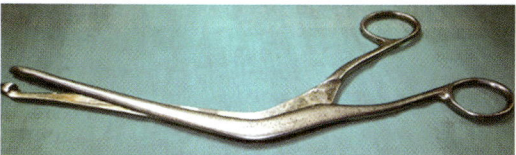

Fig. 37.4a: Punch biopsy forceps

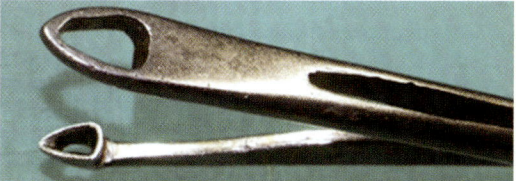

Fig. 37.4b: Tip of punch biopsy forceps

5. Hysterosalpingography (HSG) Cannula
(Figs 37.5a to c)

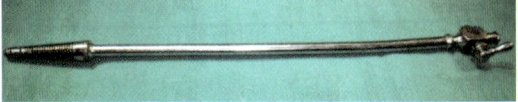

Fig. 37.5a: HSG cannula

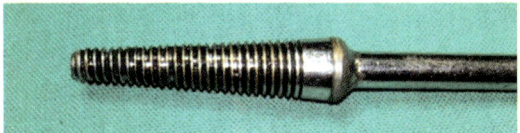

Fig. 37.5b: Open ended metal HSG cannula tip—this conical end is introduced in cervical canal

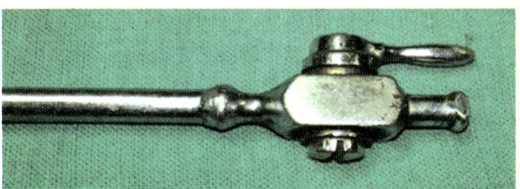

Fig. 37.5c: Outer cannula end—this end is fitted with 10 ml syringe to push radio-opaque dye inside uterine cavity

Uses
- HSG cannula is used to inject contrast medium (iodine containing radio-opaque dye-urograffin) into the endometrial cavity during hysterosalpingography.
- It can also be used to inject methylene blue dye into endometrial cavity during laparoscopic chromopertubation.
- May be used during hydrotubation. In hydrotubation medicated solution (dexamethasone 4 mg and 80 mg gentamycin in 10 ml normal saline) is instilled transcervically in conditions such as following tuboplasty operation.

6. Multiple Teeth Vulsellum (Fig. 37.6)

Uses: The instrument is used to hold and steady the cervix in operations like D&C, Cervical biopsy, insertion of Cu T, Fothergill's operation, vaginal hysterectomy, anterior colporrhaphy. Usually the anterior lip of the

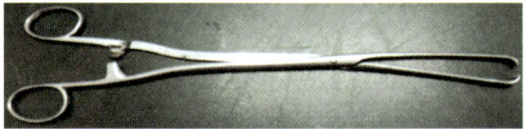

Fig. 37.6: Multiple teeth vulsellum

cervix is grasped but posterior lip of cervix is also grasped in conditions like posterior colpotomy, growth in anterior lip of cervix, during vaginal hysterectomy when posterior cervicovaginal mucosa is incised. It is not used in pregnancy as teeth are sharp and may cause laceration. Instead sponge holding forceps is used to hold the cervix in pregnancy.

7. Single Tooth Vulsellum (Figs 37.7a and b)

Uses
- To hold the left out cervical stump after (Figs 37.7a and b) amputation of cervix and during Fothergill's operation.
- Sometimes to hold anterior lip of cervix in Nulliparous women during D&C operation.

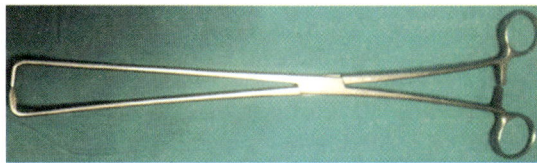

Fig. 37.7a: Single tooth vulsellum

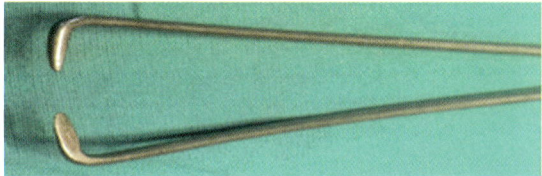

Fig. 37.7b: Tip of single tooth vulsellum

8. Sponge Holding Forceps (Figs 37.8a and b)

Uses
- For holding sponge or gauge piece during antiseptic dressing in abdominal and vaginal operations
- To hold polyp during polypectomy operation

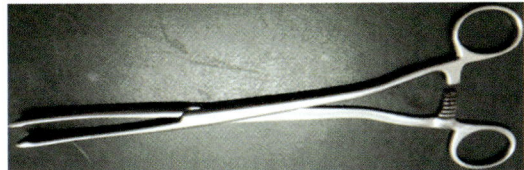

Fig. 37.8a: Sponge holding forceps

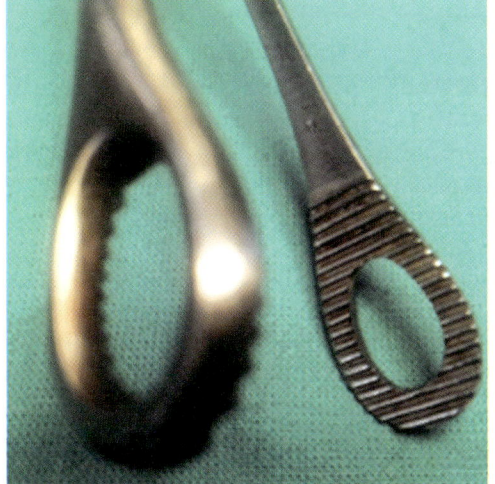

Fig. 37.8b: Tip of sponge holding forceps

- For tissue dissection when used as sponge on holder
- To hold the cervix in pregnancy, e.g. during circlage operation, exploring cervix after forceps delivery (3 sponge holding forceps are required), during second trimester MTP at the time of Foley catheter insertion or check curettage following expulsion of products.

9. Long Straight Hemostatic Forceps (Fig. 37.9)

Uses

- Used as a clamp in hysterectomy, salpingectomy, salpingo-oophorectomy

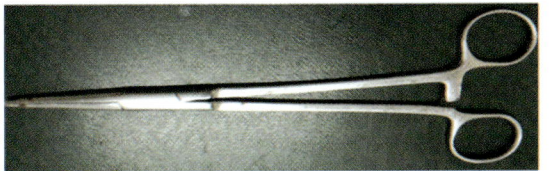

Fig. 37.9: Long straight hemostatic forceps

- To catch a bleeding vessel deep into the pelvis.

10. Sims' Double Bladed Posterior Vaginal Speculum

The instrument was designed by James Marion Sims. The blades are of unequal breadth. Small blade is used in nulliparous vagina and large blade is used in parous vagina (Fig. 37.10).

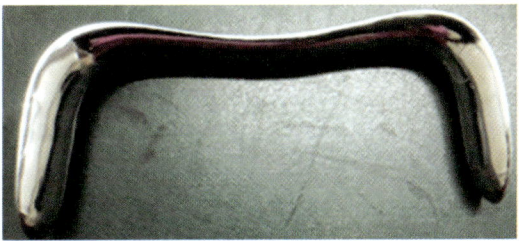

Fig. 37.10: Sims' double bladed posterior vaginal speculum

Uses

- Sims' speculum is used to depress perineum for inspection of vagina and cervix in OPD. Lesions in anterior vaginal wall that can be diagnosed are cystocele, VVF, Gartner duct cyst
- During gynecological operation to retract the perineum, e.g. D&C, Cervical biopsy, Vaginal hysterectomy, PFR, Fothergill's operation, repair of VVF, etc.
- During gynecological minor procedures like taking Pap smear, insertion and removal of Cu T, colposcopy, taking swabs.
- In obstetrics: (a) for inspection of local cause for APH, (b) for presence of dribbling in PROM, (c) during encirclage operation, D&E operation, S & E operation, etc (d) for inspection of cervix during traumatic PPH.

11. Ayer's Spatula (Fig. 37.11)

Use: Used for taking pap smear for screening of cervical cancer.

Ayer's spatula is made up of wood so that cells can adhere to its porous surface. During

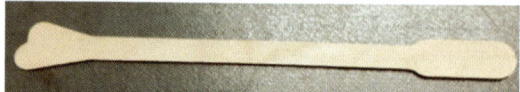

Fig. 37.11: Ayer's spatula

collection of cervical cells for pap smear, the long projected end of spatula is inserted into the cervical canal and rotated by 360°. The other end is used for collection of vaginal cells from fornices for the hormonal status.

12. Allis Tissue Forceps (Fig. 37.12)

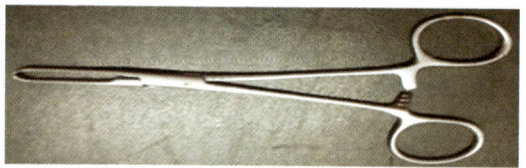

Fig. 37.12: Allis tissue forceps

Uses

- To hold cut margins of rectus sheath during abdominal operations like abdominal hysterectomy, laparotomy
- To hold the margins of vaginal wall during colporrhaphy operation, vaginal hysterectomy
- To hold the margins of vagina during abdominal hysterectomy after opening vault of vagina
- To hold the anterior lp of cervix during D&C, cervical biopsy, HSG operations.
- To hold the torn ends of sphincter ani externus during CPT repair operation.

13. Anterior Vaginal Wall Retractor (Fig. 37.13)

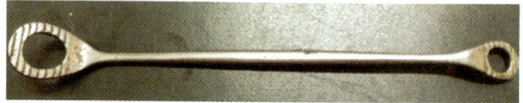

Fig. 37.13: Anterior vaginal wall retractor

Use: To elevate the anterior vaginal wall during inspection of cervix in case of cystocele.

14. Deaver's Retractor (Fig. 37.14)

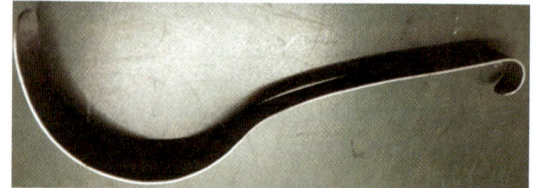

Fig. 37.14: Deaver's retractor

Use: To retract the abdominal viscera such as intestines, bladder during abdominal operations like abdominal hysterectomy, laparotomy.

15. Uterine Dressing Forceps (Fig. 37.15)

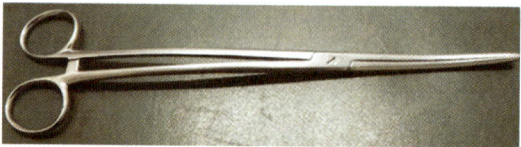

Fig. 37.15: Uterine dressing forceps

Use: To swab the uterine cavity with sterile gauge and antiseptics in D&E operation.

16. Cusco's Bivalve Self Retaining Adjustable Vaginal Speculum (Fig. 37.16)

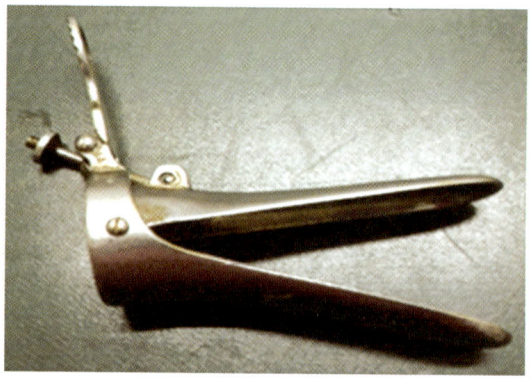

Fig. 37.16: Cusco's speculum

Uses

- Cusco's speculum is used in OPD for routine examination of cervix and vault of vagina.

- Can be used for taking cervical and vaginal smear for cytology and bacteriology.
- Can be used during insertion and removal of Cu T.

17. Myoma Screw (Fig. 37.17)

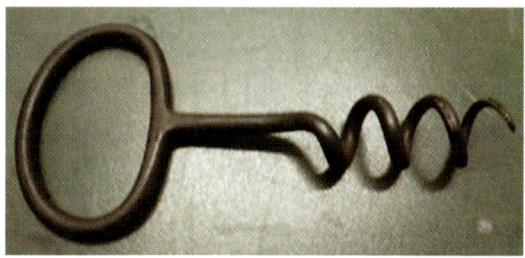

Fig. 37.17: Myoma screw

Uses

- To fix the myoma and give traction during enucleation of myoma at myomectomy operation
- To give traction in a big fibroid uterus requiring hysterectomy

18. Doyen's Retractor (Fig. 37.18)

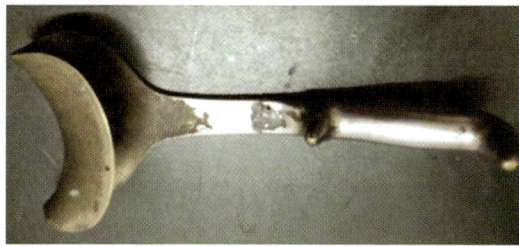

Fig. 37.18: Doyen's retractor

Use: It is used to retract the bladder during abdominal operations like hysterectomy, laparotomy, LSCS.

19. Olive Pointed Graduated Malleable Metallic Uterine Sound (Fig. 37.19)

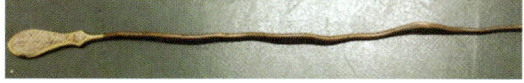

Fig. 37.19: Uterine sound

It is a long instrument with blunt tip (olive pointed) to avoid perforation. It has markings for measurement of length of uterine cavity. About 5 cm from the tip it can be bend (malleable) to make an angle of 30°.

Uses

- In D&C operation—It is used to confirm position of uterus, to measure length of uterocervical canal and acts as first dilator.
- To feel the IUCD in case of missing thread.

20. Simple Rubber Catheter (Fig. 37.20)

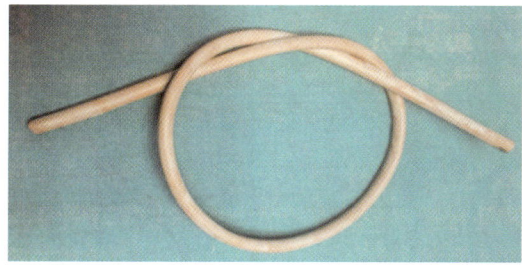

Fig. 37.20: Simple rubber catheter

Uses

- For continuous drainage of urine during abdominal hysterectomy, laparotomy.
- To empty the bladder in retention of urine
- To administer oxygen
- As tourniquet during myomectomy operation.

21. Foley Catheter (Figs 37.21a to c)

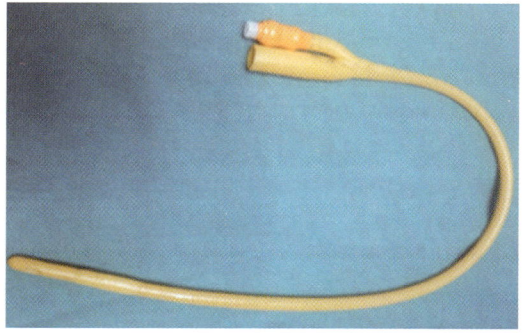

Fig. 37.21a: Foley catheter

Uses

- Self retaining catheter for continuous drainage of urine following operations like

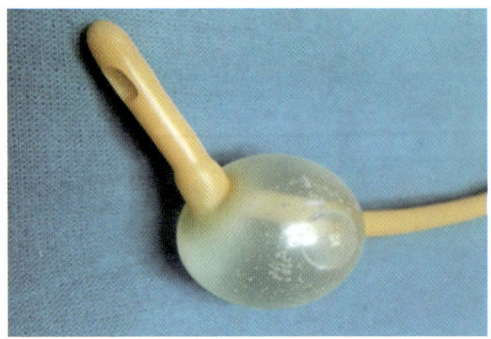

Fig. 37.21b: Tip of Foley catheter with balloon inflated with distilled water

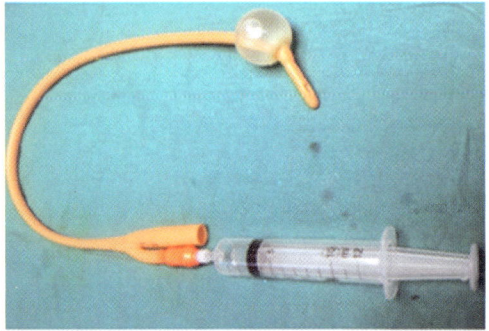

Fig. 37.21c: There are two channels—one for inflating the balloon with water and has a valve, the other channel is for drainage of urine to which urobag is attached

vaginal hysterectomy, radical hysterectomy, VVF repair, abdominal hysterectomy. No 14 or 16 F foley catheter is commonly used.

- For instillation of extra-amniotic ethacridine lactate for second trimester MTP.
- For introduction of normal saline inside uterine cavity during sonosalpingography. No 8F Foley catheter is commonly used.

22. Babcock's Forceps (Figs 37.22a and b)

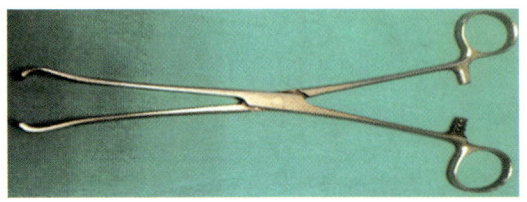

Fig. 37.22a: Babcock's forceps

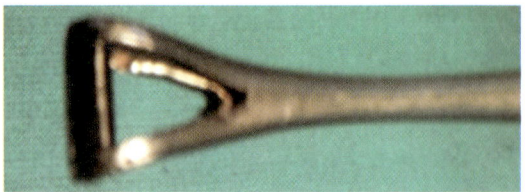

Fig. 37.22b: Tip of Babcock's forceps

Uses: To hold tubular structures like fallopian tube, ureter, appendix during operations like tubectomy/tuboplasty, radical hysterectomy and appendicectomy respectively.

23. Landon's Retractor (Fig. 37.23)

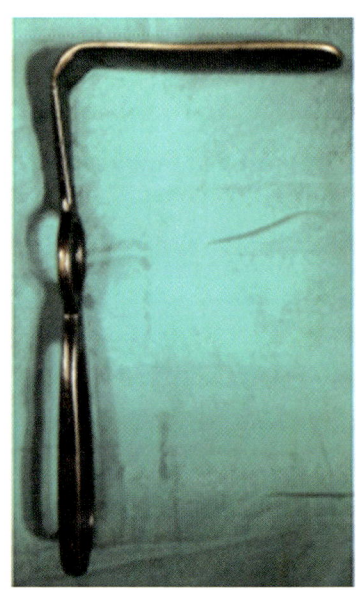

Fig. 37.23: Landon's retractor

Use: To retract urinary bladder during vaginal hysterectomy, Ward Mayo's operation.

24. Carman's Suction Cannula
(Figs 37.24a and b)

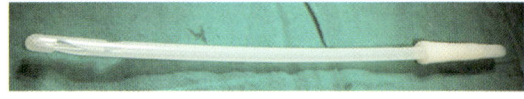

Fig. 37.24a: Carman's plastic suction cannula—disposable single use cannula

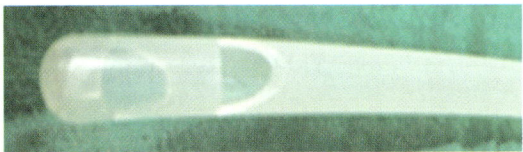

Fig. 37.24b: Tip of Carman's suction cannula

Use: Used during suction evacuation operation to aspirate product of conception.

25. Ovum Forceps (Figs 37.25a to c)

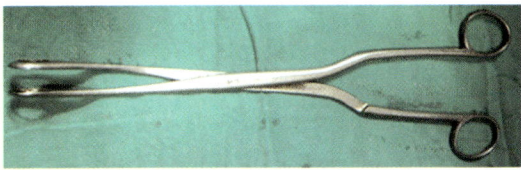

Fig. 37.25a: Ovum forceps

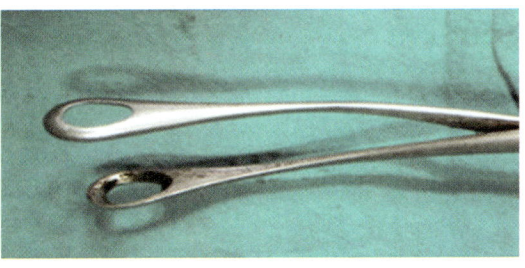

Fig. 37.25b: Tip of ovum forceps

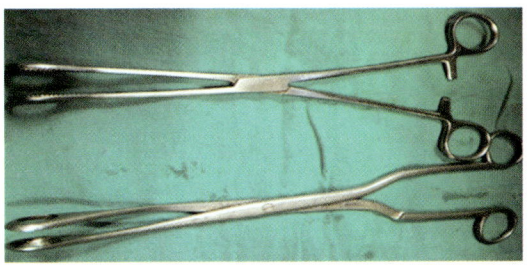

Fig. 37.25c: Sponge holding forceps (upper one) and ovum forceps (lower one)—note the similarities in appearance of the two instruments. Sponge holding forceps has catch but ovum forceps has no catch to minimise trauma if accidentally uterine wall is grasped

Use: To remove the products of conception during D&E operation.

26. Kocher's Hemostatic Forceps (Figs 37.26a and b)

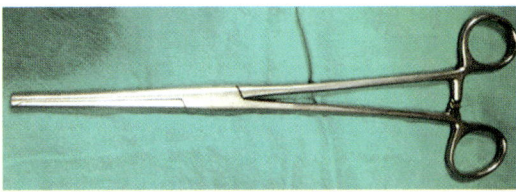

Fig. 37.26a: Kocher's straight hemostatic forceps

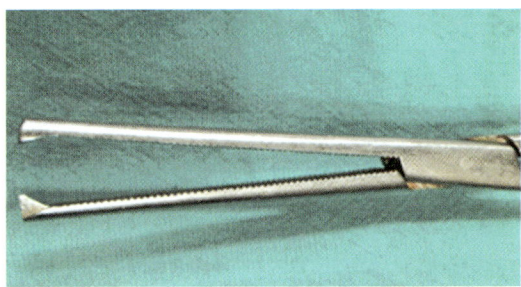

Fig. 37.26b: Tip of Kocher's hemostatic forceps—note the tip of the blades have teeth so that tissue does not slip. The blades can be straight or curved

Uses

- Used as clamp to grasp the pedicle during hysterectomy operation
- It can also be used as clamp during salpingectomy and oophorectomy operation.

SPECIMENS

Identification of Organ

Uterus

Uterus is identified by:
- Pear shaped
- Attachments of fallopian tubes and ovaries
- Presence of cervix identified by external os. In nulliparous women external os is circular and in parous women external os is transverse slit like.

Anterior surface of uterus is identified by:

Attachment of round ligament and presence of loose attachment of uterovesical peritoneum and cut margin is reflected at a higher level than in posterior surface of uterus.

Posterior surface of uterus is identified by attachment of ovarian ligament and cut margin of posterior peritoneum is firmly attached and placed at a lower level than cut margin of anterior peritoneum.

Fallopian Tube

Tubular structure with presence of fimbrial end and attachment of mesosalpinx containing blood vessels.

Ovary

Fallopian tube may be attached. If fallopian tube is not attached it is identified by its typical appearance as no other structure in pelvis resembles its appearance.

Description of specimen: To describe a specimen you will have to identify the organs and then to describe the pathology as seen in naked eye appearance.

Specimen 1 (Fig. 37.27)

Description: This is a surgically removed specimen of uterus. The uterus is uniformly enlarged to around 8 weeks size of pregnant uterus.

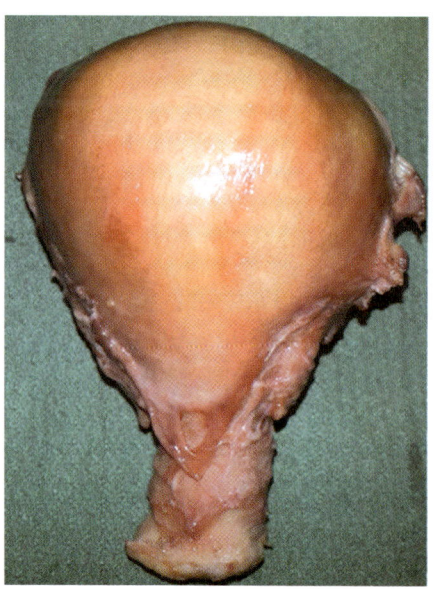

Fig. 37.27: Specimen of uterus

Diagnosis: Adenomyosis or uterine leiomyoma.

Operation done: Total hysterectomy.

Specimen 2 (Fig. 37.28)

Description: This is a surgically removed specimen of uterus and right sided tube and ovary. The uterus is hugely enlarged with smooth surface, the fallopian tube and ovary are normal.

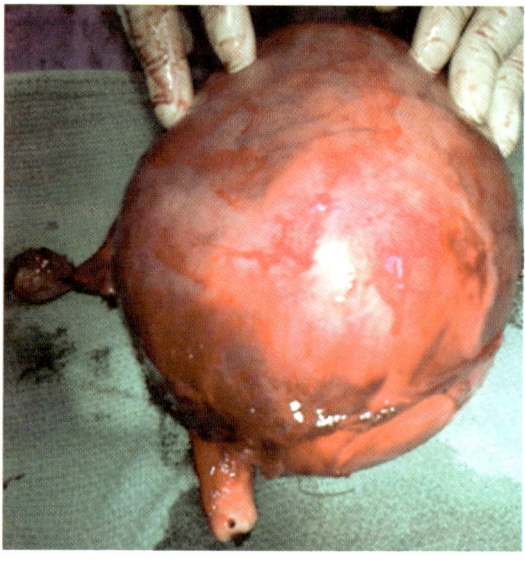

Fig. 37.28: Specimen of uterus and right tube and ovary

Diagnosis: Uterine leiomyoma in body of uterus.

Operation done: Total hysterectomy with right sided salpingo-oophorectomy

Specimen 3 (Fig. 37.29)

Description: This is a surgically removed specimen of uterus, left sided fallopian tube and ovary. Uterus is enlarged with presence of multiple nodular structures of different sizes over body of uterus, left fallopian tube and ovary are normal.

Diagnosis: Multiple leiomyoma of body of the uterus.

Operation done: Total hysterectomy with left sided salpingo-oophorectomy.

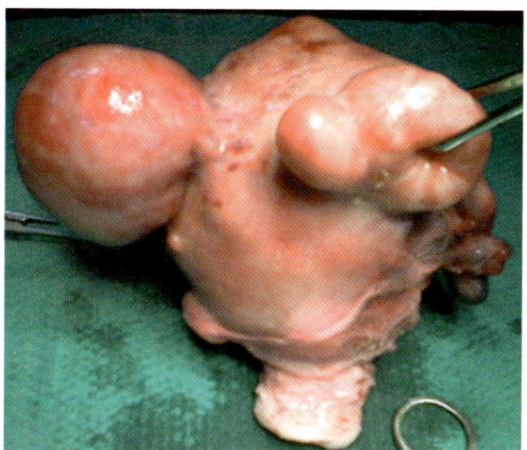

Fig. 37.29: Multiple leiomyoma

Specimen 4 (Fig. 37.30)

Description: This is a surgically removed specimen of uterus. Uterus is uniformly enlarged to 10 weeks size of pregnant uterus. The anterior surface of uterus is cut open. On cross-section, the haphazardly distributed hypertrophied muscular trabeculae is seen with scattered brown staining spots.

Diagnosis: Adenomyosis

Operation done: Total hysterectomy.

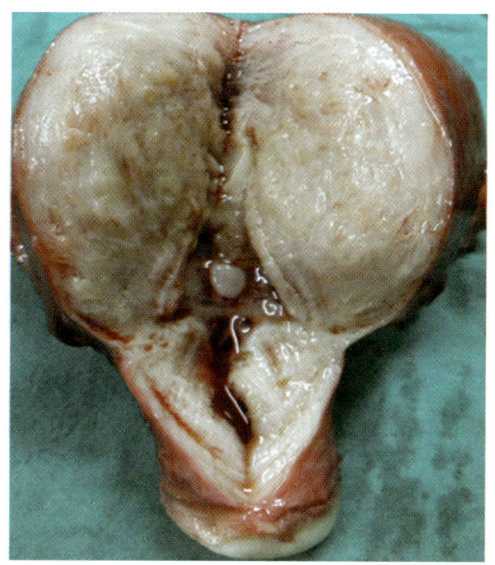

Fig. 37.30: Adenomyosis of uterus

Specimen 5 (Fig. 37.31)

Description: This is a surgically removed specimen of uterus. The uterus is uniformly enlarged to 8 weeks size of pregnant uterus. A large polypoid mass is comeing out of the cervix.

Diagnosis: Fibroid polyp

Operation done: Total hysterectomy.

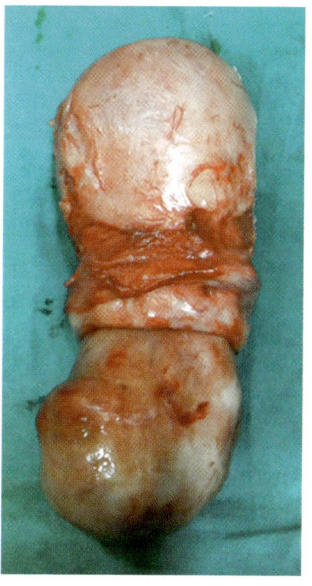

Fig. 37.31: Fibroid polyp (*Courtesy:* Dr Samaresh Malo, Assistant Professor, NRS Medical College)

Specimen 6 (Fig. 37.32)

Description: This is a surgically removed specimen of uterus. The anterior surface of uterus is cut open and showing a large pedunculated mass originating from posterior wall of uterus and coming out of the cervix. A small nodular mass is seen in front of the polypoid mass. Cut section of the uterine wall shows hypertrophy of the uterine muscle.

Diagnosis: Multiple fibroid polyp.

Specimen 7 (Fig. 37.33)

Description: This is a surgically removed specimen of uterus, both fallopian tubes and

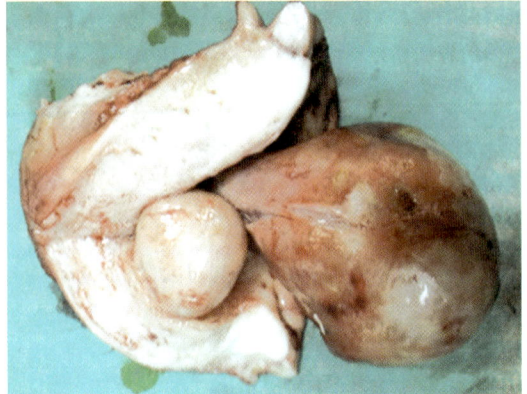

Fig. 37.32: Fibroid polyp-same specimen of Fig. 37.31. Anterior surface is cut to open endometrial cavity

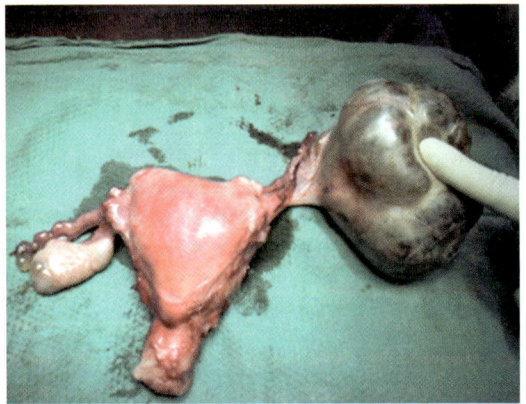

Fig. 37.33: Ovarian cyst

ovaries. The left ovary is hugely enlarged, multi-loculated, cystic with bluish tinge. Both fallopian tubes, right ovary and the uterus are normal .

Diagnosis: Left ovarian cyst-likely mucinous cyst adenoma

Operation done: Total hysterectomy with bilateral salpingo-oophorectomy.

Specimen 8 (Fig. 37.34)

Description: This is a surgically removed specimen of uterus, both ovaries and fallopian tubes. Left ovary is hugely enlarged with uneven surface and cut open to show partly solid and partly cystic areas inside with bluish

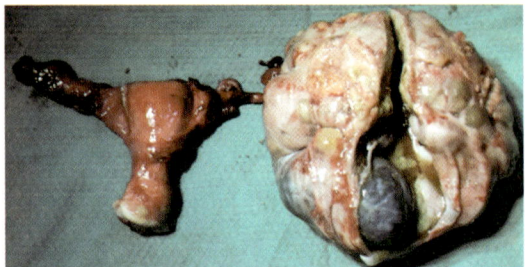

Fig. 37.34: Ovarian tumor

tinge at places. Uterus and other tube and ovary are normal.

Diagnosis: Left sided malignant ovarian tumour likely mucinous cyst adenocarcinoma.

Operation done: Total hysterectomy with bilateral salpingo-oophorectomy.

Specimen 9 (Fig. 37.35)

Description: This is a surgically removed specimen of uterus, both ovaries and fallopian tubes. The uterus is mildly enlarged and the uterus is cut open to expose endometrial cavity. There is an irregular growth arising out of endometrium and extending towards the cervix. The growth has invaded the myometrium also.

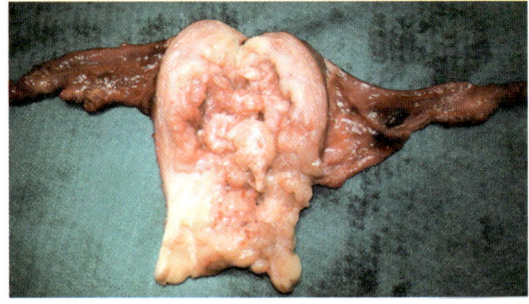

Fig. 37.35: Endometrial carcinoma

Diagnosis: Endometrial carcinoma.

Operation done: Total hysterectomy with bilateral salpingo-oophorectomy.

Specimen 10 (Fig. 37.36)

Description: This is surgically removed specimen of uterus, both fallopian tubes,

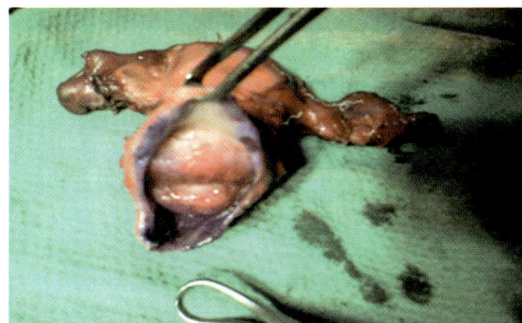

Fig. 37.36: Carcinoma cervix

ovaries, parametrium of either side with portion of vagina. The cervix is hypertrophied with ulcerative growth over both anterior and posterior lip of cervix.

Diagnosis: Cervical carcinoma

Operation done: Radical hysterectomy

Specimen 11 (Fig. 37.37)

Description: This is a surgically removed specimen of fallopian tube. The fallopian tube is markedly enlarged with a typical "retort shape".

Diagnosis: Hydrosalpinx

Operation done: Salpingo-oophorectomy.

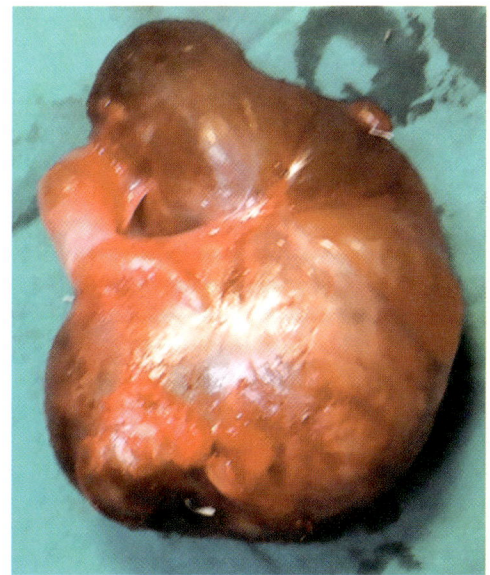

Fig. 37.37: Hydrosalpinx (*Courtesy:* Dr Samaresh Malo, Assistant Professor, NRS Medical College)

X-RAY PLATES

Hysterosalpingogram 1 (Fig. 37.38)

Description: This is a hysterosalpingogram showing the shadow of radio-opaque dye delineating the uterine cavity and both fallopian tubes. There is spillage of dye in peritoneal cavity in both sides.

Diagnosis: Bilateral patent fallopian tubes with normal uterine cavity.

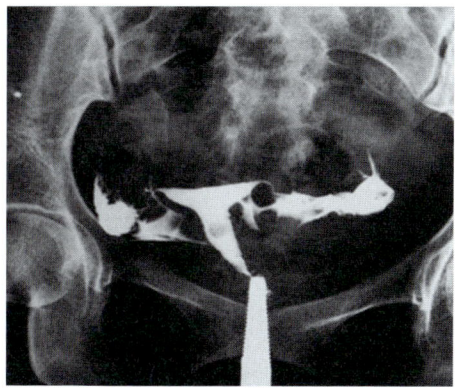

Fig. 37.38: Hysterosalpingogram showing bilateral spillage of dye

Hysterosalpingogram 2 (Fig. 37.39)

Description: This is a hysterosalpingogram showing shadow of radio-opaque dye dileneating the uterine cavity and both

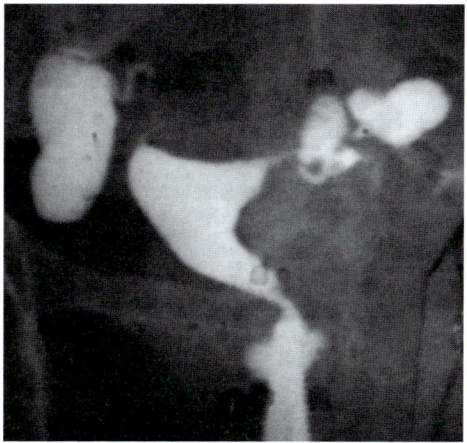

Fig. 37.39: Hysterosalpingogram showing bilateral hydrosalpinx and no spillage of dye on either side

fallopian tubes. Both the fallopian tubes are dilated and there is no spillage of dye on either side.

Diagnosis: Bilateral hydrosalpinx with tubal block at fimbrial end on both sides.

Hysterosalpingogram 3 (Fig. 37.40)

Description: This is a hysterosalpingogram showing shadow of radio-opaque dye delineating two uterine horns and both fallopian tubes. There is spillage of dye on either side.

Diagnosis: Bicornuate uterus with patent fallopian tubes.

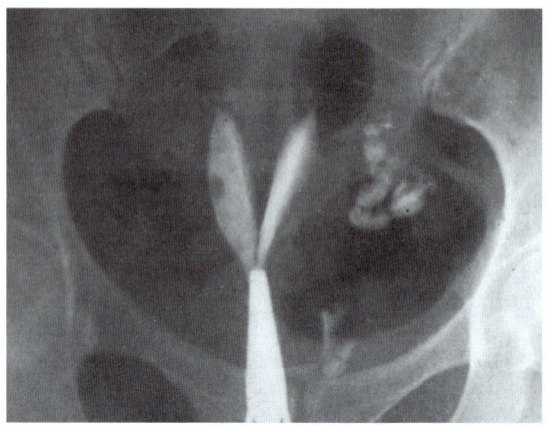

Fig. 37.40: Hysterosalpingogram showing bicornuate uterus

Index